Practical Obstetrics and Gynaecology Handbook

For O&G Clinicians and General Practitioners

Third Edition (2024)

PRACTICAL OBSTETRICS AND GYNAECOLOGY HANDBOOK

For O&G Clinicians and General Practitioners

Third Edition (2024)

Dr. Tan Kim Teng
KK Women's and Children's Hospital, Singapore

Dr. Ng Qiu Ju
KK Women's and Children's Hospital, Singapore

A/Prof. Tan Thiam Chye
Duke-NUS Medical School, Singapore
KK Women's and Children's Hospital, Singapore
Mount Elizabeth Novena Hospital, Singapore

KK Women's and Children's Hospital
SingHealth

World Scientific

NEW JERSEY • LONDON • SINGAPORE • BEIJING • SHANGHAI • HONG KONG • TAIPEI • CHENNAI • TOKYO

Published by

World Scientific Publishing Co. Pte. Ltd.
5 Toh Tuck Link, Singapore 596224
USA office: 27 Warren Street, Suite 401-402, Hackensack, NJ 07601
UK office: 57 Shelton Street, Covent Garden, London WC2H 9HE

British Library Cataloguing-in-Publication Data
A catalogue record for this book is available from the British Library.

PRACTICAL OBSTETRICS AND GYNAECOLOGY HANDBOOK FOR O&G CLINICIANS AND GENERAL PRACTITIONERS
Third Edition

ISBN 978-981-12-7645-3 (hardcover)
ISBN 978-981-12-7722-1 (paperback)
ISBN 978-981-12-7646-0 (ebook for institutions)
ISBN 978-981-12-7647-7 (ebook for individuals)

For any available supplementary material, please visit
https://www.worldscientific.com/worldscibooks/10.1142/13414#t=suppl

Printed in Singapore

Foreword to the 3rd Edition by Prof. Tan Hak Koon

The 2nd edition of the Practical Obstetrics and Gynaecology (O&G) Handbook for O&G Clinicians and General Practitioners serves as a reference text for many clinicians managing O&G patients. Deservedly, the authors' work was fêted by the British Medical Association (BMA) in 2015. Still, they have not rested on their laurels. After all, new drugs have been developed; with ongoing research, guidelines are updated and clinical environments have changed irrevocably. Therefore, it is to no one's surprise that the celebrated 2nd edition sowed the seeds for its successor, the book you hold in your hands today.

The authors have distilled their decades of clinical experience into a handbook that is brief, clear, informative, evidence-based and easy to read. Many of their formative years have been spent in KK Women's and Children's Hospital (KKH), the largest tertiary institution in Singapore, catering to the needs of women and children. You will benefit from their combined wisdom and insiders' perspective on what will happen after you refer your patients to them.

This handbook is only made possible with the joint effort and commitment of many doctors and allied healthcare professionals in KKH and farther afield. On behalf of the authors, I would like to thank everyone involved in this grand undertaking. We could not have done this without all of you.

For you, the reader, I hope you have a space for this handbook on the shelf in your clinic. I expect you will find this handbook valuable and helpful when managing O&G conditions and that it may even benefit the rest of your practice.

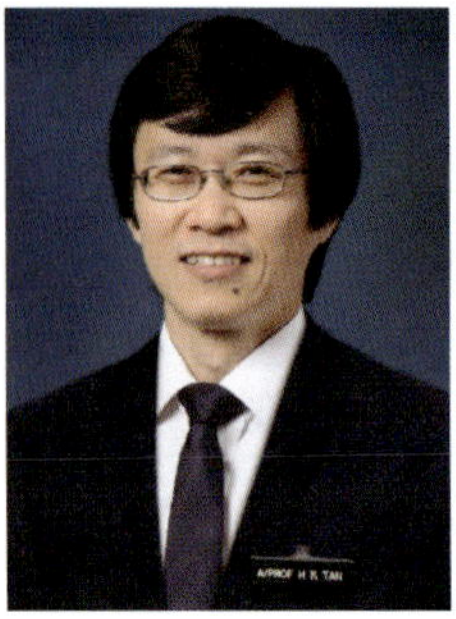

Professor Tan Hak Koon

Designated Institutional Official
SingHealth Residency

Chairman, OBGYN, Academic Clinical Programme
SingHealth Duke-NUS Academic Medical Centre

Chairman and Senior Consultant
Division of Obstetrics & Gynaecology
KK Women's and Children's Hospital

Preface to the 3rd Edition

It has been 18 years since the 1st edition of this handbook was published and 10 years since the second. In 2015, the latter received outstanding reviews by the British Medical Association (BMA) and won the "Highly Commended" award in the Obstetrics and Gynaecology (O&G) category at the BMA Book Awards.

This handbook is immensely popular among students, junior and senior colleagues and general practitioners (GPs), of whom many have requested an update to the 2nd edition. With new evidence and evolving guidelines, we have kept abreast of developments in the O&G field in the 10 years since.

With much time and effort going through multiple edits, we have updated and reorganised all the chapters in the handbook according to the latest international guidelines and other references. These references include the Royal College of Obstetrics and Gynaecology (RCOG), National Institute for Health and Care Excellence (NICE), the UK Faculty of Sexual and Reproductive Healthcare (FSRH), American College of Obstetricians and Gynecologists (ACOG), Centers for Disease Control and Prevention (CDC) and UpToDate.

Moreover, we have added several new chapters, such as Approach to Management of Red Cell Antibodies in Pregnancy, Fetal Hydrops, Intrauterine Growth Restriction, Ultrasonography and Fetal Doppler in Obstetrics, Gynaecological Emergencies and Surgical Complications and Pre-Operative Anaesthetic Information. Furthermore, for this edition, specialists in their fields were invited to update the contents of the chapters of their expertise. Finally, we thank all the contributing authors for their work in making this 3rd edition possible.

Our newest edition of this handbook seeks to empower O&G clinicians and GPs to practise up-to-date and evidence-based medicine, particularly when managing common O&G conditions. You will find this handbook helpful in deciding which investigations to perform to be cost effective with minimal hassle.

We hope this handbook can continue to serve as a quick reference text in your practice, and we welcome any feedback.

Wishing you the best in your clinical practice in the years ahead.

Dr. Tan Kim Teng
Dr. Ng Qiu Ju
Associate Professor Tan Thiam Chye

History of KK Women's and Children's Hospital (KKH) and Services Available

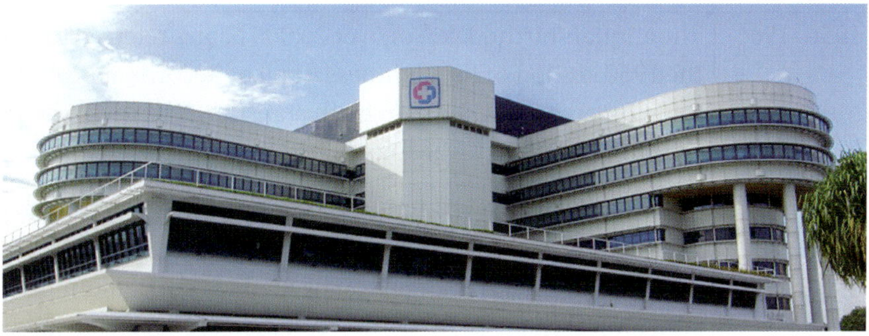

History of KKH

KK Women's and Children's Hospital (KKH) has evolved over the decades, becoming a regional leader in Obstetrics & Gynaecology (O&G), Paediatrics and Neonatology since its founding in 1858.

The story of KK Women's and Children's Hospital is the story of maternal and fetal care in Singapore. It is also a story of how KKH has led the advancement of frontiers in O&G in Singapore.

Before KK Hospital became a maternity hospital, it was a General Hospital in the Kandang Kerbau district.

Year	Milestone
1924	On 1 October 1924, Kandang Kerbau Hospital (KKH) opened with 30 beds and 12 children's cots. The hospital was led by Professor J. S. English, Singapore's first Professor of O&G. The hospital's mission then was to provide good maternity care and midwifery training for medical students and pupil midwives to reduce maternal and infant mortality rates.
1952	The School of Midwifery was set up.
1956–1966	The annual "birthquake" of over 26,000 babies referred to in the 1960 edition of the Guinness Book of Records appeared to be based on KKH's 1956 birth statistics. KKH was then the busiest maternity hospital in the world. KKH broke this record until 1966, when it achieved a peak delivery number of 39,856.
1963	Over the years, the undergraduate medical curriculum has seen radical changes. Partial accreditation of KKH's postings for membership examinations for the Royal College of Obstetricians and Gynaecologists (RCOG) was given.
1967	Full accreditation of KKH's postings for membership examinations for the RCOG was awarded.
1978	Until 1978, KKH was the only training hospital in O&G. As a result, it has a unique concentration of clinical material.
1983	KKH produced Asia's first *in vitro* fertilisation (IVF) baby.
1990	KKH ended its 132-year history as a Government Hospital and became a Restructured Hospital on 1 April 1990.
1997	KKH shifted its premises to 100 Bukit Timah Road, where it currently stands, with state-of-the-art facilities.
1999–2019	The Department of General Obstetrics & Gynaecology (GOG) in KKH was created under Associate Professor John Tee Chee Seng to focus on enhancing service commitments to patients. The department was led subsequently by Dr. KT Tan, Prof. Bernard Chern and Prof. Tan Thiam Chye.

(*Continued*)

Year	Milestone
2001	The first RCOG Part 2 Examination course was held at KKH. This was the first time the RCOG co-hosted an examination course in Asia to develop and accredit aspiring O&G trainees from the region.
2004	KKH received the Asian Hospital Management Award for advancements in patient safety and risk management with a perinatal mortality rate of 4.92 per 1,000 births and an eclampsia rate of 6.9 per 100,000 deliveries — one of the lowest in the world for a tertiary maternity hospital.
2011	KKH led the formation of the SingHealth Duke-NUS Obstetrics and Gynaecology (OBGYN) Academic Clinical Program (OBGYN ACP) — a strategic partnership in Academic Medicine between SingHealth and the Duke-NUS Graduate Medical School.
2015	KKH launched Singapore's first large-scale pre-conception study, S-PRESTO (Singapore PREconception Study of long-term maternal and child Outcomes). S-PRESTO investigates the effects that nutrition, lifestyle, mental health and other environmental factors may have before and during pregnancy on the mother's and baby's health and socio-emotional outcomes. KKH O&G Clinicians published the 2nd edition of the "Practical Obstetrics and Gynaecology Handbook for O&G Clinicians and General Practitioners". The book received outstanding reviews by the British Medical Association (BMA) and won the "Highly Commendable" Award at the BMA Medical Book Award 2015. Only the top four books in the O&G category were awarded the prize amongst 630 competing books. It was also the first Asian book to receive this prestigious award.

(*Continued*)

(*Continued*)

Year	Milestone
2017	The Integrated Platform for Research in Advancing Metabolic Health Outcomes in Women and Children (IPRAMHO) was established to conduct research towards lowering the risk of metabolic health issues such as gestational diabetes mellitus in future generations.
2018	Singapore's first clinical guideline on managing gestational diabetes mellitus was launched to improve health outcomes for pregnant women and their children.
2020	Inaugural guidelines on physical activity and exercise during pregnancy were launched. KKH clinicians established a novel clinical protocol to screen and triage women for threatened miscarriages. By using a single blood test (serum progesterone), the safe and effective clinical protocol can be readily adapted for use in other healthcare institutions.
2021	The SingHealth Duke-NUS Maternal and Child Health Research Institute (MCHRI) was launched at KKH to advance maternal and child health through a life-course approach to research and innovation in reproductive, metabolic and mental health, cognitive development and cures for cancer and critical diseases.
2023	KKH, together with SGH and NCCS, is the first institution outside of Europe to be recognised by the prestigious RCOG, as a joint subspeciality training centre in gynaecological oncology. KKH is also a RCOG accredited joint subspeciality training centre in maternal fetal medicine.
2024	The 3rd edition of the highly acclaimed "Practical Obstetrics and Gynaecology Handbook for O&G Clinicians and General Practitioners" is published.

Services in KKH

As the largest tertiary hospital for O&G patients in Singapore, KKH provides 24/7 in-house specialist coverage for women and children with urgent conditions.

The Urgent O&G Centre (UOGC) was started in 2018 by Associate Professor Tan Thiam Chye. It is a 24-hour walk-in centre that provides round-the-clock services for:

1. Acute problems in early pregnancy (less than 22 weeks of gestation), such as abdominal pain and bleeding.
2. Post-pregnancy related conditions.
3. Acute gynaecological complaints, e.g., acute vaginal bleeding and severe pelvic (lower abdominal) pain.

Pregnant women under 16 weeks who experience minimal vaginal bleeding, mild abdominal pain or would like to have an early pregnancy scan can book an appointment with the Early Pregnancy Assessment Unit (EPAU) or can call KKH hotline (62944050) to be seen by O&G specialists on the same or the next working day.

Similarly, pregnant patients 22 weeks of gestation or above can walk into our 24/7 delivery suite triage area, where our doctors will assess them.

The Children's Emergency provides initial evaluation, stabilisation and treatment for ill or injured infants and children.

Obstetrics

Being the largest maternity facility in Singapore, KKH cares for more than 12,000 obstetric patients annually. The Neonatal Intensive Care Unit (NICU) and Children's Surgery Centres are also the largest facilities in Singapore for premature infants and children, respectively. The NICU provides level 3 neonatal care and is equipped to perform major surgeries and procedures, including extra corporeal membrane oxygenation (ECMO) on newborn babies. With vastly experienced perinatal, neonatal and paediatric surgical teams, KKH serves as a one-stop referral centre for complicated pregnancies and the management of fetal anomalies. As a result, KKH has one of the lowest infant mortality rates in the world, at 1.99 deaths per 1,000 live births in 2022.

The hospital is recognised for its Integrated Labour Ward Risk Management Programme, a comprehensive programme that features speedy staff mobilisation, constant reviews and audits, training and a computerised early-warning system. The programme identifies and manages potential risks in the delivery suite, thus improving women's safety in labour and their newborns. As a result, our perinatal mortality rate has remained low, ranging from 3.3 to 5.6 per 1,000 births.

Since 1997, KKH established a protocol named "Code Green" for extremely urgent caesarean section ("crash" CS). Once the decision for "crash" CS is made, a public announcement system is used to activate the obstetrician, the anaesthetist, the neonatologist and the operating theatre staff that a "crash" CS is required. Delivery of the baby is achievable within minutes once "Code Green" is activated.

In 2014, KKH was the first hospital in Singapore to have a dedicated response code for maternal cardiac arrest, "Code Red", activating a multidisciplinary team trained in the resuscitation of pregnant women. The team will then perform prompt and effective interventions, including a perimortem CS, to improve the maternal response to resuscitation and optimise outcomes.

Maternal Fetal Medicine

The Department of Maternal Fetal Medicine specialises in managing high-risk pregnancies and screening and managing fetal anomalies. Patients enjoy a high level of coordinated care by a multidisciplinary team including the neonatologists, paediatric surgeons, genetic counsellors and clinical nurses. KKH is also a Teaching and Training Centre for the International Society of Ultrasound in Obstetrics and Gynecology (ISUOG) and is accredited by the Fetal Medicine Foundation.

Gynaecology and Subspecialties

The hospital provides comprehensive gynaecology services for women with general gynaecological conditions and sub-speciality care for gynaecological cancers, urogynaecological and fertility problems. In addition, KKH has various specialities under one roof to provide multidisciplinary care, including dermatology, psychiatry, plastic, reconstructive & aesthetic surgery and breast surgery.

Dedicated services are also available at the KK Women's Health and Wellness Centre for women who need specialised management. These include the Vulva Clinic, Menopause Clinic and Sexual Health Clinic.

Gynaecological Oncology

The KK Gynaecological Cancer Centre (GCC) harnesses the latest technology and medical innovations in the prevention and treatment services offered. As the only centre in Asia to participate in the HPV Vaccine Trial — FUTURE II Study, the hospital played a significant role in obtaining approval for the world's first cervical cancer vaccine.

In 2016, KKH GCC was the first cancer centre in Singapore to introduce the indocyanine green and near-infrared imaging (ICG-NIR) sentinel lymph node (SLN) biopsy services for endometrial cancers.

Reproductive Medicine

KKIVF Centre (KKIVF) is one of Singapore's largest infertility centres and offers a wide range of testing, diagnostic and treatment procedures. In addition, there is a paediatric and adolescent gynaecology service which manages the gynaecological health of adolescents aged 19 years and below.

Urogynaecology

The KK Urogynaecology Centre provides services for investigating and managing urinary tract disorders and pelvic floor dysfunction. These include urinary incontinence, overactive bladder, voiding dysfunction, recurrent urinary tract infection and pelvic organ prolapse.

Today, KKH continues to raise the bar on clinical excellence while providing quality care for patients. More than 400 specialists adopt a multidisciplinary and holistic approach to treatment and harness the latest innovations and technology for the best medical care possible for our patients.

As an academic healthcare institution, KKH believes that world-class training and research are imperative in raising the standard of patient care. Since then, KKH has built on its leading role in patient care and safety, teaching, training and research. In addition, it continues to produce most O&G specialists in Singapore.

(Source: https://www.kkh.com.sg/about-kkh/corporate-profile/medical-highlights)

About the Authors/Editors

1. Dr. Tan Kim Teng (Dr. K. T. Tan)

"Teaching is a great way to keep learning" — Matthea Harvey

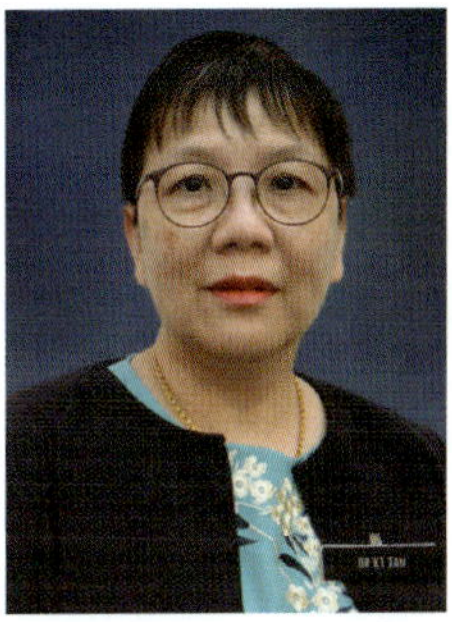

Dr. Tan Kim Teng has been a Senior Consultant in the Division of Obstetrics & Gynaecology (O&G) at KK Women's and Children's Hospital (KKH) since 2004. She previously served as the Head of the Department of General O&G in KKH from 2005 to 2007.

She enjoys doing clinical work, teaching and training the junior doctors in the Division of O&G. In order to impart up-to-date knowledge to her students, she keeps herself abreast of the latest evidence and guidelines by attending numerous Continuing Medical Education (CME) programmes and reading up regularly. In addition, she places a special emphasis on patient safety and satisfaction and seeks to find ways to improve them.

With over three decades of clinical experience from her clinical workload, she continues to keep up with the latest developments in her field, blending the theory and practice of evidence-based medicine. Furthermore, she places a deep emphasis on teaching and mentorship in various forms, such as serving as an Adjunct Assistant Professor at the Duke-NUS Graduate Medical School. In addition, she mentors the junior doctors and residents in the Division of O&G KKH for their Member of the Royal College of Obstetricians and Gynaecologists (MRCOG) examinations and the local O&G Exit Examinations for O&G specialists.

Her academic work has been published in international journals, e.g., the British Medical Journal. In addition, she has published (three) books: "The New Art and Science of Pregnancy and Childbirth" and "Practical Obstetrics and Gynaecology Handbook for O&G Clinicians and General Practitioners" (1st and 2nd editions), the latter of which was lauded as the Most Commended British Medical Association medical book award in 2015.

She takes pride in her daily work and continues to work very hard. For instance, she has spent the last 24 months writing, editing, coordinating and completing the production of this very comprehensive and updated 3rd edition of the "Practical Obstetrics and Gynaecology Handbook". She achieves great satisfaction from completing such projects successfully; the same applies when she witnesses good outcomes for the patients under her care.

2. Dr. Ng Qiu Ju

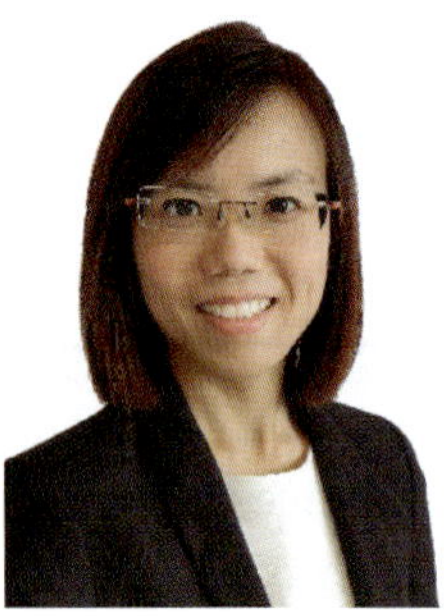

Dr. Ng Qiu Ju is a Consultant with the Department of Gynaecological Oncology at KKH. In 2015, she broadened her knowledge by obtaining the Member of the Royal College of Surgeons of Edinburgh (MRCSEd) qualification. She is also an accredited colposcopist.

In recognition of her outstanding performance during training, Dr. Ng received the Outstanding Resident Award from 2015 to 2017. In addition, she was awarded the SingHealth Quality Service Award in 2020, 2022 and 2023 and Service From the Heart Award for her excellent patient care. Dr. Ng is a strong advocate of patient-centred care and provides individualised and evidence-based management for her patients. She is passionate about Well Women's Screening, especially cervical cancer screening and diagnosing and treating gynaecological cancers.

In addition to her clinical practice, Dr. Ng has published in various scientific journals and has done many oral and poster presentations at local and international conferences. She was awarded the Outstanding Young Investigator Award in 2015 by the SingHealth Duke-NUS Obstetrics and Gynaecology Academic Clinical Programme (ACP) for her research contributions. In addition, Dr. Ng is a contributing author to the 3rd edition of the "Management of High-Risk Pregnancy: A Practical Approach". She also educates and mentors juniors and medical students from local medical schools.

3. Associate Professor Tan Thiam Chye

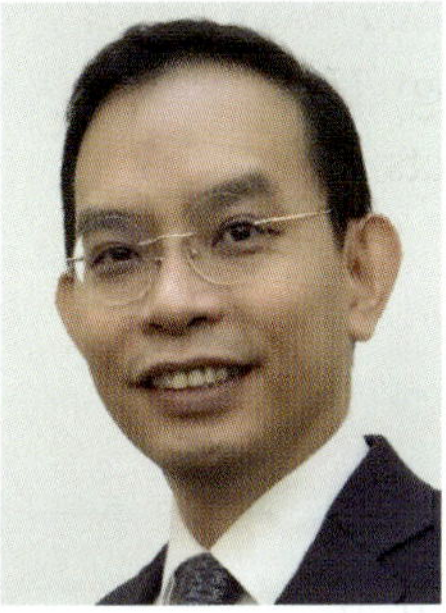

Associate Professor Tan Thiam Chye is currently the Medical Director at O&G The Women's Medical Specialist. He is also a Visiting Senior Consultant at KK Women's and Children's Hospital and Adjunct Associate Professor at Duke-NUS Medical School. He was the immediate past Head of the Department for General Obstetrics and Gynaecology in KK Women's and Children's Hospital.

He was conferred several teaching and clinician awards in his career, including the inaugural SingHealth Golden Apple Award for Outstanding Educator (2011) and SingHealth Distinguished Educator Award (2018). His research interest is in reproductive endocrinology in first-trimester miscarriages. He has received two National Medical Research Council (NMRC) national research grants and two patents.

He co-authored the book "Practical Obstetrics and Gynaecology Handbook for O&G Clinicians and General Practitioners" (1st and 2nd editions), of which the latter was awarded the prestigious British Medical Association Book Award in 2015.

Professor Tan strongly advocates using healthcare technology to enhance patient experience and education. In 2016, he co-developed the HealthHub Pregnancy Track, a new web portal and mobile app with Health Promotion Board. In 2018, he founded and is currently the Chief Editor for Pregnancy Singapore (www.pregnancy.com.sg), a one-stop pregnancy information web portal to provide bite-size content to Asian mothers. In 2019, he collaborated with the Public Service Division on Moments of Life (Families) and SG Life app to connect parents digitally with ease.

Acknowledgements – Contributors and Sponsors

"Success is best when it is shared" — *Howard Schultz*

Authors/Editors

1. **Dr Tan Kim Teng**
   Senior Consultant, Obstetrician & Gynaecologist
   Division of Obstetrics & Gynaecology,
   KK Women's & Children's Hospital
2. **Dr Ng Qiu Ju**
   Consultant, Obstetrician & Gynaecologist
   Department of Gynaecological Oncology,
   KK Women's & Children's Hospital
3. **Associate Professor Tan Thiam Chye**
   Duke-NUS Medical School
   Visiting Senior Consultant, Department of Obstetrics & Gynaecology,
   KK Women's & Children's Hospital
   Senior Consultant, Obstetrician & Gynaecologist
   Mount Elizabeth Novena Hospital

We would not have been able to complete this 3rd edition without the help and commitment of the contributors, as stated below.

We want to thank everyone for their contributions to the successful publication of the 3rd edition of the *Practical Obstetrics & Gynaecology Handbook.*

Contributors from the Division of Obstetrics & Gynaecology, KK Women's & Children's Hospital

1. **Associate Professor John Tee Chee Seng**
   Senior Consultant, Obstetrician & Gynaecologist,
   Division of Obstetrics & Gynaecology
2. **Clinical Associate Professor Ang Seng Bin**
   Senior Consultant, Family Medicine Service & Menopause Unit,
   Treasurer of International Menopause Society
3. **Dr Kazila Bhutia**
   Consultant, Department of Urogynaecology
4. **Dr Namuduri Ramapadmuvathi Devi**
   Senior Staff Physician, Department of Gynaecological Oncology
5. **Dr Anju Bhatia**
   Senior Staff Physician, Department of Maternal-Fetal Medicine
6. **Dr Boricha Yash Bhanji**
   Staff Physician, Department of General Obstetrics & Gynaecology
7. **Dr Michelle Loh Jia Min**
   Consultant, Department of Reproductive Medicine
8. **Dr Chuah Theng Theng**
   Consultant, Department of Obstetrics & Gynaecology
9. **Dr Kwek Lee Koon**
   Associate Consultant, Department of Obstetrics & Gynaecology
10. **Dr Mok Zhun Wei**
    Associate Consultant, Department of Obstetrics & Gynaecology
11. **Dr Li Mingyue**
    Associate Consultant, Department of Maternal-Fetal Medicine
12. **Dr Wang Wanxuan**
    Associate Consultant, Department of Obstetrics & Gynaecology
13. **Dr Sandra Lynn Jaya-Bodestyne**
    Resident, Division of Obstetrics & Gynaecology
14. **Dr Lee Ai Xin**
    Medical Officer, Department of Obstetrics & Gynaecology,
    KK Women's & Children's Hospital

15. **Ms Christina Choi Tien Hui**
    Senior Principal Genetic Counsellor,
    Department of Maternal-Fetal Medicine
16. **Ms Ong Phei Hong**
    Senior Executive, Division of Obstetrics & Gynaecology

Invited Contributors from Other Specialties/Hospitals

1. **Associate Professor Helen Chen**
   Director, Postnatal Depression Intervention Programme,
   Senior Consultant Psychiatrist,
   Department of Psychological Medicine,
   KK Women's & Children's Hospital
2. **Associate Professor Law Hai Yang**
   Deputy Director, National Thalassemia Registry,
   KK Women's & Children's Hospital
3. **Dr Luke Toh Han Wei**
   Head & Senior Consultant Radiologist,
   Diagnostic & Interventional Radiology,
   KK Women's & Children's Hospital
4. **Associate Professor Eileen Lew**
   Senior Consultant Anaesthetist, Women's Anaesthesia,
   Chairman, Division of Clinical Support Services,
   KK Women's & Children's Hospital
5. **Professor Alex Sia Tiong Heng**
   Senior Consultant Anaesthetist, Women's Anaesthesia,
   Chief Executive Officer,
   KK Women's & Children's Hospital
6. **Dr Mark Koh Jean Aan**
   Head and Senior Consultant Dermatologist,
   Department of Dermatology,
   KK Women's & Children's Hospital

7. **Dr Pamela Partana**
   Associate Consultant,
   Department of Obstetrics & Gynaecology,
   Singapore General Hospital
8. **Dr Tan Yah Yuen**
   Senior Consultant,
   General Surgeon (Breast),
   Solis Breast Care & Surgery Centre
9. **Ms Jamie Stephanie**
   Principal Drug Information Pharmacist,
   KK Women's & Children's Hospital
10. **Ms Lim Kae Shin**
    Principal Drug Information Pharmacist,
    KK Women's & Children's Hospital
11. **Dr Lee Kwok Hao**
    Presidential Fellow,
    Department of Strategy and Policy,
    Business School National University of Singapore
12. **Ms Danielle Grace Yap** — Handbook Cover Designer

Sponsors

1. **Abbott Educational Grant**
2. **Bayer (South East Asia) Pte Ltd**

List of Abbreviations

17-OHP	17 hydroxyprogesterone
2D echo	2-dimensional echocardiography
ABC	airway, breathing, circulation
ABG	arterial blood gas
aBME	antenatal breastmilk expression
AC	abdominal circumference
ACC	agenesis of corpus callosum
ACEi	angiotensin-converting enzyme inhibitors
ACL	anticardiolipin
ACOG	American College of Obstetricians and Gynecologists
ACR	albumin creatinine ratio
ACTH	adrenocorticotrophic hormone
AD	autosomal dominant
ADNEX	Assessment of Different NEoplasias in the adnexa
AEDF	absent end-diastolic flow
AEDs	anti-epileptic drugs
AEP	atopic eruption of pregnancy
AFB	acid fast bacilli
AFC	antral follicle count
AFF	atypical femoral fractures
AFI	amniotic fluid index
AFLP	acute fatty liver of pregnancy
AFP	alpha fetoprotein/α fetoprotein
AGEP	acute generalised exanthematous pustulosis
AGC	atypical glandular cells
AGUS	atypical glandular cells of unknown significance
AIDS	acquired immunodeficiency syndrome

AIS	androgen insensitivity syndrome or adenocarcinoma-in-situ
ALP	alkaline phosphatase
ALT	alanine aminotransferase
AMA	advanced maternal age
AMH	anti mullerian hormone or asymptomatic microscopic haematuria
AMI	acute myocardial infarction
ANA	antinuclear antibody
ANC	absolute neutrophil count
AP	anterior posterior
APH	antepartum haemorrhage
APS	antiphospholipid syndrome
APTT	activated partial thromboplastin time
ARB	angiotensin receptor blockers
ARDS	acute respiratory distress syndrome
ARM	artificial rupture of membranes
ART	assisted reproductive technology or antiretroviral therapy
ARU	acute retention of urine
AS	aortic stenosis
ASA	American Society of Anaesthesiologists
ASAP	as soon as possible
ASB	asymptomatic bacteriuria
ASC-H	atypical squamous cells cannot exclude high-grade squamous intraepithelial lesion
ASCUS	atypical squamous cells of undetermined significance
ASD	atrial septal defect
ASRM	American Society for Reproductive Medicine
ATD	antithyroid drugs
ATN	acute tubular necrosis
AUB	abnormal uterine bleeding
AV	atrioventricular
AVM	arteriovenous malformation
AXR	abdominal x-ray

BA	bile acids
BASHH	British Association for Sexual Health and HIV
BCC	basal cell carcinoma
BCG	bacillus calmette-guerin
BD	twice a day
BMD	bone mineral density
BMI	body mass index
BML	benign metastasising leiomyoma
BP	blood pressure
BPD	biparietal diameter
BPS	bronchopulmonary sequestration
BRCA	breast cancer gene
BSA	body surface area
BSE	breast self-examination
BSO	bilateral salpingo-oophorectomy
C&S	culture and sensitivity
CA	cancer antigen or cancer or carcinoma
CA125	cancer antigen 125
CAH	congenital adrenal hyperplasia
cART	combined antiretroviral therapy
CAUTI	catheter-associated urinary tract infection
CBT	cognitive behavioural therapy
CCF	congestive cardiac failure
CD4	clusters of differentiation 4 T lymphocytes
CDC	Centers for Disease Control and Prevention
CDH	Congenital Diaphragmatic Hernia
CEA	carcinoembryonic antigen
cfDNA	cell free DNA
cFTS	combined first trimester screening
CFU/ml	colony forming unit per millilitre
CHB	congenital heart block
CHC	combined hormonal contraception
CHD	congenital heart disease
CIED	cardiac implantable electrical devices
CIN	cervical intraepithelial neoplasia
CISC	clean intermittent self-catheterisation

CKD	chronic kidney disease
CMA	chromosomal microarray analysis
CMIA	chemiluminescent microparticle immunoassay
CMV	cytomegalovirus
CNB	central neuraxial block
CNS	central nervous system
COA	certificate of attendance
COC/COCP	combined oral contraceptive pill
COPD	chronic obstructive pulmonary disease
CPAM	congenital pulmonary airway malformation
CPAP	continuous positive airway pressure
CPP	central precocious puberty
CPR	cardiopulmonary resuscitation or cerebroplacental ratio
CrCl	creatinine clearance
CRL	crown rump length
CRP	c-reactive protein
CS	caesarean section
CSF	cerebrospinal fluid
CSP	caesarean scar pregnancy
CT	computed tomography
CT TAP	computed tomography scan of the thorax abdomen and pelvis
CTG	cardiotocography
CTPA	computed tomography pulmonary angiogram
Cu	copper
CUS	complex duplex ultrasound
CVA	cerebrovascular accident
CVC	central venous catheter
CVP	central venous pressure
CVS	chorionic villus sampling or cardiovascular system
CXR	chest x-ray
CZS	congenital zika syndrome
D&C	dilation and curettage
D&E	dilation and evacuation
DC	dichorionic

DCDA	dichorionic diamniotic
DCIS	ductal carcinoma in situ
DCM	dilated cardiomyopathy
DEET	N,N-diethyl-meta-toluamide
DES	diethylstilbestrol
DEXA scan	dual x-ray absorptiometry
DHA	docosahexaenoic acid
DHEA-S	dehydroepiandrosterone-sulfate
DI	diagnostic imaging
DIC	disseminated intravascular coagulation
DIF	direct immunofluorescence
DKA	diabetic ketoacidosis
DM	diabetes mellitus
DMPA	depot medroxyprogesterone acetate
DNA	deoxyribonucleic acid
DO	detrusor overactivity
DOAC	direct oral anticoagulants
DRESS	drug reaction with eosinophilia and systemic symptoms
DS	Down syndrome
DV	ductus venosus
DVP	deepest vertical pocket
DVT	deep vein thrombosis
E2	oestradiol
EBV	Epstein-Barr virus
EC	emergency contraception
ECC	endocervical curettage or curettings
ECG	electrocardiogram
ECT	electroconvulsive therapy
ECV	external cephalic version
EDD	estimated date of delivery
EDF	end-diastolic flow
EFI	endometriosis fertility index
EFW	estimated fetal weight
EH	endometrial hyperplasia
EIA	enzyme immunoassay

EID	enzyme-inducing drug
EM	early menopause
EMPD	extramammary Paget disease
EP	ectopic pregnancy
EPDS	Edinburgh postnatal depression scale
ER	oestrogen receptor
ERCP	endoscopic retrograde cholangiopancreatography
ESBL	extended-spectrum beta-lactamases
ESR	erythrocyte sedimentation rate
ESS	endometrial stromal sarcoma
ET	endometrial thickness or embryo transfer
ETT	epithelioid trophoblastic tumour or endotracheal tube
EUA	examination under anaesthesia
FA	fetal anomaly
FAI	free androgen index
FAQ	frequently asked questions
FAS	fetal alcohol syndrome
FAST scan	focused assessment with sonography for trauma
FBC	full blood count
FBS	fetal blood sampling
FDA	food and drug administration
FDG	fluorodeoxyglucose
FETO	fetoscopic endoluminal tracheal occlusion
FGM	female genital mutilation
FGR	fetal growth restriction
FH	fetal heart
FHR	fetal heart rate
FIGO	The International Federation of Gynecology and Obstetrics
FL	femur length
FMC	fetal medicine clinic or family medicine clinic
FMH	fetomaternal haemorrhage
FRAX	fracture risk assessment tool
FSH	follicle-stimulating hormone
FSRH	Faculty of Sexual and Reproductive Healthcare
FTR	fallopian tube recanalisation

FTS	first trimester screening
FVS	fetal varicella syndrome
G6PD	glucose-6-phosphate dehydrogenase deficiency
GA	general anaesthesia or gestational age
GAS	group A streptococcus
GBS	group B streptococcus
GCS	glasgow coma scale OR graduated compression stockings
GCSF	granulocyte colony stimulating factor
GCT	germ cell tumour
GDM	gestational diabetes mellitus
GE	gastroenteritis
GERD	gastro-oesophageal reflux disease
GFR	glomerular filtration rate
GGT	gamma-glutamyl transferase
GI	gastrointestinal or granuloma inguinale
GIT	gastrointestinal tract
GnRH	gonadotrophin-releasing hormone
GnRHa	gonadotrophin-releasing hormone agonist
GP	general practitioner
GRAS	generally recognised as safe
GS	general surgery
GSM	genitourinary syndrome of menopause
GT	gestational thrombocytopenia
GTD	gestational trophoblastic disease
GTN	gestational trophoblastic neoplasia
GXM	group and crossmatch
H1N1	influenza A virus subtype H1N1
HA	hypothalamic amenorrhoea
HAART	highly active antiretroviral therapy
HAS	Health Science Authority
Hb	haemoglobin
HbA1c	glycated haemoglobin
HbIg	hepatitis B immune globulin
HBS	hepatobiliary system
HBV	hepatitis B virus

HC	head circumference
HCG	human chorionic gonadotrophin
HCM	hypertrophic cardiomyopathy
HCQ	hydroxychloroquine
HCT	haematocrit
HCV	hepatitis C virus
HDFN	haemolytic disease of the fetus and newborn
HDL	hyperlipidaemia
HDU	high dependency unit
HELLP syndrome	haemolysis, elevated liver enzymes and low platelets
HER2	human epidermal growth factor receptor 2
HF	heart failure
HFI	hormone free interval
HFMD	hand foot and mouth disease
HG	hyperemesis gravidarum
HH	hypogonadotrophic hypogonadism
HHS	hyperosmolar hyperglycaemic state
HIE	hypoxic ischaemic encephalopathy
HIT	heparin-induced thrombocytopenia
HIV	human immunodeficiency virus
HLD	hyperlipidaemia
HMB	heavy menstrual bleeding
HOD	head of department
HP	hypopituitarism
HPB	hepatopancreatobiliary
HPF	high power field
HPO	hypothalamic-pituitary-ovarian
HPV	human papillomavirus
HR	heart rate
hrHPV	high-risk human papillomavirus
HRT	hormone replacement therapy
HSA	human sperm assay or semen analysis or Health Science Authority
HSG	hysterosalpingogram
HSIL	high grade squamous intraepithelial lesion
HSV	herpes simplex virus

HTN	hypertension
HUS	haemolytic uraemic syndrome
HUSLS	high uterosacral ligament suspension
HyFoSy	hystero-salpingo foam contrast sonography
I&D	incision and drainage
I/O	input/output
IBD	inflammatory bowel disease
IBS	irritable bowel syndrome
ICH	intracranial haemorrhage
ICP	intrahepatic cholestasis of pregnancy
ICS	inhaled corticosteroids
ICSI	intracytoplasmic sperm injection
ICU	intensive care unit
ID	infectious disease
IDA	iron deficiency anaemia
IDC	indwelling catheter
IE	infective endocarditis or impending eclampsia
IgG	immunoglobulin G
IgM	immunoglobulin M
IGRA	interferon-gamma release assays
IHC	immunohistochemistry
IHD	ischaemic heart disease
IM	intramuscular
IMB	intermenstrual bleeding
INR	international normalised ratio
IOL	induction of labour
IOM	Institute of Medicine
IOTA	International Ovarian Tumour Analysis group
IPC	intermittent pneumatic compression
IPL	intense pulsed light
IQ	intelligence quotient
IR	interventional radiology
ITP	immune thrombocytopenia
IUCD	intrauterine contraceptive device
IUD	intrauterine death or intrauterine device
IUGR	intrauterine growth restriction

IUGS	intrauterine gestational sac
IUI	intrauterine insemination
IUP	intrauterine pregnancy
IUS	intrauterine system
IUT	intrauterine transfusion or in-utero transfer
IV	intravenous
IVC	inferior vena cava
IVF	in-vitro fertilisation
IVIG	intravenous immunoglobulin
IVU	intravenous urogram
KIV	keep in view
KKH	KK Women's and Children's Hospital
KUB	kidneys, ureters and bladder
LABA	long-acting beta agonists
LAC	lupus anticoagulant
LARC	long-acting reversible contraception
LBW	low birth weight
LDA	low dose aspirin
LDH	lactate dehydrogenase
LEEP	loop electrosurgical excision procedure
LFT	liver function test
LGTI	lower genital tract infection
LGV	lymphogranuloma venereum
LH	luteinising hormone
LHC	left hypochondrium
LHR	lung heart ratio
LIF	left iliac fossa
LLETZ	large loop excision of the transformation zone
LMP	last menstrual period
LMWH	low molecular weight heparin
LNG-IUS	levonorgestrel-releasing intrauterine system
LP	lichen planus
LS	lichen sclerosus
LSC	lichen simplex chronicus
LSCS	lower segment caesarean section
LSIL	low grade squamous intraepithelial lesion

LUNA	laparoscopic uterosacral nerve ablation
LV	left ventricle
LVEF	left ventricular ejection fraction
LVS	low vaginal swab
MAO inhibitors	monoamine oxidase inhibitors
MAP	mean arterial pressure
MBL	menstrual blood loss
MBRRACE-UK	mothers and babies: reducing risk through audits and confidential enquiries across the UK
MC	monochorionic
MCA	middle cerebral artery
MCA-PSV	middle cerebral artery peak systolic velocity
MCDA	monochorionic diamniotic
MCMA	monochorionic monoamniotic
MCV	mean corpuscular volume
MDT	multidisciplinary care
MESA	microsurgical epididymal sperm aspiration
MF	maternal fetal
MHT	menopausal hormone therapy
MI	myocardial infarction
MIS	minimally invasive surgery
MMF	mycophenolate mofetil
MMG	mammogram
MMMT	malignant mixed mullerian tumour of the uterus (uterine carcinosarcoma)
MMR	mumps, measles, rubella
MOD	mode of delivery
MOH	Ministry of Health
MoM	multiple of the median
MR	mitral regurgitation
MRCP	magnetic resonance cholangiopancreatography
MRI	magnetic resonance imaging
MRKH	mayer-rokitansky-küster-hauser
mRNA	messenger ribonucleic acid
MRP	manual removal of the placenta
MRSA	methiciliin-resistant staphylococcus aureus

MS	mitral stenosis
MSM	men who have sex with men
MSS	maternal serum screening
mSv	millisievert
MSW	medical social worker
MTCT	mother to child transmission
MTPT	mid-trimester termination of pregnancy
MTX	methotrexate
NAAT	nucleic acid amplification tests
NB	nasal bone
NBM	nil by mouth
NEC	necrotising enterocolitis
NGT	nasogastric tube
NGU	non-gonococcal urethritis
NICE	National Institute for Health and Care Excellence
NICU	neonatal intensive care unit
NIPT	noninvasive prenatal testing
NNJ	neonatal jaundice
NOS	not otherwise specified
NPU	not passed urine
NPV	negative predictive value
NRFS	non-reassuring fetal status
NSAID	non-steroidal anti-inflammatory drug
NT	nuchal translucency
NTD	neural tube defects
NTR	National Thalassaemia Registry
NYHA	New York Heart Association
O&G/OBGYN	obstetrics & gynaecology
OAB	overactive bladder
OASIS	obstetric anal sphincter injuries
OATS	oligoasthenoteratozoospermia
OC	obstetric cholestasis
OGD	oesophago-gastro-duodenoscopy
OGTT	oral glucose tolerance test
OHGA	oral hypoglycaemic agent
OHSS	ovarian hyperstimulation syndrome

OI	ovulation induction
OM	once every morning
ON	once every night
ONJ	osteonecrosis of the jaw
OPS	outpatient services (polyclinics)
OPU	oocyte pick-up
ORADS	Ovarian-Adnexal Imaging Reporting Data System
OSA	obstructive sleep apnoea
OSTA	osteoporosis self-assessment tool for Asians
OTC	over-the-counter
OTM	ovarian tumour markers
PA	posterior anterior
PAND	paraaortic lymph node dissection
PAP smear	papanicolaou smear
PAPP-A	pregnancy-associated plasma protein-A
PARP	poly (ADP-ribose) polymerase
PAS	placenta accreta spectrum
PAT	preadmission testing
PBF	peripheral blood film
PCA	patient controlled analgesia
PCB	postcoital bleeding
PCN	percutaneous nephrostomy
PCOS	polycystic ovarian syndrome
PCR	polymerase chain reaction or protein-creatinine ratio
PCT	packed cell transfusion
PDA	patent ductus arteriosus
PDHM	pasteurised donor human milk
PE	pulmonary embolism or pre-eclampsia
PEG	percutaneous endoscopic gastrostomy
PEP	post-exposure prophylaxis
PET-CT	positron emission tomography-computed tomography
PFE	pelvic floor exercise
PFO	patent foramen ovale
PGS	preimplantation genetic screening

PGT	preimplantation genetic testing
PICC	peripherally inserted central catheter
PID	pelvic inflammatory disease
PJS	peutz-jeghers syndrome
PlGF	placental growth factor
PLLR	pregnancy and lactation labelling
PLND	pelvic lymph node dissection
Plt	platelet
PMB	postmenopausal bleeding
PND	postnatal depression
PO	per oral
POC	products of conception
POD	pouch of douglas
POI	primary ovarian insufficiency
POP	pelvic organ prolapse or progestogen-only pill
PPCM	peripartum cardiomyopathy
PPE	personal protective equipment
PPH	postpartum haemorrhage
PPI	proton pump inhibitors
PPROM	preterm prelabour rupture of membranes
PPT	postpartum thyroiditis
PPV	positive predictive value
PR	per rectal or progesterone receptor
PRES	posterior reversible encephalopathy syndrome
PROM	prelabour rupture of membranes
PS	pulmonary stenosis
PSN	placental site nodules or presacral neurectomy
PSTT	placental site trophoblastic tumour
PT	prothrombin time
PTD	preterm delivery
PTDS	post-traumatic stress disorder
PTEN	phosphatase and tensin homolog
PTL	preterm labour
PTNS	percutaneous tibial nerve stimulation
PTU	prophylthiouracil
PU	pass urine

PUL	pregnancy of unknown location
PUPPP	pruritic urticarial papules and plaques of pregnancy
PUQE	pregnancy-unique quantification of emesis
PUV	pregnancy of unknown viability
PV	per vaginal
PVA	polyvinyl alcohol
PVB	per vaginal bleeding
PVRU	postvoid residual urine
QDS	four times a day
QUS	quantitative ultrasound
RA	regional anaesthesia or rheumatoid arthritis
RAST	radioallergosorbent test
RBC	red blood cells
RCOG	Royal College of Obstetricians and Gynaecologists
RDA	recommended dietary allowance
RDS	respiratory distress syndrome
REDF	reverse end-diastolic flow
Rh	rhesus
RHC	right hypochondrium
RIF	right iliac fossa
RNA	ribonucleic acid
RPL	recurrent pregnancy loss
RPOC	retained products of conception
RR	respiratory rate
RR BSO	risk-reducing bilateral salpingo-oophorectomy
RT	radiotherapy
RTA	road traffic accident
rTPA	recombinant tissue plasminogen activator
RT-PCR	reverse transcription polymerase chain reaction
RV	right ventricle
RVOT	right ventricular outflow tract
SA	semen analysis
SABA	short-acting beta agonists
SB	stillbirth
SC	subcutaneous
SCA	sex chromosome aneuploidy

SCAR	severe cutaneous adverse reaction
SCC	squamous cell carcinoma
SCCO	squamous cell carcinoma of the ovary
SCN	special care nursery
SCT	sacro-coccygeal teratoma
SD	standard deviation
SDA	same day admission
SERM	selective estrogen receptor modulators
SF	serum ferritin
SFH	symphysial fundal height
SGA	small for gestational age
SGLT2i	sodium-glucose Cotransporter-2 inhibitors
SHBG	sex hormone binding globulin
SIDS	suddent infant death syndrome
SIL	squamous intraepithelial lesion
SIS	saline infusion sonohysterography
SJS	Steven Johnson Syndrome
SLE	systemic lupus erythematosus
SNHL	sensorineural hearing loss
SNP	single nucleotide polymorphism
SNRI	serotonin and norepinephrine reuptake inhibitors
SNS	sacral nerve stimulation
SO	salpingo-oophorectomy
SOB	shortness of breath
SO-IUI	superovulation and intrauterine insemination
SPD	symphysis pubis dysfunction
SpO2	oxygen saturation
SR	sustained release
SROM	spontaneous rupture of membranes
SSF	sacrospinous fixation
SSRI	selective serotonin reuptake inhibitors
STI	sexually transmitted infection
SUA	single umbilical artery
SUDEP	sudden unexpected death in epilepsy
SUI	stress urinary incontinence
SVC	superior vena cava

SVT	supraventricular tachycardia
T&S	type and screen
T13	Trisomy 13/Patau Syndrome
T18	Trisomy 18/Edward Syndrome
T21	Trisomy 21/Down Syndrome
TA	transabdominal
TAT	turnaround time
TB	tuberculosis
TCA	tricyclic antidepressants
TCRE	transcervical resection of endometrium
TCRM	transcervical resection of myoma
Tdap	Diphtheria, Tetanus, and Pertussis
TDS	thrice a day
TED	thrombo-embolus deterrent
TEN	toxic epidermal necrolysis
TESA	testicular sperm aspiration
TFT	thyroid function test
TGA	transposition of the great arteries
THBSO	total hysterectomy bilateral salpingo-oophorectomy
TIA	transient ischaemic attack
TOA	tuboovarian abscess
TOC	trial off catheter or test of cure
TOF	tetralogy of fallot
TOP	termination of pregnancy
TPHA	treponema pallidum haemagglutination
TPN	total parental nutrition
TPO Ab	thyroid peroxidase antibodies
TPPA	treponema pallidum particle agglutination assay
TR	tricuspid regurgitation or transrectal
TRAB	TSH receptor antibody
TSH	thyroid stimulating hormone
TSS	toxic shock syndrome
TSST	type-specific serological test
TST	tuberculin skin test
TT	total testosterone
TTC	trying to conceive

TTP	thrombocytopenic purpura
TV	transvaginal
TVT	tension-free vaginal tape
TW	total white cell count
TXA	tranexamic acid
TZ	transformation zone
U/E/Cr	urea, electrolytes and creatinine
UA	umbilical artery
UAE	uterine artery embolisation
uE3	unconjugated estriol
UFEME	urine microscopy
UFH	unfractionated heparin
UG	urogynaecology
UKMEC	UK Medical Eligibility Criteria for Contraceptive Use
UPA	ulispristal
UPSI	unprotected sexual intercourse
UPT	urine pregnancy test
UROGYN	urogynaecology
URTI	upper respiratory tract infection
US	ultrasound
USI	urodynamic stress incontinence
UtA	uterine artery
UTI	urinary tract infection
UV	umbilical vein
UVB	ultraviolet B
VACTERL	vertebral defects, anal atresia, cardiac defects, tracheo-esophageal fistula, renal anomalies, and limb abnormalities
VAIN	vaginal intraepithelial neoplasia
VAMA	very advanced maternal age
VBAC	vaginal birth after caesarean section
VDRL	venereal disease research laboratory
VE	vaginal examination
VEGF	vascular endothelial growth factor
VFA	vertebral fracture assessment

VHD	valvular heart disease
VIN	vulval intraepithelial neoplasia
VP3	Gram stain, wet mount or nucleic acid probe test (VP3) for detection of vaginal candidiasis, trichomoniasis or bacterial vaginosis
VQ scan	ventilation-perfusion scan
VSD	ventricular septal defect
VTE	venous thromboembolism
VUS	variant of uncertain significance
VVA	vulvovaginal atrophy
VZIG	varicella-zoster immune globulin
VZV	varicella-zoster virus
WBC	white blood cell
WES	whole genome sequencing
WHI	women health initiative
WHO	World Health Organisation
WLE	wide local excision
βHCG	β human chorionic gonadotrophin

Contents

Part 1

Obstetrics

CHAPTER 1

Pre-Conception Preparation

Objectives: To Improve Pregnancy Outcomes

1. Health screening, education and promotion
2. Risk assessment for pregnancy
3. Optimising chronic medical conditions
4. Medication review — Avoid teratogenic drugs
5. Contraception: Avoid unplanned pregnancies
6. General pre-conception advice

Pre-Conception Visit

History:

- Gynaecological history, menstrual history
- Cervical cancer screening: Is it up to date?
- Family history of genetic conditions or congenital fetal anomalies
- Environmental exposure to toxins
- Screening for domestic violence and counselling

Physical examination. Body mass index (BMI), blood pressure (BP), abdominal, speculum and vaginal examination, relevant investigations.

Start pre-conception folic acid every morning.

Vaccinations. Measles, mumps and rubella (MMR); influenza; varicella; hepatitis B; tetanus, diphtheria, pertussis (Tdap).

Medications. Review long-term medications. Use the lowest dose possible or switch to safer alternatives. Stop teratogenic medications. Refer to Chapter 18: *Medications in Pregnancy and Lactation.*

Optimising medical conditions. Refer to respective specialists to optimise chronic medical conditions.

Diabetes mellitus (DM). Target HbA1c <6.5%.

Hypertension. Target BP <135/85.

Epilepsy. Use the lowest dose of anti-epileptic drugs (AEDs). Switch to monotherapy if possible. Start high-dose folic acid 5 mg OM pre-conception and continue throughout the first trimester of pregnancy.

Renal disease. Multidisciplinary team (MDT) care. Stabilise the condition. Optimise the BP, monitor proteinuria, review medications, optimise glycaemic control in diabetics, make treatment plans during hyperemesis gravidarum, and reduce the risk of disease exacerbation/relapse in pregnancy.

Cancer. Breast cancer — Avoid pregnancy within the first 2 years of completion of cancer treatment.

Overweight/obesity or underweight. Target ideal BMI between 18.5 and 24.9 kg/m^2. Refer dietician.

General Lifestyle Modifications

Recommend regular moderate exercise.

Advise to avoid hyperthermia (hot tubs, overheating).

Advise to be cautious of being obese or underweight.

Assess nutritional deficiencies (vegan/pica/milk intolerance/calcium and iron deficiency).

Low-Dose Aspirin (LDA) for Pre-Eclampsia Prophylaxis in Pregnancy

- The UK National Institute for Health and Care Excellence (NICE) guidelines recommend aspirin 75–150 mg/day until delivery.
- American College of Obstetricians and Gynecologists (ACOG) guidelines recommend 81 mg/day of aspirin to be started between 12 and 28 weeks (best started before 16 weeks) and continued until delivery.
- Since 2022, we have been adopting the following regime for pre-eclampsia prophylaxis in KKH (aspirin 150 mg ON from 11–14 weeks to 36 weeks of gestation) as per the ASPRE (Combined Multimarker

Screening and Randomised Patient Treatment with Aspirin for Evidence-Based Pre-eclampsia Prevention) Trial. The administration of aspirin compared to placebo resulted in a 62% reduction in incidence of preterm pre-eclampsia but no significant effect in term pre-eclampsia.

<table>
<tr><th>NICE Guidelines 2019: Hypertension in pregnancy: Planning care for women at moderate- and high risk of pre-eclampsia</th><th>ACOG Guidelines July 2018: LDA use during pregnancy</th></tr>
<tr><td>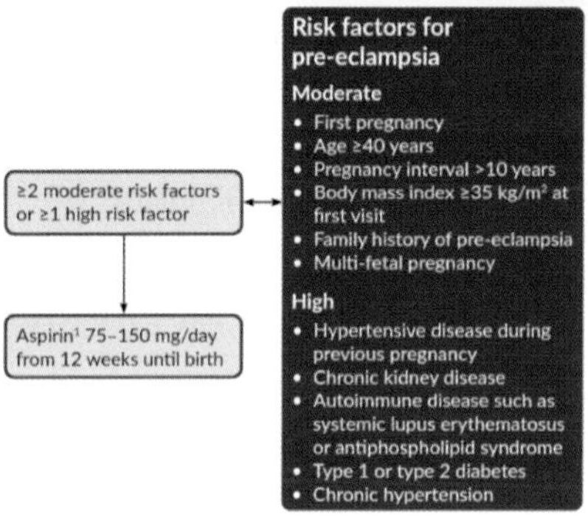
</td><td><u>≥2 Moderate-risk factors:</u>
- Age ≥35
- BMI ≥30
- Family history of pre-eclampsia
- Socio-demographic characteristics (African American, low socio-economic status)
- Personal history of low birth weight or small for gestational age (SGA), previous adverse pregnancy outcomes, >10-year pregnancy interval
<u>≥1 High-risk factor:</u>
- History of pre-eclampsia
- Multi-fetal pregnancy
- Chronic hypertension
- Type 1 and type 2 DM
- Renal disease
- Autoimmune condition [systemic lupus erythematosus (SLE), anti-phospholipid syndrome (APS)]</td></tr>
</table>

Optimising Medical Conditions Before Pregnancy — To Improve the Outcomes for Mother and Baby

Diabetes Mellitus

- <u>Multidisciplinary care team</u>: Maternal-fetal specialist, endocrinologist, general practitioner (GP), dietician, diabetic nurse educator.
- Baseline full blood count (FBC), urea, electrolytes and creatinine (UECr), urine protein–creatinine ratio (PCR).

- Eye and foot screen. Refer to an ophthalmologist for retinopathy.
- 2D echocardiogram if there is a history of poorly controlled DM. Refer to a cardiologist if there is any cardiac issue.
- Refer to a nephrologist if serum creatinine is ≥120 mmol/L or proteinuria is >0.5 g/day or albumin to creatinine ratio (ACR) >30 mg/mmol.
- Aim for HbA1c <6.5% to reduce the risk of miscarriage, congenital anomalies and stillbirth.
- If HbA1c is >10%, avoid pregnancy until DM control is optimised. Use effective contraception until optimal glucose control is achieved.
- Counsel on the risks of DM in pregnancy and pregnancy on DM, follow-up and the need for close monitoring.
- Prescribe folic acid 5 mg/day from 3 months pre-conception till 12 weeks of gestation.
- Metformin, glibenclamide and insulin can be used for glycaemic control in pregnancy.
- Refer to Chapter 11: *Medical Disorders in Pregnancy.*

Hypertension (HTN)

- Ensure optimal BP control (target BP <135/85).
- Ensure compliance to taking anti-hypertensives as required.
- **Stop** ACE inhibitors, angiotensin II receptor antagonists, thiazide diuretics and statins.
- Switch to safe anti-hypertensives (e.g., labetalol, nifedipine, methyldopa).
- Since 2022, we have been adopting the following regime for pre-eclampsia prophylaxis in KKH (aspirin 150 mg ON from 11–14 weeks to 36 weeks of gestation) as per ASPRE Trial.
- Refer to Chapter 11: *Medical Disorders in Pregnancy.*

Cardiac Disease in Pregnancy

- Optimise maternal status. Assess according to the New York Heart Association (NYHA) class.
- MDT care team: Cardiologist and maternal-fetal specialist.
- Perform a complete evaluation, including a 2D echocardiogram.

- Counsel on the maternal and fetal risks.
- Cardiac surgery improves fertility. Repair cardiac defects before pregnancy if indicated. Make necessary medication adjustments. If the cardiac condition can be treated, rectify it pre-pregnancy [atrial septal defects (ASDs), patent ductus arteriosus (PDA), some forms of coarctation]. If the condition can be ameliorated, rectify it pre-pregnancy [mitral stenosis (MS), mitral regurgitation (MR), atrial stenosis (AS), tetralogy of Fallot, ventricular septal defect (VSD) with mild pulmonary hypertension, pulmonary stenosis (PS)]. Advise to avoid pregnancy before prosthetic valve replacement is performed.
- Women with valve replacements should be counselled on the need for close monitoring and therapeutic anticoagulation. Women on long-term warfarin planning to conceive must do a pregnancy test once they miss their menses. This is to ensure prompt adjustment of anticoagulation therapy. For example, to change to heparin pre-conception or as soon as they are pregnant. Warfarin should be avoided between 6 and 12 weeks of gestation to minimise the risk of warfarin embryopathy.
- Refer to Chapter 11: *Medical Disorders in Pregnancy.*

Thyroid Disorders

- Co-manage with endocrinologist.
- Optimise thyroid control. Advise to defer pregnancy until a stable euthyroid state is achieved.
- Definitive therapy, e.g., radioactive iodine or surgery, should be considered for women with Graves' disease before pregnancy.
- Advise to avoid pregnancy for at least 6 months after radioactive iodine therapy or thyroidectomy for thyroid cancer.
- Refer to Chapter 11: *Medical Disorders in Pregnancy.*

Epilepsy

- Co-manage with neurologist.
- Refer to a geneticist for counselling if there is a risk of inheritance of epilepsy.

  - If the *mother* has epilepsy, there is a 5% risk the child will have epilepsy.
  - If the *father* has epilepsy, there is a 3% risk the child will have epilepsy.
  - If *both parents* have epilepsy, there is a 10–15% risk the child will have epilepsy.
- Assess the type of epilepsy. A woman is **not** considered to have epilepsy if she has been seizure-free for at least 10 years, of which the last 5 years have been off AEDs or a woman with childhood epilepsy but has remained seizure-free and treatment-free in adulthood.
- Counsel on the maternal risks, e.g., sudden unexpected death in epilepsy (SUDEP) and fetal risks, e.g., congenital anomalies. SUDEP is the sudden, unexpected death of someone with epilepsy who was otherwise healthy. Explain the risk of self-discontinuation of AED and the effect of seizures on the woman and her fetus.
- One-third of women will have deterioration of their epilepsy during pregnancy. Pre-pregnancy seizure-free duration is the most important factor in the risk of deterioration.
  - If the woman has been seizure-free for 1 year before pregnancy, she would mostly be seizure-free during pregnancy.
  - If the woman has stopped her AED and has been seizure-free for at least 6 months, she can try to conceive.
- Folic acid 5 mg/day at least 3 months pre-conception till the end of the first trimester.
- Optimise AED treatment by a neurologist.
  - Considerations for stopping AED:
    - May consider stopping AED if the woman has been seizure-free for 2–4 years.
    - Individualised management depending on the woman's condition and preference.
    - Need to balance the risk of seizure recurrence.
  - If unable to stop AED, use monotherapy, if possible, at the lowest possible dose. The risk of fetal anomalies depends on the type, dose and number of AEDs.
  - Lamotrigine and carbamazepine are associated with facial clefts and cardiac defects, but the lowest dose of monotherapy has the lowest rate of fetal anomalies.

  - o Avoid teratogenic drugs, e.g., sodium valproate (risk of neural tube and cardiac defects, cleft lip/palate, poor cognition and long-term adverse effects on neurodevelopment) and Lithium (Ebstein anomaly).
  - o However, if the risk of epilepsy deterioration from changing the AED is high, some women will need to continue sodium valproate or AED polytherapy in consultation with the neurologist.
- Regarding the use of AEDs in pregnancy, refer to Chapter 18: *Medications in Pregnancy and Lactation.*

Major Psychiatric Disorders (Including Alcohol or Substance Abuse)

- Co-manage with psychiatrist.
- The use of benzodiazepines may be associated with anomalies like cleft lip/palate and neonatal withdrawal syndrome.
  - o Exposure to tricyclic antidepressants (TCA) and selective serotonin reuptake inhibitors (SSRI) in late pregnancy may be associated with neonatal withdrawal syndrome (adaptation syndrome).
- Refer to Chapter 18: *Medications in Pregnancy and Lactation* for the use of psychotropic drugs.

Malignant Disorders

- Refer to a fertility specialist for counselling immediately after the diagnosis of cancer, especially in young patients who still desire fertility, to discuss the possibility of fertility preservation.
- Consider embryo/semen/oocyte/ovarian tissue cryopreservation before cancer treatment (e.g., chemotherapy, radiotherapy, surgery).
- Advise to avoid pregnancy for 2 years after completion of breast cancer treatment.

Obesity

- Optimise maternal weight (ideal BMI: 18.5–24.9 kg/m^2).
- Refer to a dietician — Maintenance diet of 1,800 calories/day pre-conception.
- Exercise.
- Refer to weight management clinics.

- Refer for bariatric surgery if the BMI is >40 or >35 with medical co-morbidities [e.g., type 2 DM, hypertension (HTN), hyperlipidaemia (HLD), obstructive sleep apnoea (OSA)].
- Advise to avoid pregnancy for 12–18 months post-bariatric surgery to stabilise weight and optimise nutrition.
- Counsel on anovulatory cycles, subfertility, lower IVF success rates, miscarriage risk and other obesity-related pregnancy complications, e.g., gestational diabetes mellitus (GDM) and pre-eclampsia.

Underweight (BMI <18.5 kg/m^2)

- Optimise weight (ideal BMI: 18.5–24.9 kg/m^2).
- Refer to a dietician.
- Counsel on ovulatory dysfunction, risk of hypothalamic amenorrhoea, nutritional deficiencies, osteoporosis, preterm birth, small for gestational age (SGA) and low-birth-weight babies.

Venous Thromboembolism (VTE)

Refer to Chapter 11: *Medical Disorders in Pregnancy.*

1. **Avoid teratogenic drugs** — Refer to Chapter 18: *Medications in Pregnancy and Lactation.*
2. **Screen for infections and genetic disorders.**
   Treat, immunise and counsel.
   - Full blood count with red cell indices — If the mean corpuscular volume (MCV) is low <80, screen for thalassaemia. Refer to Chapter 23: *Approach to Prenatal Screening for Thalassaemia.*
   - Syphilis screening.
   - Hepatitis B surface antigen.
   - Human immunodeficiency virus (HIV) testing and counselling.
   - Rubella IgG antibody level — check rubella immunity.
   - Varicella (in women with no known history of chickenpox).

Pre-conception vaccinations — Measles, mumps and rubella (MMR); influenza; varicella; hepatitis B; tetanus, diphtheria, pertussis (Tdap).
Vaccinate before pregnancy if non-immune.

Avoid pregnancy within 4 weeks of vaccination with live vaccines (e.g., rubella/varicella vaccines).

Miscellaneous Tests

Screening for sexually transmitted infections (STIs), e.g., chlamydia and gonorrhoea in high-risk groups.

Cervical cancer screening — PAP smear (25–29 years old) or primary HPV testing (≥30 years old).

Ultrasound scan (US) of pelvis to exclude pelvic pathology (fibroids, ovarian cysts, etc.).

Precautions to Avoid Infections in Pregnancy

Toxoplasmosis

- Avoid cat faeces in home and garden (avoid clearing cat litter box).
- Keeping cats indoors.
- If gardening or handling soil, wear gloves and wash hands afterwards.

Cytomegalovirus/Parvovirus B19

- Frequent hand washing — universal precautions for childcare and healthcare workers.

Salmonella

- Avoid raw/undercooked eggs. Use pasteurised eggs.
- Avoid home-made mayonnaise, salad dressings, ice cream, raw cake batter.

Listeriosis

Refer to Chapter 15: *Infections in Pregnancy.*

Check dental hygiene

— Refer to a dentist for a dental assessment.

Gum and dental infections have been shown to increase the risk of preterm labour.

Appropriate Counselling Sessions

Genetic Counselling Can Be Offered to Women With

- ✓ A family history of a known or suspected genetic disorder
- ✓ A known carrier of a genetic condition
- ✓ Consanguinity
- ✓ A history of exposure to teratogens
- ✓ A history of recurrent pregnancy losses
- ✓ Abnormal results of first-trimester aneuploidy screening (FTS)/non-invasive prenatal test (NIPT)
- ✓ Abnormal diagnostic testing results — chorionic villus sampling (CVS)/amniocentesis
- ✓ Fetal structural anomalies on the 20-week screening ultrasound scan
- ✓ Request for more information on genetic screening or testing options

Avoid High-Risk Activities

Refer to Chapter 11: *Medical Disorders in Pregnancy.*

Alcohol is associated with fertility issues, miscarriages, fetal anomalies, fetal alcohol syndrome (FAS), and adverse neuropsychological outcomes in newborns. Therefore, women should be treated through interventional counselling. In addition, refer them to a support group and treatment programmes.

Smoking is associated with miscarriage, intrauterine growth restriction (IUGR), preterm labour, placental abruption and attention deficit disorders in children.

Smoking cessation:

- Behavioural techniques, support groups and family help.
- Nicotine patches or gum may be helpful before conception. Strict supervision by a doctor is recommended.
- Second-hand smoke can also affect fertility and the perinatal period.

Substance Abuse — Recreational drugs such as heroin, cocaine, opiates and marijuana are associated with miscarriage, IUGR, preterm labour, placental abruption, and neurobehavioural abnormalities.

- MDT management with the psychiatrist and medical social worker.
- Refer to the Substance Abuse Treatment Programme.
- For women with heroin abuse, refer to a supervised withdrawal programme pre-conception.

An alternative is a supervised methadone maintenance programme, i.e., if the woman cannot complete/tolerate the withdrawal programme.

Exercise

Regular **moderate** exercise is generally beneficial. Aim for at least 150 minutes of moderate-intensity exercise every week. In addition, women are encouraged to do muscle-strengthening exercises at least twice a week.

Benefits of exercise during pregnancy: Reducing excessive weight gain, improving health, mood, sleep and fitness and reducing the risk of hypertension and GDM.

Pregnant women should limit vigorous exercises to avoid an increase in core body temperature (≥39°C), which can increase the risk of neural tube defects (NTDs) during the first 4–6 weeks of pregnancy. It is unlikely to reach such high core temperatures during typical exercise.

Nutrition

Dietary and Vitamin Supplementation

Starting folic acid pre-conception and for the first 3 months of pregnancy effectively reduces NTDs in the fetus. (Dose of folic acid for women at low risk of NTD is 400–800 μg/day, while for women at high risk is 5 mg/day.)

Advise high-dose folic acid 5 mg/day for women:

- With a history of NTDs.
- **With maternal conditions:** Diabetes, epilepsy (on AEDs, e.g., sodium valproate, carbamazepine), obesity, malabsorption disorders, e.g., inflammatory bowel disease or HIV.

- On anti-folate drugs, e.g., sulphonamides, methotrexate, anti-epileptics, anti-retrovirals.
- Who smoke.

In KKH, we routinely prescribe folic acid 5 mg/day pre-conception and for the first trimester.

Strict vegans may be deficient in amino acids, zinc, calcium, iron, vitamin D and B12. Refer to the dietician for advice.

Women with *milk intolerance* can benefit from taking lactose-reduced milk, lactose tablets or calcium supplements.

Avoid overdose of:

Vitamin A (limit to 3,000 IU/day). Teratogenic if >10,000 IU/day.

Vitamin D (limit to 2,000 IU/day or 50 μg/day). Do not exceed 4,000 IU/day (or 100 μg/day).

Vitamin D >10,000 IU/day can cause vitamin D toxicity resulting in hypercalcaemia and hypercalciuria.

Women with the following parameters/conditions/lifestyle are at higher risk of vitamin D deficiency. They need a higher dose of vitamin D at 1,000 IU/day:

- ✓ Pigmented skin
- ✓ BMI ≥30 kg/m^2
- ✓ Housebound or remaining covered
- ✓ Vegan diet
- ✓ Malabsorption
- ✓ Multiparity with short inter-pregnancy intervals
- ✓ Liver or renal disease
- ✓ On AEDs, anti-retroviral treatment, rifampicin
- ✓ Alcohol abuse

- Women at risk of pre-eclampsia should have oral calcium and vitamin D 800 IU/day.

- Screen for vitamin D deficiency if the patient is symptomatic (e.g., bone pain, fragility fractures), has a history of vitamin D deficiency, malabsorption disorders, multiple sclerosis, chronic renal disease or is a high-risk woman as listed above.
- **Vitamin D deficiency** — serum 25-hydroxyvitamin D level <12 ng/ml (30 nmol/L).

  Women need a higher oral dose of 4,000 IU/day or 20,000 IU/week for 6 weeks and then repeat serum vitamin D levels.

  Once they are treated, women should be on regular maintenance of vitamin D 1,000 IU/day.
- **Vitamin D insufficiency** — serum 25-hydroxyvitamin D level 12 to <20 ng/ml (30 to <50 nmol/L).

  Women should be on vitamin D 2,000 IU/day.

Caffeine (limit to 200 mg caffeine/day ~1 cup/day) — High caffeine intake may increase the risk of miscarriage and low-birth-weight babies.

Iron — Recommended dietary allowance (RDA) in pregnancy = 30 mg of elemental iron/day.

Elemental calcium — RDA in pregnancy = 1,200 mg/day.

- For women at high risk of pre-eclampsia: Assess dietary calcium intake from 20 weeks of gestation.

  If <900 mg/day, start calcium supplementation (≥500 mg/day).

  Aim 1.5–2.0 g of elemental calcium/day. This can have a 50% reduction in the risk of pre-eclampsia.

Avoid Environmental Toxins

- **Radiation**, e.g., during imaging scans with ionising radiation risks, e.g., computed tomography (CT) or PET scans — Refer to Chapter 62: *Imaging Modalities in Obstetrics and Gynaecology.*
- Metals like lead and mercury.
- Pesticides (2,4,5-T and 2,4-D organophosphates).
- Plastics (vinyl chloride).
- Solvents like trichloroethylene, benzene and toluene in paint strippers, dry cleaning fluid.

CHAPTER 2

Routine Antenatal Care

Purpose of Antenatal Visits

1. To assess maternal and fetal well-being.
2. To identify risk factors, complications and institute appropriate interventions. Refer to a maternal–fetal (MF) specialist or other specialists for multidisciplinary team management if indicated.
3. To review long-term medications and any additional medications needed, e.g., start low-dose aspirin (LDA) in women with risk factors for pre-eclampsia.
4. To provide health education, advice, reassurance and support for the woman and her family.
5. To offer Down syndrome screening to all women regardless of age, personal or family history.
   - First-trimester screening at 11–13+6 weeks of gestation.
   - Non-invasive prenatal testing (NIPT) or cell-free DNA (cfDNA) testing at ≥10+0 weeks of gestation.
   - Maternal serum screening at 15–20 weeks of gestation.
   - Diagnostic tests (chorionic villus sampling, amniocentesis) if the screening test result indicates high risk (>1:300) or other indications are present.
6. To screen for hypertension, diabetes mellitus, venous thromboembolism, mental health, domestic violence and fetal anomalies.
7. To administer antenatal vaccines — inactivated influenza and whooping cough (Tdap) vaccines.
8. To review all the investigation results promptly and act appropriately if results are abnormal.
9. To plan the birth, contraception and breastfeeding.

Recommended Routine Antenatal Follow-Up in KKH

Trimester	Weeks	Laboratory screening tests	Management
First trimester Check blood pressure (BP)/body mass index (BMI) Urine dipstick for protein and glucose	**First antenatal (booking) visit 8–12 weeks**	(Refer to Chapter 22: *Routine Antenatal Investigations*) Full blood count (FBC) thalassaemia screen Syphilis Hepatitis B surface antigen Human immunodeficiency virus (HIV) antibody testing Rubella IgG antibody level for immunity Blood group and antibody screen For women with previous gestational diabetes mellitus (GDM), screen at booking with a 2-point oral glucose tolerance test (OGTT). If it is normal, repeat a 3-point OGTT at 24–28 weeks Urine culture (midstream clean-catch specimen) to screen for asymptomatic bacteriuria Pap smear if 25–29 years old or HPV testing if ≥30 years old (if appropriate)	<u>Booking visit:</u> Take a thorough *history* to stratify risk If high risk, refer to a MF specialist or other specialists for multidisciplinary team care *Ultrasound scan (trans-abdominal/ transvaginal US)*: o Assess pregnancy location, dating and viability o The expected date of delivery (EDD) is the most accurate in the first trimester o Determine single or multiple gestation o Look for any adnexal masses or free fluid in the pouch of Douglas <u>*Manage abnormal antenatal blood results:*</u> o If an antibody is present, the patient may need close follow-up and fetal surveillance, depending on the type. (Refer to Chapter 24: *Approach to Management of Red Cell Antibodies in Pregnancy*). Take folic acid 5 mg daily Symptomatic management of nausea and vomiting in pregnancy Counsel on vaccines in pregnancy Can give influenza vaccine during the first visit. Provide pregnancy advice and antenatal follow-up
Check BP/ BMI Urine dipstick for protein and glucose	**11–13+6 weeks**	Down syndrome screening (first trimester screening) (Refer to Chapter 25: *Prenatal Screening for Chromosomal Defects and Invasive Diagnostic Tests*)	1. Combined **first trimester screening** (FTS) test, which includes a nuchal translucency (NT) scan + maternal serum screening (PAPP-A and free βHCG) — done at **11–13+6 weeks of gestation** 2. NIPT or cfDNA test using maternal blood — done at **≥10 weeks of gestation**
Second trimester Check BP/ BMI Urine dipstick for protein and glucose	**15–20 weeks**	Down syndrome screening (if not done earlier) Can offer NIPT versus maternal serum screening (triple test) — AFP, hCG and unconjugated estriol in KKH	Administer Tdap vaccines between 16 and 32 weeks of gestation

(*Continued*)

(*Continued*)

Trimester	Weeks	Laboratory screening tests	Management
Check BP/BMI Urine dipstick for protein and glucose	**18–20+6 weeks**	Discuss the mode of delivery and identify any obstetric indications for a caesarean section	20-week screening ultrasound scan to exclude fetal structural anomalies and determine fetal biometry, presentation, placental location and amniotic fluid volume. Perform uterine artery Doppler.
Third trimester Check BP/BMI Urine dipstick for protein and glucose	**24–28 weeks**	Universal GDM screening in Singapore using 75 g 3-point OGTT at 24–28 weeks of gestation Repeat FBC, blood group and antibody screen Document delivery plans by 28 weeks if possible	For Rh-negative women with Rh-positive partner, test for Rh antibody. – If Rh antibody is negative, administer routine antenatal anti-D prophylaxis (RAADP) at 28–30 weeks. – If Rh antibody is positive, manage as a Rh-isoimmunised pregnancy. Refer to a MF specialist. (Refer to Chapter 24: *Approach to Management of Red Cell Antibodies in Pregnancy*.) Interval growth scans to identify intrauterine growth restriction (IUGR) or macrosomia.
Subsequent antenatal visits Check BP/BMI Urine dipstick for protein and glucose	**32–35 weeks**	Routine follow-up	Refer for anaesthetic review at about 32 weeks for singletons and twins at an earlier gestation (if indicated)
	35–37 weeks (weekly follow-up)	Ultrasound scan to determine presentation, estimated fetal weight (EFW) and amniotic fluid index (AFI). Re-check the placenta if there is a history of low-lying placenta. We perform universal group B *Streptococcus* (GBS) screening in KKH for women planned for vaginal delivery. A swab from the lower vagina/anorectum is usually done at 35–37 weeks or 3–5 weeks before EDD. For *twins*, swab at 32–34 weeks. If tested positive for GBS, the woman will require intrapartum antibiotics prophylaxis (IAP) for vaginal	Confirm the mode and timing of delivery. Any birth plans or preferences? Any cord blood banking? Educate women on the signs and symptoms of labour and when to go to the hospital for delivery. Also, to monitor fetal movements closely and to seek medical attention *immediately* if reduced. Discuss vaginal examination and membrane sweeping at term.

(Continued)

Trimester	Weeks	Laboratory screening tests	Management
		delivery or if she has a spontaneous rupture of membranes (SROM). Women with GBS in a previous pregnancy can either opt for IAP without repeat testing (as the likelihood of maternal GBS colonization in the present pregnancy is 50%) or request repeat testing, and IAP is required only if tested positive. **Exclusion criteria for GBS Testing** **These women will need IAP:** a. Women with GBS bacteriuria detected in the current pregnancy. b. Women with a previous infant with early- or late-onset GBS disease.	
	37–39+6 weeks (weekly follow-up)	For women who need caesarean delivery. Arrange for elective caesarean section at term, usually done around 39 weeks of gestation. However, earlier delivery may be indicated for maternal and fetal indications.	Educate women to monitor fetal movements, signs and symptoms of labour and when to go to the hospital for delivery. Discuss vaginal examination and membrane sweeping. Discuss induction of labour if indicated.
	40 weeks onwards	Cardiotocography (CTG) ultrasound scan to assess EFW and AFI	Discuss induction of labour or await spontaneous labour if post-dates. Counsel on risks of post-dates. Do vaginal examination

NICE recommends 10 routine antenatal appointments for *nulliparous* women and 7 routine antenatal appointments for *multiparous* women (NICE Guidelines, 19 August 2021).

Warning Symptoms in Pregnancy

Symptoms	Action for woman
Abdominal contractions or pain To exclude preterm delivery, which occurs in about 10% of women	Exclude labour by assessment of cervical dilatation **Refer to OBGYN** if in labour Braxton Hicks contractions are common in the third trimester. Unlike labour pains, they are irregular in intensity, unpredictable, non-rhythmic and usually taper off and disappear.
Vaginal discharge or leaking liquor	Perform a sterile speculum examination: 1. Definite pool of liquor seen → Diagnosis of pre-labour rupture of membranes (PROM) 2. If no amniotic fluid is seen, use the following tests to diagnose PROM a. **Actim® PROM** [detects insulin-like growth factor-binding protein 1 (IGFBP-1)] or b. **AmniSure®** [detects placental alpha microglobulin-1 (PAMG-1) test of vaginal fluid] **Amnicator is **not** recommended as it can result in a false-positive result with blood.* Perform low vaginal/anorectum swabs for GBS screening if indicated If the GBS test is positive, the woman will need intrapartum antibiotics (IAP) to prevent early-onset GBS infection (EOGBS).
Reduced fetal movements (after 24 weeks of gestation)	**Refer to OBGYN immediately** for assessment of fetal well-being Instruct the woman on Cardiff "count-to-10" fetal movement chart. Alternatively, advise the woman to lie on her left side and focus on fetal movements for 2 hours. If she does not feel >10 discrete movements in 2 hours, she should seek medical attention immediately (RCOG 2011 Guidelines on reduced fetal movements).

How to instruct your patient on Cardiff "count-to-10" fetal movement chart?
This method uses an 8–12 hour period to record 10 of your baby's movements. The time you choose is preferably your baby's most active period, for example, in the evenings.
When charting, start your timing at around the same time each day. The first time you feel your baby move, record the time, and write it on your graph. Try to count every movement or kick until your baby has moved 10 times. When you feel your 10th movement, note the time.
If your baby has at least 10 movements within this 12-hour period, he/she is thought to be well. If your baby has not moved 10 times in 12 hours or you have any concerns about the baby's well-being, you should see your doctor **immediately**.

Warning Signs in Pregnancy

	Action for woman
General	
Blood pressure (BP) To look out for signs and symptoms of pre-eclampsia	Repeat if ≥140/90. Check for proteinuria **Refer to OBGYN** if BP is still elevated Start anti-hypertensives as indicated — safe anti-hypertensives in pregnancy include labetalol and nifedipine Start LDA 150 mg ON from 11 to 14 weeks till 36 weeks in women with risk factors for pre-eclampsia (New KKH 2022 protocol)
Maternal weight	**Aim for a normal maternal weight increase based on BMI** *WHO International Classification of BMI* *Ideal weight gain in a singleton pregnancy* BMI <18.5 Underweight Weight gain 12.5–18.0 kg BMI 18.5–24.9 Normal weight Weight gain 11.5–16.0 kg BMI 25.0–29.9 Overweight Weight gain 7.0–11.5 kg BMI ≥30.0 Obese Weight gain 5–9.0 kg
Urinalysis	***Positive urine albumin*** Exclude urinary tract infection (UTI), vaginal discharge, pre-eclampsia or renal disease Check BP and do blood/urine tests to exclude pre-eclampsia Do urine protein creatinine ratio (urine PCR): PCR is abnormal if ≥0.3 g/day ***Glycosuria*:** To exclude DM if persistent (≥2 episodes). Do 75 g 2-point OGTT if in the first trimester. Do 75 g 3-point OGTT if in the second or third trimester. **Refer to OBGYN** if the results are abnormal.
Examination	
Symphysial fundal height (smaller or larger than dates)	**Refer to OBGYN** to exclude small for gestational age (SGA)/ intrauterine growth restriction (IUGR) or macrosomia (if the first trimester dating was accurate). Can do growth scans ± Doppler scans for IUGR.
Malpresentation	Repeat ultrasound scan for presentation at 34–36 weeks of gestation. **Refer to OBGYN** if the fetal presentation is non-cephalic.
Bedside doptone (>12 weeks of gestation)	**Refer to OBGYN** if doptone is negative to rule out a late miscarriage/intrauterine death (IUD) or if there are any other concerns about fetal well-being. The normal fetal heart ranges from 110 to 160 beats/min, although variations can occur due to numerous causes.

CHAPTER 3

Vaccination in Pregnancy

General Principles

Maternal immunisations may be recommended during pregnancy to protect the mother and fetus from the morbidity of certain infections.

The benefits of vaccinating pregnant women outweigh the potential risks when the likelihood of disease exposure is high or when infection poses a risk to the mother or fetus, and the vaccine is unlikely to cause harm. The healthcare provider should ensure that all vaccines administered are fully documented in the patient's medical record.

There is no evidence of risks to the fetus from vaccinations due to inactivated vaccines, toxoids or immune globulin preparations (i.e., passive immunisation), but these should only be administered if indicated and when the benefits outweigh the risks.

Live Vaccines

Live vaccines are **contraindicated** in pregnancy due to the theoretical risk of transmission to the fetus via placental transfer. The recommended interval between live vaccine administration, e.g., measles, mumps and rubella (MMR), varicella, or measles, mumps, rubella and varicella (MMRV), and the start of conception is 28 days.

If a live vaccine is inadvertently given within 28 days of conception or during pregnancy, counsel the patient on the theoretical risk for the fetus. However, this should **not** be an indication to terminate the pregnancy. It is important to counsel women on the 2–4% background risk of birth defects in the general population.

Immunosuppressives should not be started until at least 4 weeks after the live vaccines were given to women.

Vaccines During Pregnancy

Two vaccines are routinely recommended during ***each*** pregnancy — the inactivated influenza vaccine and the tetanus, diphtheria and acellular pertussis (Tdap) vaccine.

COVID-19 vaccines are recommended for pregnant women and those trying to conceive.

Most other vaccines are not indicated during pregnancy but may be required if pregnant women are at increased risk of infections or are travelling to endemic areas.

Pregnant women are advised against travelling to Saudi Arabia for Hajj or Umrah. If they choose to travel, they should receive meningococcal vaccination (quadrivalent ACWY vaccine, either conjugate or polysaccharide). Travellers need to be up to date with their vaccinations, and other vaccinations may also be indicated.

Travelling to areas where certain diseases may be endemic, such as typhoid fever or yellow fever, is **not recommended**.

Breastfeeding and Vaccinations

Breastfeeding does not adversely affect immunisation and is not a contraindication for vaccination.

Neither inactivated nor live vaccines (except for smallpox and yellow fever vaccination) affect the safety of breastfeeding for mothers or infants.

COVID-19 vaccines are recommended for people who are breastfeeding. Breastfeeding mothers can continue to breastfeed immediately after the vaccination. However, due to evolving evidence, please refer to the latest local guidance before vaccination.

Guidance for Vaccine Recommendations in Pregnancy

Recommendation	Vaccine	Type of vaccine	Remarks
Vaccines that are recommended in pregnancy	COVID-19	mRNA/ inactivated (depending on the brand)	Pregnant or recently pregnant women have an increased risk of severe illness from COVID-19 compared with non-pregnant women. None of the currently available COVID-19 vaccines crosses the placenta. The COVID-19 vaccine may be administered at any trimester. ***Please refer to your latest local guidance as the recommendations may change due to evolving evidence.***
	Influenza	Inactivated	Pregnant and postpartum women are at increased risk of severe illness and influenza-related complications if not vaccinated, due to changes in their immune system, heart and lungs during pregnancy. Inactivated influenza vaccines may be administered at any trimester. They provide positive protection to infants in the first few months after birth when they cannot be vaccinated themselves. **Live attenuated influenza vaccine is not recommended in pregnancy**.
	Tdap	Inactivated	Tdap vaccine prevents pertussis (whooping cough) in the newborn baby via the transplacental transfer of antibodies to the fetus. It provides passive protection for infants up to 3 months of age as the Tdap vaccine can only be administered to infants 2 months old and above. In Singapore, a single dose is administered between 16 and 32 weeks of ***each*** pregnancy, regardless of the interval since the previous Tdap vaccination. If given earlier in pregnancy (e.g., in the first trimester), it should *not* be repeated later in pregnancy. For pregnant women after 32 weeks of gestation, vaccination may still be considered to protect the mother from pertussis infection and reduce the risk of exposure to the infant.

Vaccines that are recommended only in specific situations in pregnancy	Hepatitis A	Inactivated	Vaccination is indicated if the pregnant woman has a high risk of exposure to hepatitis A.
	Hepatitis B	Inactivated	Vaccination is indicated for pregnant women who are identified as being at risk of hepatitis B infection during pregnancy, e.g., having >1 sexual partner during the previous 6 months, having been evaluated or treated for a sexually transmitted infection (STI), recent or current injection drug use, or having had an HBsAg-positive sex partner.
	Meningococcal (MenACWY/ MPSV4)	Inactivated	Vaccination is indicated only for pregnant women at high risk of meningococcal disease (e.g., travel to Hajj).
	Pneumococcal conjugate/ polysaccharide	Inactivated	The indications for administration of the pneumococcal vaccine in a non-pregnant adult are not altered by pregnancy, i.e., pregnant women may require vaccination if they have a very high risk of invasive pneumococcal disease. Administration from the second trimester onwards can be considered if required during pregnancy. There is limited to no safety information available on the use in the first trimester.
	Rabies	Inactivated	Vaccination is indicated for pregnant women if there is a significant risk of exposure (pre-exposure prophylaxis) or following rabies exposure (post-exposure prophylaxis).
	Typhoid	Inactivated	No data are available in pregnancy, but inactive typhoid Vi polysaccharides may be considered for pregnant women travelling to typhoid-affected areas. **Live attenuated typhoid vaccine is *not* recommended in pregnancy.**

(*Continued*)

(*Continued*)

Recommendation	Vaccine	Type of vaccine	Remarks
Vaccines that are *not* recommended in pregnancy	Bacillus Calmette–Guerin (BCG)	Live	Live vaccines are contraindicated in pregnancy (refer to section *General Principles*). Although no harmful effects of BCG vaccination on the fetus have been observed, further studies are required to prove its safety.
	Human papillomavirus (HPV)	Inactivated	Limited safety data in pregnancy. If a woman gets pregnant after initiating the vaccination series, the remaining doses should be delayed until the completion of pregnancy.
	Mumps measles rubella (MMR)	Live	Live vaccines are contraindicated in pregnancy (refer to section *General Principles*). Postpartum women previously unimmunised and seronegative should be vaccinated **after** delivery. To avoid pregnancy for 28 days post MMR. Theoretical risk of congenital rubella syndrome. However, data have not shown an increased risk of fetal anomalies or adverse outcomes in fetuses of women inadvertently vaccinated with MMR. Termination of pregnancy (TOP) is not indicated due to a lack of proven harm.
	Polio	Inactivated	Not recommended in pregnancy unless at increased risk of infection and immediate risk of polio.
	Varicella zoster (chickenpox)	Live	Live vaccines are contraindicated in pregnancy (refer to section *General Principles*). For post-exposure prophylaxis, pregnant women without immunity who are exposed should be strongly considered for **varicella-zoster immune globulin** (VZIG). VZIG is effective when given up to 10 days after contact. In the case of continuous exposures, it is defined as 10 days from the appearance of the rash in the index case (RCOG).
	Yellow fever	Live	In contrast to other live vaccines, the yellow fever vaccine is not contraindicated in pregnancy but rather a precaution. Pregnant women should avoid travelling to areas where yellow fever is endemic; however, vaccination should be considered if travel is unavoidable and the woman is at significant risk of exposure.

CHAPTER 4

Approach to Bleeding in Early Pregnancy

Around 20–25% of women have some bleeding in the first 12 weeks of pregnancy.

50% of women with bleeding in pregnancy will have a healthy baby.

Check if bleeding occurred after sexual intercourse, pelvic examination, cervical smear test or transvaginal ultrasound scan.

It is essential to do an ultrasound scan [transabdominal (TA)/ transvaginal (TV)] in women with bleeding or pain in early pregnancy — to locate the pregnancy, date and assess fetal viability, assess the adnexa and look for free fluid in the pouch of Douglas.

Causes

1. Miscarriage — Threatened/missed/inevitable /incomplete/complete/ septic.
2. Ectopic pregnancy — It is important not to miss a diagnosis of an ectopic pregnancy as it is potentially life-threatening.
3. Local causes — Cervical polyps (common)/ectropion/infection/ cervical cancer (rare).
4. Molar pregnancy (rare).
5. Implantation bleeding — Occurs 1–2 weeks after fertilisation.
6. Subchorionic haematoma — Bleeding beneath the chorionic membranes that enclose the embryo in the uterus.
7. Biochemical pregnancy — Absence of an identifiable pregnancy on ultrasound scan despite a positive urine or serum βHCG test.

Approach to Bleeding in Early Pregnancy

Fig. 4.1 PBAC chart.

PBAC Score	Pads
1	Lightly soaked
2	Moderately soaked
3	Heavily soaked
4	Clots (Small or large)

History

Menstrual history
Weeks of amenorrhoea, regularity of menstrual cycles.

Vaginal bleeding
Onset, quantity, trigger factors. Assess the amount using the pictorial blood loss assessment (PBAC) chart.

Associated symptoms
Lower abdominal pain, giddiness.

↓

Physical examination

Vital parameters
Assess if haemodynamically stable.
Haemodynamic instability is usually associated with a ruptured ectopic pregnancy, severe haemorrhage from miscarriage, gestational trophoblastic disease.

Abdomen
Abdominal tenderness.
Signs of acute abdomen, e.g., guarding and rebound tenderness, usually associated with ruptured ectopic pregnancy.

Vaginal examination
Amount of ongoing bleeding.
Cervical or vaginal lesions such as polyps, ectropion, cancer.
Products of conception.
Cervical dilatation, cervical excitation.

↓

Investigations

Ultrasound pelvis – TA/TV scan

Consider **serum progesterone** to distinguish early viable from non-viable pregnancy if ultrasound findings are inconclusive.

A serum progesterone level of 35 nmol/L in patients with threatened miscarriage can be used to differentiate women at high risk from those at low risk of subsequent miscarriage.

Women with first trimester bleeding + serum progesterone <19 nmol/L(6ng/ml) reliably predicts a non-viable pregnancy.

In our hospital, patients with a serum progesterone level of <35 nmol/L will be offered progesterone supplementation.

Consider **cervical smear** if not up to date/suspicious of cervical cancer.

Transabdominal/Transvaginal Ultrasound Scan (TA/TV US)

- To assess pregnancy location, number, viability, adnexa and free fluid in the pouch of Douglas.
- An intrauterine gestational sac (IUGS) seen on a TVUS may be identified as early as 5 weeks when β-HCG >1,500 IU/L. (In KKH, we use serum β-HCG of 1,500 IU/L as the discriminatory level.)
- A double decidual sign indicates an intrauterine pregnancy.
- The yolk sac is usually visualised by 5–6 weeks of gestation and usually disappears by 10 to 12 weeks.
- Identify the fetal cardiac activity if a fetal pole is present.
  - Measure the **crown-rump length (CRL)** — If there is no visible fetal cardiac activity.
    - If CRL <7 mm on TVUS, repeat the US scan at least 7 days later.

      If the repeat CRL is still <7 mm and fetal cardiac activity is absent — miscarriage is confirmed.
    - If CRL ≥7 mm and fetal cardiac activity is absent, likely a miscarriage, advise repeating the US scan at least 7 days later before making a miscarriage diagnosis.
  - Measure the **mean sac diameter (MSD)** if a fetal pole is absent.
    - If MSD <25 mm on TVUS, repeat the US scan at least 7 days later.

      If the repeat MSD is still <25 mm and no fetal pole is seen, miscarriage is confirmed.
    - If MSD ≥25 mm on TVUS and no yolk sac or fetal pole is seen, advise repeating the US scan at least 7 days later before making a miscarriage diagnosis.
- If **missed miscarriage** is confirmed, discuss with the patient the 3 management options, i.e., expectant, medical or surgical.
- If **incomplete miscarriage** is diagnosed, identify any retained products of conception (RPOC) and measure the endometrial thickness to determine further management options.
- **Ectopic pregnancy** is suspected if an IUGS is absent. Efforts should be made to look for adnexal masses or free fluid in the pouch of Douglas.
- ***Complete molar pregnancy*** has the classic image of a cystic "snowstorm" appearance, whereas a ***partial molar pregnancy*** is often diagnosed retrospectively by histology after an evacuation of the uterus, as it may often mimic a miscarriage on an ultrasound scan.

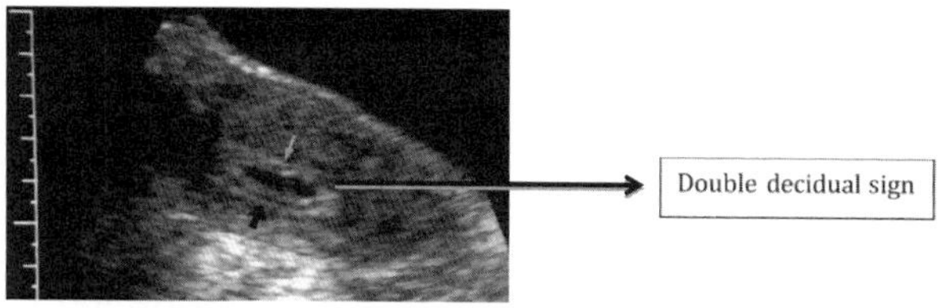

Fig. 4.2 Intrauterine gestational sac (IUGS).

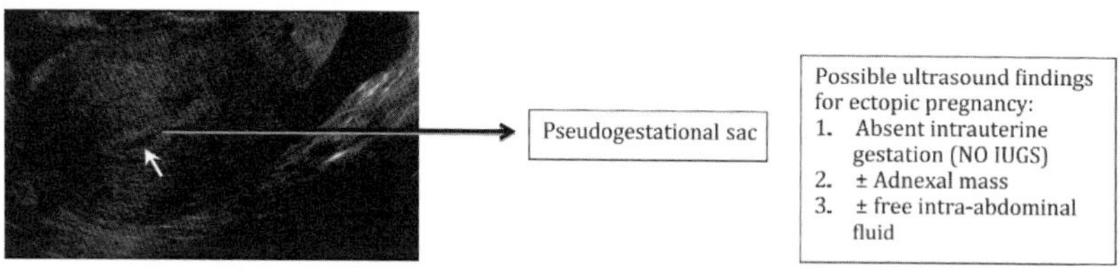

Fig. 4.3 Pseudogestational sac in an ectopic pregnancy.

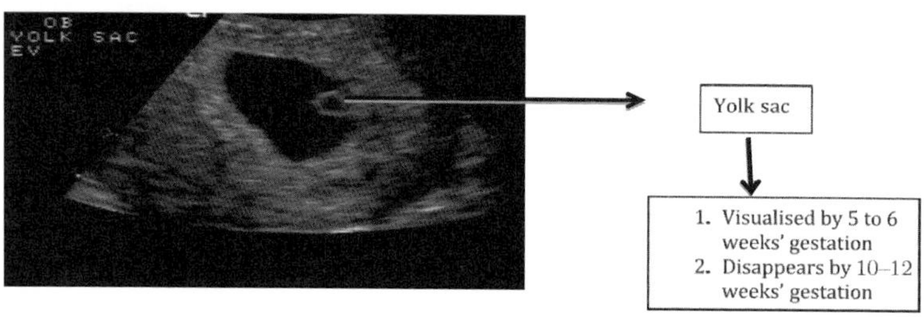

Fig. 4.4 IUGS with yolk sac.

Indications for anti-D prophylaxis in <12 week pregnancy in rhesus negative women. ***(Adapted from BCSH 2014 Guidelines for the use of anti-D immunoglobulin for the prevention of haemolytic disease of the fetus and newborn.)***

Potentially sensitising events:

- For pregnancies <12 weeks + miscarriage/threatened miscarriage: Give anti-D Ig if there is heavy or repeated vaginal bleeding or bleeding associated with abdominal pain
- Termination of pregnancy (medical/surgical)
- Molar pregnancy
- Ectopic pregnancy

A minimum anti-D Ig 250 IU must be administered within 72 hours of the event.

In KKH, a standard dose of 1,500 IU (=300 mcg) is used for these sensitising events as this is the only formulation available in our pharmacy.

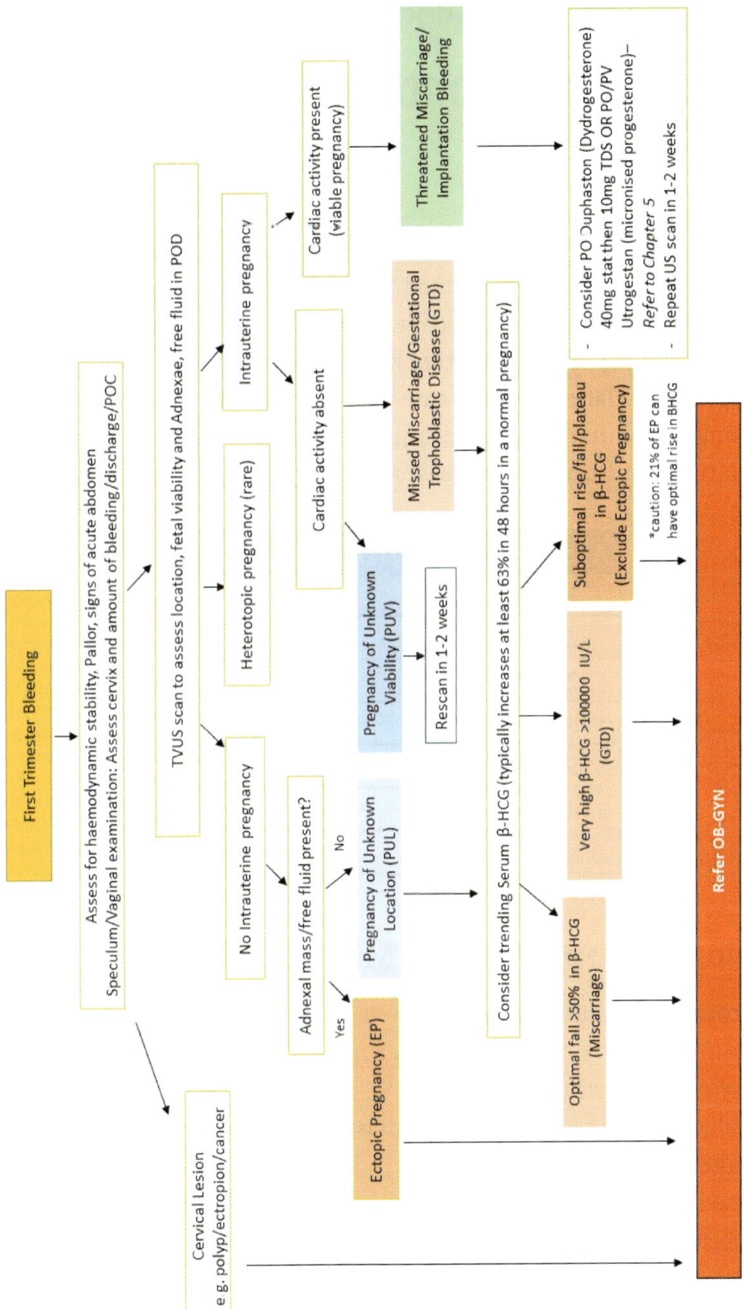

Fig. 4.5 Management of early pregnancy bleeding.

CHAPTER 5

Approach to Spontaneous Miscarriage

Spontaneous miscarriage is defined as the loss of a clinically recognised pregnancy before the 24th week of gestation.

The incidence of spontaneous miscarriage averages around 15% in the general population, with a rate of 8–20% in the first trimester and decreasing to about 3% in the second trimester.

The risk of miscarriage increases with increasing maternal age.

Age (years)	Miscarriage Rate (%)
12–19	13
20–24	11
25–29	12
30–34	15
35–39	25
40–44	51
≥ 45	93

Aetiologies of Spontaneous Miscarriage

1. **Chromosomal abnormalities**
   Account for 50% of first-trimester miscarriages and 30% of second-trimester miscarriages.
   Usually due to aneuploidies, mosaicism and structural abnormalities.
2. **Congenital anomalies**
   Caused by genetic, chromosomal abnormalities or extrinsic factors such as teratogens.

3. **Endocrine disorders**
   Poorly controlled diabetes mellitus, thyroid disorders, polycystic ovarian syndrome.
4. **Hypercoagulable disorders**
   Autoimmune: Antiphospholipid syndrome, systemic lupus erythematosus.
5. **Maternal infections**
   Listeriosis, toxoplasmosis, parvovirus B19, rubella, herpes simplex virus, cytomegalovirus infection.
6. **Structural uterine abnormalities**
   Congenital: Uterine septum, uterine didelphys.
   Acquired: Submucosal fibroids.
7. **Unexplained**

Different Types of Spontaneous Miscarriages

	Threatened	Incomplete	Complete	Missed	Septic
History	PV staining Mild abdominal pain	Heavy PV bleeding Abdominal pain Incomplete passage of POC	PV bleeding Abdominal pain Complete passage of POC	PV staining No abdominal pain May be asymptomatic – Incidental finding on a routine US scan	PV bleeding/discharge Abdominal/pelvic pain Fever Foul-smelling vaginal discharge Can follow spontaneous miscarriage, medical or surgical evacuation of the uterus
Physical exam	Cervical os closed PV bleeding, usually minimal	Cervical os open PV bleeding Some POC seen	Cervical os closed ± PV bleeding	Cervical os closed ± PV bleeding	Haemodynamic instability Fever Cervical os open PV bleeding Uterine tenderness
Transvaginal ultrasound scan (TVUS)	FH activity present Viable intrauterine pregnancy	FH activity absent Irregular IUGS RPOC	Empty uterus Thin ET	CRL ≥7 mm without FH activity **or** MSD ≥25 mm (without yolk sac or fetal pole) Empty irregular IUGS	FH activity absent RPOC
Management	**Expectant** — Reassure 97% have a normal outcome Consider serum progesterone versus progesterone supplementation (*Refer to our protocol on first trimester threatened miscarriage*) Avoid strenuous activity/ sexual activity Repeat US in 1–2 weeks	**Expectant** — Analgesia ± antibiotics **Medical** — Single-dose 600 μg PV misoprostol **Surgical** — Evacuation of the uterus (vacuum aspiration)	**Expectant**	**Expectant** **Medical** — Single dose 800 μg PV misoprostol **Surgical** — Evacuation of the uterus (vacuum aspiration in the first trimester)	Resuscitation IV fluids Broad spectrum **IV antibiotics** followed by **surgical** evacuation of the uterus (vacuum aspiration under ultrasound guidance to reduce the risk of uterine perforation)

PV — per vaginal, FH — fetal heart, RPOC — retained products of conception, US — ultrasound, TV — transvaginal, IUGS — intrauterine gestational sac, CRL — crown-rump length, MSD — mean sac diameter, ET — endometrial thickness.

Management of Incomplete/Missed Miscarriage

<table>
<tr><th>Expectant management</th><th>Medical management</th><th>Surgical management</th></tr>
<tr><td>First-line management strategy for 7–14 days
• Efficacy rates ~70–80%
• Alternative treatment options if unsuccessful despite expectant management after 4 weeks due to risk of DIC</td><td>Indicated if:
▪ Expectant management is not acceptable/suitable
▪ Pain/bleeding has not started during 7–14 days of expectant management (suggesting that the miscarriage process has not begun)
▪ If bleeding and pain persist or increase (suggestive of incomplete miscarriage)

Offer US pelvis
Explain risks of bleeding, infection, retained products of conception</td><td>Indicated if:
▪ Bleeding and medical management are not acceptable/suitable
▪ Haemodynamic instability
▪ Signs of infection
▪ Woman's preference

Explain surgical procedure — Evacuation of the uterus: (vacuum aspiration in the first trimester) under general anaesthesia in operating theatre.
Explained risks of bleeding, uterine perforation, infection, retained products of conception, Asherman syndrome and surgical cost.</td></tr>
<tr><td colspan="2">Contraindications
• Increased risk of haemorrhage (late first-trimester)
• Previous adverse traumatic experience (previous stillbirth, miscarriage or antepartum haemorrhage)
• Increased risk from the effects of bleeding (severe anaemia/coagulopathies/unable to have a blood transfusion)
• Evidence of infection</td><td></td></tr>
</table>

(Continued)

(*Continued*)

Expectant management	Medical management	Surgical management
***Follow-up*:** If bleeding/pain does not occur after 7–14 days of expectant management, advise medical or surgical management. If a spontaneous complete miscarriage occurs, do a urine pregnancy test (UPT) after 3 weeks and ensure that it is negative.	Offer *vaginal misoprostol* — a single dose of 800 µg. Oral administration is acceptable if this is the woman's preference. Oral mifepristone can be given 24–48 hours before vaginal misoprostol for cervical priming (KKH protocol). Offer analgesia and anti-emetics as needed.	Take consent for surgery Full blood count Type & screen (T&S) Vaginal misoprostol for cervical priming, if indicated
	***Follow-up*:** Seek medical attention if bleeding does not occur 24 hours after treatment. If a miscarriage occurs and is complete, do a UPT after 3 weeks and ensure negative. If an incomplete miscarriage occurs, the woman may need a repeat dose of medical treatment or the surgical option.	
For women with regular menstrual cycles, menses usually return 4–6 weeks following treatment of the miscarriage.		

When to Try to Conceive Again after a Miscarriage?

Provide emotional support to women after miscarriage.
Refer to mental wellness or miscarriage support groups.
Ensure that the woman is physically and psychologically ready for her next pregnancy.

Ensure lifestyle modifications, e.g., lose weight, quit smoking, reduce alcohol and caffeine intake, if required.
Advise folic acid pre-conception.

Women who conceive within the first 6 months of an initial miscarriage have the best reproductive outcomes and the lowest complication rates in a subsequent pregnancy.

Our Suggested Protocol for Management of First-Trimester Threatened Miscarriage

Clinical Assessment + Ultrasound Scan (US) showing viable intrauterine pregnancy (up to 12 weeks gestation) *with* **abdominal pain** *and/or* **vaginal bleeding**

Threatened Miscarriage

EXCLUDE
Pregnancy of Unknown Location (PUL) / Ectopic Pregnancy
Multiple /IVF Pregnancy
Bleeding from local causes
Missed//Inevitable/
Incomplete /Complete miscarriage

No previous miscarriage

Discuss options with patient:

1. **Supportive care and bed rest.**
2. **Serum progesterone** to triage the risk of miscarriage
   - If < 35 nmol/L: for progesterone therapy. (risk of miscarriage 70.8%)
   - If ≥ 35 nmol/L: reassure woman. No treatment is required. (risk of miscarriage 9.6%)
3. **Progesterone treatment** if patient requests.

Types of Progesterone Therapy:

- PO Dydrogesterone with loading dose 40 mg stat followed by 10mg BD/TDS x 2/52 or
- PO micronized progesterone 200 mg ON x 2/52 or
- PV micronized progesterone 200 mg ON x 2/52

Follow-up clinic in 1-2 weeks
Return advice if increased P.V. bleeding /abdominal pain

≥ 1 previous miscarriage

- Recommend progesterone treatment to 16 weeks or until symptoms remit (whichever is later)

Types of Progesterone Therapy:*

- PO Dydrogesterone 40 mg stat followed by 10mg BD/TDS (if active bleeding) or
- PV micronized progesterone 400 mg BD

Follow-up clinic in 1-2 weeks
Return advice if increased P.V. bleeding /abdominal pain

**Vaginal/rectal/parenteral progesterone treatment has higher bioavailability. However, oral progesterone is likely to be more acceptable as it is less invasive and easier to administer.*

Evidence Supporting Our Protocol

Since 2016, there are 4 systemic reviews (Lee HJ *et al., Biomed Res Int* 2017:3616875; Wahabi. HA *et al., Cochrane Database Syst Rev* 2018; 8(8):Cd005943; Wang XX *et al., J Obstet Gynaecol Res* 2019; 45(4):794-802; Li L *et al.*, BJOG 2020; 127(9):1055-1063) which showed a decrease in miscarriage with oral dydrogesterone.

NICE Guidelines 2021

— There is no benefit of Progesterone supplementation for women with early pregnancy bleeding but without a history of miscarriage
— Recommends vaginal micronised progesterone 400 mg twice a day once pregnant in the first trimester until 16 weeks of gestation for women with a viable intrauterine pregnancy, vaginal bleeding, and a previous miscarriage.

ROCG Recurrent Miscarriage Guidelines 2023

— Consider progestogen supplementation in women with recurrent miscarriages who present with bleeding in early pregnancy.
— For example, 400 mg micronised vaginal progesterone twice daily at the time of bleeding until 16 weeks of gestation.
— However, it is unclear which formulations, routes and timings of administration of progesterone may confer the most positive outcomes and whether these factors may affect the outcomes of asymptomatic women and people with unexplained recurrent miscarriages.

FIGO Good Practice Recommendations 2023 for reeurrent first-trimester miscarriages

— Consider oral progesterone supplementation during pregnancy as there may have been a beneficial impact on first-trimester recurrent miscarriages. An optimal dose is 20 mg oral progesterone daily, but there are limited trials and studies regarding the dose.

— Vaginal and rectal progesterone supplementation during pregnancy is <u>not</u> recommended as there is no beneficial impact on first-trimester recurrent miscarriages.
— Injectable progesterone supplementation during pregnancy is <u>not</u> recommended as there is no beneficial impact on first-trimester recurrent miscarriages.
— In KKH, we usually prescribe oral dydrogesterone 40 mg loading dose followed by 10 mg 3 times a day for 2 weeks or till bleeding stops.

CHAPTER 6

Approach to Recurrent Pregnancy Loss (RPL)

Definition

There are various definitions of recurrent pregnancy loss (RPL), also referred to as recurrent spontaneous miscarriage.

RCOG definition: The occurrence of three or more consecutive losses of clinically recognised pregnancies before the 24th week of gestation.

The updated ESHRE RPL 2018 guidelines state that it could be considered RPL after losing two or more pregnancies. It includes biochemical pregnancies, resolved or treated pregnancies of unknown location. Ectopic and molar pregnancies are ***not*** part of the definition.

Primary RPL — RPL without a previous viable pregnancy beyond 24 weeks of gestation.

Secondary RPL — RPL after one or more previous pregnancies progressing beyond 24 weeks of gestation.

RPL affects 1% of couples trying to conceive.

It is estimated that 1–2% of second-trimester pregnancies miscarry before 24 weeks of gestation.

Risk Factors/Aetiologies for RPL

- **Age**
  - The risk of pregnancy loss is much higher if the maternal age is ≥40 years, ranging from 50% at 40–44 years to 93% if ≥45 years.
  - Advancing paternal age >40 years old increases the risk of miscarriage, although not as significant as advancing maternal age.

- **Previous pregnancy loss**
  - The general risk of miscarriage is ~10% in the first pregnancy, 15–20% after the first miscarriage, 24–29% after the second miscarriage and 31–33% after the third miscarriage.
  - The risk of miscarriage may be higher depending on the cause of the pregnancy loss.
- **Genetic**
  - <u>*Embryonal chromosomal abnormalities*</u> account for 30–57% of miscarriages.
  - <u>*Parental chromosomal abnormalities:*</u> In 2–5% of couples with recurrent miscarriage, one of the partners carries a balanced structural chromosomal anomaly, most commonly a balanced reciprocal or Robertsonian translocation.
- **Anatomic**

  <u>*Structural abnormalities/congenital uterine malformation*</u> *(1.8–37.6%)*
  - The **septate uterus** is the congenital uterine malformation associated with the worst reproductive outcomes and most commonly associated with RPL. Bicornuate uterus is also associated with an increased risk of miscarriage.
  - Submucosal fibroids can affect normal implantation.
  - Adenomyosis has been associated with higher pregnancy loss and is thought to be due to an inflammatory state in the endometrium from adenomyosis or associated endometriosis.
  - Intrauterine synechiae can cause RPL.
  - Endometrial polyps *have **not*** been shown to be associated with RPL.
- **Endocrine**
  - Poorly controlled diabetes mellitus (DM) — high HbA1c levels in the first trimester increases the risk of miscarriage and fetal malformation.
  - Poorly controlled thyroid disease. Subclinical hypothyroidism or presence of thyroid autoantibodies are associated with an increased risk of miscarriage.
  - Polycystic ovarian syndrome — insulin resistance, hyperinsulinaemia and hyperandrogenaemia likely to have a role in RPL.
  - Hyperprolactinaemia.
- **Autoimmune [e.g., antiphospholipid syndrome (APS) or SLE]**
  - ***APS*** refers to the association between antiphospholipid antibodies such as lupus anticoagulant (LAC), anticardiolipin antibodies

  (ACL), anti-β2 glycoprotein-I antibodies and adverse pregnancy outcomes or vascular thrombosis.
  - It is a form of *acquired* thrombophilia.
  - Adverse pregnancy outcomes include:
    1. Three consecutive miscarriages before 10 weeks of gestation.
    2. One morphologically normal fetal loss after 10 weeks of gestation.
    3. One preterm birth <34 weeks of gestation due to placental malfunction.
  - Antiphospholipid antibodies are present in 15% of women with RPL versus 2% in women with no history of miscarriage.
  - Live birth rates with no pharmacological intervention can be as low as 1%.
  - Treatment with aspirin and low-molecular-weight heparin (LMWH) improves pregnancy outcomes in this group of women. These treatments may be initiated pre-conception or once urine pregnancy test is positive.
- **Hereditary thrombophilias**
  - There are conflicting data on the association of maternal hereditary thrombophilias with RPL. Some studies have shown a weak or no association between *inherited* thrombophilias, including activated protein C resistance (most commonly due to factor V Leiden mutation), deficiencies of protein C/S, antithrombin III and prothrombin mutation, and RPL.
- **Cervical incompetence**
  - Usually causes second-trimester miscarriages.
  - Preceded by rupture of membranes or painless cervical dilatation.
  - Risk factors include previous cervical excisional procedures (e.g., cone biopsy of the cervix), connective tissue disorders (e.g., Ehlers–Danlos syndrome), prior cervical lacerations and Müllerian duct abnormalities.
- **Infections**
  - Usually, infections are isolated events that cause sporadic miscarriages instead of RPL.
  - There is a limited role of infections as a causative factor in RPL.
- **Others**
  - A high body mass index (BMI) increases the risk of sporadic miscarriages and RPL.

- o Lifestyle — the role of caffeine and excessive exercise is less clear. Alcohol and smoking increase the risk of sporadic miscarriages in a dose-dependent manner.
- o Stress is associated with RPL, but there is **no** evidence that it directly causes RPL.

- **Idiopathic**
  - o Up to 50% of RPL will not have an identified cause.

The evaluation of women with RPL is often challenging as they often seek definitive reasons for their condition and hope for curative measures. However, the aetiology of RPL may not always be identified and there are few evidence-based treatment strategies.

Detailed History and Physical Examination for RPL

History:

- Obstetric history
- Consanguinity/Change in partners?
- **Number** of spontaneous miscarriages and gestational age of miscarriages
- **Features** of prior miscarriages
- **Gynaecological history**: Menstrual history. Any abnormalities?
- History of galactorrhoea/thyroid dysfunction/hirsutism?
- Known uterine abnormalities — uterine didelphys/bicornuate or septate uterus
- Evidence of vaginal discharge
- History of congenital/genetic abnormalities
- **Past medical/surgical history**
- Previous painless cervical dilatation
- History of uterine instrumentation/evacuation of uterus/surgical termination of pregnancies
- History of VTE
- **Family history**: Thrombophilias/VTE, congenital/genetic abnormalities

- **Social history**
  - Smoking, alcohol, caffeine, illicit drug use
  - Assess mental well-being
- **Previous investigations and treatment**

RPL typically occurs at similar gestation in consecutive pregnancies
  - Miscarriages at earlier gestations may reflect an underlying chromosomal abnormality
  - Miscarriages at later gestations tend to be related to anatomical factors

Examination

- *General condition*: Vitals, BMI
- Signs of goitre/thyroid dysfunction/galactorrhoea/hirsutism
- Abdominal examination
- Speculum and vaginal examination: Müllerian abnormalities?

Investigations for RPL

Suggest to follow a graded approach

One pregnancy loss — Preconception advice and self-help support resources as needed.

Two pregnancy losses — *Limited* screening investigations.

Three pregnancy losses — *Full* screening investigations.

- ***Karyotyping — parental or products of conception (POC)***
  - Balanced reciprocal, Robertsonian translocations or mosaicism may be passed to the fetus in the unbalanced form.
  - Karyotyping should be performed on POC of the third and subsequent consecutive miscarriage(s) and in any second timester miscarriages.
  - It should be performed on peripheral blood of both partners where testing of POC reports an *unbalanced* structural chromosomal abnormality.
  - Refer for genetic counselling if patient or partner has an abnormal karyotype or abnormal fetal karyotype.
  - If the karyotype of the miscarried pregnancy is abnormal, the prognosis is better for the next pregnancy.

- Couples with *balanced translocations* have a low risk (0.8%) of pregnancies with an unbalanced karyotype surviving into the second trimester. Their chance of having a healthy child is high (83%).

- ***Uterine assessment***
  - Ultrasound pelvis ± 3D ultrasound scan: to look for uterine anomaly.

  Suspected anomalies/intrauterine adhesions may warrant tests like saline sonography, hysterosalpingography (HSG), hysterosalpingo-foam sonography and hysteroscopy ± laparoscopy.
  - Combined hysteroscopy and laparoscopy and possibly 3D ultrasound/MRI scan can be used for definitive diagnosis.
  - Ultrasound scan of the kidneys and urinary tract in women with Müllerian tract abnormality due to a 20–30% association with renal tract abnormalities.
- ***Endocrine screening***
  - HbA1c, thyroid function test (TFT), thyroid peroxidase (TPO) antibody.
  - If there is clinical suspicion of hyperprolactinaemia, do serum prolactin.
  - ESHRE does not recommend assessing for PCOS.
- ***Autoimmune screening***
  - Test for ACL, LAC and anti-β2 glycoprotein-I antibodies to screen for APS.

  Diagnosis of APS:
  - Mandatory for two positive tests at least 12 weeks apart (and at least 6 weeks post miscarriage) for either LAC or ACL.
  - Antibodies of immunoglobulin G and/or immunoglobulin M class — medium or high titre over 40 GPL or MPL or >99th percentile.
- ***Hereditary thrombophilia***
  - Test for inherited thrombophilias are factor V Leiden, prothrombin gene mutation (or factor II mutation or prothrombin G20210A), antithrombin deficiency, protein C and S deficiency.
  - RCOG suggests screening for factor V Leiden, prothrombin gene mutation and protein S deficiency — ideally within a research context. Women need to be informed there is limited evidence that treatment improves outcomes.

For protein C/S and antithrombin deficiency, they should be done at least 6 weeks after pregnancy loss and patients should not be on hormonal medication.
  - ESHRE suggests screening only if there are additional risk factors for thrombophilia.
- *Others*
  - Cytokine testing should **not** be used.
  - **Insufficient evidence** to advise natural killer (NK) cell testing of peripheral blood or endometrial tissues.

Investigations for RPL after 3 previous first-trimester miscarriages (RCOG)

- ➢ ACL IgG/IgM antibodies and LAC
- ➢ Ultrasound of the pelvis for uterine anomalies, ideally with 3D ultrasound
- ➢ Karyotype for POC — parental karyotyping if indicated — genetic counselling if abnormal karyotype detected (1.9–3.5%)
- ➢ Offer TFT with TPO antibody

Management of RPL

1. **Multidisciplinary care:**
   - o Refer to a dedicated RPL clinic.
   - o Refer to a medical social worker for psychological support. Psychological support is important for couples with RPL.
   - o Patient support group.

   Counselling and support for RPL:
   - o For unexplained RPL, the chance of a live birth after RPL is about 75%, with supportive care alone.
2. **Preconception counselling:**
   - o Advise couples to aim for a normal BMI (18.5–24.9 kg/m^2).
   - o Avoid alcohol and illicit drug use. Limit caffene to 200 mg/day
   - o Quit smoking.
   - o Peri-conception folic acid daily for at least 3 months.
   - o Consider vitamin D supplements.

3. **Treat the underlying cause and optimise any pre-existing medical conditions.**
   - ***Parental karyotype anomalies***

     Refer for genetic counselling.

     Reproductive options in couples with chromosomal rearrangements include:

     a. Continuing to try and conceive naturally with or without a prenatal diagnostic test.

     b. Preimplantation genetic testing (PGT).

        <u>For translocation carrier:</u>

        - Preimplantation genetic testing for structural rearrangements (PGT-SR) is a possible treatment option and improves pregnancy outcomes. It reduces the miscarriage rate and time to conceive a pregnancy which results in a live birth.
        - PGT necessitates that the couple undergoes IVF. There are costs involved; it takes a longer time and requires freeze-all cycles.
        - It can differentiate between euploid and aneuploid embryos. However, it may take a few cycles before an embryo with balanced chromosomes is found.

        <u>For unexplained RPL:</u>

        - IVF-PGT-A (preimplantation genetic testing for aneuploidy = previously known as preimplantation genetic screening, PGS) does not improve live birth rates or decrease conception time.
        - For IVF-PGT-A, the aim is to identify aneuploidies in embryos. However, couples need to be counselled on the possibility of no normal embryos, and not all pregnancies result in a live birth.
        - Offer if the couple has subfertility factors.

     c. Gamete (egg/sperm) donation.

     d. Surrogacy.

     e. Adoption.

     f. Child-free life.
   - ***Uterine anomalies***
     - Surgery if the anomaly is potentially correctable, e.g., uterine septum, intrauterine adhesions and submucosal fibroids, although evidence is not strong for surgical removal of polyps and fibroids in RPL management.

- Metroplasty is **not** recommended for a bicornuate uterus.
- Uterine reconstruction is **not** recommended for women with a hemi-uterus.

- ***Endocrine***
  - Refer to an endocrinologist, e.g., hyperprolactinaemia, DM, thyroid disorders.
  - There is a lack of consensus regarding the normal upper limit of TSH. There is no strong evidence that treating subclinical hypothyroidism would be useful in RPL.
  - Most will advise a TSH <2.5 before trying to conceive.
  - TFT should be checked during pregnancy at the booking visit and every 4 weeks.
  - There is **insufficient** evidence to evaluate the effect of metformin in pregnancy to prevent a miscarriage in women with RPL.
- ***APS***
  - May benefit from aspirin and heparin once the urine pregnancy test is positive. (Refer to Chapter 18: *Medications in Pregnancy and Lactation*.) Low-dose aspirin (LDA) and LMWH throughout pregnancy reduce the risk of miscarriage by 54% and maternal thrombosis. (Continue until at least 34 weeks of gestation (RCOG).)
  - ***Side effects of APS treatment:***

    LDA: There are no adverse fetal outcomes.

    LMWH:

    - *Fetal complications* — There is **no** potential to cause fetal haemorrhage or teratogenicity (as heparin does not cross the placenta).
    - *Maternal complications* include bleeding, hypersensitivity, heparin-induced thrombocytopenia, osteopenia and vertebral fractures with long-term use.

    LMWH is as safe as unfractionated heparin and has potential advantages during pregnancy since it causes less heparin-induced thrombocytopenia.
- ***Cervical incompetence***
  - Perform *cervical length surveillance* during pregnancy for women with a history of second-trimester miscarriages or cervical incompetence.

 - Offer *cervical cerclage* if serial cervical length measurement shows a cervical length of ≤25 mm by transvaginal ultrasound scan from 16 weeks at 2 weekly intervals until 24 weeks (recommendation does not apply to multiple pregnancies).
 - Offer *oral/vaginal progesterone* 200 mg ON/BD from 16 weeks until 34 weeks for cervical shortening with no cerclage or after cerclage has been placed.
- ***Thrombophilia***
 - ESHRE suggests the use of anticoagulation for the indication of VTE prevention. RCOG recommends considering thromboprophylaxis for women with Factor V Leiden, Protein S Deficiency and prothrombin mutation when there are risk factors for thrombosis and/or a history of second trimester miscarriage, especially with evidence of placental thrombotic lesions.
 - Heparin treatment during pregnancy may improve the live birth rates of women with *second*-trimester miscarriages associated with inherited thrombophilias.
 - However, there is **insufficient** evidence for the association of recurrent *first*-trimester miscarriages with inherited thrombophilia.
- ***Use of progesterone***
 - For RPL, consider progestogens.

 ***For women with early-pregnancy bleeding and a history of miscarriage*:**
 - Recent data showed an improvement in live birth rates when vaginal micronised progesterone was given to women with a history of ≥1 miscarriage and vaginal bleeding.
 - There is **no** benefit of progesterone supplementation for women with early-pregnancy bleeding but without a history of miscarriage.
 - ***NICE guidelines 2021*** recommend vaginal micronised progesterone 400 mg twice a day once pregnant in the first trimester until 16 weeks of gestation for women with a viable intrauterine pregnancy with vaginal bleeding and a previous miscarriage.
 - ***RCOG guideline 2023*** recommends progestogen supplementation in women with recurrent miscarriages who present with bleeding

in early pregnancy, However, it is unclear which formulation, route and timing of progesterone confers the best outcomes.

- ***FIGO Good Practice Recommendations 2023*** advise oral progesterone supplementation during pregnancy due to possible beneficial impact on first-trimester recurrent miscarriages.
- There is **no** evidence of fetal abnormalities or short-term harm with progesterone use.

- ***Idiopathic***
  - Almost 50% of RPLs remain unexplained. Women with unexplained RPLs have an excellent prognosis for future pregnancy outcomes without pharmacological intervention. Support in the setting of a dedicated RPL clinic is recommended for patients with idiopathic RPL.

CHAPTER 7

Abdominal Pain in Pregnancy

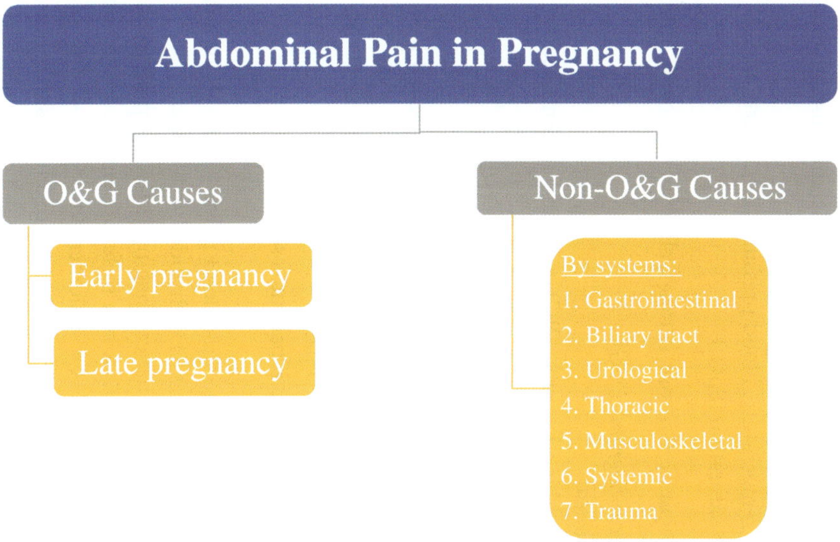

<table>
<tr>
<td>Approach to Abdominal Pain in Pregnancy
1. SOCRATES (for pain assessment)
• Site of pain
• Onset
• Character-stabbing/sharp/ache?
• Radiation
• Associations, e.g., nausea, vomiting, fever, urine, or bowel complaints
• Time course — does the pain follow any pattern?
• Exacerbating or relieving factors
• Severity of pain — pain score (0–10)</td>
<td rowspan="2">3. Investigations (guided by differential diagnosis/clinical presentation)
Examination:
Vitals: Temperature, blood pressure (BP), heart rate (HR), respiratory rate (RR), oxygen saturation (SpO_2)

Urine dipstick: Glucose, ketones, albumin, leucocyte, nitrites

Electrocardiogram (ECG)
Biochemical
• Full blood count (FBC), type and screen (T&S) or group and crossmatch (GXM)
• Urea, electrolytes and creatinine (UECr)
• Liver function test (LFT)
• Partial thromboplastin time (PTT)/activated partial thromboplastin time (aPTT)
• C-reactive protein (CRP)
• Serum amylase/lipase
• Septic work-up if patient is septic
Imaging
• Ultrasound scan abdomen ± pelvis — transabdominal/transvaginal (TA/TV).
• Chest X-ray (CXR) with abdominal shield.
• Magnetic resonance imaging (MRI) — preferred imaging modality as no ionising radiation risk to fetus compared to computer tomography (CT) scan. Risk with CT abdomen and pelvis — dose of radiation exposure can be as high as 30–50 mGy. Risk to fetus is small, but risk of childhood cancer is increased by 0.1% and fatal adult cancers by 0.3%.</td>
</tr>
<tr>
<td>2. Clinical red flags
• Re-admission/multiple admissions
• Repeated doses of analgesia without ascertaining cause
• New onset anxiety/confusion attributed to a psychiatric cause rather than an underlying (undiagnosed) organic disease
*Requires senior clinician evaluation</td>
</tr>
</table>

4. Management

Anaesthesia/medical/surgical considerations:

Multidisciplinary team approach. airway, breathing, circulation, disability, exposure (ABCDE) prioritised approach.

Broad-spectrum antibiotics for sepsis.

Involve surgical and medical teams early. *Do not delay surgical interventions because of pregnancy.*

Obstetric considerations:

In case of operative intervention for non-obstetric condition — no increased risk of miscarriage/preterm labour (counsel on the background risk of miscarriage and preterm labour). Benefits outweigh the risks of surgery.

Laparoscopy can be performed at any gestation if indicated.

- ≥20 weeks of gestation — left lateral position to minimise aortocaval compression.
- Steroids for fetal lung maturity if preterm delivery is indicated.
- ≥24 weeks of gestation: perform fetal heart rate monitoring. Confirm fetal viability pre- and post-surgery.
- Post-op VTE prophylaxis.
- No manipulation of the uterus.
- Administer anti-D in rhesus negative mothers (with rhesus positive partners).

O&G Causes: Simple Approach by Site of Pain

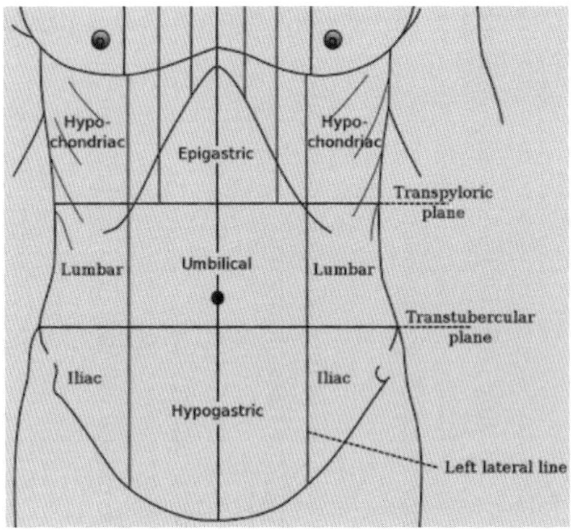

Nine quadrants of abdomen
Adapted from Study.com

O&G Causes: Simple Approach by Site of Pain

Right hypochondrium *Late pregnancy* Acute fatty liver of pregnancy Impending eclampsia	**Epigastrium** *Late pregnancy* – Acute fatty liver of pregnancy – Impending eclampsia	**Left hypochondrium**
Right lumbar *Late pregnancy* – Polyhydramnios	**Umbilical** *Late pregnancy* – Polyhydramnios – Uterine rupture – Chorioamnionitis	**Left lumbar** *Late pregnancy* – Polyhydramnios
Right iliac fossa (RIF) *Early pregnancy* – Stretching of right round ligament – Right ectopic pregnancy – Right adnexal torsion – Right ovarian cyst rupture, haemorrhage, infection – Incarcerated cyst or fibroid – Fibroid degeneration – Ovarian hyperstimulation syndrome (OHSS) – Deep vein thrombosis (DVT) in pelvic vessels	**Hypogastrium/suprapubic** *Early pregnancy* – *Miscarriage*: Threatened, inevitable, incomplete, complete, septic – Fibroid degeneration – Acute retention of urine (ARU) due to acute uterine retroversion/incarcerated fibroids/cysts *Late pregnancy* – Labour – Placental abruption – Uterine rupture – Chorioamnionitis – Braxton Hicks contractions – Symphysis pubis dysfunction (SPD) – Rectus abdominis rupture – Fibroid degeneration	**Left iliac fossa (LIF)** *Early pregnancy* – Stretching of left round ligament – Left ectopic pregnancy – Left adnexal torsion – Left ovarian cyst rupture, haemorrhage, infection – Incarcerated cyst or fibroid – Fibroid degeneration – OHSS – DVT in pelvic vessels

Non-O&G Causes: Simple Approach by Site of Pain

1. **Right Hypochondrium** **Thoracic** – Right lower lobe pneumonia – Right pleural effusion **Biliary** – Cholecystitis – Biliary colic – Cholangitis **Gastrointestinal** – Peptic ulcer **Hepatic** – Hepatitis – Hepatic abscess **Musculoskeletal** – Costochondritis	2. **Epigastrium** **Gastrointestinal** – Oesophagitis – Gastritis – Peptic ulcer disease – Gastroesophageal reflux – Pancreatitis	3. **Left hypochondrium** **Thoracic** – Left lower lobe pneumonia – Left pleural effusion – Referred pain from pulmonary embolism **Gastrointestinal** – Peptic ulcer disease – Pancreatitis – Diverticulitis **Musculoskeletal** – Costochondritis
4. **Right lumbar** **Biliary** – Cholecystitis – Cholelithiasis – Cholangitis **Urological** – Pyelonephritis – Hydronephrosis – Renal calculi **Gastrointestinal** – Appendicitis **Musculoskeletal** – Strain	5. **Umbilical** **Gastrointestinal** – Early appendicitis – Bowel obstruction – Sickle cell crisis – Gastroenteritis – Inflammatory bowel disease – Colitis **Systemic** – Diabetic keto acidosis (DKA) **Trauma Musculoskeletal** – Umbilical hernia	6. **Left lumbar** **Urological** – Pyelonephritis – Hydronephrosis – Renal calculi **Musculoskeletal** – Strain **Gastrointestinal** – Colitis – Constipation
7. **RIF** **Gastrointestinal** – Appendicitis – Mesenteric adenitis – Colitis – Hernia – Inflammatory bowel disease	8. **Hypogastrium/Suprapubic** **Urological** – Cystitis – Urinary tract infection – ARU – Bladder calculi	9. **LIF** **Gastrointestinal** – Constipation – Diverticulitis – Colitis – Hernia – Inflammatory bowel disease

***Others*:** Drug abuse or withdrawal, psychological cause.

O&G Causes of Abdominal Pain in Early Pregnancy

- **Exclude *miscarriage*:** Refer to Chapter 5: *Approach to Spontaneous Miscarriage.*
- **Exclude *ectopic pregnancy*:** Refer to Chapter 8: *Approach to Ectopic Pregnancy.*

Condition	Symptoms	Signs	Investigations	Management
Ruptured /haemorrhage from ovarian cyst *Risk factors*: • History of ovarian cysts • Pain may be preceded by strenuous physical activity • Rupture of mucinous cystadenoma may cause pseudomyxoma peritonei	• Acute onset of lower abdominal pain • Pain is usually unilateral • Pain radiates along the inner aspect of the thigh down to the knee (referred pain along the cutaneous distribution of the obturator nerve) • Pain may subside after the acute presentation or may become generalised	• Low-grade fever • May have signs of shock: hypotension, tachycardia • Acute abdomen • Cervical excitation • Adnexal tenderness	• *US pelvis*: Adnexal mass, free fluid in the pelvis • FBC, UECr, GXM • May test for factor VIII deficiency/Von Willebrand disease in cases of massive haemorrhage in young girls • Ovarian tumour markers (OTM) (Refer to Chapter 60: *Tumour Markers in Gynaecology and Pregnancy*) • Fetal monitoring	• Advise conservative management for uncomplicated cyst rupture • Analgesia • Antibiotics if suspect sepsis • Correct electrolyte imbalance • Monitor symptoms • Monitor FBC • Surgical management if haemodynamically unstable or suspected acute abdomen
Adnexal torsion *Risk factors*: • History of ovarian cysts (mature cystic teratomas are the most common cysts to tort, followed by cystadenomas) • Most common in the first trimester	• Twisting/colicky abdominal pain, which may wax and wane • Sudden onset of severe abdominal pain • Nausea, vomiting • Pain radiates along the inner aspect of the thigh down to the knee	• Low-grade fever • May have signs of shock: hypotension, tachycardia • Acute abdomen ± peritonism • Cervical excitation • Adnexal tenderness/ tender mass	• *US pelvis*: Adnexal mass with absent or impaired ovarian venous flow on Doppler scan, twisted pedicle, free fluid • FBC, UECr, GXM • OTM (Refer to Chapter 60: *Tumour Markers in Gynaecology and Pregnancy*) • Fetal monitoring	• Surgical evaluation of ovarian viability, detorsion with/without cystectomy with/without salpingo-oophorectomy • Analgesia • Anti-emetics • Antibiotics • Correct electrolyte imbalance

(*Continued*)

(Continued)

Condition	Symptoms	Signs	Investigations	Management
Infected ovarian cyst *Risk factors*: • Endometriotic cyst • Immunocompromised	• Nausea, vomiting • Lower abdominal pain • Fever • Confusion (sepsis)	• Low-/high-grade fever • May have signs of shock: hypotension, tachycardia • Acute abdomen ± peritonism • Cervical excitation • Adnexal tenderness/ tender mass	• *US pelvis*: Adnexal mass with hyperechoic collection/pus in pouch of Douglas (POD) • FBC, UECr, GXM, CRP, lactate blood cultures • Fetal monitoring	• Sepsis bundle • Fluid resuscitation • Broad-spectrum intravenous (IV) antibiotics • IR-guided aspiration/drainage • Surgical evaluation if unresponsive to conservative measures • Correct electrolyte imbalance
Fibroid degeneration *Risk factors*: • History of fibroids • Higher risk if the fibroid is >5 cm	• Constant localised pain over fibroid • Nausea, vomiting	• Low-grade fever • Tenderness over fibroid	• *US pelvis*: Fibroid with degenerative cystic changes may be present • FBC, UECr, GXM • Fetal monitoring	• Conservative management • Give analgesia, anti-emetics • Correct any electrolyte imbalance
ARU • Usually between 10 and 14 weeks of gestation (especially with a retroverted uterus)	• Abrupt inability to pass urine • Lower abdominal/ suprapubic discomfort	• Palpable bladder • Suprapubic tenderness	• FBC, UECr • Urine FEME, urine culture • *US pelvis* to exclude pelvic mass, e.g., fibroid	• Insertion of an indwelling catheter • Antibiotics if UTI • Correct electrolyte imbalance
OHSS *Risk factors*: • Recent treatment with gonadotrophin stimulation to induce ovulation • Recent treatment with assisted reproductive technology, e.g. IVF	• Abdominal pain, distension • Nausea, vomiting, diarrhoea • Shortness of breath • Rapid weight gain • Oliguria • Lower limb swelling	• Tachypnoea • Pleural effusion • RIF or LIF tenderness • Ascites • Peripheral oedema	**Mild OHSS** – FBC – US pelvis **Moderate OHSS** – FBC (twice weekly) – UECr (twice weekly) – LFT (weekly) – PT/PTT (weekly) – US pelvis	**Mild OHSS** – Outpatient monitoring – Increase oral fluids – Bed rest – Analgesia (paracetamol/ codeine) – No contraindication to luteal support with progesterone **Moderate OHSS** – Inpatient monitoring – Daily measurement of abdominal girth and weight

(*Continued*)

Condition	Symptoms	Signs	Investigations	Management
• **Grade 1 (mild OHSS)** Affects 33% of IVF cycles • **Grade 2 (moderate OHSS)** Affects 3–8% of IVF cycles • **Grade 3 (severe OHSS)** • **Critical OHSS**	• Abdominal pain and bloating • Bilateral ovarian enlargement • Ovarian size <8 cm^3 • Moderate abdominal pain. Nausea, vomiting • Ultrasound shows evidence of ascites • Ovarian size 8–12 cm^3 • Clinical ascites, oliguria, haemoconcentration, haematocrit >45%, hypoproteinaemia • Ovarian size >12 cm^3 • Tense ascites, large hydrothorax, haematocrit >55% • White cell count >25,000/ml • Oliguria/anuria • Thromboembolism • Acute respiratory distress syndrome (ARDS)		**Severe OHSS** – FBC (daily) – UECr (daily) – LFT (twice weekly) – PT/PTT (twice weekly) – Arterial blood gas (ABG) – US pelvis – Consider CT pulmonary angiogram (if pulmonary embolism is suspected) – ECG and echocardiogram (if suspect pericardial effusion)	– Input/output monitoring and fluid management – Correct electrolyte imbalance – Consider IV 20% albumin 100 ml 6–12 hourly – Anti-emetics **Severe OHSS/Critical OHSS** – Inpatient monitoring – Admission to ICU if necessary – Refer to an anaesthetist – Consider central venous pressure monitoring – Daily measurement of abdominal girth and weight – Input/output monitoring and fluid management – Correct electrolyte imbalance – Consider IV 20% albumin 100 ml 6–12 hourly – VTE prophylaxis: TED anti-embolic stockings, low molecular weight heparin (LMWH, e.g., Clexane®-weight adjusted) – Paracentesis under ultrasound guidance

O&G Causes of Abdominal Pain in Late Pregnancy

Condition	Symptoms	Signs	Investigations	Management
1. Labour	**Latent** phase • Irregular contraction pain **Active** phase • Regular painful contractions (increasing in frequency and intensity) ± Leaking liquor ± Vaginal bleeding (show)	• Dilated ± effaced cervix • Ruptured membranes • Liquor (clear/meconium-stained) • Show	• Cardiotocography (CTG) • ± Bedside ultrasound of the fetus: presentation, estimated fetal weight, placenta location, amniotic fluid volume **Preterm labour** • **Actim® Partus** – Used to rule out the risk of preterm delivery from 22+0 weeks of gestation – Detects the presence of the phosphorylated form of insulin-like growth factor binding Protein1 (phIGFBP-1) – phIGFBP-1 is produced by maternal decidual cells and leaks into cervical secretions when labour occurs – 98% negative predictive value for preterm delivery in the next 1–2 weeks	• **Term active labour** Admit to labour ward for monitoring and delivery • **Preterm labour** Check the availability of neonatal intensive care unit (NICU) beds. Consider *in utero* transfer if NICU beds are *not* available, the mother's condition is stable for transfer and delivery is not imminent. Admit to labour ward for monitoring. Intramuscular (IM) corticosteroids for fetal lung maturity (<34+0 weeks) Tocolysis till 24 hours post-steroids completion. IV magnesium sulphate ($MgSO_4$) <30–32 weeks for fetal neuroprotection if at high risk of delivery within 24 hours. IV $MgSO_4$: – Reduces risk of cerebral palsy (RR 0.71) – IV loading dose of 4 g over 15 minutes followed by 1 g/hour, with a minimum of 4 hours and up to 24 hours. – Discontinue at delivery or if delivery is no longer imminent. Delivery should *not* be delayed for $MgSO_4$ administration if there are maternal or fetal indications for immediate delivery. – Stop tocolysis when on IV $MgSO_4$ – There is insufficient evidence to recommend a repeat course *Contraindications of* $MgSO_4$: myasthenia gravis, women with myocardial compromise or cardiac conduction defects. *Use* $MgSO_4$ *with caution in women with renal impairment* — doses have to be adjusted.

(Continued)

Condition	Symptoms	Signs	Investigations	Management
2. Placental abruption *Risk factors* • Increasing maternal age and parity • ART pregnancies • Hypertension/pre-eclampsia • Maternal thrombophilia • IUGR • Abdominal trauma • Drugs, e.g., cocaine use (10% risk), amphetamines • Smoking • Preterm pre-labour rupture of membranes • Intrauterine infection • *Previous placental abruption* • 5% recurrence risk with one previous abruption • 20–25% recurrence with two previous abruptions • Polyhydramnios • Multiple pregnancy	• Constant periumbilical, suprapubic, or lower abdominal pain • Per vaginal bleeding	• May have *signs of Hypovolaemic shock*: tachycardia, hypotension • Vaginal bleeding • Abdominal tenderness • Tense and woody hard uterus on abdominal palpation • Non-reassuring fetal status or intrauterine death (IUD) • Retroplacental clot on the US of the placenta • Couvelaire uterus (seen during caesarean section)	• CTG • Bedside US of the fetus • FBC • UECr • LFT • GXM • Coagulation panel: PT/PTT ± disseminated intravascular coagulation (DIC) screen (including serum fibrinogen level) *After delivery:* • Paired cord blood gases • ± Placenta for histology, especially for preterm deliveries	• *Resuscitation and stabilisation* — airway, breathing, circulation (ABC) • Expedite delivery if there are maternal/fetal indications, e.g., haemodynamic instability, massive bleeding or fetal distress • Delivery is usually by caesarean section unless vaginal delivery is imminent • Multidisciplinary team care • Neonatal standby at delivery • Active management of the third stage of labour/postpartum haemorrhage (PPH) prophylaxis and management • Correct DIC with transfusion of blood and blood products • Administer anti-D if the woman is Rhesus negative • VTE prophylaxis post-delivery once bleeding has been controlled • Counsel on recurrence risk • If there is massive PPH, watch for Sheehan syndrome. *Complications of placental abruption:* (a) Maternal: Severe haemorrhage DIC Severe anaemia and its complications, e.g., cardiac events Transfusion reactions and complications Caesarean section Hysterectomy Hypotensive shock, acute renal failure Postnatal depression, post-traumatic stress disorder (PTSD)

(Continued)

(Continued)

Condition	Symptoms	Signs	Investigations	Management
				Sheehan syndrome Maternal mortality (b) <u>Fetal:</u> Prematurity risks Fetal anaemia — may require blood transfusions Birth asphyxia/IUD/neonatal death
3. Uterine rupture *Risk factors*: • Previous caesarean section – Elective lower segment caesarean section (LSCS) has a risk of scar rupture <0.02%, similar to an unscarred uterus – Trial of vaginal birth after caesarean section (VBAC): 0.5% risk of scar rupture. Induction of labour/ augmented labour increases rupture risk by 2–3 times • Previous uterine surgery, e.g., myomectomy, uterine perforation • Grand multiparity • Trauma	• Sudden onset of severe abdominal pain, especially between contractions • Pain at the caesarean scar site • Per vaginal bleeding	• May have *signs of hypovolemic shock*: tachycardia, hypotension • Uterine tenderness • Acute abdomen with rebound/guarding • Fetal parts may be palpable per abdomen • Change in abdominal contour • Scar tenderness • Per vaginal bleeding on speculum exam • Loss of fetal station on vaginal exam • Blood-stained liquor • Haematuria • CTG abnormalities: – e.g., Acute bradycardia, late decelerations – Cessation of uterine activity	• CTG • FBC • Coagulation panel: PT/PTT, ± DIC screen, GXM • UECr <u>*After delivery*</u>: • Paired cord blood gases	• *Resuscitation and stabilisation* — ABC • Expedite delivery • Caesarean section keep in view (KIV) hysterectomy in life-threatening PPH (about 1 in 3 women requires hysterectomy following uterine rupture) • Neonatal standby at delivery • PPH management • VTE prophylaxis post-delivery • In case of maternal collapse and there is no response by 4 minutes of the collapse, *a perimortem caesarean section* should be performed to assist maternal resuscitation The baby should be delivered within 5 minutes of maternal cardiac arrest. • Activate code red in KKH for maternal collapse.

(Continued)

Condition	Symptoms	Signs	Investigations	Management
• Excessive/ injudicious use of oxytocin • Shoulder dystocia • Difficult instrumental delivery • Maternal connective tissue disorders, e.g., Ehlers–Danlos syndrome				
4. Intra-amniotic infection/ chorioamnionitis	Refer to Chapter 11: *Medical Disorders in Pregnancy*			
5. Severe pre-eclampsia/ eclampsia				
6. Acute fatty liver of pregnancy				
7. Gynaecological causes of pain in pregnancy *Causes* • Ovarian cyst accidents, e.g., torsion • Acute degeneration of uterine fibroid • Pelvic inflammatory disease (PID)/tubo-ovarian abscess (TOA)	• Lower abdominal pain • Nausea • Vomiting • Fever • Foul-smelling vaginal discharge	• Signs of shock • Abdominal tenderness • May have signs of acute abdomen	• FBC, CRP • UECr • LFT • PT/PTT, T&S • SEPSIS bundle • US pelvis • ± MRI pelvis	• Broad-spectrum IV antibiotics • Analgesia • Treat the underlying cause • If ovarian cyst accident/torsion occurs, the woman will require emergency surgical intervention. Consider an open approach if late gestation. • Weigh the pros and cons of expediting delivery in the same setting as the surgery versus treating the source of infection first • Delivery at the same setting as the surgery may be required if the mother is critically ill, in preterm labour and requires a caesarean section for obstetric indication or fetal distress

(Continued)

(*Continued*)

Condition	Symptoms	Signs	Investigations	Management
				• If preterm delivery is required, consider antenatal steroids and IV $MgSO_4$. • Perform a Doptone/ultrasound scan of the fetus to check fetal viability before and after surgery if the fetus is not delivered yet • VTE prophylaxis
8. Braxton Hicks contractions "False labour pains"	• Irregular, infrequent, non-rhythmic, no increase in intensity or frequency, discomfort rather than pain • Painless tightenings • No leaking liquor or show	• No cervical change	• Nil	• Reassurance • Change in position
9. Symphysis Pubis Dysfunction (SPD) The average symphysis pubis gap is 7.7 mm in the last 2 months of pregnancy **Symphysis pubis diastasis** Symphysis pubis gap is >10 mm Incidence of Symphysis pubis diastasis 1:800 *Risk factors*: • *Pelvic instability* — pelvic asymmetry/ lordosis/increased load	• Pain localised to pubic symphysis: shooting, stabbing, burning, grinding, audible clicking, persistent discomfort • Pain radiating to the lower abdomen, groin, perineum, thigh, leg and back • Pain worsens with movement while walking, ascending/descending stairs, rising from a chair, turning in bed, etc.	• Tenderness over symphysis pubis and sacroiliac joints • Anterior posterior (AP) or superoinferior displacement of the upper border of the symphysis pubis • Unilateral or bilateral tenderness of iliopsoas muscle, sacrotuberous ligaments and sacroiliac joints • Limited hip movement during abduction and lateral rotation	Imaging to assess misalignment of the pelvic bones postnatally • Pelvic X-ray usually first-line • Other imaging modalities include ultrasound, MRI and CT scan	• Physiotherapy to teach safe exercises: avoid activities that trigger discomfort, straddling and squatting, bending/twisting, rolling out of bed and breaststroke while swimming. • Ozzlo pillow for support of the pregnant abdomen • Water gymnastics/aqua-natal classes from 20 weeks • Analgesia • Ice packs • Aids to assist stability Pelvic support, bath board and elevated toilet seat • Reassurance • Outpatient follow-up • **Delivery**: May require induction of labour (IOL) if there is persistent pain • Vaginal delivery is not contraindicated.

(Continued)

Condition	Symptoms	Signs	Investigations	Management
• *Enzymatic* — increased hyaluronidase/ decreased collagen • *Hormonal* — Progesterone/ oestrogen/relaxin • *Metabolic* — decreased calcium/ vitamin D • *Traumatic* — Parturition • *Inflammatory* — Sacroiliitis/ symphysitis • *Degenerative* — Arthritis of symphysis pubis • *Pregnancy-related* — Strenuous exercise, weight gain, multiparty, increased maternal age • *Previous difficult delivery* -shoulder dystocia		• **Limited active straight leg raising test (ASLR)** • Waddling gait • Palpation of symphysis pubis anterior surface with woman supine — elicits pain that persists for >5 seconds after removal of the hand • **Trendelenburg** • When the woman stands on one leg — The inability to maintain the pelvis in the horizontal plane and the opposite buttock drops • **Patrick/Faber test** One iliac spine held fixed with the woman in the supine position, placing her opposite heel on the ipsilateral knee with the leg falling passively outwards — Elicits pain in either sacroiliac joint.		• Keep leg separation to the minimum during the second stage of labour • Support during the postnatal period — Usually rest in bed for 24–48 hours • **VTE prophylaxis** — TEDs stockings/LMWH • Gradual mobilisation • A recurrence rate of 68–85% in future pregnancies

Non-O&G Causes of Abdominal Pain in Pregnancy

- There may be atypical presentation of conditions (non-classical signs/symptoms).

There should be a high index of suspicion, taking into account anatomical changes in pregnancy.

Condition	Symptoms	Signs	Investigations	Management
Urological				
Cystitis	– Suprapubic pain – Frequency – Urgency – Dysuria – Haematuria	– Suprapubic pain – Haematuria	– UFEME, urine culture	– Antibiotics, e.g., PO cefalexin 500 mg TDS – Encourage oral fluid intake – Encourage post-coital voiding and good perineal hygiene
Pyelonephritis	– Loin pain – Fever, chills – Frequency – Urgency – Dysuria – Haematuria – Nausea, vomiting	– Fever – Renal punch positive	– UFEME, urine culture – FBC, CRP, UECr – Blood cultures – US kidneys, ureter and bladder (KUB)	– Inpatient treatment – IV Antibiotics – IV Hydration – Analgesia
Urinary tract calculi	– Loin to groin pain – Nausea, vomiting – Haematuria – Passage of stones – May present with Cystitis/ pyelonephritis	– Suprapubic tenderness – Renal punch positive – Haematuria	– UFEME, urine culture – FBC, UECR – US KUB – X-ray KUB is NOT routinely done in pregnancy	– Consider inpatient treatment – IV fluids – Analgesia – Antibiotics if an infection is present – Refer to urology if signs of urinary tract obstruction

(Continued)

Condition	Symptoms	Signs	Investigations	Management
Gastrointestinal				
Gastritis, peptic ulcer disease, gastro-oesophageal reflux disease (GERD)	– Epigastric pain – Burning sensation related to meals – Nausea, vomiting – Abdominal bloating	– Epigastric tenderness		– Advise regular meals – Antacids, H2-receptor antagonists (famotidine), proton pump inhibitors (PPIs) – Refer to a gastroenterologist/general surgeon – KIV oesophagogastroduodenoscopy (OGD) if severe or persistent symptoms
Appendicitis Appendix location migrates cephalad with the enlarging uterus; hence the location of pain may be atypical	– Periumbilical pain radiating to RIF – Loss of appetite – Nausea, vomiting – Fever	– Fever – Tachycardia – RIF tenderness maximum at McBurney's point – ± rebound, tenderness, guarding	– FBC, CRP – GXM, PT/PTT if preparing for operation (PFO) – US abdomen and pelvis (may be inconclusive in up to 80% of cases) – MRI pelvis (avoid prolonged supine position in the third trimester)	Inpatient treatment – Serial abdominal examinations – Refer to a general surgeon KIV laparoscopic or open appendicectomy. A laparoscopic approach is preferred. – Conservative management of uncomplicated appendicitis is not advisable due to the higher risk of peritonitis, fetal loss, shock and VTE. – Immediate surgical management is recommended for complicated appendicitis, e.g., perforated appendicitis ± abscess/peritonitis – Keep nil-by-mouth – IV fluids – IV antibiotics
Intestinal obstruction (IO) *Causes*: • Previous abdominal surgery- adhesions • Volvulus • Crohn's disease • Malignancy • Intussusception	– Colicky abdominal pain – Nausea, vomiting – Constipation – Bloating or distension	Abdomen: – Distension – Tenderness – ± rebound, guarding – Tinkling bowel sounds	– FBC, UECr – Ca/Mg/PO4 – ABG – Judicious use of abdominal X-rays in pregnancy (supine/erect)	Inpatient treatment – Refer to a general surgeon – Keep nil-by-mouth – IV fluids – NG tube insertion – Correct electrolyte imbalance

(Continued)

(Continued)

Condition	Symptoms	Signs	Investigations	Management
Pancreatitis High maternal and fetal morbidity and mortality *Risk factors* • Gallstones • Hyperlipidaemia • Alcohol • Autoimmune	– Epigastric pain radiating to the back – Nausea, vomiting – Loss of appetite	– Fever, tachycardia – Epigastric tenderness	– Amylase, lipase – FBC, UECr, LFT, lactate – Calcium (Ca)/ magnesium (Mg)/ phosphate (PO_4) – ABG – US abdomen	Inpatient treatment — KIV ICU care – Refer to a general surgeon – Keep nil-by-mouth – IV fluids – Analgesia – Anti-emetics – Strict I/O monitoring – KIV endoscopic retrograde cholangiopancreatography (ERCP) if cholangitis or biliary duct obstruction – Monitor for possible complications of multi-organ failure in severe pancreatitis
Biliary colic	– Epigastric/RHC pain after meals – Nausea/vomiting – Bloating	– Epigastric/RHC tenderness	– LFT – US hepatobiliary system (HBS)	Inpatient treatment – Refer to a general surgeon – Analgesia – Anti-emetics – Antibiotics – Conservative management – Consider cholecystectomy, preferably after delivery – Laparoscopic cholecystectomy in the second trimester and ERCP can be performed if indicated
Liver				
Acute viral hepatitis A, B, C, D, E • Pregnant women are likely to progress to fulminant hepatitis	– RHC pain – Nausea/vomiting – Jaundice – Anorexia – Fatigue – Myalgia – Dark urine – Fever	– Febrile – Jaundice – RHC tenderness – May have Hepatosplenomegaly	– FBC, UECr, LFT, PT/PTT – Hepatitis screen – HIV screen	Inpatient supportive treatment – Universal precautions – Refer to a gastroenterologist – IV fluids – Analgesia Refer to Chapter 15: "*Infections in Pregnancy*" *for more details on Hepatitis in pregnancy.*

(Continued)

Condition	Symptoms	Signs	Investigations	Management
Liver abscess *Risk factors* – Recent travel history – DM – Immunocompromised	– RHC pain – Swinging fever, chills – Nausea, vomiting – Anorexia – Jaundice – Diarrhoea – Dark urine	– Febrile – Jaundice – RHC tenderness – Hepatomegaly – Rarely, may be in septic shock	– FBC, UECr, LFT, PT/PTT, CRP – Blood cultures – US abdomen or US HBS	Inpatient treatment – Refer to GS – KIV refer to an interventional radiologist (IR) for the feasibility of drainage of abscess – IV antibiotics – IV fluids – Analgesia
Thoracic				
Pneumonia	– Fever, chills – Cough, SOB – Chest pain – Anorexia	– Fever – Tachycardia – Tachypnoea – Inspiratory crepitations – If severe, confusion can occur	– FBC, CRP, UECr – ABG – Respiratory multiplex swab, including for coronavirus (COVID-19) – Sputum for acid-fast bacilli (AFB), tuberculosis culture – CXR with abdominal shield – Blood cultures	Inpatient treatment – SpO_2 monitoring – Supplemental O_2, if required – IV fluids – Oral (PO)/IV antibiotics
Systemic				
DKA	Refer to Chapter 11: *Medical Disorders in Pregnancy*			
Sickle cell crisis *Risk factors* • History of sickle cell disease with triggers for painful crises, e.g., dehydration, stress, over-exertion, infection	– Abdominal pain – Nausea/vomiting – Painful joints/bones – Chest pain, SOB – Palpitations	– Fever, tachycardia – Dry mucous membranes, Capillary refill time >2 seconds – Pallor – Abdominal tenderness	– FBC, CRP, UECr, LFT – GXM – ECG – ± CXR with abdominal shield – ± Blood, urine and sputum cultures	Inpatient treatment if in severe pain – IV fluids – Supplemental oxygen – Analgesia — *avoid pethidine* – VTE prophylaxis with TEDS stockings – Treat precipitating causes, e.g., infection, dehydration – Early recognition of complications, e.g., acute coronary syndrome, acute stroke – ± Blood transfusion

(Continued)

(Continued)

Condition	Symptoms	Signs	Investigations	Management
Trauma				
Road traffic accident (RTA) *Primary survey* Identify and treat life-threatening injuries *Secondary survey* Head-to-toe examination Take brief targeted history Exclude major injuries *Tertiary survey* A patient evaluation that identifies and catalogues all injuries after the initial resuscitation and operative intervention.	– Abdominal pain – ± contractions – ± leaking liquor – ± per vaginal bleeding – Other symptoms depend on injuries sustained	*Primary survey:* ABC, neurological evaluation *Secondary survey:* – To determine obstetric and non-obstetric injuries and fetal well-being – Speculum – Vaginal examination – Focused assessment with sonography for trauma (FAST) scan – Check gestational age and fetal viability	– FBC, UECr, PT/PTT – GXM – CTG – Appropriate imaging depending on injuries sustained – FAST scan	Multidisciplinary team care Maternal resuscitation takes priority over fetal care — *Focus on the mother* – Resuscitation and stabilisation of mother – Left lateral tilt of the body to reduce uterine compression on the inferior vena cava – Chest tube insertion (may need to insert 1–2 intercostal spaces higher than usual due to the elevated diaphragm in pregnant women) – Early recognition of penetrating abdominal trauma – *Complications* include haemorrhage, placental abruption, preterm labour, spontaneous rupture of membranes, uterine rupture, intrauterine death, amniotic fluid embolism, maternal morbidity and mortality – Perform a *maternal Kleihauer–Betke test* in all women at >12 weeks of gestation → anti-D administration if the patient is Rhesus negative and her partner is Rhesus positive/unknown. – Fetal monitoring (CTG) after maternal stabilisation if >24 weeks of gestation → CTG monitoring for a minimum of 6 hours affer RTA → Continue CTG monitoring if there are uterine contractions for ≥1 in 10 minutes, non-reassuring fetal status, vaginal bleeding, significant uterine tenderness/irritability, serious maternal injury OR leaking liquor. – Consider the Tdap vaccine if not given yet in the present pregnancy – KIV perimortem caesarean to aid maternal resuscitation in severe cases

(Continued)

Condition	Symptoms	Signs	Investigations	Management
Rectus abdominis rupture ± Rupture of epigastric vessels	– Sudden-onset abdominal pain – Usually precipitated by coughing or vomiting	– Signs of shock – Abdominal tenderness – Deranged hypocount – Abdominal tenderness – May have an acute abdomen – Haematoma in rectus sheath	– FBC – PT/PTT ± DIC screen – GXM – UECr – CTG	– Analgesia – Conservative management – Refer to a general surgeon for surgical exploration and drainage (if the haematoma is expanding)

CHAPTER 8

Approach to Ectopic Pregnancy (EP)

Ectopic pregnancy (EP) is the leading cause of pregnancy-related maternal deaths in the first trimester. It occurs in ~1% of pregnancies.

A high clinical index of suspicion should be present if a patient complains of vaginal bleeding and abdominal pain in early pregnancy.

A transabdominal (TA) and transvaginal (TV) ultrasound scan (US) should be performed to rule out an EP, as it can be a life-threatening condition if not detected early.

A ruptured EP can cause massive haemoperitoneum and maternal collapse.

In addition, there may be medico-legal implications if the diagnosis is missed.

Some conditions can mimic an EP, e.g., ruptured corpus luteal/haemorrhagic cyst.

Natural progression of EP:

- Tubal abortion
- Tubal rupture
- Spontaneous resolution

Fig. 8.1. Possible sites of EP.

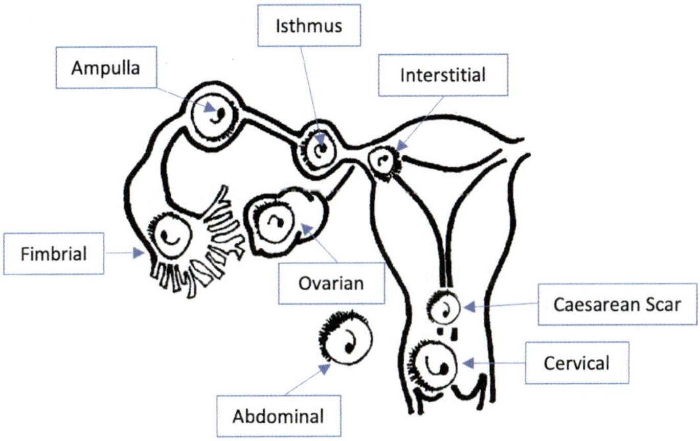

<u>**Incidence of EP**</u>

- Fallopian tube — Majority in fallopian tube (96%)
  - Ampulla — 70%
  - Isthmus — 12%
  - Fimbrial — 11%
  - Interstitial — 2.4%

  } Locations of EP within the fallopian tube
- Abdominal — 1.3%
- Ovarian — 3.2%
- Cervical
- Caesarean scar (1 in 2,000 pregnancies)
- Cornual — 1 in 76,000 pregnancies
- Heterotopic
  - 1.5 per 1,000
  - <1/30,000 (natural conception)
  - 1 in 100–500 (assisted reproductive techniques)
  - 5% of all pregnancies after IVF

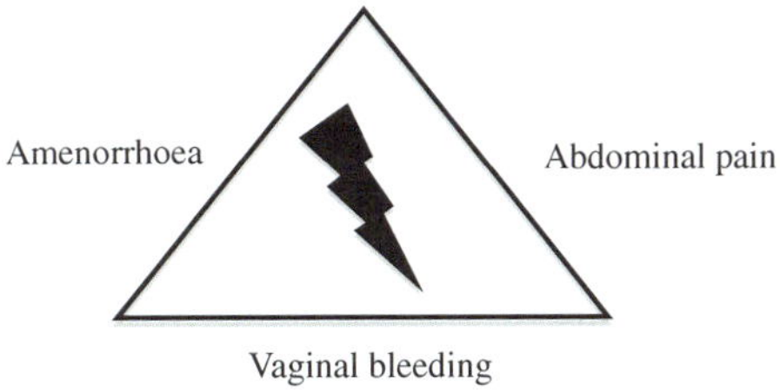

Fig. 8.2. Classical triad of an EP.

Risk Factors for EP

About 50% of patients with EP have no risk factors.

1. Tubal factors:
- *Previous tubal surgery* — tubal ligation/tubal re-anastomosis/neo-salpingostomy.
- *Previous pelvic inflammatory disease:* Chronic salpingitis, salpingitis isthmica nodosa (10%).
- Tubal anatomical distortions/adhesions.
- Previous EP — risk is higher in women with a previous salpingostomy.
  - *Risk of recurrence after one previous EP: 7–10%.*
  - *Risk of recurrence after two previous EPs: 30%.*

2. Uterine factors:
- Uterine anomalies/Asherman syndrome.
- Presence of an intrauterine contraceptive device (IUCD).
  - Women using IUCDs have a lower incidence of pregnancy than those who do not use contraceptive devices, as IUCDs prevent fertilisation and implantation.
  - IUCD users are at higher risk of having an EP if a pregnancy occurs. However, the overall risk of an EP with an IUCD is still lower than without contraception.
  - The risk of EP with Mirena® (a levonorgestrel-releasing intrauterine system) is lower than with copper IUCDs.

3. Procedure-related:
- Previous caesarean section (look out for caesarean scar pregnancy)/ uterine surgery.
- Previous pelvic or abdominal surgery.
- Assisted reproductive techniques (ARTs), e.g., *In vitro* fertilisation (IVF).

4. Others:
- Traditional progestogen-only pill (POP): The overall risk of pregnancy is reduced, but if a pregnancy does occur, 10% of them may be EP. A previous EP is *not* a contraindication to POP use.
- Smoking.
- Advanced maternal age.
- History of infertility for >2 years.

History of Presenting Complaints

- Amenorrhoea, lower abdominal pain, per-vaginal (PV) bleeding

***Other symptoms of* EP *include*:**

- Gastrointestinal symptoms
- Breast tenderness
- Dizziness/fainting/syncope
- Shoulder tip pain
- Urinary symptoms
- Passage of tissues per vagina
- Rectal pressure/pain on defaecation/diarrhoea
- Back pain, usually in the lower back

Physical Examination

Vital signs:
Assess for haemodynamic instability, which may indicate a ruptured EP.
- Pallor/tachycardia/hypotension/shock/collapse.

Abdominal examination:
Assess for signs of an acute abdomen — distension, tenderness, guarding and rebound tenderness.

Vaginal examination:
Assess for cervical excitation, adnexal tenderness, which may indicate free fluid in the pouch of Douglas (POD).

Investigations

Findings on TA/TVUS of the pelvis:

- Empty uterus
- No IUGS seen except in a heterotopic pregnancy
- Pseudo-sac or decidual cyst in 10–20% of EP
- Normal/thickened endometrial thickness (ET)
  ± Adnexal mass, moving separately from the ovary
  ± A tubal ring/sonolucent sac about 5 mm in size, ± yolk sac, ± a live embryo that appears by 6 weeks ("**Bagel sign**")
- Doppler flow around the EP — typical "**ring of fire**" appearance (may not be easy to differentiate from a corpus luteal cyst)
  ± Free intra-abdominal fluid
  ± Heterogeneous masses in the POD due to blood clots

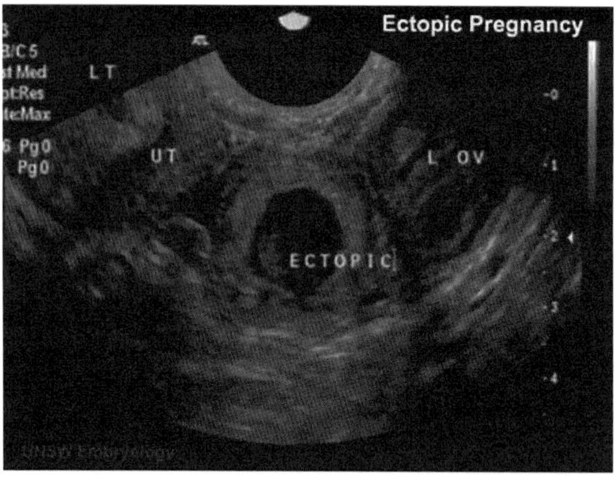

Fig. 8.3. TVUS image of a left tubal Ectopic Pregnancy.

Ultrasound Features of an Early Normal Intrauterine Pregnancy (IUP)

Intra-decidual sign: Gestational sac located within the endometrial cavity and deviates the endometrial lining. Seen at 4 weeks + 5 days of gestation.

Double decidual sign: Two concentric echogenic rings surrounding an IUGS, which is visible at 4–6 weeks of gestation. IUGS may contain a fetal pole and a yolk sac.

+

Blood investigations:

Serum βHCG

- Discriminatory zone
  - Gestational sac should be seen via TVUS when serum βHCG ≥1,500 IU/L
- Serum βHCG increases by at least >63% over 48 hours in an IUP ("doubling time")
- Suboptimal rise/fall/plateau in βHCG are commonly seen in ectopic pregnancies

Algorithm for Management of EP

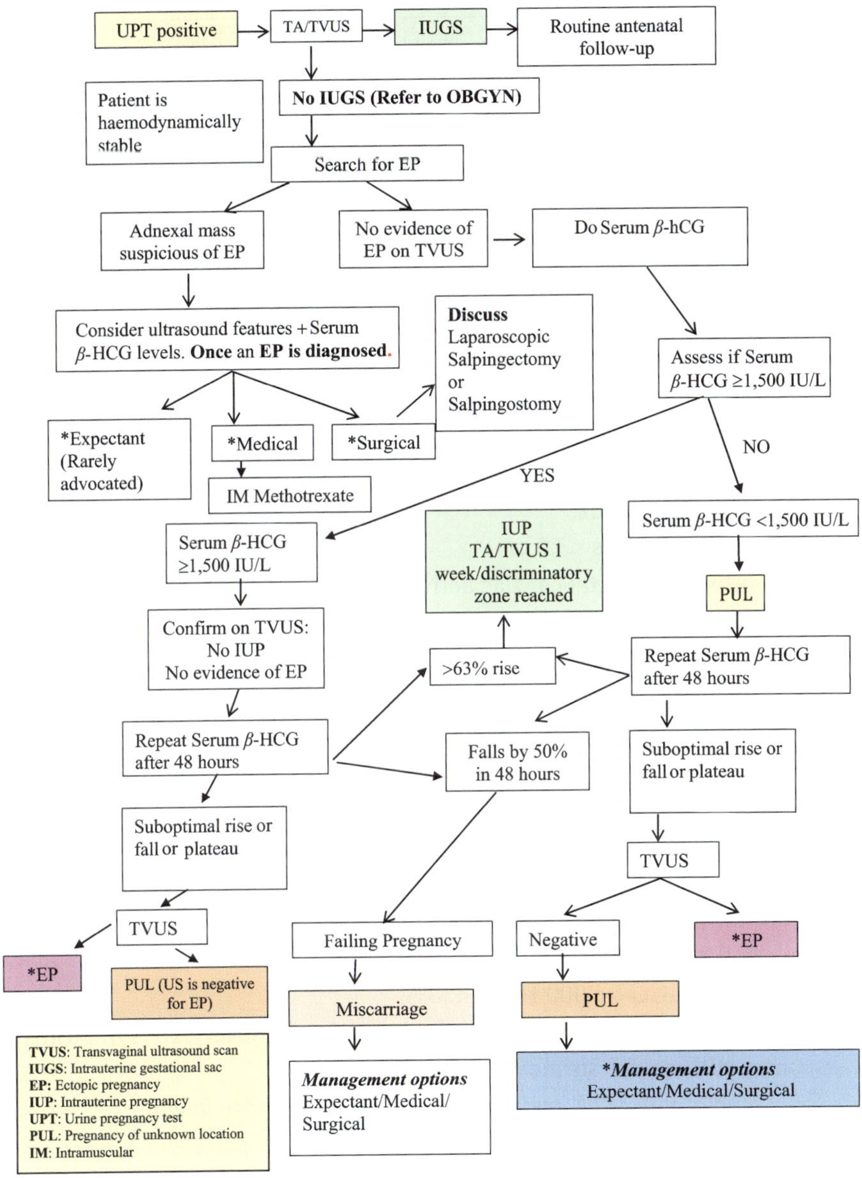

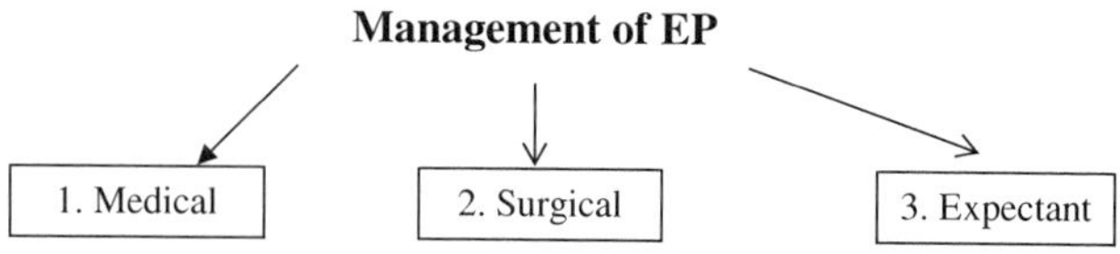

Management depends on the clinical situation and shared decision-making with the patient. It should be decided after thoroughly discussing the pros and cons of the above treatment options.

Medical Management of EP

Intramuscular methotrexate (MTX) — MTX is a folate antagonist

- **Criteria for MTX treatment**
  - ✓ No intrauterine pregnancy
  - ✓ Stable vital parameters
  - ✓ No evidence of acute abdomen
  - ✓ Unruptured EP
  - ✓ Adnexal mass <3.5 cm
  - ✓ Absence of fetal cardiac activity
  - ✓ Serum β-HCG <5,000 IU/L
  - ✓ *No contraindications to MTX:* Deranged FBC, renal function, LFT, pre-existing blood dyscrasias, pulmonary disease, peptic ulcer disease and immunodeficiency
  - ✓ Must be compliant to follow-up
- **Failure rate 15–25%.**

  The success rate with a *single dose of MTX* is 65–95%.

  The success rate depends on **the** β-HCG level at the time of MTX administration.

  For β-HCG <1,000 IU/L: 88%.

  For β-HCG >4,000 IU/L: <50%.

  Treatment failure (persistently elevated β-HCG levels or symptoms) may still require surgical intervention.

  Single-dose MTX regime is associated with the following:

  Risk of rupture — 7%.

  Need for second dose of MTX — 3 to 27% of patients.

  Need for surgery — 7%.

  To avoid pregnancy for 3 months after MTX due to its teratogenic risks.

Advantages of MTX treatment:

Less invasive/cheaper.

The risk of recurrent EP with MTX treatment is similar to that of surgery.

Note of caution:

MTX should ***not*** be offered at the first consultation.

Inadvertent administration of MTX in pregnancy can lead to complications such as miscarriage and teratogenicity.

Therefore, offer MTX **only** at the first consultation if the diagnosis of EP is confirmed and an intrauterine pregnancy has been confidently excluded.

MTX is associated with teratogenic effects such as:

- *Central nervous system (CNS) abnormalities*, e.g., spina bifida, hydrocephalus, anencephaly and mental retardation
- *Skeletal abnormalities*, e.g., synostosis of lambdoid sutures, partial or absent ossification of bones, micrognathia, cleft lip or palate, broad depressed nasal bone, hypertelorism, short limbs, syndactyly, absent digits and clubfoot
- *Cardiac abnormalities*, e.g., dextrocardia

The minimal maternal dose of MTX needed to induce birth defects was >10 mg/week. The postulated critical period was between 6 and 8 weeks after conception, corresponding to the time that a woman presents with a suspected EP.

Dose of IM MTX: **50 mg/m^2 of body surface area (BSA)**

Contraindications to MTX Treatment:

1. Haemodynamic instability
2. Ruptured EP -evidence of haemoperitoneum
3. Heterotopic pregnancy
4. Breastfeeding
5. Non-compliance to follow-up
6. Immunodeficiency
7. Acute peptic ulcer disease
8. Active pulmonary illness
9. Renal disease with creatinine clearance <50 ml/min/1.73 m^2
10. Haematologic dysfunction — bone marrow hypoplasia/leukopenia/thrombocytopenia/severe anaemia

11. Deranged blood tests: FBC, renal panel, LFT
12. Hypersensitivity to methotrexate

Side effects of IM MTX:
Increased flatulence, abdominal pain, conjunctivitis, stomatitis, xerostomia, alopecia, dermatitis, pneumonitis, impaired liver function, gastritis, enteritis, nausea, diarrhoea, neutropenia, fever, malaise.

Follow-up after IM MTX:
Serum βHCG on day 4 and day 7 (day 1 being the day of MTX administration)

- If serum βHCG declines by 15% between days 4 and 7, do weekly serum βHCG till negative.
- If serum βHCG declines by <15%, assess for further management.

Precautions to take after IM MTX:

1. Avoid foods and vitamins rich in folic acid (fortified cereal/peanuts/orange juice/beans/dark green leafy vegetables).
2. Avoid sun exposure, alcohol and vigorous physical activities.
3. Avoid non-steroidal anti-inflammatory drugs (NSAIDs): Bone marrow, gastrointestinal toxicity.
4. To return if severe abdominal pain/increased bleeding/fever, etc.
5. Avoid new conception for a minimum of 3 months post MTX treatment.

When can the woman expect her next menstrual period?
Usually, within 4–6 weeks, though this may vary.

The first menses may be heavier or lighter than her previous menses.

Advise the woman to seek medical attention if she has heavy vaginal bleeding.

Surgical Management of EP

Laparoscopy Versus Laparotomy (Salpingectomy/Salpingostomy)

The type of surgery is guided by clinical status, desire for future pregnancy, the extent of fallopian tube damage and patient's preference, where feasible.

<u>Indications for Surgical Management:</u>

1. Haemodynamic instability
2. Ruptured EP
3. Serum βHCG >5,000 IU/L
4. Known tubal disease with planned IVF in future
5. Failed medical therapy
6. Size of adnexal mass >3.5 cm and presence of a fetal heartbeat (live ectopic)

- Ensure haemodynamic stability by active resuscitation.
- Laparoscopic Salpingectomy (tube removal) is the gold standard management. In the presence of haemodynamic instability, the access should be by the most expedient method. It is also dependent on the surgical expertise available.
- *<u>Alternative</u>* — salpingostomy (tube preserved)
  - Salpingostomy is performed when the contralateral fallopian tube is diseased and the patient desires future fertility.
  - Follow-up with serum βHCG on day 7 and if decreasing, repeat weekly until negative. The rate of persistent trophoblastic tissue is 5–15%. About one in five women will require additional treatment (MTX or surgery — salpingectomy).
  - However, salpingostomy is *not* possible if the tubal EP has ruptured.
- No difference in subsequent fertility rates between salpingostomy and salpingectomy.

Reproductive outcomes of laparoscopic <u>salpingectomy</u>

IUP — 40%
Recurrent ectopic risk — 10%

Reproductive outcomes of laparoscopic <u>salpingostomy</u>

IUP — 60%
Recurrent ectopic risk — 15% if contralateral tube absent/abnormal

Recommendations for salpingectomy

1. Uncontrolled bleeding
2. Severely damaged fallopian tube
3. Large EP (>5 cm)
4. Recurrent ipsilateral EP

5. Women who require IVF due to tubal factor (salpingectomy improves success rate in women with hydrosalpinx)
6. Women who do not desire fertility

Counselling for Surgery

Complications: Bleeding, infection, injury to bladder, bowels, blood vessels, ureters, nerves.

Possibility of a negative laparoscopy — requires correlation with serum βHCG.

Evacuation of the uterus is **not** routinely performed but may be done to reduce post-surgical vaginal bleeding, which may occur due to decidual reaction.
Consider evacuation of the uterus and sending the uterine curettings for histology if an EP is not found on laparoscopy, provided a viable intrauterine pregnancy has been confidently excluded.

Expectant Management of EP

Criteria

- ✓ Haemodynamically stable
- ✓ Asymptomatic women with low βHCG <1,000 IU/L
- ✓ Declining serum βHCG levels
- ✓ Adnexal mass absent or <3.5 cm in size
- ✓ The patient is compliant to follow-up
- ✓ Absence of free fluid in the POD

The success rate of expectant management is 80–90% if the above criteria are met.

Follow-up for women who opt for expectant management
Do serum βHCG on days 2/4/7 after the initial test. If serum βHCG decreases by ≥15% from the previous value on days 2, 4 and 7, repeat weekly until a negative βHCG result.

If serum βHCG levels do not fall as expected, seek senior review and management.

***Patient counselling should include*:**

No difference between expectant versus medical management with regard to:

1. Rate of natural resolution
2. Risk of rupture
3. Need for additional treatment

Different Sites of EPs

1. ***Fallopian tube EP*:**
   a. Isthmic EP
      The narrow, compact portion of the fallopian tube
      EP invades quickly into the muscularis of the tube — EP ruptures early
   b. Ampullary EP — the *most common site* of EP
   c. Fimbrial EP

2. ***Interstitial EP*:**
   - Occurs in the interstitial part of the tube, ~1 to 2 cm, which transverses the myometrium and enters the uterine cavity via the ostia.
   - Difficult to diagnose → higher mortality rate.
   - Late rupture (12–14 weeks) — a higher rate of catastrophic haemorrhage.
     Risk factor for interstitial EP — prior ipsilateral salpingectomy (in residual stump).

   Ultrasound diagnosis:
   - Empty uterine cavity.
   - Gestational sac is located in the interstitial part of the fallopian tube and is surrounded by <5 mm of myometrium in all planes.
   - *Interstitial "line" sign* — an echogenic line between the sac and cavity.
   - Can perform a 3D US scan or MRI scan to confirm the pregnancy location.

   Treatment:
   Medical MTX — higher risk of treatment failure.
   Surgical resection (cornual resection) is the mainstay of management. However, this has a small risk of uterine rupture in subsequent pregnancies.

3. ***Cornual EP***:
   A pregnancy that is implanted in one horn of a septate/bicornuate uterus or rudimentary horn of a unicornuate uterus.
   Treatment:
   Medical MTX.
   Excision of the rudimentary horn.
4. ***Ovarian EP***:
   Risk factors: Previous PID, endometriosis, ART.
   Diagnosis:
   "*Spiegelberg criteria*"
   - The fallopian tube is intact and distinct from the ovary on the affected side.
   - Gestational sac implants on the ovary on the affected side.
   - Ovary and gestational sac are connected to the uterus by ovarian ligament.
   - Ovarian tissue in the wall of the gestational sac as confirmed on histology.

   Ultrasound:
   - Wide echogenic ring with internal echolucent area on ovarian surface.
   - Presence of ovarian cortex, follicles and corpus luteum around this mass.
   - Negative "sliding organ" sign — unable to separate gestational sac from the ovary.
   - Differentiate from distal tubal EP and haemorrhagic cyst.

   Treatment: Enucleating the products of conception (POC), ovarian wedge resection/cystectomy/oophorectomy.

5. ***Abdominal EP***:
   Sites — POD, mesosalpinx, omentum, bowel, mesentery, liver and spleen.
   Diagnosis:
   - Empty uterus.
   - Very mobile gestational sac.
   - "*Studdiford*" *criteria*.
     - Normal fallopian tubes and ovaries — no evidence of recent or remote trauma.
     - Absent utero-peritoneal fistula.

- o A pregnancy that is attached exclusively to the peritoneal surface and is diagnosed early enough that a possibility of a secondary abdominal pregnancy is excluded.

MRI scan — useful adjunct in advanced abdominal pregnancy to plan surgical management.

Treatment of abdominal pregnancy

Early gestation — MTX or surgery (can consider laparoscopic rather than laparotomy approach).

Advanced gestation — Laparotomy and delivery of the fetus. The placenta may have to be left *in situ* if it involves major vessels or vital structures and cannot be removed safely. Complications of leaving the placenta *in situ* include bleeding, peritonitis, fistula formation, ileus and bowel obstruction.

6. ***Cervical EP*:**

Pregnancy is implanted within the cervical canal, beneath the internal os of the cervix.

Risk factors for cervical EP

History of dilatation and evacuation, IVF, anatomic anomalies, e.g., myoma/synechiae, IUCD use.

Presentation — Painless vaginal bleeding.

Diagnosis: To differentiate from an impending miscarriage — a negative "sliding sac" sign is indicative of a cervical EP.

Ultrasound scan findings of cervical EP:

- Empty uterine cavity.
- Barrel-shaped enlarged cervix.
- Endometrial stripe with gestational sac *below* the internal os of the cervix.
- *Colour Doppler* — vascular flow around the gestational sac.
- Hour-glass appearance of the uterus.

Treatment of cervical EP: **High risk of haemorrhage for cervical EP**

- *MTX*: Systemic/intra-gestational sac MTX injection.
- *Uterine artery embolisation (UAE)* followed by evacuation of the uterus or in combination with systemic/intra-gestational sac MTX injection.
- *Dilatation and evacuation, hysteroscopic resection* — can use Foley's catheter to tamponade the bleeding.

- *Cervical artery ligation (descending branches)* followed by cervical suction evacuation and balloon tamponade.
- *Hysterectomy* — only in the event of a massive haemorrhage.

7. ***Caesarean scar pregnancy (CSP):***
A pregnancy that is implanted into a myometrial defect at the site of a previous uterine incision.
Risk factors: Previous caesarean section/myomectomy, previous manual removal of the placenta (MRP), IVF.
Ultrasound findings of CSP
   - Empty uterine cavity and cervical canal.
   - Gestational sac embedded within the myometrium and fibrous tissue of caesarean scar at the lower uterine segment, at the level of the internal cervical os.
   - The gestational sac fills the niche of the caesarean scar.
   - Thin/absent myometrium between the bladder and gestational sac.
   - *Doppler scan* — high-velocity, low-impedance vascular flow around the gestational sac.
   - Negative "sliding sign."
   - Consider MRI scan if diagnosis of CSP is equivocal

   Types of CSP:
   1. *Type 1 or endogenic:* Gestational sac that implants on the scar and progresses into the cervico-isthmic or uterine cavity. There is potential to reach a viable gestational age, but there is a risk of massive bleeding from the implantation site.
   2. *Type 2 or exogenic:* Gestational sac is deeply embedded in the scar and the surrounding myometrium. It progresses deeper towards the uterine serosal surface or bladder with a risk of first-trimester uterine rupture and bleeding.

   Treatment for CSP:
   Multidisciplinary team management
   It is vital that the woman is counselled on the morbidity and mortality of a CSP. There is a high risk of severe bleeding, uterine rupture, risk of developing into placenta accreta spectrum (PAS), caesarean hysterectomy and maternal/fetal mortality.
   Current literature supports a surgical rather than medical approach as surgery is the most effective.

MTX (intra-gestational sac or systemic or combination)
- Risk of bleeding as the trophoblast degenerates.
- *Systemic MTX:* The complication rate is higher as it may require a second dose if the pregnancy progresses. This can make subsequent treatment more difficult if MTX fails.
- *Intra-gestational sac MTX*: The complication rate is lower.

Local injection of potassium chloride (KCl) — can be in combination with MTX or surgery.

UAE — used in combination with MTX or surgery.

Surgery
- *Evacuation of the uterus*: Suction evacuation/hysteroscopic resection under ultrasound or laparoscopic guidance. Can use a Foley catheter to treat and control bleeding.
- *Excision of CSP with the repair of the defect* via laparoscopy/laparotomy.
- Higher risk of uterine perforation, injury to the bladder, ureters or uterine vessels with a residual myometrial thickness of <3 mm.
- If the caesarean scar niche is <u>not</u> repaired, there is a risk of symptoms due to the niche, e.g., intermenstrual bleeding, adverse obstetric outcomes, e.g., PAS, uterine rupture.
- *Hysterectomy* may be required for women with life-threatening haemorrhage.

After CSP treatment, the woman will need βHCG monitoring to check for declining levels.

8. ***Heterotopic EP*:**

Simultaneous intrauterine and extrauterine pregnancy.

Rising incidence due to ART.

<u>*Treatment of Heterotopic EP:*</u>

Surgical
- *Salpingectomy* is the mainstay of treatment.
- However, salpingostomy can be considered in women with fertility-reducing factors (e.g. previous EP, contralateral tubal damage, previous abdominal surgery or history of PID.
- Must counsel patient regarding the small risk of requiring further treatment with salpingostomy.
- MTX is *contraindicated* for heterotopic pregnancy.

Additional Information Following the Management of EP

1. Administer anti-D immunoglobulin (IM Rhogam) to all *rhesus-negative* women with EP and have rhesus-positive partners. (If they have surgical treatment or repeated heavy bleeding or associated with abdominal pain).
2. *Subsequent pregnancy outcomes following an EP*:
   - About 30% of women have difficulty conceiving after an EP.
   - The overall conception rate is about 77% regardless of management option.
   - The recurrent EP rate is 7–10% and increases to 30% in women with two consecutive EP compared to just over 1% in the general population.
3. Avoid pregnancy for 3 months after MTX treatment — counsel on the need for effective contraception.
   - Ensure that the patient is physically and emotionally ready before trying for another pregnancy.
   - Folic acid pre-conception if future pregnancy is desired.
   - Refer to a fertility specialist for ART if the patient still desires fertility and has bilateral tubal damage, bilateral salpingectomy or is of advanced maternal age.
   - Advise early booking for future pregnancies.

CHAPTER 9

Approach to Gestational Trophoblastic Disease (GTD)

Gestational trophoblastic disease (GTD)is a type of tumour of trophoblastic cells. It is caused by abnormalities in the fertilisation process.

GTD is of the following subtypes:

a. **Molar pregnancy** (complete or partial hydatiform mole)
b. **Gestational trophoblastic neoplasia (GTN)** = malignant form of GTD
   - Invasive mole
   - Choriocarcinoma
   - Placental site trophoblastic tumour (PSTT) — rare
   - Epithelioid trophoblastic tumour (ETT) — extremely rare
c. **Atypical placental site nodules (PSNs):** malignant potential remains *unclear*

GTN can be related to hydatiform moles but is almost always cancerous.

Risk Factors for GTD

1. Extremes of age: <15 years old or >40 years old
2. Race: Asian and American Indian ancestry
3. Previous molar pregnancy
   - Overall recurrence risk after one mole is <1%
   - Two previous moles: recurrence risk is 1 in 6
   - Three previous moles: recurrence risk is 1 in 2
4. Smoking/hypertension — associated with partial mole
5. Vitamin A deficiency and low dietary carotene — associated with complete mole
6. Genetic syndromes — there are rare familial clusters and recurrent moles

	Complete mole	Partial mole	Choriocarcinoma
Karyotype	Diploid – 46XX (75–80%) – 46XY	Triploid – 69 XXY (90%) – Tetraploid or mosaic conceptions	Aneuploid – X – Y
Pathophysiology	• Most are due to the duplication of a single sperm following fertilisation of an "empty" ovum • 20–25% are a result of dispermic fertilisation of an "empty" ovum • Very rarely, there is biparental origin — worse prognosis	• Almost all are due to dispermic fertilisation of an ovum	• Neoplastic change
Histology	• Extensive hydropic villi • No fetal tissues • Hyperplasia of trophoblastic tissue	• Less hydropic villi • Evidence of fetal tissues/red blood cells (RBCs) • Less hyperplasia of trophoblastic tissue	• Malignant cytotrophoblasts, syncytiotrophoblasts without villi
Presenting symptoms	• Per vaginal (PV) bleeding • Abdominal pain • Nausea and vomiting	• PV bleeding • Abdominal pain • Nausea and vomiting	• ± Symptoms of distant metastases, *e.g., respiratory symptoms*
Examination findings	• Uterus *larger* than dates • Abdominal tenderness • PV bleeding • Grape-like vesicles at the introitus	• Uterus *smaller* than dates • Abdominal tenderness • PV bleeding • Products of conception (POC) or grape-like vesicles at the introitus	• Uterus *larger* than dates • ± Signs of distant metastases
Investigations	• Pelvic scan – Pathognomonic changes, e.g., "snowstorm" or Swiss cheese appearance – Bilateral functional ovarian cysts (theca lutein cysts) are seen in <20% due to high βHCG stimulation	• US pelvis – Cystic appearance of the placenta, a deformed gestational sac, scan findings like those of a miscarriage or retained products of conception (RPOC) – May have a fetus	• Pelvic scan + chest X-ray (CXR) to exclude distant metastases or • Computer tomography (CT) scan of thorax, abdomen and pelvis (TAP) ± brain
Malignant sequelae	• 15% risk of invasive mole	• 0.5% risk of invasive mole	• Malignant condition

Presentation of Molar Pregnancy

A positive urine pregnancy test with any of the signs and symptoms as stated below:

Symptoms	Signs
– Asymptomatic via incidental finding on ultrasound scan in pregnancy – Vaginal bleeding – Pelvic pain or pressure – Hyperemesis gravidarum – Pre-eclampsia – Hyperthyroidism – Chest pain/shortness of breath – Headache	– Haemodynamic instability – Tachycardia – Hypertension – Anaemia – Dyspnoea, respiratory distress – Signs of hyperthyroidism – Uterus larger than dates – Adnexal masses, e.g., ovarian theca lutein cysts – Vaginal masses are usually in the fornices or sub-urethral region – **Abnormally high βHCG levels** – **Ultrasound findings, as stated above**

Investigations for Molar Pregnancy

Blood tests	βHCG, FBC, PT/PTT, U/E/Cr, LFT, TFT Blood group and antibody screen, group and crossmatch (GXM)
Radiological	Ultrasound scan of the pelvis: transabdominal/transvaginal CXR ± ECG

Management of Molar Pregnancy

- Evacuation of the uterus is the standard of treatment → send products of conception (POC) for histological confirmation.
- Multidisciplinary care involving the consultant and anaesthetist.
- Intravenous plug; ensure that GXM 2 pints of packed cells transfusion (PCT) are valid and on standby.
- Perform investigations as stated above.

- Arrange for evacuation of the uterus under ultrasound guidance to reduce the risk of uterine perforation and retained POC (RPOC).
- Cervical priming immediately before the evacuation of the uterus is safe.
- Oxytocin can be given for life-threatening bleeding, as the benefits outweigh the risk of tissue embolisation.
- Give anti-D (IM Rhogam) if the woman is **Rhesus (Rh) negative** and the partner is Rh positive to prevent Rh isoimmunisation.

Once Histology Confirms the Diagnosis of Molar Pregnancy

- The woman needs regular follow-up, ideally in a dedicated molar clinic.
- Patient information leaflet and education regarding the need for compliance to follow-up.
- Patient counselling.
  - Request multidisciplinary team (MDT) review if histology is *unclear*.
  - Inform regarding diagnosis and need for follow-up due to the risk of GTN.
  - Avoid pregnancy until follow-up is completed.
  - The fertility rate is not affected by GTD.
  - Risk of recurrent GTD.
  - The woman will need an early dating ultrasound scan for future pregnancies at 6–8 weeks.
  - Serum βHCG is *no longer required* after future pregnancies unless the woman has received chemotherapy (RCOG Guideline 2020).
- **βHCG trending**
  - There are different protocols for follow-up of GTD depending on the institution
  - In KKH: we perform weekly serum βHCG till it normalises.
  - *RCOG Guidelines*:
    - For *partial mole*: Follow-up is concluded once the βHCG has normalised on two blood samples, at least 4 weeks apart.

  - For <u>*complete mole*</u>: Perform monthly UPT. If βHCG normalises within 56 days of the evacuation of the uterus, complete monitoring at 6 months post-evacuation.
    If βhCG normalises >56 days post-evacuation of the uterus, complete monitoring at 6 months after the first normal βHCG.

- **Contraception**
  - Advise the woman to delay pregnancy until surveillance for the molar pregnancy is completed.
  - Oestrogen and progestogen taken before βHCG normalises do not appear to increase the risk of an invasive mole or choriocarcinoma.

Contraceptive Options for GTD Patients

	Combined hormonal contraception (CHC)	Progestogen-only pill (POP)	Depot medroxyprogesterone acetate (DMPA)	Progestogen-only implant, e.g., Implanon®	Copper intrauterine device	Levonorgestrel-releasing intrauterine system (Mirena®)
Undetectable βHCG levels	1	1	1	1	1	1
Decreasing βHCG levels	1	1	1	1	3*	3*
Persistently elevated βHCG levels or malignant disease	1	1	1	1	4	4

*Insertion of IUCD is *best avoided* until βHCG level normalised due to the risk of uterine perforation.

Based on the UK medical eligibility criteria for contraceptive use (UKMEC) guidance

UKMEC 1: A condition for which there is no restriction for the use of the method
UKMEC 2: A condition where advantages outweigh the risks
UKMEC 3: A condition where the risks outweigh the advantages
UKMEC 4: A condition that represents an unacceptable health risk

Co-Existing Twin Pregnancy and a Molar Pregnancy

Rarely, a molar pregnancy can co-exist with a viable twin.

- MDT care involving the maternal-fetal medicine specialist.
- 40–60% chance of live birth, but there is an increased risk of morbidity: 30–40% risk of fetal loss, 35% risk of preterm delivery and 4–20% risk of pre-eclampsia.
- Close monitoring of the pregnancy.
- Send placenta for histology.
- The risk of GTN in a co-existing molar and normal pregnancy is higher at 27–46%.

Following Diagnosis of GTN

Refer to GYNAE-oncologist if:

1. Histological diagnosis of invasive mole, choriocarcinoma, PSTT or ETT
2. **FIGO criteria for diagnosis of post-molar GTN:**
   - βHCG plateau of four values ± 10% over 3 weeks (days 1, 7, 14, 21)
   - βHCG increase of >10% of three values over 2 weeks (days 1, 7, 14)
     ***Consider the possibility of a new pregnancy if serum βHCG rises.**
   - If there is a histological diagnosis of choriocarcinoma
3. **Other criteria for chemotherapy for GTN:**
   - Brain, liver, gastrointestinal (GI) or lung metastases >2 cm on chest X-ray
   - Histological evidence of choriocarcinoma
   - Heavy PV bleeding or GI/intraperitoneal bleeding
   - Pulmonary, vulval or vaginal metastases unless the βHCG level is falling
   - Serum βHCG >20,000 more than 4 weeks after evacuation of uterus

Management Plan for GTN

- MDT
- List for tumour board discussion.
- Abdominal and pelvic examination, especially to look for vagina metastasis.
  - The most common metastatic sites of GTN are the lungs and vagina.

- Arrange for a CT scan of the thorax, abdomen and pelvis to rule out distant metastasis.
- Other investigations: βHCG, FBC, U/E/Cr, LFT, PT/PTT.
- The GTN staging and risk stratification system is a combination of the FIGO staging system and WHO prognostic scoring system.
  - A score of ≤6 is low risk and ≥7 is high risk.
  - *For low-risk women, single-agent chemotherapy* is given. This is usually intramuscular Methotrexate alternating daily with folinic acid for 1 week, followed by 6 rest days.
  - *For high-risk women, multi-agent chemotherapy* is given, commonly EMACO — etoposide, methotrexate, dactinomycin, cyclophosphamide and vincristine.
  - Continue treatment in all cases until the βHCG level has normalised and then for another 6 consecutive weeks.
- Most GTNs are highly chemo-sensitive and respond well to chemotherapy with a good prognosis and survival. High cure rate at 98–100%.
- PSTT /ETT are not as chemosensitive as the other GTN subtypes. *Treatment* is usually by surgery, i.e., hysterectomy ± chemotherapy.
- *For atypical PSN*, MDT review of the histology and perform staging investigations.
- Consider hysterectomy for women who have completed family due to the risk of transformation to PSTT/ETT.

WHO Prognostic Scoring System (Adapted by FIGO)

Scores	0	1	2	4
Age (Years)	<40	≥40	—	—
Antecedent pregnancy	Mole	Abortion	Term	—
Interval months from index pregnancy	<4	4–6	7–12	>12
Pre-treatment serum βHCG (IU/L)	$<10^3$	10^3–10^4	10^4–10^5	$>10^5$
Largest tumour size (including the uterus)	<3 cm	3–4 cm	≥5 cm	—
Site of metastases, including the uterus	Lung	Spleen, kidney	Gastrointestinal tract	Liver, brain
Number of metastases	—	1–4	5–8	>8
Previous failed chemotherapy	—	—	Single drug	≥2 drugs

FIGO 2000 Staging for GTD

Stage	Description
I	Gestational trophoblastic tumours strictly confined to the uterine corpus
II	Gestational trophoblastic tumours extending to the adnexa or the vagina, but limited to the genital structures
III	Gestational trophoblastic tumours extending to the lungs, with or without genital tract involvement
IV	All other metastatic sites

CHAPTER 10

Termination of Pregnancy (TOP)

Indications for Termination of Pregnancy (TOP)

1. Social reasons
2. Medical reasons
   a. Maternal, e.g., chorioamnionitis, sepsis, maternal medical conditions for which pregnancy is contraindicated
   b. Fetal, e.g., fetal anomalies (FA)

It is necessary to fulfil any of the criteria of the following under the TOP act in Singapore for a woman to have a TOP in Singapore:

- Singapore citizen/permanent resident or wife of a Singapore citizen
- Work permit/employment pass holder or wife of work permit/ employment pass holder
- Person who has resided in Singapore for ≥4 months

***UNLESS** the TOP is immediately necessary to save the pregnant woman's life or prevent grave permanent injury to the physical or mental health of the pregnant woman.

Legal Limits of the TOP Act in Singapore

- <24 weeks of gestation.
- The pregnancy duration can be determined by calculation from the first day of the last menstrual period or by clinical examination.

Mandatory Abortion Counselling in Singapore

- All women requesting TOP, regardless of nationality, educational level and parity, must undergo mandatory counselling by an accredited abortion counsellor.

- If unmarried and <16 years old (except for rape victims), it is mandatory to refer the patient for pre-abortion counselling at the Health Promotion Board Counselling Centre. A certificate of attendance (COA) will then be issued to the girl. Without the COA, abortion cannot be legally carried out.
- After counselling, the woman has to wait for at **least 48 hours** before she can give written consent and proceed with the TOP.

Evaluation During Consultation for TOP

1. **History**
   - Gynaecological code
   - *Menstrual history*: Last menstrual period, duration of amenorrhoea
   - Obstetric history
   - Past medical and surgical history
   - Drug allergies
   - Cervical cancer screening
   - Breast cancer screening (if ≥40 years old)
   - Smoking status
   - Any contraception use
   - Sexually transmitted infection (STI) risk assessment
   - Enquire the reason for the TOP
2. **Examination**
   - Vitals, BMI
   - Heart/lungs examination
   - Abdominal examination: the size of the uterus
   - Speculum and vaginal examination, if indicated
   - Others, e.g., breast examination
3. **Investigations**
   - Ultrasound scan of the pelvis: transabdominal/transvaginal
     - Confirm the location, dating and viability of the pregnancy:
       - Ensure that it is intrauterine and not an ectopic pregnancy.

  - o If no fetal heart activity or a miscarriage is confirmed after the ultrasound scan, it will no longer be considered a TOP. Instead, the woman will be offered the three management options for miscarriage, i.e., expectant, medical, or surgical evacuation of the uterus.
- FBC
- Blood group and antibody screen — to check Rhesus (Rh) status
- Perform a STI risk assessment
  - o Screen if high risk for STI: urine chlamydia/gonorrhoea and for blood-borne viruses, e.g., HIV and syphilis
  - o Treat women with symptoms or signs of STI
- Other tests — **ONLY** if clinically indicated
  - Renal panel
  - Thyroid function test
  - PT/PTT
  - ECG
  - Chest X-ray

4. **Management**

   Counsel on various options for the pregnancy:

   1. Continue with the pregnancy
   2. Put the child up for adoption
   3. Proceed with TOP: either medical or surgical TOP (depending on the gestation)
      - o Explain the methods of TOP available in Singapore
      - o Risks of TOP (refer to flowcharts below)
      - o Implications on future fertility
        - ▪ Safe and uncomplicated TOPs generally do not affect fertility or the chance of having normal pregnancies in the future. It also does not increase the risk of pregnancy complications.
        - ▪ However, illegal, repeated or complicated abortions, e.g., resulting in pelvic inflammatory disease (PID), can affect fertility.

- If TOP was complicated by uterine perforation, there may be a very small risk of uterine rupture in subsequent pregnancies.

Once the Patient Has Decided to Proceed With TOP

Pre-Abortion

- Mandatory abortion counselling
- Discuss contraception
- Refer to anaesthetist for review, if required
- Venous thromboembolism (VTE) risk assessment

On the Day of Initiating TOP — Medical/Surgical TOP

- Confirm the patient's decision to proceed with TOP.
  - The medications used can have adverse fetal effects if the patient changes her mind midway through TOP.
  - *Mifepristone*: Associated with spontaneous miscarriage, limited data do not show an association with fetal anomalies.
  - *Misoprostol*: Associated with fetal anomalies, e.g., limb reduction defects, Möbius syndrome (type of congenital cranial nerves palsy associated with limb anomalies and craniofacial defects), hemifacial microsomia, arthrogryposis and microtia.
- Ensure ≥48 hours have passed post-TOP counselling.
- Complete the consent form for TOP.
- If gestation is 22+0 to 23+6 weeks, perform fetocide before commencing the mid-trimester pregnancy termination (MTPT).
  - Feticide involves an intracardiac injection of potassium chloride (KCl) into the fetal heart-performed by MF specialists in KKH.

Management of TOP With Gestation Under 16 Weeks

1. Patient decides to proceed with TOP
2. Ensure ≥48 hours after TOP counselling
3. Complete the consent for TOP

Medical TOP

Contraindications to Medical TOP:

- IUCD-*in situ*
- Suspected/confirmed ectopic pregnancy
- Known coagulopathy/on anticoagulants
- Allergy/intolerance to mifepristone/misoprostol
- Severe renal/liver/respiratory distress
- Uncontrolled hypertension/cardiovascular disease
- Severe uncontrolled asthma (avoid mifepristone due to possible risk of exacerbation. But can use misoprostol)
- Chronic adrenal failure
- Inherited porphyria

Methods:

PO mifepristone 200 mg STAT dose followed by vaginal misoprostol 24–48 hours after.

Will need repeated vaginal misoprostol 4 hourly until expulsion if > 10 weeks.

Dosage/frequency of vaginal misoprostol can vary based on institution's practice, presence of a scarred uterus and gestational age.

Procedure and risks:

Success rate ~90%

Risks of pain, bleeding, infection (10%), *side effects from medications* (nausea, vomiting, fever, diarrhoea, giddiness), retained products of conception/failed TOP (10%), need for surgical TOP (10%), uterine rupture (<0.1% for second-trimester TOP), toxic shock syndrome, psychological and psychiatric issues, e.g., depression, implications on future fertility, death (<1 in 100,000)

If failed/incomplete medical TOP → Consider repeat course of medication versus surgical TOP

Surgical TOP

Methods:

1. Vacuum aspiration <12 weeks
2. Dilatation & evacuation (D&E) if ≥ 12 and <16 weeks

Procedure and risks:

Pre-TOP cervical priming with cervagem/misoprostol is recommended to reduce the risk of uterine perforation and cervical laceration.

Performed under general anaesthesia

Ultrasound-guided especially for D&E

Risks of pain, bleeding, infection (10%), failed TOP (<1%), retained products of conception, risk of requiring further intervention/repeated surgery (3–5%), uterine perforation (0.1–0.4%), cervical injury (1%), cervical stenosis or incompetence, intrauterine adhesions/Asherman syndrome, psychological and psychiatric issues, e.g., depression, implications on future fertility, death (<1 in 100,000)

Risks are higher in second-trimester TOP >12+0 weeks than first trimester TOP

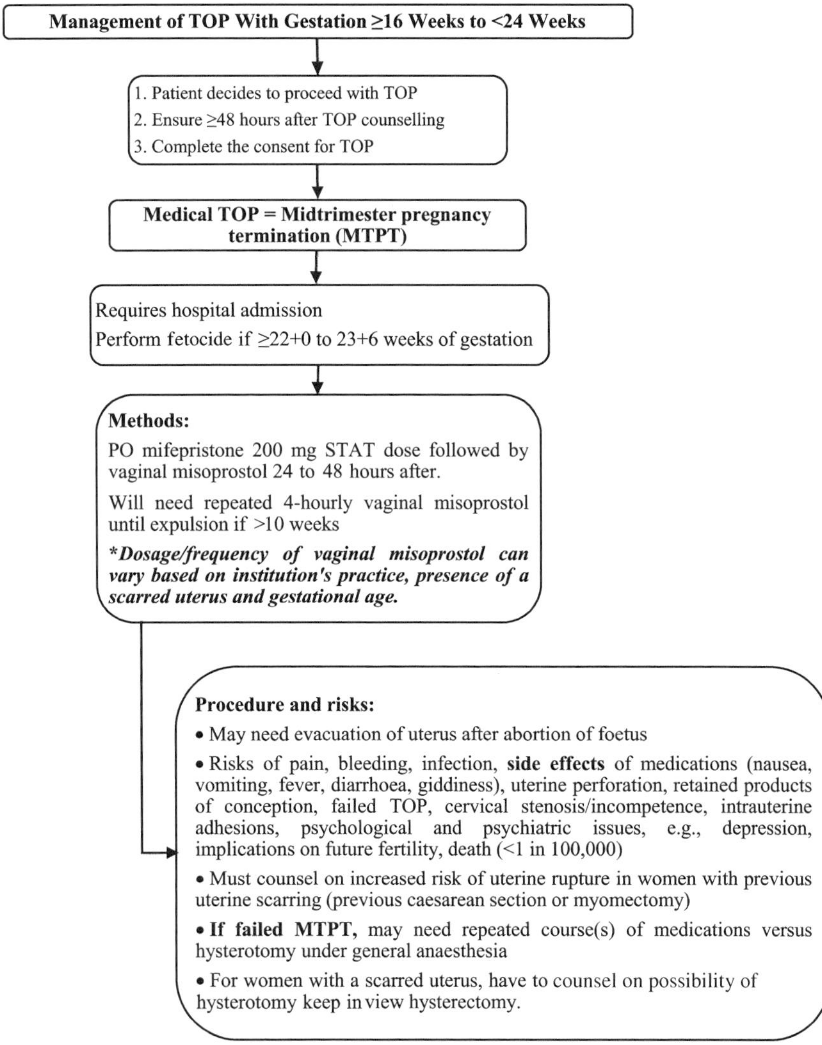

Post-TOP Care:

- Analgesia for pain relief
- Antibiotic prophylaxis
  - Prophylactic antibiotics are not required for medical TOP but are required for surgical TOP (WHO Guidelines 2022, RCOG Best Practice in Abortion Care 2022)

- This can vary based on the institution's antibiogram
- **KKH's protocol (for abortion)**
  - Oral azithromycin 1 g STAT and oral metronidazole 400 mg BD for 1 week.
  - **If allergic to azithromycin**, give oral doxycycline 100 mg BD and oral metronidazole 400 mg BD for 1 week.
  - **If allergic to metronidazole**, give oral azithromycin 1 g STAT and oral clindamycin 300 mg BD for 1 week.
  - If membranes are ruptured, start intravenous (IV) ceftriaxone 2 g OM and IV metronidazole 500 mg q8H OR I.V. clindamycin 900 mg q8H.
- **RCOG guideline**
  - PO doxycycline 100 mg BD for 3–7 days, starting within 2 hours of the procedure

- Anti-D administration
  - Rh D negative unsensitised women with Rh (D) positive partners should receive I.M. Anti-D immunoglobulin (Rhogam) 1,500 IU post-abortion (standard dose of anti-D available in KK Hospital).
  - There are limited studies that suggest that anti-D may not be required if <12 weeks of gestation (WHO Guidelines 2022, RCOG Best Practice in Abortion Care 2022).
- Lactation suppression for patients >20 weeks gestation — give P.O. cabergoline 1 mg stat
- Perform post-TOP investigations
  - For TOP:
    - Histology of products of conception — sent in selected patients
  - For TOP due to maternal/fetal reasons:
    - If there is an infection, e.g., chorioamnionitis: send placental swabs for culture
    - Placental histology
    - If there is a fetal anomaly: karyotype/chromosome microarray (CMA) of the fetus, post-mortem examination of the fetus
- Discuss and provide contraception if the patient is keen
  - Encourage long-acting reversible contraception (LARC).
  - *Oral hormonal contraception/patch/IM Depo Provera* — can be given at the time of medical/surgical TOP.

- *Implanon* — can be inserted at the time of medical/surgical TOP.
- *IUCD* — can be inserted at the time of surgical TOP except after septic abortions/presence of sepsis. Post-medical TOP, IUCD can be inserted after the expulsion of pregnancy and after ensuring that TOP is complete.
- If contraception is started immediately or within 5 days of TOP, the woman does <u>not</u> require any additional contraception precautions.

- Return advice for patient
  - Educate regarding red flag symptoms or signs that warrant urgent medical attention:
    - Heavy per vaginal bleeding, e.g., soaking ≥2 maxi-size sanitary pads per hour for ≥2 hours
    - Foul-smelling vaginal discharge
    - Worsening/severe abdominal pain or pain not relieved by analgesics
    - Fever/malaise/lethargy/unwell
    - Symptoms of ongoing pregnancy (may or may not suggest a failed TOP)
    - No bleeding with medical management of abortion
- Provide follow-up for the patient
  - For medical TOP
    - If *<u>incomplete</u>*: Review 1 week later with an ultrasound scan on arrival
    - If *<u>complete</u>*: Review 3 weeks later with a urine pregnancy test on arrival
  - For surgical TOP
    - Review 2–3 weeks later.

During the follow-up visit

- Assessment of patient
  - History
  - Vitals, examination
- Ensure that TOP is complete.

- If *incomplete*, discuss options of:
  - Medical management with misoprostol

    If uterus <14 weeks:
    - Misoprostol 400 micrograms — buccal/sublingual/vaginal or
    - Misoprostol 600 or 800 micrograms orally or
  - Surgical management
    - Either evacuation of the uterus under ultrasound guidance or hysteroscopic evacuation of the uterus
    - Surgical management is advised in the presence of sepsis

- Review relevant investigations, e.g., histology
- Check the return of menses (may be disrupted if the patient is on contraception)

  Generally, menses should return 4 to 6 weeks after abortion.
- Contraception
  - Advise on contraception if the patient has not yet started on it
  - If the patient has started on the contraception, assess usage and any side effects
- Assess the mood and need for psychosocial support
- Cervical cancer screening, if not up to date
- Mammogram if not up to date (for women ≥40 years old)

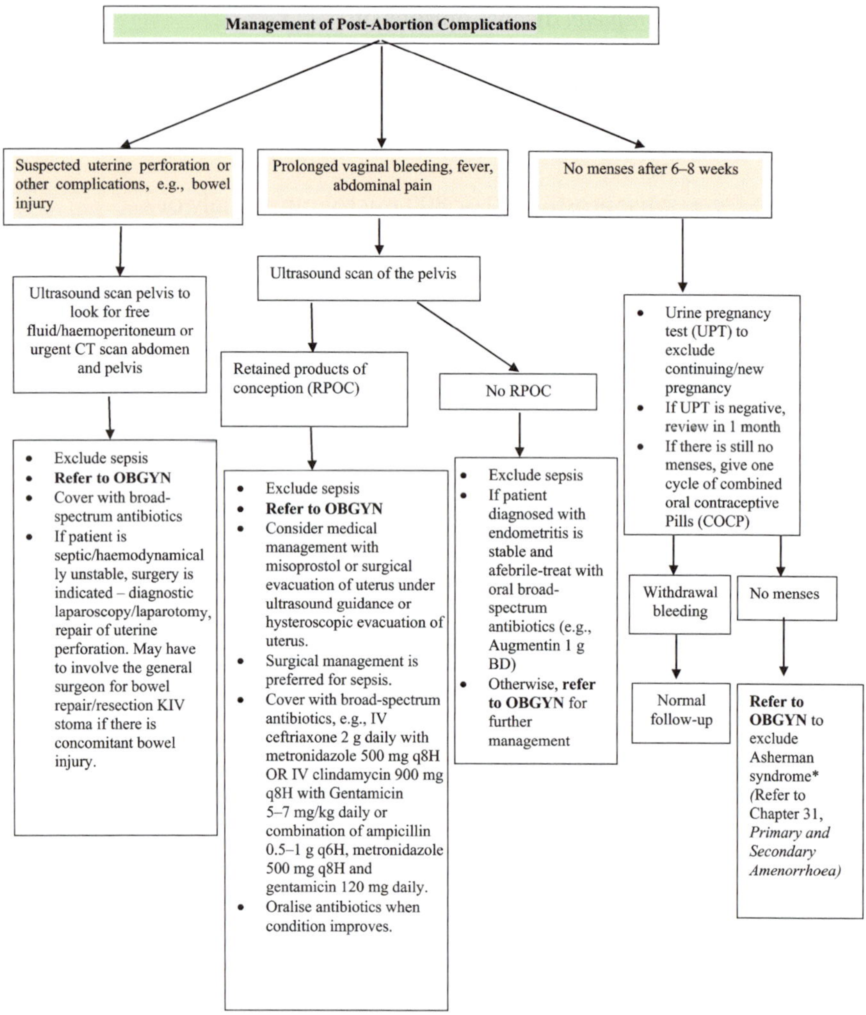
Management of Post-Abortion Complications
Suspected uterine perforation or other complications, e.g., bowel injury
Prolonged vaginal bleeding, fever, abdominal pain
No menses after 6–8 weeks
Ultrasound scan pelvis to look for free fluid/haemoperitoneum or urgent CT scan abdomen and pelvis
Ultrasound scan of the pelvis
Retained products of conception (RPOC)
No RPOC
• Urine pregnancy test (UPT) to exclude continuing/new pregnancy
• If UPT is negative, review in 1 month
• If there is still no menses, give one cycle of combined oral contraceptive Pills (COCP)
• Exclude sepsis
• Refer to OBGYN
• Cover with broad-spectrum antibiotics
• If patient is septic/haemodynamically unstable, surgery is indicated – diagnostic laparoscopy/laparotomy, repair of uterine perforation. May have to involve the general surgeon for bowel repair/resection KIV stoma if there is concomitant bowel injury.
• Exclude sepsis
• Refer to OBGYN
• Consider medical management with misoprostol or surgical evacuation of uterus under ultrasound guidance or hysteroscopic evacuation of uterus.
• Surgical management is preferred for sepsis.
• Cover with broad-spectrum antibiotics, e.g., IV ceftriaxone 2 g daily with metronidazole 500 mg q8H OR IV clindamycin 900 mg q8H with Gentamicin 5–7 mg/kg daily or combination of ampicillin 0.5–1 g q6H, metronidazole 500 mg q8H and gentamicin 120 mg daily.
• Oralise antibiotics when condition improves.
• Exclude sepsis
• If patient diagnosed with endometritis is stable and afebrile-treat with oral broad-spectrum antibiotics (e.g., Augmentin 1 g BD)
• Otherwise, refer to OBGYN for further management
Withdrawal bleeding
No menses
Normal follow-up
Refer to OBGYN to exclude Asherman syndrome* (Refer to Chapter 31, Primary and Secondary Amenorrhoea)

CHAPTER 11

Medical Disorders in Pregnancy

1. Anaemia in Pregnancy
2. Asthma in Pregnancy
3. Antiphospholipid Syndrome (APS) in Pregnancy
4. Systemic Lupus Erythematosus (SLE) in Pregnancy
5. Cardiac Disease in Pregnancy
6. Patients with Prosthetic Valves in Pregnancy
7. Cardiomyopathy in Pregnancy
8. Hyperglycaemia in Pregnancy
9. Pre-Existing Diabetes in Pregnancy
10. Diabetic Ketoacidosis (DKA) in Pregnancy
11. Gestational Diabetes Mellitus (GDM)
12. Hypertensive Disorders in Pregnancy/PE Screening in Pregnancy
13. Chronic Hypertension (HTN)
14. Gestational HTN
15. Pre-Eclampsia (PE)
16. Severe Pre-Eclampsia (SPE)
17. HELLP Syndrome
18. Eclampsia
19. Previous Severe Pre-Eclampsia
20. Hyperthyroidism in Pregnancy
21. Thyroid Storm (Thyroid Crisis)
22. Hypothyroidism in Pregnancy
23. Postpartum Thyroiditis (PPT)/Indications for TFT in Pregnancy
24. Role of Thyroid Antibodies
25. Liver Disease in Pregnancy
26. Diagnostic Modalities for Liver Diseases in Pregnancy and Lactation
27. Hyperemesis Gravidarum (HG)
28. Obstetric Cholestasis/Intrahepatic Cholestasis in Pregnancy (ICP)
29. Acute Fatty Liver of Pregnancy (AFLP)

30. Acute Kidney Injury (AKI) in Pregnancy
31. Chronic Kidney Disease (CKD) in Pregnancy
32. Pregnancy in Women on Dialysis
33. Urinary Tract Infections (UTIs) in Pregnancy (Asymptomatic Bacteriuria, Acute Cystitis and Acute Pyelonephritis)
34. History of Second-Trimester Fetal Loss
35. Preterm Labour (PTL)
36. Preterm Prelabour Rupture of Membranes (PPROM)
37. Chorioamnionitis/Intra-Amniotic Infection
38. Thrombocytopenia in Pregnancy
39. Previous Caesarean Sections (CS) (≥2)
40. Advanced Maternal Age (AMA) (≥35 years old) at Expected Date of Delivery (EDD)
41. Teenage/Adolescent Pregnancy
42. Grand Multiparity (Parity ≥5)
43. Obesity in Pregnancy (BMI ≥30)
44. Low Body Mass Index (BMI) in Pregnancy (BMI <18.5)
45. Alcohol Consumption in Pregnancy
46. Cigarette Smoking in Pregnancy
47. Venous Thromboembolism (VTE) Prophylaxis in Pregnancy/Venous Thromboembolism (VTE) in Pregnancy
48. Intrauterine Death (IUD) and Stillbirth

1. Anaemia in Pregnancy

<table>
<tr><th>Risk factors</th><th>Signs/symptoms and implications</th><th>Action</th></tr>
<tr>
<td>
Anaemia in pregnancy RCOG criteria:
• First trimester
Hb <110 g/L (<11.0 g/dl)
• Second and third trimesters
Hb <105 g/L (<10.5 g/dl)
• Postpartum
Hb <100 g/L (<10.0 g/dl)
Diagnosis of iron deficiency anaemia (IDA):
• Serum ferritin (SF) <30 g/L or <30 ng/ml (reduced iron stores)

Exclude other causes of anaemia:
• Thalassaemia — Hb electrophoresis, alpha gene probe
• Megaloblastic anaemia — serum vitamin B12
• Folate deficiency — serum folate

Causes of anaemia in pregnancy:
• IDA — the most common cause
• Physiological anaemia of pregnancy
• Thalassaemia
• Folate deficiency
• Vitamin B12 deficiency
</td>
<td>
Symptoms of anaemia:
• Fatigue
• Dyspnoea/palpitations
• Anorexia/sore mouth/ dysphagia
• Headache/vertigo
• Dizziness/fainting
• Leg cramps
• Hair loss
• Poor concentration
• Irritability
• Low mood

Signs of anaemia:
• Pallor
• Tachycardia
• Systolic flow murmur

Complications of anaemia:
Maternal risks
• Preterm labour (PTL)
• Susceptibility to infections
• Cardiovascular risk
• Eclampsia
• Prolonged/abnormal labour
• Postpartum haemorrhage
• Blood transfusion and its risks
• Poor wound healing
• Postpartum depression
• Decreased breast milk production
• Maternal mortality
</td>
<td>
<u>Prevention:</u>
Primary prevention
• Iron-rich diet and food that enhances iron absorption
• Start low-dose peroxidase (PO) elemental iron supplements (60–120 mg/day) at the booking visit
Secondary prevention
Screen for anaemia at booking visit

Investigations:
• Full blood count (FBC) at booking and 28 weeks: Hb, mean corpuscular volume (MCV), mean corpuscular haemoglobin (MCH), peripheral blood film (PBF)
– If PBF shows microcytic, hypochromic red blood cells (RBCs) — do Hb electrophoresis and serum ferritin (SF) to differentiate between thalassaemia and iron deficiency.
• Serum ferritin (SF)
Serum iron and total iron-binding capacity (TIBC) saturation have lower diagnostic accuracy in pregnancy.

Management:
1. Dietary advice
2. Oral iron:
• Iron salts — ferrous sulphate/ferrous gluconate/ferrous fumarate
• Dose: 100–200 mg/day (elemental iron 60–100 mg daily)
<table>
<tr><th>Form</th><th>Formulation (brand name)</th><th>Elemental Fe</th><th>Dosage</th></tr>
<tr><td>Ferrous fumarate</td><td>324 mg tablet</td><td>106 mg</td><td>1 tab BD</td></tr>
<tr><td rowspan="2">Ferrous gluconate</td><td>300 mg tablet</td><td>35 mg</td><td>1–2 tabs BD/TDS</td></tr>
<tr><td>250 mg tablet (Sangobion)</td><td>30 mg</td><td>2 tabs OM</td></tr>
<tr><td rowspan="2">Ferrous sulphate</td><td>325 mg tablet</td><td>65 mg</td><td>1 tab TDS</td></tr>
<tr><td>525 mg tablet (Iberet)</td><td>105 mg</td><td>1 tab OM</td></tr>
<tr><td>Iron poly-maltose</td><td>370 mg tablet or syrup (Maltofer)</td><td>100 mg (tablet)
50 mg/ml (drops)</td><td>1 tab OM
2 ml OM</td></tr>
<tr><td></td><td>100 mg (Floron)</td><td>30 mg</td><td>2 tabs OM</td></tr>
</table>
BD, twice a day; TDS, thrice a day; OM, every morning.
</td>
</tr>
</table>

(Continued)

Risk factors: • Adolescents • Short inter-pregnancy interval (<18 months) • Multiple pregnancy • Nausea and vomiting • Malnutrition • History of anaemia before pregnancy (women with abnormal uterine bleeding due to fibroids, endometriosis, adenomyosis) • History of chronic illness [e.g., systemic lupus erythematosus (SLE)/inflammatory bowel disease (IBD)/chronic renal failure] • History of bariatric surgery • Infections, e.g., schistosomiasis, parasites • Pregnancy and labour related: Bleeding in first trimester/ placenta praevia/abruption/ uterine rupture **Iron requirements in pregnancy** First trimester: 0.8 mg/day Second trimester: 4–5 mg/day Third trimester: 3–7.5 mg/day	**Fetal risks:** • Intrauterine growth restriction (IUGR) • Low birth weight (LBW) • Preterm birth • Intrauterine death (IUD) • Neonatal depression, developmental delay • Neonatal anaemia • Poor cognitive, motor, social and emotional performances	• One hour before meals on an empty stomach with orange juice/other vitamin C formulation. • Repeat Hb after 2–3 weeks — if normal, continue 3–6 months till serum ferritin >30 ng/mL. • Common supplements (refer to Chapter 18: *Medications in Pregnancy and Lactation*) • *Side effects of oral iron*: Nausea, heartburn, constipation, black stools. **3. Parenteral iron:** ***Indications:*** – After second trimester and intolerance/non-compliance to oral iron – >34 weeks with iron deficiency and Hb <10 g/dl – Women with malabsorption disorders ***Contraindications:*** – First trimester of pregnancy (unknown fetal effects) – Previous hypersensitivity to IV iron – Acute infection/sepsis • *IV Ferinject dose:* 1,000 mg (body weight ≥35 kg) 500 mg (body weight <35 kg) Administer at 100–500 mg/min over 15 minutes **4. Blood transfusion:** ***Indications:*** Patients with risk of further bleeding, imminent cardiac compromise, symptomatic anaemia, Hb <8 g/dl in late pregnancy. If asymptomatic — keep Hb at least 8 g/dl. **Aim for Hb >10 g/dl at delivery**. ***Special consideration*** for blood objectors, e.g., Jehovah's witness. Consider cell salvage in selected cases. **5. Management of labour:** Intravenous (IV) access Active management of third stage of labour Postpartum haemorrhage (PPH) prophylaxis and management (uterotonics and tranexamic acid) *Postpartum* — continue 100–200 mg of elemental iron for 3 months

2. Asthma in Pregnancy

Risk factors	Implications	Action
Asthma in pregnancy • 7% require emergency treatment, 1.5% require hospitalisation in pregnancy. • 1/3 — asthma worsens 1/3 — no change 1/3 — improves • The symptoms peak in the late second trimester and early third trimester (24 to 36 weeks) • Symptoms return to pre-pregnancy ~3 months postnatal **Asthma triggers:** • Allergens • Smoking • Exercise • Occupational exposure • Pollution • *Drugs* — aspirin, beta-blockers • Food and drinks — dairy, alcohol, peanuts, orange • Rhinitis • Gastric reflux	**Maternal risks:** • Gestational hypertension (HTN) • Pre-eclampsia • Gestational diabetes mellitus (GDM) • PTL • Worsening of asthma — respiratory failure and need for mechanical ventilation **Fetal risks:** • Preterm birth • IUGR • LBW • Neonatal morbidity (e.g., transient tachypnoea of newborn, neonatal seizures) • Neonatal intensive care unit (NICU) admissions • Neonatal death • Asthma in the child (6–30%)	**Management:** • Aim to maintain good asthma control • *Multidisciplinary team care* involving a respiratory physician, general practitioner (GP), obstetrician, neonatologist and pharmacist • Patient education — the importance of optimal control for maternal and fetal health, avoiding triggers, correct use of inhalers, compliance to medications, the safety of medications, regular follow-up • Address co-morbidities, e.g., rhinitis and gastric reflux • In active asthma cases — serial growth scans • Avoid smoking and alcohol • *Avoid drugs*, e.g., prostaglandin F2α (carboprost), ergot derivatives, non-steroidal anti-inflammatory drugs (NSAIDs), beta-blockers • Review asthma control every 4 weeks during pregnancy • Administer influenza/COVID-19 vaccinations • Chest X-ray (CXR), if required, with an abdominal shield • Encourage exclusive breastfeeding for ≥6 months **Pharmacologic management:** *"Advantages of active treatment of maternal asthma outweigh potential risks of asthma medication use in pregnancy" (GINA 2020 guidelines)*

(Continued)

	Differential diagnosis: • Anxiety • Gastro-oesophageal reflux disease (GERD) • Postnasal drip • Vocal cord dysfunction • Hyperventilation syndrome [secondary to diabetic ketoacidosis (DKA), renal disease] • Cardiac disease • Pulmonary embolism	Use inhalational rather than oral route where possible 1. *Reliever for mild intermittent asthma*: Inhaled short-acting $\beta2$ agonist (SABA) when needed 2. *Regular prevention*: Add inhaled corticosteroids (ICS) 200–800 mcg/day 3. *Initial add-on therapy*: Inhaled long-acting $\beta2$ agonist (LABA): – If there is a good response — continue LABA + steroids. – If suboptimal control — stop LABA and increase the inhaled steroid dose. – If still poorly controlled — consider sustained-release (SR) theophylline. 4. *Persistent poor control*: Increase dose of inhaled steroid + SR theophylline/$\beta2$ agonist tablets. Consider oral steroids. **Continuous or frequent use of oral corticosteroids:** Previous studies showed a small increased risk (<0.3%) of fetal cleft lip/palate in the first trimester. However, more extensive prospective studies have refuted this risk. There is no evidence to demonstrate an increased miscarriage, stillbirth or other congenital abnormalities to steroid use. **Consider IV stress steroids intrapartum:** If the patient has been on >3 weeks of systemic steroids. – Indicated if the woman has been on >5 mg prednisolone or equivalent, e.g., 0.8 mg dexamethasone daily for >3 weeks. – This is to prevent adrenal suppression. – Refer to Chapter 64 — for regime for stress steroids.

3. Antiphospholipid Syndrome (APS) in Pregnancy

<table>
<tr><th>Risk factors</th><th>Implications</th><th>Action</th></tr>
<tr>
<td>APS in pregnancy
– An <u>acquired</u> autoimmune disorder associated with thrombotic events, pregnancy failure and other presentations involving organs such as central nervous system (CNS), cardiovascular system (CVS) and skin.
– Antiphospholipid antibodies (aPL) are a major cause of recurrent miscarriages and adverse pregnancy outcomes when other causes cannot be found.
– aPL includes:
• Lupus anticoagulant (LAC).
• Anti-cardiolipin (ACL).
• Anti-β2 glycoprotein I.
Sydney criteria (modified Sapporo criteria)
≥1 clinical and 1 laboratory criteria.

Clinical criteria
1) Vascular thrombosis
• ≥1 episode of arterial, venous, or microvascular thrombosis in any tissue or organ.
• Confirmed by imaging or biopsy.
2) Pregnancy morbidity (≥1 of the following):
• ≥1 unexplained death of a morphologically normal fetus ≥10 weeks.
• ≥1 premature birth (<34 weeks) of morphologically normal neonate due to eclampsia, severe pre-eclampsia, or placental insufficiency.
• ≥3 consecutive spontaneous miscarriages <10 weeks otherwise unexplained.</td>
<td>Maternal risks:
• Thrombosis
a. Venous
– Deep vein thrombosis (DVT) in 30–50%
– Pulmonary embolism in 5% of patients with APS
– Sites: cerebral/retinal/splanchnic/axillary veins
b. Arterial
Sites:
o CNS — transient ischaemic attack (TIA) accounts for 50%
o CVS — Myocardial infarction (MI) accounts for 20% of arterial events
o Others: Lungs/retina/gut/spleen/extremities
• Obstetric APS
Gestational HTN
Pre-eclampsia
PTL
Placental abruption
Postpartum syndrome
Pleuro-pulmonary disease/fever/cardiac manifestations
• <u>Catastrophic APS (rare)</u>
– Multiorgan failure involving ≥3 different organ systems, e.g., lungs, brain and kidneys
– Triggers:
Infections or surgery</td>
<td>Management:
• Multidisciplinary team care, e.g., rheumatologist, obstetricians, haematologist and neonatologists.
• A detailed history of past thrombotic events (arterial/venous, spontaneous/provoked).
• Stratify risk.
– High-risk: Triple positivity, LAC positivity, co-existing SLE with LAC positivity, thrombotic APS, previous adverse pregnancy outcomes.
– Determine clinical phenotype: Recurrent pregnancy loss/ischaemic placental complications/maternal thrombosis.
• Start low-dose aspirin (LDA) for confirmed cases before conception, and low-molecular-weight heparin (LMWH) should be added as soon as pregnancy is confirmed.

<table>
<tr><th>Clinical features</th><th>Management</th></tr>
<tr><td>APS without clinical features and previous healthy pregnancies</td><td>No treatment ± LDA (150 mg ON — KKH protocol 2022).</td></tr>
<tr><td>Primigravida with isolated aPL</td><td>LDA.</td></tr>
<tr><td>Obstetric APS</td><td>LDA + LMWH (prophylactic).</td></tr>
<tr><td>Thrombotic APS</td><td>LDA + LMWH (therapeutic). Switch to LMWH as soon as pregnancy is confirmed, before 6 weeks of gestation.</td></tr>
<tr><td>APS with recurrent thrombotic events</td><td>LDA + therapeutic LMWH ± warfarin (to avoid warfarin between 6 to 12 weeks of pregnancy).</td></tr>
</table></td>
</tr>
</table>

(Continued)

Laboratory criteria:

- Positive LAC on ≥2 occasions, ≥12 weeks apart.
- Medium- or high-titre IgG or IgM aPL (i.e., >40 GPL* or MPL*, >99th percentile) on ≥2 occasions, ≥12 weeks apart (ELISA).

**GPL denotes the result is from the IgG isotype and MPL denotes the result is from the IgM isotype.*

- Medium or high titre IgG or IgM anti-$\beta 2$ glycoprotein I antibody on ≥2 occasions, ≥12 weeks apart (ELISA).
- APS can co-exist with other autoimmune conditions like SLE, rheumatoid arthritis and autoimmune thyroiditis.
- Up to 40% of SLE patients are positive for aPL, and only 50% develop thrombosis or have miscarriages.

- Other features:
  Thrombocytopenia
  Heart valve defects
  Skin involvement-livedo reticularis
  Cerebral — epilepsy, cerebral infarction, chorea, migraine
  Renal — APS associated nephropathy, glomerulonephritis, lupus nephritis, arterial HTN, interstitial kidney sclerosis

Fetal risks:

Recurrent pregnancy loss (RPL) — all trimesters
IUGR
Preterm birth
IUD

Weight (kg)	LMWH (enoxaparin) (mg daily)
<50	20
50–90	40
91–130	60
131–170	80
>170	0.6 mg/kg/day
High prophylactic dose (50–90 kg)	40 mg BD
Therapeutic dose	1 mg/kg BD

Treatment with LDA + LMWH increased the live birth rate to 72% versus 42% with LDA alone.

Note of caution:

Change warfarin to heparin once the urine pregnancy test (UPT) is positive, before 6 weeks of pregnancy. There is a risk of **warfarin embryopathy** (5–10%) in the first trimester and later risk of fetal loss, haemorrhage and subtle neurological changes.

Antenatal management

- Early dating ultrasound scan
- Record blood pressure (BP) and urine protein at every visit
- Start LDA + LMWH — as stated above
- Regular antenatal visits
- Uterine artery Doppler at 20 weeks
- Ultrasound scans ± Doppler scans 3 to 4 weekly from 24 weeks
- Deliver at term if there are no maternal/fetal indications for earlier delivery

Postpartum:

Safe to breastfeed while on LMWH/warfarin
Avoid oestrogen-containing contraceptives
Continue venous thromboembolism (VTE) prophylaxis for 6 weeks

4. Systemic Lupus Erythematosus (SLE) in Pregnancy

Risk factor	Implications	Action
SLE – Establish good control pre-conception. – Aim for 6 months of disease remission before conception. – Continue hydroxychloroquine as it reduces the risk of systemic flares and lupus nephritis. It also reduces the risk of recurrence of congenital heart block by >50%. **Higher risk of flares in pregnancy for the following women: (from UpToDate)** • n primigravida • Have active disease 6 months before conception • Have a history of lupus nephritis • Who stop hydroxychloroquine – Anti-phospholipid antibodies may be present in up to 40% of SLE pregnancies ***Contraindications to pregnancy*:** – Severe lupus flare (including renal flare) within the last 6 months – Stroke within the last 6 months – Severe pulmonary hypertension (systolic pulmonary artery pressure >50 mmHg) – Moderate-to-severe heart failure – Severe valvulopathy – Severe restrictive lung disease – Chronic kidney disease (CKD) stage 4–5 – Uncontrolled hypertension	**Maternal risks:** • Disease exacerbation/flares in 25–65% of pregnancies. It can occur in any trimester. • Gestational HTN/pre-eclampsia in 20–30%. • Pregnancy loss. • VTE. • Placental abruption. • Caesarean section (CS). • Anaemia and blood transfusion risks. • Thrombocytopenia. • Bleeding. • Infection. • Nephritis. • Stroke. • Seizures. • Psychosis. • Mortality. **Fetal risks:** • Preterm delivery with prematurity risks. • IUGR. • IUD. *If the mother has anti-Ro/La antibodies* • Neonatal lupus (5%): 10% neonatal lupus erythematosus rash, 20% transient cytopenias, 30% mild transient transaminitis. Spontaneously resolves when the maternal antibodies disappear in the neonate. • Congenital heart block (CHB) 2% — the risk of recurrent CHB is up to 18%.	**Management:** • *Multidisciplinary team care*, e.g., rheumatologist, obstetrician, ± nephrologist and neonatologist. • Assess disease activity and stratify care based on disease activity and antibody profile. • Early recognition and management of flares/complications are important. • Manage other pre-existing co-morbidities. • Review existing medications and VTE risk assessment. • Early dating ultrasound scan. • Record BP, urine protein at every visit. • Screen for maternal anti-Ro/La antibodies — if present, screen for CHB by fetal 2D echocardiography. Monitor fetal heart rate. • Folate/vitamin D/calcium supplements. • If renal involvement, or suspect pre-eclampsia, perform urine protein-creatinine ratio (PCR). • Aneuploidy screening between 11 and 13+6 weeks. • **Low dose aspirin (LDA) 150 mg ON from 11–14 weeks to 36 weeks (KKH protocol 2022).** • Those with APS syndrome may need LDA ± LMWH therapy. • Screening scan at 20 weeks. • Oral glucose tolerance test (OGTT) at 24–28 weeks or earlier for those on steroids or previous GDM. • Visits 4 weekly till 24 weeks, 2 weekly till 34 weeks then weekly till delivery. • Serial growth scans ± Doppler scans. • ***Drugs of choice*: Hydroxychloroquine (HCQ)** — start HCQ if the patient is not currently on it. (Steroids and azathioprine can be used in pregnancy.) • ***Avoid immunosuppressants***, e.g., methotrexate, mycophenolate mofetil (MMF), cyclophosphamide and leflunomide throughout pregnancy, and NSAIDs in the third trimester. *NSAIDs risk*: It can result in the premature closure of patent ductus arteriosus (PDA).

(*Continued*)

	• Perinatal mortality. *N.B.*: Poorer outcome if the woman has concurrent chronic hypertension, APS or active disease.	• **VTE risk assessment** — anticoagulation needed for SLE patients with APL antibodies or previous VTE. • If preterm delivery, consider antenatal steroids and IV magnesium sulphate ($MgSO_4$) as appropriate. • Continuous intrapartum cardiotocography (CTG) monitoring. • IV intrapartum stress steroids if systemic steroids >3 weeks to reduce adrenal suppression. (Refer to Chapter 64 for stress steroid regime) • Postnatal — look out for flares and VTE. • Long-term follow-up for SLE. • **Infants are to avoid live vaccines for the first 6 months of life if there was *in utero* exposure to TNF inhibitors.** • ***Contraception*:** Avoid oestrogen-containing contraceptives. • **Drugs considered safe for breastfeeding:** hydroxychloroquine, prednisolone, cyclosporin, azathioprine and tacrolimus.

5. Cardiac Disease in Pregnancy

Risk factors	Signs/symptoms and implications	Action
Cardiac disease in pregnancy **Poor outcome predictors:** • New York Heart Association (NYHA) score ≥3 or cyanosis • Left ventricular outflow tract obstruction • Severe pulmonary HTN • Cardiac dysfunction • Left ventricular ejection fraction (LVEF) <40% • Previous arrhythmia requiring treatment • Previous cardiac complication Pre-pregnancy counselling and assessment are important for women with cardiac disease. • Cardiac disease is a significant cause of maternal morbidity and mortality. ***Major risk factors for cardiovascular disease:*** ➢ Advanced maternal age ➢ Obesity ➢ Diabetes mellitus ➢ Smoking ➢ Hyperlipidaemia (HLD) ➢ HTN	**Clinical features:** • Fatigue • Shortness of breath (SOB) • Oedema • Tachycardia • Raised JVP >2 cm • Fourth heart sound • Murmurs (systolic/diastolic) **Maternal risks:** • Instrumental delivery/CS • Pulmonary oedema • Arrhythmias • Stroke • Cardiac arrest • VTE • Death **Fetal risks:** • Increased risk (2–5%) of congenital heart disease (CHD) in the child if the mother has CHD • Recurrence risk varies with the specific parental defect, i.e., 50% with Marfan syndrome and DiGeorge syndrome. • *Frequent recurrent cardiac lesions include*: VSD, coarctation of the aorta, hypoplastic left heart syndrome	**Management:** • *Multidisciplinary team care*, e.g., cardiologist, maternal-fetal specialist, anaesthetist and neonatologist. • Electrocardiogram (ECG), maternal 2D echocardiogram (2D-ECHO). • *Termination of pregnancy (TOP) option for some conditions*, e.g., Eisenmenger syndrome, pulmonary hypertension, Marfan syndrome with aortic root dilatation (>4–4.5 cm), severe left ventricular outflow tract obstruction, severe left ventricular dysfunction with — LVEF <30%, previous peripartum cardiomyopathy with any residual left ventricular (LV) impairment. • **Review medications:** Stop angiotensin-converting enzyme (ACE) inhibitors/ angiotensin receptor blockers (ARBs) and avoid statins and amiodarone. Continue beta-blockers (need fetal growth surveillance due to risk of IUGR), e.g., metoprolol or bisoprolol. – For patients with pulmonary arterial hypertension: Stop endothelin receptor antagonists (ERA) but can continue phosphodiesterase type 5 inhibitor (PDE5 inhibitor), e.g., sildenafil. • Treat co-existing anaemia, arrhythmia, HTN, diabetes mellitus (DM). • Avoid or minimise aggravating factors. • Fetal echocardiography. • Growth and fetal surveillance, especially in a left-to-right shunt. • *Individualised birth plan by 28 weeks of gestation.* • Vaginal delivery is preferred. • Avoid prolonged labour. Shorten the second stage by assisted vaginal delivery for those with more severe cardiac disease (e.g., in patients with pulmonary arterial hypertension, NYHA Class 3 or 4, Marfan syndrome with aortopathy). • CS is reserved for obstetric indications and in women with Eisenmenger syndrome/ severe cardiac failure/dilatation of ascending aorta >4.5 cm/severe aortic stenosis/PTL while on anti-coagulants/pulmonary hypertension. A CS is associated with twice as much blood loss as a vaginal delivery. However, a CS may benefit women with cardiac conditions requiring planning concerning delivery timing, care coordination, and management of anticoagulation regimen. • Induction of labour (IOL) should be considered at 40 weeks if still undelivered.

(Continued)

Common cardiac disorders in pregnancy: 1. Systemic ventricular dysfunction 2. Left heart obstruction 3. Arrhythmias 4. Coronary artery disease 5. Aortopathies 6. Congenital heart disease 7. Cardiac failure	• PTL • IUGR • Fetal acidosis • Fetal death	• Prostaglandins are safe for IOL. • Oxygen administration, haemodynamic monitoring, judicious fluid management. • Encourage left lateral position during labour. • Consider epidural — low-dose epidural anaesthesia. • Continuous intrapartum CTG monitoring. • Oxytocin should be given via a slow IV infusion to minimise the impact on the CVS. • Terbutaline contraindicated in women with high-risk cardiac conditions. • Avoid ergotamines. Avoid carboprost in women with vascular disease, aortic aneurysms, pulmonary hypertension and significant shunt lesions. • Avoid fluid overload. • Strict input and output charting with IV $MgSO_4$ use. Avoid concurrent use with calcium channel blockers due to the risk of hypotension from potential synergism. • VTE thromboprophylaxis. • ***Infective endocarditis prophylaxis:*** Intrapartum prophylactic antibiotics are ***not*** recommended routinely. **American Heart Association (AHA) guideline**. *Prophylactic antibiotics for high-risk cardiac lesions, e.g.,* – Previous history of IE – Prosthetic heart valves – Cyanotic heart disease – Cardiac transplant recipients with valvulopathy *Preferred prophylactic antibiotics:* Routine antibiotic prophylaxis for obstetric indications, e.g., CS, will also cover endocarditis prophylaxis. **1. IV** — IV ampicillin 2 g OR IV cefazolin 2 g (<120 kg) or 3 g (≥120 kg) before LSCS. **2. If allergic to penicillin:** IV vancomycin 1 g over 1–2 hours or IV clindamycin 900 mg. **Note: For infective endocarditis prophylaxis, recommended to use IV clindamycin 600 mg.** • **Contraception:** Avoid oestrogen-containing contraceptives. Postpartum — monitor for at least 72 hours in women with high-risk cardiac conditions.

6. Patients with Prosthetic Valves in Pregnancy

Risk factors	Implications	Action
Patients with prosthetic valves in pregnancy ***Types:*** **1. Bioprosthetic:** – Less thrombogenic – Finite lifespan – Pregnancy may accelerate valvular degeneration/failure **2. Mechanical:** – More thrombogenic – Longer lifespan – Requires life-long anticoagulation	**Maternal risks:** • *Bioprosthetic valves* – Structural valve failure • *Mechanical* valves: – Stroke – Valvular thrombosis – MI ***Other risks:*** • Anticoagulation risks • Heart failure (HF) • *Heparin risks*: Osteoporosis/ thrombocytopenia **Fetal risks:** • Miscarriage • Prematurity • Stillbirth • Fetal haemorrhage • Risk of warfarin embryopathy (5–10% risk between 6 and 12 weeks,<5% if <5 mg warfarin daily): o Nasal hypoplasia o Choanal stenosis o Stippled epiphysis o Optic nerve atrophy	**Management:** • *Multidisciplinary team care*, e.g., cardiologist, maternal–fetal specialist, anaesthetist, haematologist and neonatologist. • Patient education — excellent dental hygiene/ensure regular follow-up/medication compliance/side effects. • Low dose aspirin (LDA) in addition to LMWH/warfarin. *Three possible therapeutic options*: 1. Therapeutic dose LMWH throughout pregnancy. 2. Therapeutic dose LMWH between 6 and 12 weeks of pregnancy, then continue with warfarin. 3. Warfarin throughout pregnancy. ***Patients on heparin:*** • Doses have to be adjusted based on anti-factor Xa levels. The 4–6 hours peak anti-factor Xa level should be at 0.8–1.2 U/ml or pre-dose trough levels of >0.6 U/ml. • Reduce LMWH dose in renal impairment. • *Antidote for heparin*: Protamine sulphate. ***Patients on warfarin:*** • Aim for therapeutic INR of 2–3-INR: 2.5–3.5 for mechanical heart valves. • Stop warfarin and start LMWH at 36 weeks or 10–14 days before delivery to allow fetal warfarin clearance. • Prothrombinase complex and vitamin K can be used to reverse the effects of warfarin. • Aim delivery at term. CS is for obstetric indication. • The timing of delivery depends on the maternal and fetal condition and should be decided by a multidisciplinary team discussion. • Regional anaesthesia should not be undertaken until **≥12 or 24 hours** after the last prophylactic or therapeutic LMWH dose, respectively. • LMWH should not be given for 4 hours after spinal anaesthesia or after the epidural catheter removal. The catheter should not be removed <12 hours after the most recent injection. • Consider re-starting LMWH 4–6 hours after vaginal delivery and 6–12 hours after caesarean delivery if there is a low risk of haemorrhage → if previously on warfarin, consider resuming warfarin only 5–7 days after delivery (RCOG). • Infective endocarditis prophylaxis intrapartum as per AHA guidelines. • Standby blood and blood products. PPH prophylaxis and management.

7. Cardiomyopathy in Pregnancy

Risk factor	Signs/symptoms and implications	Action
Cardiomyopathy in pregnancy ***Definition:*** • Development of HF in the last month of pregnancy or within 5 months of delivery. • Absence of demonstrable heart disease before the last month of pregnancy. • **2D-ECHO:** LVEF <45%. ***Common types of cardiomyopathy:*** • Hypertrophic cardiomyopathy (HCM) • Dilated cardiomyopathy (DCM) • Peripartum cardiomyopathy (PPCM) ***Risk factors for cardiomyopathy:*** • Advanced maternal age • Obesity • Smoking • Alcohol • Multiple pregnancy • Pre-eclampsia • Malnutrition • History of myocarditis	**Clinical features:** • Fatigue • Palpitations • Orthopnoea • Dizziness • Syncope • Oedema • Low BP • Tachycardia **Maternal risks:** • Pulmonary oedema • HF • Cardiogenic shock • Arrhythmia • Ischaemic stroke • VTE • Mortality (2–50%) **Fetal risks:** • Prematurity • LBW • Respiratory distress syndrome • Low Apgar scores • NICU admission • Mortality	**Management:** • *Multidisciplinary team care*, e.g., cardiologist, maternal–fetal specialist, anaesthetist and neonatologist. • Maternal 2D-ECHO, ECG. • **For DCM/PPCM:** o Optimise preload. o Adequate oxygenation. o ***Drugs:*** Bisoprolol/carvedilol/nitrates/hydralazine/diuretics/digoxin. o If the patient is *not* stable — add inotropes ± vasopressors. o Expedite delivery. o *Postnatally*, consider bromocriptine + anticoagulation. • VTE thromboprophylaxis. • Instrumental delivery is preferred in stable patients. • CS for obstetric indications or maternal instability (severe HF). • Consider wearable cardioverter-defibrillator if LVEF ≤35% postnatally. • Avoid breastfeeding in NYHA Class III–IV patients due to high metabolic demands. • The likelihood of normalisation of cardiac function is higher in women with LVEF >30% at diagnosis. About 50% recover within 6 months after delivery. Continue HF therapy for ≥12 months after recovery of symptoms and LVEF. ***Relapse of PPCM:*** • *If LVEF has recovered,* 14–44% risk of relapse. • *If LVEF has not recovered,* 16–56% risk of relapse, 50% worsening cardiac failure and 25% risk of death in future pregnancies.

8. Hyperglycaemia in Pregnancy

1 in 6 women has hyperglycaemia in pregnancy.

Hyperglycaemia in pregnancy is divided into either **pre-existing diabetes in pregnancy or GDM**.

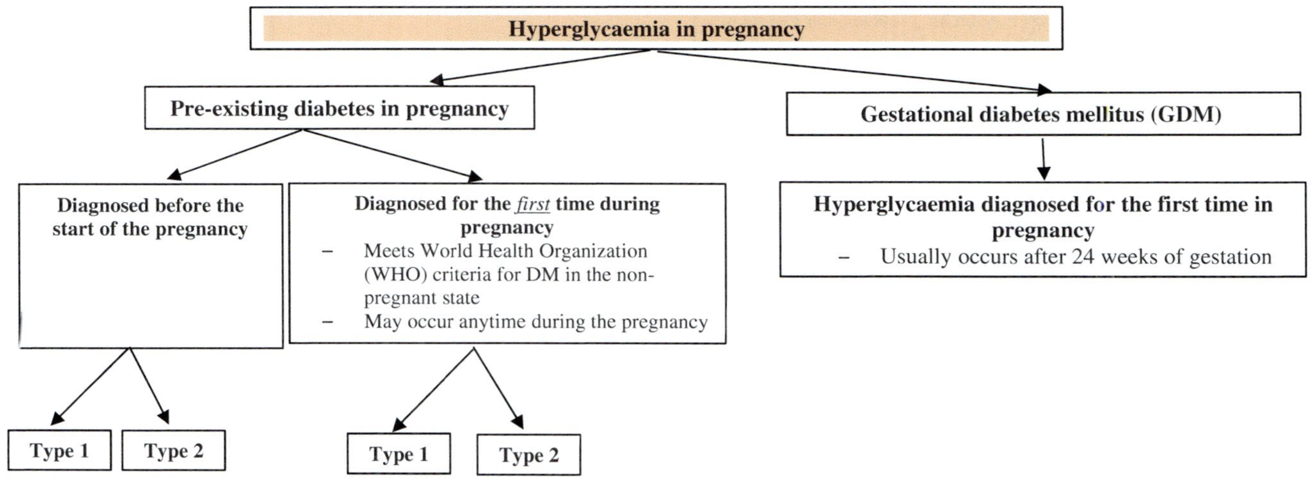

9. Pre-Existing Diabetes in Pregnancy

Definition	Implications	Management
Pre-existing diabetes in pregnancy This can refer to pre-existing type 1 or type 2 DM diagnosed before pregnancy. OR It can refer to the first diagnosis of DM at any time during the pregnancy. The OGTT results meet the World Health Organization (WHO) criteria for DM in non-pregnant women. ***WHO — DM diagnostic criteria*** When ≥1 of the criteria is met: o Fasting plasma glucose (PG) ≥7.0 mmol/L o 2-hour PG ≥11.1 mmol/L following a 75 g oral glucose load o Random PG ≥11.1 mmol/L in the presence of diabetes symptoms o HbA1c ≥6.5%	***Effect of pregnancy on DM*** 1. ***Retinopathy*** • The risk of diabetic retinopathy progression is doubled. • It may develop for the first time during pregnancy. • Progression of retinopathy is dependent on the duration and severity of diabetes, any associated hypertensive disorders, the degree of DM control and the retinal blood flow. 2. ***Nephropathy*** • Renal function may deteriorate. Depending on the severity of pre-existing nephropathy, it can be transient or permanent. 3. ***Neuropathy*** • Pregnancy does not worsen neuropathy, except in women with pre-existing carpal tunnel syndrome, advanced autonomic neuropathy or severe gastroparesis (severe gastroparesis is a *relative contraindication* to pregnancy). 4. The insulin requirements will increase in pregnancy. 5. Risk of "hypoglycaemia unawareness." 6. Diabetic emergencies: DKA, hyperosmolar hyperglycaemic syndrome (HHS). ***<u>Effect of DM on pregnancy</u>*** ***<u>Maternal risks:</u>*** ***Antenatal*** • Miscarriage • Gestational HTN/pre-eclampsia • Polyhydramnios • Infections, e.g., UTI	• *Multidisciplinary team care:* Maternal–fetal specialist, endocrinologist, ophthalmologist, nephrologist, GP, cardiologist, dietician, diabetic nurse educator, anaesthetist and neonatologist. • DM diet, 7-point blood sugar profile. ***At booking visit:*** • Optimise DM control — counsel patient on hypoglycaemia and hyperglycaemia. • Educate on the prevention and identification of DKA and hypoglycaemia (especially in hyperemesis gravidarum) and the importance of diet and exercise. • Review medications for other co-morbidities, e.g., to stop ACE inhibitors, ARBs and statins. Omega-3 can be continued. • Start anti-hypertensive if BP >140/90 and aim to target BP <135/85. Maintain BP >110/70 to avoid impairing fetal growth. • Screen for other autoimmune diseases associated with type 1 DM, e.g., autoimmune thyroiditis or coeliac disease. • Check BMI, BP, urine dipstick for protein, glucose and ketones. • Aim for HbA1c <6.5%. • Metformin, glibenclamide and insulin are safe in pregnancy. • Screen for DM complications. • Baseline FBC, urea, electrolytes and creatinine (UECr), urine PCR. • Eye and foot screen. Eye screen may be required every trimester, depending on the severity of retinopathy. • 2D-ECHO if there is a history of poorly controlled DM. • Refer to a nephrologist if serum Cr ≥120 mmol/L or protein leak >0.3 g/day or albumin creatinine ratio (ACR) >30 mg/mmol. • VTE prophylaxis in pregnancy. Start LMWH if nephrotic-range proteinuria (urine PCR >300 mg/mmol or 3 g/day or ACR >250 mg/mmol). • Optimise control of co-morbidities, e.g., HTN/HLD. • LDA 150 mg ON for pre-eclampsia prophylaxis from 11–14 weeks till 36 weeks of gestation (KKH protocol 2022). • Patient education.

Definition	Implications	Management
Pre-existing diabetes in pregnancy	***Intrapartum and postpartum*** • PTL • Prolonged labour • Instrumental delivery • Traumatic delivery • Perineal trauma, obstetric anal sphincter injuries (OASIS) • CS • Postpartum infection • PPH • VTE ***Puerperium*** • Failure to initiate and/or maintain breastfeeding ***Long term outcomes*** • Weight retention • GDM in future pregnancies • Future DM, cardiovascular disease ***Fetal risks:*** ***Antenatal*** • Congenital anomalies, e.g., cardiac and neural tube defects (associated with pre-existing DM): The more poorly controlled the DM, the higher the risk of fetal anomaly. • Macrosomia. • Stillbirth. ***Delivery*** • Shoulder dystocia and associated birth trauma, e.g., soft tissue, fractures or nerve injury, e.g., Erb's palsy.	• Lifestyle and dietary advice — low glycaemic index and high fibre foods, avoid sweet and highly processed food, individualised meal plan. • Regular moderate low-risk exercise. • Importance of optimal glucose control. • Avoid hypoglycaemia and hyperglycaemia. • Folic acid 5 mg daily for the first trimester to reduce the risk of neural tube defects. **Antenatal management:** • Accurate dating ultrasound scan. • Check BMI, BP and urine for protein every visit. • Target BP <135/85. • VTE prophylaxis. • 7-point blood sugar profile. Consider measuring HbA1c every 4–6 weeks, especially in high-risk women. • Aneuploidy screening at 11–13+6 weeks. DM may affect the interpretation of some serum analytes. • Fetal anomaly scan and 2D-ECHO at 20 weeks. • Serial growth scans especially estimated fetal weight (EFW) and amniotic fluid index (AFI). • Timing and mode of delivery are dependent on maternal/fetal wellbeing. • The mode of delivery is based on obstetric indications. However, if the EFW is >4,500 g in women with DM, the risk of shoulder dystocia is >15%. Elective CS should be considered. • Offer delivery between 37+0 and 38+6 weeks if DM is well-controlled. • Earlier delivery <37 weeks if there are maternal/fetal complications. **Intrapartum management:** • Continuous intrapartum CTG monitoring. • Hourly hypocount monitoring while nil by mouth. • Aim: Hypocount 4–7 mmol/L. • Insulin sliding scale or IV insulin infusion with dextrose drip. • If antenatal steroids were given, monitor the blood sugar profile closely.

(*Continued*)

(Continued)

Pre-existing diabetes in pregnancy	***Neonatal*** • Respiratory distress syndrome (RDS). • NICU/SCN admission. • Prematurity. • Hypoglycaemia. • Hypothermia. • Polycythaemia. • Neonatal jaundice. • Electrolyte disturbances: hypocalcaemia, hypomagnesaemia. • Cardiomyopathy. • Hypoxic ischaemic encephalopathy (HIE). • Perinatal mortality. ***Long-term outcomes*** Higher risk of diabetes, obesity, HTN and metabolic syndrome due to epigenetic imprinting. ***Effect of antenatal steroids on glucose levels:*** Blood glucose levels usually rise 4–6 hours after a steroid injection. The main effect on blood glucose levels occurs in the first 24 hours after the injection. After that, there may be a diminishing effect on blood glucose levels for up to 5 days (usually, the insulin dose is increased by 25–40%). Thus, glucose monitoring and control are essential after administering antenatal corticosteroids.	• Avoid salbutamol for tocolysis as it can cause hyperglycaemia. Use nifedipine instead. • Shoulder dystocia precautions. **Postpartum management:** • Reduce insulin dose as compared to pregnancy dose. • The risk of hypoglycaemia is increased postpartum. • Encourage breastfeeding. • Contraception — avoid oestrogen-containing contraception if there is nephropathy, retinopathy, neuropathy or other vascular diseases. • Follow-up with GP/endocrinologist.

10. Diabetic Ketoacidosis (DKA) in Pregnancy

DKA in pregnancy

Rare, life-threatening medical emergency.
More common in type 1 diabetes.
There should be a high index of suspicion.

Risk factors:

- Hyperemesis gravidarum
- Poor oral intake
- Infection
- Medications, e.g., beta sympathomimetic agents
- Steroids use
- Non-compliance to diabetic medications/failure of insulin pump
- Diabetic gastroparesis
- Major illnesses, e.g., myocardial infarction (MI), pancreatitis

In total, 30% of DKA cases during pregnancy are euglycaemic.

Women should check their blood ketone levels if their blood glucose levels are persistently elevated in pregnancy, e.g., ≥15 mmol/L, even if they feel well.

Maternal mortality: *<1%.*
Perinatal mortality after 1 episode of DKA: *9–35%.*

Patient education is crucial in preventing DKA.

Signs and symptoms:

- Abdominal pain
- Nausea/vomiting
- Poor oral intake
- Muscle weakness
- Lethargy
- Polyuria and polydipsia
- Tachypnoea
- Kussmaul breathing
- Tachycardia
- Hypotension
- Blurring of vision
- Drowsiness, confusion or disorientation
- Signs of shock
- Deranged hypocount
- Abnormal CTG

Investigations:

- FBC, UECr, glucose, liver function test (LFT), PT/PTT, GXM
- Urine/serum ketones
- Serum lactate
- Arterial blood gas
- C-reactive protein (CRP), septic workup
- CTG monitoring

Management of DKA:

- *Multidisciplinary team care*: Anaesthetist, endocrinologist, maternal–fetal specialist, neonatologist
- Monitor the patient in HDU/intensive care unit (ICU)
- Insert indwelling catheter
- Strict input and output charting
  - Maintain urine output >50 ml/hour
- Aggressive IV fluid replacement
- IV insulin therapy
- Correct electrolytes — potassium (K), calcium, phosphate, magnesium
- Replace bicarbonate if needed
- Monitor fetal status via continuous CTG
- Identify and treat the underlying cause of DKA
- Monitor the maternal response to the above treatment

Recovery from DKA:

– Serum ketone <0.6 mmol/L
– pH >7.3
– Serum HCO_3 >15 mmol/L
– Anion gap ≤12 mEq/L

11. Gestational Diabetes Mellitus (GDM)

Definition	Implications	Management of GDM
GDM In Singapore, we perform universal screening for GDM as Asians generally have a higher prevalence of GDM. We screen with a 75 g 3-point OGTT between 24 and 28 weeks of gestation unless they have pre-existing DM. *Diagnosis of GDM — based on IADPSG criteria* GDM is diagnosed if any one of the following is met: • *Fasting*: Serum glucose ≥5.1 mmol/L • *First-hour post-OGTT*: Serum glucose ≥10 mmol/L • *Second-hour post-OGTT*: Serum glucose ≥8.5 mmol/L ***Screening for DM in the first trimester*** We screen women with risk factors for pre-existing DM in the **first trimester** with a 75 g **2-point** OGTT. If the initial OGTT results are normal, repeat a 75 g **3-point** OGTT at 24–28 weeks of gestation. ***Risk factors for DM include:*** • Age ≥40 years • Pre-pregnancy BMI >30 • Previous GDM	***Effects of GDM on pregnancy*** • As above Not associated with fetal anomalies. ***Definition of pre-diabetes:*** First trimester OGTT screening results: o Fasting serum glucose ▪ 6.1–6.9 mmol/L OR o 2-hour post-OGTT ▪ 7.8–11.0 mmol/L ***Management:*** – Diet control – Blood glucose profile monitoring	– *Multidisciplinary team care*, e.g., maternal–fetal specialist, endocrinologist, GP, anaesthetist, dietician, diabetic nurse educator and neonatologist – Patient education – Lifestyle and dietary advice – Low-glycaemic-index foods – Regular moderate- to low-risk exercise – Importance of optimal glucose control – Avoid hypoglycaemia and hyperglycaemia – Accurate dating scan – GDM diet – 7-point blood sugar profile – Optimise glucose control **Glycaemic targets:** – **Fasting**: 4.4–5.5 mmol/L AND **2 hours postprandial**: 5.5–6.6 mmol/L. – **If fasting glucose is ≥7.0 mmol/L at diagnosis,** consider starting metformin and/or insulin. – **If fasting glucose is 6.0–6.9 mmol/L but with concomitant complications** such as macrosomia or polyhydramnios, consider metformin and/or insulin. **Antenatal management:** – Serial growth scans. – Timing and mode of delivery are dependent on maternal and/or fetal well-being. – Mode of delivery is based on obstetric indications. – Deliver no later than 40+6 weeks if diabetes is well controlled. – Expedite delivery if there are maternal or fetal complications. Deliver no later than 38 weeks.

Definition	Implications	Management of GDM
• History of PCOS • History of pre-diabetes • Previous macrosomia ≥4 kg • Family history of DM (first-degree relatives)		**Intrapartum management:** – Continuous intrapartum CTG monitoring. – Hourly hypocount monitoring while on nil by mouth. Aim: 4–7 mmol/L. – Insulin sliding scale or IV insulin infusion with dextrose drip. – If antenatal steroids were given, monitor the blood sugar profile closely. – Avoid salbutamol for tocolysis as it can cause hyperglycaemia. Use nifedipine instead. **Postpartum management** – Monitor hypocount. – Stop all medications post-delivery. – Encourage breastfeeding — reduces the risk of obesity and DM in the offspring. – Contraception. – Follow-up postnatally in 6 weeks with a 2-point 75 g OGTT (done in KKH). If OGTT is normal, continue DM screening 1–3 yearly. – Treat any diagnosed pre-DM or DM. – Explain long-term complications of DM: ▪ GDM recurrence: 33–55% risk of developing type 2 DM: 40–60% within 10–15 years of delivery. ▪ Risk of developing cardiovascular disease and metabolic syndrome. ▪ A healthy diet and increased exercise reduce the risk of pre-diabetes to diabetes by 35% over 10 years in women with GDM.

12. Hypertensive Disorders in Pregnancy

Methods to Prevent Pre-Eclampsia (PE)

- **Moderate exercise** ≥140 min/week throughout pregnancy → ~40% reduction in pre-eclampsia.
- **Aspirin initiation** ≥100 mg/day before 16 weeks of gestation → ~60% reduction in preterm pre-eclampsia.
- Assess **dietary calcium intake:** If <900 mg/day, initiate calcium supplementation ≥500 mg/day → ~50% reduction in pre-eclampsia.
- **Timed birth** → ~35% reduction in pre-eclampsia after 39+0 weeks of gestation.

Pre-eclampsia (PE) Screening in Pregnancy

- Using risk factors to screen for risk of pre-eclampsia in pregnancy has a detection rate of 40% and a screen positive rate (SPR) of 10%.
- The addition of other factors, e.g. patient's mean arterial pressure (MAP), uterine artery pulsatility index (UtA-PI), and biomarkers such as pregnancy-associated plasma protein-A (PAPP-A) and placental growth factor (PlGF) increases detection rate.

Risk of Pre-eclampsia <37 weeks	Detection rate (%) at 10% SPR
History + MAP + UtA-PI	67
History + MAP + UtA-PI + PAPP-A	67
History + MAP + UtA-PI + PlGF	74

(Source: Mazer Zumaeta A, Wright A, Syngelaki A, Maritsa VA, Dasilra AB, Nicolaides KH. Screening for pre-eclampsia at 11-13 weeks, gestation: use of pregnancy associated plasma protein A, placental growth factor or both. Ultrasound Obstet Gynecol 2020; 56(3): 400–407.)

13. Chronic Hypertension (HTN)

Definition	Implications	Management
Chronic hypertension: – Some women have known chronic HTN – BP ≥140/90 mmHg OR – Use of anti-hypertensives before pregnancy OR – HTN diagnosed during pregnancy (BP ≥140/90 mmHg before 20 weeks of gestation) or persisting beyond 12 weeks postpartum Significant proteinuria is when urine PCR ≥0.3. It may be essential HTN or due to an underlying renal condition. 1 in 4 develops superimposed pre-eclampsia in pregnancy.	• Increased risk of adverse maternal and fetal outcomes. • With optimal control, good pregnancy outcomes are possible. **Maternal risks:** • Placenta abruption • Exacerbation of HTN • Superimposed pre-eclampsia 25%: the risk increases with poorly controlled chronic HTN • PTL in 25% • Disseminated intravascular coagulation (DIC) • Cerebrovascular accidents/ cortical blindness • Acute myocardial infarction (AMI) • Cardiac failure • Acute kidney injury (AKI) • Pulmonary oedema • Acute respiratory distress syndrome (ARDS) • Maternal mortality **Fetal risks:** • IUGR • LBW in 15% • IUD	• *Multidisciplinary team care*, e.g., maternal–fetal specialist, physician/GP, anaesthetist, pharmacist, cardiologist, intensivist, neonatologist. • Patient education — the importance of compliance to follow-up and medications and the safety of medications. **At booking visit** • **Optimise hypertension control.** • Target BP ≤135/85 mmHg. • Review pre-pregnancy medications for safety. • <u>*Stop* medications, e.g., statins *(potentially teratogenic)*, ACE inhibitors, angiotensin II receptor blockers (ARBs)</u> *(risk of fetal anomalies, e.g., hypocalvaria, decreased skull ossification, neonatal renal failure-renal tubular dysgenesis, oligohydramnios, IUGR and death).* • <u>*Avoid:*</u> Diuretics *(potential for teratogenicity and intravascular volume depletion → reduced placental perfusion).* • <u>*Avoid*</u> *beta-blockers*, e.g., atenolol — which may cause IUGR. **Safe oral antihypertensives:** • **First line**: Labetalol (PO 100 mg BD to maximum 500 mg QDS). **Avoid in**: Asthma, cardiac failure. • Nifedipine (long-acting dose: PO 30 mg OM/BD, max 120 mg/day). • **Second line**: Methyldopa (PO 250 mg BD to maximum 1 g TDS) — ***Contraindication***: **Depression** → to stop postnatally due to the risk of postpartum depression. • <u>***Screen for complications***</u> • *Bloods*: FBC/UECr — repeat later in pregnancy as indicated. • Urine PCR. • 2D-ECHO for women with poorly controlled HTN. **Antenatal management:** • Check BMI, BP and urine dipstick. • Folic acid 5 mg in the first trimester. • Dating ultrasound scan. • VTE prophylaxis.

(Continued)

(Continued)

	• Prematurity (spontaneous/ iatrogenic) • Increased perinatal mortality **Long-term risks:** • Cardiovascular disease • Stroke • Mortality ***Interventions to reduce risks:*** • Lifestyle modifications: • DASH (dietary approaches to stop hypertension) diet and optimal weight (BMI: 18.5–24.9) • Exercise • Avoid smoking • Optimise BP control • LDA for pre-eclampsia prophylaxis in pregnancy (start 11–14 weeks gestation)	***Pre-eclampsia prophylaxis*** • LDA 150 mg ON from 11–14 weeks till 36 weeks of gestation (KKH protocol 2022). • Assess dietary calcium intake. If intake is <900 mg/day, initiate calcium supplementation ≥500 mg/day. • *Aneuploidy screening*: 11–13+6 weeks of gestation. • Fetal anomaly and uterine artery Doppler scan at 20 weeks. • OGTT from 24 to 28 weeks. • Serial growth scans 2–4 weekly from 26 to 28 weeks depending on maternal and fetal condition ± Doppler scans. • Timing and mode of delivery are dependent on maternal and fetal well-being. • Prostaglandins can be used for the IOL. • If a patient has well-controlled chronic HTN and is *not on* medications, aim for delivery between 38+0 and 39+6 weeks. • If the patient has well-controlled chronic HTN *on* medications, aim for delivery between 37+0 and 39+6 weeks. • If the patient has *poorly controlled* chronic HTN, advise for delivery between 36+0 and 37+6 weeks. **Severe HTN:** • Do blood tests (FBC/UECr/LFT/PT/PTT/uric acid) and urine PCR to diagnose if it is severe chronic HTN versus pre-eclampsia. • Offer placental growth factor (PIGF) testing between 20–35 weeks of gestation to exclude pre-eclampsia. • Antenatal steroids are recommended for up to 34+6 weeks. Discuss benefits and risks of antenatal steroids from 35+0 to 36+6 weeks. ***Dosing of antenatal corticosteroids:*** • IM betamethasone 12 mg × 2 doses, 24 hours apart. • IM dexamethasone 12 mg × 2 doses 12 hours apart (KKH) or 6 mg × 4 doses 12 hours apart (ACOG). ***Indications for IV magnesium sulphate:*** • Fetal neuroprotection if delivery is imminent <32+0 weeks (KKH) (RCOG from 24+0 and 29+6 weeks). • Maternal eclampsia/prophylaxis for severe pre-eclampsia/impending eclampsia. Expedite delivery if there are maternal/fetal indications.

Definition	Implications	Management
		Intrapartum management: • Judicious fluid management • Continuous CTG monitoring • Measure BP hourly/every 15–30 minutes till BP <160/110 • Avoid ergot alkaloids in third stage of labour (risk of worsening HTN) **Postnatal management:** • BP surveillance. *Not on anti-hypertensives:* • Monitor QDS inpatient/once between days 3 and 5. • Check BP on alternate days till normal if BP on days 3–5 was high. *On anti-hypertensives:* • Monitor QDS inpatient/every 1–2 days after transfer to community care for up to 2 weeks post-delivery till BP normalised. • Anti-hypertensives that are **safe** for breastfeeding: o Labetalol. o Nifedipine. o Enalapril/captopril — monitor UECr, especially potassium (K) levels. o Atenolol/metoprolol. o ± Amlodipine. • ***Drugs to avoid*:** Diuretics, methyldopa, ARBs in breastfeeding mothers. • ***Contraception*:** Avoid oestrogen-containing contraceptives. • **Refer to a general medicine specialist** to exclude secondary causes of HTN if not investigated previously.

(*Continued*)

14. Gestational HTN

Definition	Risks of condition	Management
Gestational HTN – New-onset HTN with BP ≥140/90 mmHg on two occasions ≥4 hours apart, after 20 weeks of gestation ***without*** proteinuria and ***no*** evidence of maternal organ dysfunction/fetal growth restriction. – It resolves by 12 weeks postpartum. – This could be a temporary diagnosis in the following women: • Women who have pre-eclampsia but have not yet developed proteinuria OR • Chronic HTN that is only diagnosed during pregnancy — if high BP persists >12 weeks postpartum. About 50% of women diagnosed with gestational HTN between 24–35 weeks ultimately develop pre-eclampsia.	**Maternal risks:** • Pre-eclampsia/haemolysis, elevated liver enzymes, low platelets (HELLP) syndrome/eclampsia • Placenta abruption • PTL • DIC • Cerebrovascular accidents/cortical blindness • Posterior reversible encephalopathy syndrome (PRES) – A constellation of vision deficit, seizure, headache, altered sensorium or confusion • AMI • Cardiac failure • AKI • Pulmonary oedema • ARDS • Maternal mortality **Fetal risks:** • IUGR • LBW • IUD • Prematurity (spontaneous/iatrogenic) • Increased perinatal mortality	• *Multidisciplinary team care*, e.g., maternal–fetal specialist, physician, anaesthetist and neonatologist. **Antenatal management:** • Baseline pre-eclampsia blood tests (FBC/UECr/LFT/PT/PTT/uric acid), urine PCR. • Patient education. Optimise BP control. • **First line:** *Labetalol* (PO 100 mg BD to maximum 500 mg QDS). **Avoid in:** Asthma, cardiac failure. • *Nifedipine* (long-acting dose: PO 30 mg OM/BD, max 120 mg/day). • **Second line:** *Methyldopa* (PO 250 mg BD to maximum 1 g TDS) — ***Contraindication:*** **Depression** → to stop after delivery due to the risk of postpartum depression. • Regular monitoring → monitor for progression to pre-eclampsia. • PIGF testing between 20–35 weeks of gestation to exclude pre-eclampsia. • Fetal surveillance via serial growth scans ± Doppler scans. • CTG monitoring at diagnosis of severe gestational HTN. Repeat CTG if clinically indicated. • The mode of delivery is based on obstetric indications. • The timing of delivery is dependent on maternal/fetal well-being. Deliver at 37+0 to 38+6 weeks or earlier if there are maternal/fetal indications. • Prostaglandins can be used for the IOL. • For severe gestational HTN ≥160/110, to deliver at 34+0 weeks or at diagnosis. **Intrapartum management:** • Judicious fluid management. • Continuous CTG monitoring. • Measure BP hourly/every 15–30 minutes till BP <160/110. • Avoid ergot alkaloids in third stage of labour (risk of worsening HTN). **Postnatal management:** • Inpatient BP monitoring and then outpatient. • Stop anti-hypertensives after delivery and monitor BP.

<table>
<tr><th>Definition</th><th>Risks of condition</th><th>Management</th></tr>
<tr>
<td></td>
<td>Long-term risks:
• Cardiovascular disease — risk increases 1.5–3 times after pre-eclampsia/gestational HTN)
• Cardiovascular (CVS) mortality — risk increases 2 times after pre-eclampsia
• Stroke — risk increases 2–3 times</td>
<td>• Re-start anti-hypertensives that are safe for breastfeeding if BP ≥150/100.
o Labetalol.
o Nifedipine.
o Enalapril/captopril — monitor UECr, especially K levels.
o Atenolol/metoprolol.
o ± Amlodipine.
• Drugs to avoid: Diuretics, methyldopa, ARBs in breastfeeding mothers.
• Contraception: Avoid oestrogen containing contraceptives.
• VTE prophylaxis.
• Recurrence rates: Explain recurrence risk and long-term implications. The overall recurrence rate is 20%.
<table>
<tr><th>Prevalence</th><th>Any HTN</th><th>Pre-eclampsia</th><th>Gestational HTN</th></tr>
<tr><td>Any HTN</td><td colspan="3">1 in 5</td></tr>
<tr><td>Pre-eclampsia</td><td>1 in 7</td><td>Overall, 1 in 6
– If delivered <28 weeks: 40%
– If delivered at 28–34 weeks: 1 in 3
– If delivered at 34–37 weeks: 1 in 4</td><td>1 in 14</td></tr>
<tr><td>Gestational HTN</td><td>1 in 11</td><td>1 in 8</td><td>1 in 7</td></tr>
<tr><td>Chronic HTN</td><td>—</td><td>1 in 50</td><td>1 in 34</td></tr>
</table>
</td>
</tr>
</table>

15. Pre-Eclampsia (PE)

Definition	Risks of condition	Management
Pre-eclampsia New-onset HTN with BP ≥140/90 mmHg on two occasions ≥4 hours apart, after 20 weeks of gestation and co-existence of ≥1 of the following new-onset conditions: A. *Proteinuria* ➢ Urine protein: Creatinine ratio (uPCR) ≥0.3 mg/dl or ➢ 24-hour urine total protein (UTP) ≥0.3 g/24 hours or ➢ Urine albumin: creatinine ratio (ACR) ≥8 mg/mmol or ➢ At least 2+ protein on urine dipstick (needs to be confirmed by spot uPCR ≥0.3 mg/dl or 24 hours ≥0.3 g/24 hours) B. *Other maternal dysfunction:* ➢ Renal insufficiency (creatinine ≥90 μmol/L) ➢ Impaired liver function — elevated transaminases ≥2× upper limit of normal or severe right upper quadrant/epigastric pain ➢ Pulmonary oedema ➢ Thrombocytopenia — platelet count <100,000/μl ➢ Neurological complications, e.g., eclampsia, altered mental status, blindness, persistent visual scotomata, stroke, hyperreflexia with clonus or severe headaches, not accounted for by alternative diagnosis	**Maternal risks:** • HELLP syndrome/eclampsia • Placenta abruption • PTL • Oligohydramnios • Caesarean Section (CS) • Disseminated intravascular coagulopathy (DIC) • Cerebrovascular accidents/ cortical blindness • PRES – A constellation of vision deficit, seizure, headache and altered sensorium or confusion • AMI • Cardiac failure • Hepatic failure or rupture • AKI • Pulmonary oedema • ARDS • Maternal mortality **Fetal risks:** • IUGR • LBW • Non-reassuring fetal status (NRFS) • IUD • Prematurity (spontaneous/ iatrogenic) • Increased perinatal mortality	– *Multidisciplinary team care*, e.g., maternal–fetal specialist, physician, anaesthetist and neonatologist. – Patient education — to understand compliance to follow-up, medications and safety of medications. – Baseline PE blood tests (FBC/UECr/uric acid/LFT/PT/PTT), urine PCR. – Optimise BP control. – Target BP ≤135/85. – **First line:** *Labetalol* (PO 100 mg BD to maximum 500 mg QDS). **Avoid in** asthma, cardiac failure. – *Nifedipine* (long-acting dose: PO 30 mg OM/BD max 120 mg/day). – **Second line:** *Methyldopa* (PO 250 mg BD to maximum 1 g TDS) — ***Contraindication*: Depression** → to stop after delivery due to the risk of postpartum depression. – Regular BP monitoring. – Blood tests for pre-eclampsia (i.e., FBC/UECr/LFT/PT/PTT/uric acid) and urine PCR — repeat as indicated, e.g., 1–2 weekly or have signs and symptoms of severe pre-eclampsia. – Fetal surveillance via serial growth scans ± Doppler scans. – CTG monitoring at diagnosis of pre-eclampsia. Repeat CTG if clinically indicated. – The mode of delivery is based on obstetric indications. – The timing of delivery depends on maternal/fetal well-being. – Need to balance the risk of prematurity against worsening pre-eclampsia. – Prostaglandins can be used for the IOL. – Deliver at 37+0 weeks or at diagnosis if pre-eclampsia is only diagnosed at term. – Preterm pre-eclampsia <34 weeks: Expectant management if the patient is stable. – Preterm pre-eclampsia diagnosed between 34+0 and 36+6 weeks. – Discuss expectant management till 37+0 weeks if the patient is stable versus earlier delivery. There should be a low threshold for delivery if there is maternal/fetal indication.

Definition	Risks of condition	Management
C. *Uteroplacental dysfunction* ➢ IUGR, abnormal uterine artery Doppler scan, stillbirth ***Hyperuricaemia is <u>not</u> diagnostic of pre-eclampsia*** ***Risk factors for pre-eclampsia*:** Refer to Chapter 1: *Pre-Conception Preparation* — indications for LDA 150 mg ON for pre-eclampsia prophylaxis — from 11–14 weeks to 36 weeks of pregnancy (ideally start before 16 weeks) *Prediction of complications from pre-eclampsia*: • FullPIERS (use anytime in pregnancy) — to predict adverse outcomes from pre-eclampsia or • PREP-S (use only ≤34 weeks) These are validated risk prediction models.	**Long-term risks:** • Cardiovascular disease — risk increases 1.5–3 times after pre-eclampsia/gestational HTN • CVS mortality — risk becomes 2-fold after pre-eclampsia • Stroke — risk increases 2–3 times	**Intrapartum management:** – Similar to gestational HTN. **Postpartum management:** – Similar to gestational HTN. – **Explain the risk of recurrence and long-term implications:** • Increased risk of cardiovascular disease [hypertension, myocardial infarction (MI), congestive cardiac failure, cerebrovascular events (stroke), peripheral arterial disease and cardiovascular mortality later in life].

16. Severe Pre-Eclampsia (SPE)

Definition	Goals of treatment	Management
SPE Signs and symptoms of impending eclampsia (IE) include: • BP ≥160/110 mmHg • <u>Neurological symptoms:</u> Headache/visual disturbances, photopsia, scotomata, blindness • <u>Liver dysfunction:</u> Severe right hypochondrial/epigastric pain, elevated transaminases ≥2 times upper limit of normal or >70 IU/L • <u>Thrombocytopenia</u> <100,000/μl • <u>Renal insufficiency</u> (creatinine ≥90 μmol/L or a doubling in the absence of renal disease) • Pulmonary oedema *<u>Prediction for complications from pre-eclampsia:</u>* • FullPIERS (use anytime in pregnancy) OR • PREP-S (use only ≤34 weeks) – Validated risk prediction models	Treatment goals for severe pre-eclampsia include: 1. Fluid management 2. Prevention of seizures 3. Lowering BP to prevent maternal end-organ damage 4. Expediting delivery based on gestation and severity of disease **Once severe hypertension is diagnosed (KKH protocol):** ▪ Monitor BP every 15 minutes. ▪ Give anti-hypertensives. ▪ Ensure adequate fluid loading to minimise hypotensive episodes. ▪ Adhere to fluid protocol. ▪ Aim to keep BP <150/80–100 mmHg. ▪ Concomitant use of $MgSO_4$ and nifedipine can cause severe hypotension. Thus, close monitoring is recommended.	• *Multidisciplinary team care*, e.g., maternal–fetal specialist, physician, anaesthetist and neonatologist. • Monitor in HDU/ICU. • Stabilise the patient. • Vitals monitoring (BP, HR, RR, SpO_2) every 15–30 minutes. • Hourly urine monitoring. • Strict input and output charting with an indwelling catheter. • Judicious fluid management — limit maintenance fluids to 80 ml/hour (unless there is ongoing fluid loss, e.g., haemorrhage) • Pre-eclampsia blood tests: FBC/UECr/LFT/PT/PTT/uric acid, urine PCR. • **Treat severe HTN as per the institution's protocol** – Aim BP: 140–150/90–100. Excessive lowering of BP may lead to uteroplacental insufficiency. – Monitor response to treatment every 15 minutes. *<u>Anti-hypertensives used:</u>* – Labetalol (PO/IV). – Nifedipine (PO fast-acting) — if no IV access. – Hydralazine (IV). ***<u>KKH protocol for severe pre-eclampsia 2022</u>*** ***<u>First line</u>* (if no contraindications to labetalol):** – If there is *<u>no IV access:</u>* **PO labetalol** 200 mg STAT dose can be given and repeat another 200 mg dose after 30 minutes if there is no response. – *Once there is <u>IV access:</u>* Give IV labetalol 10–20 mg bolus over 10 minutes, then repeat 10 mg bolus every 10 minutes until MAP <140 mmHg (maximum cumulative dose of IV labetalol is 300 mg). – Start IV labetalol infusion 250 mg in 50 ml, infuse at 1–2 mg/minutes with a syringe pump, then titrate every 30 minutes according to the BP **OR** ***<u>Second line:</u>*** – **PO nifedipine** 10 mg stat dose and repeat another 10 mg dose 20 minutes later if BP >160/90 mmHg. – If BP is still high, give 10–20 mg every 2–6 hours to a maximum daily dose of 180 mg. *Side effects*: reflex tachycardia and headaches.

Definition	Goals of treatment	Management

	Contraindications for IV $MgSO_4$:
	1. Myasthenia gravis
	2. Hypocalcaemia
	3. Moderate to severe renal failure
	4. Cardiac ischaemia
	5. Heart block
	6. Myocarditis
		– Consider **nifedipine LA 30 mg,** but it takes 1 hour for the onset of action.
		– Monitor BP closely if nifedipine and IV $MgSO_4$ are used concomitantly due to the risk of severe hypotension.
		Third line: (Needs anaesthetist/maternal-fetal medicine consultant review first)
		– **IV hydralazine** 5 mg bolus over 20 minutes.
		– Can repeat second dose of IV 5 mg bolus over 20 minutes if BP is still severely high.
		– Can repeat third dose of IV 5 mg bolus over 20 minutes if BP is still severely high.
		– After 3 boluses, start IV hydralazine maintenance infusion at 5 mg/hour, up to a maximum of 10 mg/hour.
		– *Side effects*: Maternal hypotension, headache, NRFS.
		• **Start IV magnesium sulphate.**
		• Antenatal steroids are recommended for up to 34+6 weeks. Discuss benefits and risks of steroids from 35+0 to 36+6 weeks.
		• VTE prophylaxis.
		• Continuous CTG monitoring.
		• **Stabilise and deliver if the patient is ≥34+0 weeks.**
		• **If <34+0 weeks,** expedite delivery if there are maternal/fetal indications as stated below:
		  – Severe HTN not responding to treatment, despite 3 or more classes of anti-hypertensive medications.
		  – Worsening biochemistry ± haematology, e.g., progression to HELLP syndrome, coagulopathy, DIC, worsening liver or renal function.
		  – Impending eclampsia/eclampsia.
		  – Abnormal neurological features.
		  – Other complications, e.g., acute pulmonary oedema.
		  – Fetal indications, e.g., NRFS, IUGR with stagnant growth or abnormal Dopplers.
		• The mode of delivery is based on obstetric indications. If there is a need to expedite delivery, then a CS is required unless vaginal delivery is imminent.
		
		Intrapartum management:
		• PPH prophylaxis and management.
		• Avoid ergot alkaloids in third stage of labour (risk of worsening HTN).

17. HELLP Syndrome

Definition	Risks of condition	Management
HELLP *Diagnosis (Tennessee classification)*: • Haemolysis: Severe anaemia Raised bilirubin >20 μmol/L, lactate dehydrogenase (LDH) 2 times upper limit of normal, low serum haptoglobin ≤25 mg/dl • Elevated transaminases, i.e., aspartate aminotransferase (AST) and alanine aminotransferase (ALT), ≥2 times upper limit of normal • Low platelets (PLT) — <100,000 μ/L *HELLP can be subclassified based on the Mississippi classification*: It measures the severity of the syndrome using the lowest observed PLT count along with the other two main clinical criteria (LDH and AST). This allows us to prognosticate and determine the bleeding risk. *Class I is the most severe*, with relatively high morbidity and mortality risk compared to the other two classes. • ***Class 1:*** PLT count <50,000/μl + LDH >600 IU/L + AST or ALT ≥70 IU/L • ***Class 2:*** PLT count >50,000/μl but ≤100,000/μl + LDH >600 IU/L + AST or ALT ≥70 IU/L • ***Class 3:*** PLT count >100,000/μl but ≤150,000/μl + LDH >600 IU/L + AST or ALT ≥40 IU/L	**Maternal risks:** Pulmonary oedema ARDS Renal failure DIC Caesarean section (CS) Transfusion of blood and blood products ICU/HDU admission Mortality **Fetal risks:** Prematurity NICU/SCN admission Perinatal mortality	• **Multidisciplinary team care,** e.g., maternal–fetal specialist, physician, anaesthetist and neonatologist. • Monitor in HDU/ICU. • Supportive care — stabilise the patient. • Vitals monitoring (BP, HR, RR, SpO_2) every 15–30 minutes. • Hourly urine monitoring. • Strict input and output charting with an indwelling catheter. • Judicious fluid management. • Pre-eclampsia blood tests (FBC/UECr/LFT/PT/PTT/uric acid), urine PCR ± DIC screen. • Treat severe HTN as per the institution's protocol. • Antenatal steroids if <34 weeks. • Start IV $MgSO_4$. • Correct any anaemia or coagulopathy via transfusion of blood or blood products. • Regional anaesthesia can be used if there is no coagulopathy and the platelet count is >80,000 μ/L. • Expedite delivery. • If the patient is ≥34 weeks: Stabilise the patient and deliver. • If <34 weeks: Deliver after antenatal steroids completion if the patient is stable. • A low threshold to expedite the delivery if there is maternal/fetal deterioration. • The mode of delivery is usually via CS unless vaginal delivery is imminent or the patient is stable for IOL. ***Intrapartum management:*** • PPH prophylaxis and management. • Avoid ergot alkaloids in third stage of labour (risk of worsening HTN). ***Postnatal management:*** • Similar to pre-eclampsia. • Postnatal BP surveillance and management. • *Contraception*: Avoid oestrogen-containing contraceptives. • Explained recurrence rate and long-term complications. • 5% risk of recurrence of HELLP. • 20% risk of gestational HTN or pre-eclampsia. • Class I HELLP syndrome has the highest recurrence rate.

18. Eclampsia

Definition	Risks of condition	Management
Eclampsia: Life-threatening emergency which can occur: 1. Antepartum — 53%. 2. Intrapartum — 19%. 3. Postpartum — 28%. Seizures can occur without features of severe pre-eclampsia and with a normal BP. ***Eclampsia*** is defined as new-onset tonic-clonic, focal or multifocal seizures in the absence of other conditions, e.g., epilepsy, cerebral arterial ischaemia/infarction, intracranial haemorrhage or drug use. Post-ictal confusion, agitation or combativeness may follow. The fetus may demonstrate hypoxia-related bradycardia during the seizure, but it usually recovers.	**Maternal risks:** Maternal hypoxia. Maternal trauma. Aspiration pneumonia. Morbidity-impaired memory and cognitive function, especially after recurrent seizures. Mortality. **Fetal risks:** **CTG changes** — recurrent decelerations, tachycardia, reduced variability, bradycardia. Maternal resuscitation is usually followed by normalisation of the CTG trace. Neonatal mortality.	• **"Code Blue" — it is an obstetric emergency.** • *Multidisciplinary team care*, e.g., maternal–fetal specialist, intensivist, neurologist, anaesthetist, haematologist, blood bank and neonatologist. • Stabilise patient's airway, breathing and circulation. • Placement in the lateral decubitus position. • Prevent aspiration or injuries. • PE blood tests, urine PCR. • Strict input and output charting with an indwelling catheter. • CTG monitoring. • Control hypertension. • **Start IV magnesium sulphate (KKH protocol 2022).** – **Loading dose** of IV $MgSO_4$ of 4 g over 5 minutes (dilute 8 ml $MgSO_4$ with 12 ml of 0.9% normal saline) followed by **maintenance** $MgSO_4$ infusion at 1 g/hour for 24 hours. – *If no IV access: IM $MgSO_4$ 10 g (IM 5 g in each buttock), followed by IM $MgSO_4$ 5 g every 4 hours. IM $MgSO_4$ can be mixed with 1 ml of lignocaine 2% solution to reduce pain from the injection. However, IM $MgSO_4$ has a higher rate of adverse effects.* – $MgSO_4$ should be continued for at least 24 hours after a patient's last seizure or after delivery, whichever is later. – Monitor respiratory rate, SpO_2 and BP every 30 minutes, heart rate, patellar reflexes and urine output every hour. – Routine measurement of serum magnesium (Mg) level is *not* required unless there are signs of toxicity, e.g., absent reflexes, decreased urine output, SpO_2 or respiratory rate. – **Therapeutic Mg level:** 2–4 mmol/L. – ***Magnesium toxicity:*** ➢ **>3.5 mmol/L:** Flushing, nausea, weakness, feeling of warmth, ECG changes, loss of reflexes. ➢ **>5 mmol/L:** Double vision, slurred speech, respiratory rate <10/minutes, SpO_2 <92%. ➢ **6–7.5 mmol/L:** Muscle paralysis, respiratory arrest. ➢ **>12.5 mmol/L:** Cardiac arrest.

(*Continued*)

		– ***Dose adjustment based on Mg level/clinical signs:*** – <u>*Mg level >5 mmol/L:*</u> Stop maintenance dose and repeat Mg level. – <u>*Mg level 4.1–5.0 mmol/L:*</u> Decrease maintenance dose to 0.5 g/hour. – <u>*Mg level <2 mmol/L:*</u> Increase maintenance dose to 2 g/hour. – <u>*Oliguria*</u> (<0.5 ml/kg over 4 consecutive hours) or urea >10 mmol/L: Give 0.5 g/hour maintenance dose and measure Mg levels more closely. – <u>*Loss of patellar reflex:*</u> Stop maintenance infusion and urgently check serum Mg level. Withhold further Mg treatment until patellar reflexes return or the Mg level is known. Restart at 0.5 g/hour and check levels closely. – <u>*Respiratory depression or CNS depression:*</u> Stop $MgSO_4$ infusion. Administer IV calcium gluconate. Intubate the patient. – *Treatment for $MgSO_4$ toxicity:* IV 10 ml of 10% calcium gluconate over 3 minutes. ***Recurrent fits:*** – Repeat a dose of 2–4 g of IV $MgSO_4$ over 5 minutes. – If refractory to $MgSO_4$ (still seizing at 20 minutes after bolus or >2 recurrences), consider IV phenytoin infusion of 1250 mg at a rate of 50 mg/minutes and intubate the patient. – Arrange for brain imaging scans. – *For patients with contraindications to $MgSO_4$*, e.g., acute renal failure/cardiac disease/myasthenia gravis/use of calcium antagonist, IV diazepam 5 mg into a large vein over at least 2 minutes can be given. IV diazepam can be repeated 5 mg (over 2 minutes) till fits stop to a maximum of 30 mg. • Immediate delivery once the mother is stabilised. • Antenatal steroids — do not delay delivery to await administration of steroids. • PPH prophylaxis and management. • Avoid ergot alkaloids in third stage of labour (risk of worsening HTN). ***Postnatal management:*** • Admission to HDU/ICU. • As per that for pre-eclampsia.

19. Previous Severe Pre-Eclampsia

Definition	Risks of condition	Management
Previous SPE Check that patient does not have chronic HTN.		• Pre-pregnancy weight loss (if BMI >30). • Lifestyle modifications. • LDA 150 mg ON for pre-eclampsia prophylaxis from 11–14 weeks till 36 weeks of gestation (New KKH protocol 2022). • Assess dietary calcium intake: If <900 mg/day, initiate calcium supplementation ≥500 mg/day. • Monitor BP/urine albumin at each visit. • Counsel regarding risk of recurrence.

Thyroid Disorders in Pregnancy

20. Hyperthyroidism in Pregnancy

Condition	Signs/symptoms and implications	Action
Hyperthyroidism in pregnancy ***Causes:*** • Graves' disease — 85% of cases • Gestational thyrotoxicosis • Viral thyroiditis • Multinodular goitre • Solitary toxic adenoma • Molar pregnancy (rare) ***Overt* hyperthyroidism:** Elevated free T4, low thyroid stimulating hormone (TSH). ***Subclinical* hyperthyroidism:** Normal free T4, low TSH Usually not associated with adverse pregnancy outcomes.	**Clinical features:** • Tremors • Anxiety, sweating • Heat intolerance • Decreased exercise tolerance • Weight loss • Increased appetite • Vomiting/diarrhoea • Tachycardia • Atrial fibrillation • Hypertension • Proximal muscle weakness • Hyperreflexia • Goitre • Ophthalmopathy **Maternal risks:** • Miscarriage • Gestational HTN/pre-eclampsia • Polyhydramnios • PTL • Placental abruption • Obstructed labour from neck extension related to fetal goitre • Failure to gain weight • Infection • Thyroid storm • Congestive cardiac failure	**Management:** • Aim to achieve normal TSH levels according to pregnancy-specific ranges. • *Multidisciplinary team care*, e.g., endocrinologist, GP, obstetrician, neonatologist, anaesthetist and pharmacist. • Patient education — to understand control, compliance and safety of medications. • Individualised management. • TFT — 3 monthly or within 2–4 weeks of switching drugs and 4–6 weekly after target values achieved. <u>*Indications of measuring TRAb in pregnancy:*</u> – Untreated hyperthyroidism. – Currently on medications. – History of Graves' disease treated with radioactive iodine or surgery. – History of an infant with hyperthyroidism. • TRAb is *not* indicated in those who are in remission after medications. • Measure TRAb at diagnosis — if high TRAb, risk of fetal/neonatal thyrotoxicosis. If TRAb is high, repeat at 18–22 weeks; if still high, repeat at 30–34 weeks. • Monitor for fetal thyrotoxicosis and scan for fetal goitre, IUGR and oligohydramnios if TRAb is elevated. • Most patients can reduce the dose of antithyroid drugs during pregnancy, and 1/3 can stop under the supervision of an endocrinologist. • Aim to keep free T4 at the upper limit of normal to reduce the risk of fetal hypothyroidism.

<table>
<tr><th colspan="2">Condition</th><th rowspan="2">Signs/symptoms and implications</th><th rowspan="2">Action</th></tr>
<tr><th>Gestational thyrotoxicosis</th><th>Graves' disease</th></tr>
<tr><td>Non-autoimmune</td><td>Autoimmune</td><td rowspan="6">• Retrosternal pressure of the goitre can cause dysphagia and tracheal obstruction
• Recurrence/exacerbation of Graves' disease postpartum

Fetal risks:
• Miscarriage.
• Hydrops.
• IUGR.
• Prematurity.
• Fetal thyrotoxicosis
Fetal tachycardia, IUGR, excessive fetal movements, goitre, hydrops fetalis, IUD, craniosynostosis.
Obstructed labour due to goitre
• Fetal hypothyroidism-due to transplacental transfer of anti-thyroid drugs.
• If high TRAb, the risk of fetal thyroid dysfunction and neonatal thyrotoxicosis.
• Neonatal thyrotoxicosis.
– The mortality rate is 15% without treatment.
– Treatment is required until maternal auto-antibodies disappear. Regular thyroid function test (TFT).
• Stillbirth.
• Increased perinatal mortality.</td><td rowspan="6">• Thyroid function improves in third trimester but worsens postpartum.
• Serial growth scans at 28, 32 and 36 weeks.

<u>Antithyroid drugs (ATDs):</u>
1. Thionamides, e.g., carbimazole
o Up to 15 mg/day is safe for a fetus.
o Screen for fetal anomalies (2–4%): Aplasia cutis, choanal and oesophageal atresia.
o Watch for maternal agranulocytosis.
2. Propylthiouracil (PTU)
o Up to 150 mg/day is safe for the fetus.
o Screen for fetal anomalies (2–3%): Primarily face and neck cysts and urinary tract abnormalities in males. They are less severe birth defects than those associated with carbimazole.
o Watch for maternal agranulocytosis and hepatotoxicity.
3. Beta-blockers, e.g., propranolol — treat symptoms such as palpitations, tremors, anxiety.
For short-term use (<2–6 weeks) only. Usually stopped once the ATD works and there is improvement in the patient's clinical condition.
<u>Risks with long-term use of beta-blockers:</u>
• IUGR.
• Fetal bradycardia.
• Neonatal hypoglycaemia.
• Neonatal respiratory depression.
Over-treatment with ATDs may cause fetal hypothyroidism and goiter.
(Refer to Chapter 18: Medications in Pregnancy and Lactation)</td></tr>
<tr><td>1–5% of pregnant mothers</td><td>0.2% of pregnant mothers</td></tr>
<tr><td>Thyroid stimulating hormone receptor antibody (TRAb) negative</td><td>TRAb positive</td></tr>
<tr><td>Associated with hyperemesis, multiple and molar pregnancy</td><td></td></tr>
<tr><td>No prior history of thyroid disease</td><td>Prior history of thyroid disease/previous infant with thyroid dysfunction</td></tr>
<tr><td>No adverse fetal outcomes</td><td>Adverse pregnancy outcomes — if left untreated</td></tr>
</table>

(Continued)

		Role of thyroidectomy — rarely done. – Ideally done in second trimester or postpartum. <u>*Indications for thyroidectomy:*</u> • Obstructive symptoms, e.g., tracheal obstruction. • Confirmed/suspicion of malignancy. • Failure/non-compliance with medical therapy. • Allergy to ATDs. **Radioactive iodine** is contraindicated in pregnancy. ***N.B.: If women undergo radioactive iodine therapy, avoid conception for 6 months*** • Assess baby's thyroid function postnatally. • Cord blood for TSH level. • Safe to breastfeed on ATDs.

21. Thyroid Storm (Thyroid Crisis)

Thyroid storm (thyroid crisis)	Signs/symptoms and implications	Management
• Rare endocrine/metabolic emergency with high mortality. • Prompt recognition and timely intervention is crucial. • Extreme physiologic state in a spectrum of thyrotoxicosis. • **Underlying Graves'** most common cause but may occur secondary to thyrotoxicosis of any other aetiology. ***Triggers for thyroid crisis:*** • Infection • Trauma • Pregnancy, labour and delivery • CS • Surgery • DKA • MI • Abrupt cessation of antithyroid drugs **Management of thyroid crisis:** 5 Bs: 1. **B**lock synthesis (anti-thyroid drugs) 2. **B**lock release (iodine) 3. **B**lock T4 to T3 conversion (high dose PTU, propranolol, corticosteroids) 4. **B**eta-blocker (propranolol) 5. **B**lock entero-hepatic circulation (cholestyramine)	• Fever • Extreme lethargy • Profuse sweating • Agitation/profound delirium or psychosis • Abdominal pain with nausea, vomiting, and diarrhoea • Jaundice • Pedal oedema • Tachycardia **Maternal risks:** • Cardiac failure • Pre-eclampsia • Arrhythmias • DIC • Respiratory failure/pulmonary oedema • Seizures/coma • Placental abruption • Preterm labour • Multiorgan failure • Mortality (8–25%) **Fetal risks:** • Miscarriage • Preterm delivery • IUD • Fetal mortality	• *Multidisciplinary team care*, e.g., endocrinologist, obstetrician, intensivist, pharmacist and neonatologist • Manage in HDU or ICU • **Burch–Wartofsky Point Scale for diagnosis** Score ≥45 — thyroid storm Score 25–44 — impending Score <25 — storm unlikely ***Supportive/resuscitative measures:*** o IV fluids to prevent dehydration o Electrolytes replacement o Nutritional support o Treat fever — antipyretics o Ventilatory support, if needed o VTE prophylaxis • Treat the precipitating cause ***Definitive therapy*** — **PTU and propranolol** • **Iodides** — Lugol's iodine or potassium iodide solution (to give 1 hour after the first dose of thionamide to prevent iodine from being used as a substrate for new hormone synthesis). • **Steroids,** e.g., IV hydrocortisone. • **Cholestyramine.** • CTG monitoring for the fetus. • Clinical improvement is usually after 24–72 hours. • Rarely, may need plasmapheresis or plasma exchange. • Continue maintenance treatment till euthyroid. • Consider definitive treatment after the acute stage of thyroid storm, i.e., either ATDs (radio-active iodine is contraindicated in pregnancy) or surgery.

22. Hypothyroidism in Pregnancy

Hypothyroidism in pregnancy	Signs/symptoms and implications	Management
Causes: Autoimmune/Hashimoto's thyroiditis. Iodine deficiency. Iatrogenic — after antithyroid drugs. ***Overt* hypothyroidism:** Low free T4 and elevated TSH. ***Subclinical* hypothyroidism:** Normal free T4 and elevated TSH. *L-Thyroxine is needed if:* • Thyroid peroxidase antibody (TPO-Ab) positive and TSH >2.5 mU/L. • TPO-Ab negative and TSH >pregnancy-specific range and <10 mU/L. • TSH ≥10 mU/L (regardless of TPO-Ab negative or positive). No L-thyroxine is needed if TPO-Ab is negative and TSH < the upper limit of the pregnancy-specific range.	• Fatigue • Cold intolerance • Weight gain • Decreased exercise tolerance • Dry skin • Hair loss • Constipation • Bradycardia • Muscle weakness/cramps • Depression • Carpal tunnel syndrome **Maternal risks:** • Miscarriage • Anaemia • Pre-eclampsia/gestational HTN • PTL • Placental abruption • Fetal distress • CS • PPH • Postnatal depression • Cardiac failure • Myxoedema coma **Fetal risks:** • LBW • Prematurity • Congenital anomalies • Stillbirth • Congenital hypothyroidism or cretinism • Perinatal mortality • Neurodevelopmental delay	• Aim to achieve normal TSH levels according to pregnancy-specific ranges. • *Multidisciplinary team care*, e.g., endocrinologist, GP, obstetrician, anaesthetist and neonatologist. • Patient education — to understand control, compliance and safety of medications. • Make individualised plan. • Regular TFT — at booking and once in each trimester or 4–6 weekly after dose adjustment. • If TSH >2.5 mU/L, to do TPO-Abs. • L-Thyroxine (LT4): Start 100–150 mcg/day (safe in pregnancy) → adjust the dose to target TSH in the lower half of the trimester-specific range. If unavailable, target TSH <2.5 mIU/L. • Reduce T4 to pre-pregnancy doses postpartum. • Do not use other thyroid preparations, e.g., T3 or natural desiccated thyroid drugs. • Take thyroxine at the same time every morning on an empty stomach. Wait for 30 minutes to an hour before breakfast. Take thyroxine 4 hours before or after taking iron, antacids or calcium supplements as they affect the absorption of thyroxine. • Monitor for postnatal depression. • No contraindications to any form of contraception.

23. Postpartum Thyroiditis (PPT)

PPT	Clinical features	Management of PPT
• Abnormal TSH within the first 12 months postpartum in the absence of a toxic thyroid nodule/thyrotrophin receptor antibodies. • Thyroiditis induced by an autoimmune mechanism within 1 year after parturition. • Most patients are asymptomatic. • Presentation is usually 3–4 months after delivery but may be delayed up to 6 months postpartum. • PPT may also occur after pregnancy loss (miscarriage, abortion and ectopic pregnancy) and after a normal delivery. • **Important to have a high clinical index of suspicion.** **Risk factors:** • Autoimmune disease, e.g., type 1 DM. • Previous history of PPT. • Positive TPO-Ab patients. • Women on thyroid hormone replacement.	<u>*Postpartum presentation:*</u> • 32%: Transient hyperthyroidism alone • 43%: Transient hypothyroidism alone • 25% (biphasic): Transient hyperthyroidism followed by hypothyroidism and then recovery <u>*Suspect PPT in the following patients:*</u> • Fatigue postpartum • Postpartum depression • Graves' disease	• High or high-normal free T4 and T3 and low TSH during the hyperthyroid phase. • Most women do not require treatment. • Repeat TFT 4–8 weeks later to check for resolution. • If symptomatic, treat with 40–120 mg *propranolol* or 25–50 mg *atenolol* daily. • During the hypothyroid phase, free T4 is low or low-normal, and TSH is high. Treat if symptomatic with *L-thyroxine* (T4) (50–100 mcg/day). • Serum TPO-Ab — elevated. • 3–4% of women have permanent hypothyroidism. • 20–30% with TPO-Ab positive PPT have permanent hypothyroidism within 4 years. Thus, yearly screening with TFT is recommended. • **Recurrence risk of PPT:** 10–25%.

Indications for TFT in Pregnancy

- Currently on anti-thyroid treatment
- Previous history of thyroid disorders or thyroid surgery
- History of autoimmune disorder, type 1 DM, head and neck irradiation
- Presence of a goitre
- Signs and symptoms suggestive of thyroid disorders
- Family history of autoimmune or thyroid disorders
- History of PPT
- Previous infant with thyroid disorder
- Use of amiodarone, lithium or recent iodinated radiologic contrast agents

24. Role of Thyroid Antibodies

Role of thyroid antibodies	When to order thyroid antibodies	Other facts on thyroid antibodies
1) TPO-Ab • Elevated in Hashimoto's thyroiditis, Graves' disease. • Patients at increased risk of PPT.	**TPO-Ab is** ordered when: • Symptoms are suggestive of thyroid disease. • Before starting patients on medications that have risks of hypothyroidism when TPO-Abs are present, e.g., lithium, amiodarone, interferon alpha or interleukin-2.	TPO-Ab has been associated with reproductive problems, e.g., • Miscarriage • Pre-eclampsia • Pre-term delivery • *In vitro* fertilisation (IVF) failure
2) TRAb • Elevated in Graves' disease. • TRAb should be checked at booking, 18–22 weeks and again at 30–34 weeks to determine the need for postnatal and neonatal monitoring. Risk of fetal thyrotoxicosis if TRAb is increased.	**TRAb** is ordered when: • Symptoms of hyperthyroidism. • Monitor the effectiveness of anti-thyroid therapy.	

Maternal status	TSH	Free thyroxine (FT4)	Total thyroxine	Free triiodothyronine (T3)
Pregnancy	Decrease	Decrease slightly in second and third trimesters	Increase	Decrease
Hyperthyroidism	Decrease	Increase	Increase	Increase/no change
Hypothyroidism	Increase	Decrease	Decrease	Decrease/no change

Trimester-specific ranges for TFTs				
	Non-pregnant	First trimester	Second trimester	Third trimester
TSH (mIU/L)	0.3–4.3	0.1–2.5	0.2–3.0	0.3–3.0
Free T4 (ng/dl)	0.8–1.7	0.8–1.2	0.6–1.0	0.5–0.8
Free T4 (pmol/L)	7–16	11.4–19.5	10.1–15.4	8.9–14.9

25. Liver Disease in Pregnancy

***Liver disease in pregnancy* disease categories**		
Pre-existing liver disease	Viral hepatitis (Refer to Chapter 15: *Infections in Pregnancy*), autoimmune hepatitis, pre-existing cholestasis, drug-induced hepatitis, Wilson's disease, primary biliary cirrhosis, primary sclerosing cholangitis and other metabolic conditions, cirrhosis and liver transplant.	
Newly acquired liver disease in pregnancy	Viral hepatitis, gallstones, drugs, sepsis, Budd–Chiari syndrome (usually post-partum).	
Trimester	**First**	**Second/Third**
Diseases related to pregnancy	Hyperemesis gravidarum	Obstetric cholestasis (OC), pre-eclampsia/ HELLP syndrome Acute fatty liver of pregnancy (AFLP)

26. Diagnostic Modalities for Liver Diseases in Pregnancy and Lactation

Diagnostic modality	Pregnancy suitability	Lactation suitability	Other implications
Ultrasound	Acceptable modality	Acceptable modality	Safe in pregnancy and lactation.
CT scan	**Ionising radiation risk** to the fetus in pregnancy.	Acceptable modality	The greatest radiation risk is between 8 and 15 weeks of gestation.
			Oral and iodinated contrast media are not teratogenic.
			<1% of iodinated contrast is excreted in breast milk.
MRI scan (Refer to Chapter 62: Imaging Modalifies in O&G)	Acceptable modality if without contrast. No ionising radiation risk.	Acceptable modality (with and without contrast)	Gadolinium use is associated with teratogenicity in animal studies. Therefore, it should generally be avoided unless the benefits outweigh the risks. <0.04% is excreted into breast milk.
Magnetic resonance cholangiopancreatography (MRCP)	No ionising radiation risk.	Acceptable modality	Safe at any gestation in pregnancy.
Endoscopic retrograde cholangiopancreatography (ERCP)	It can be performed during pregnancy, ideally second or third trimester.	Acceptable modality	Fetal radiation between <0.1 and 0.5 mGy (which is below the threshold for malformation = 50 mGy).
Liver biopsy	It can be performed during pregnancy.	Acceptable modality	Limited data on preterm births when performed in pregnancy.
			Transjugular liver biopsy confers radiation exposure.
Transient liver elastography	Not FDA approved for use in pregnancy but can be done at any gestation if required.	Not contraindicated in lactation	There may be a small increase in liver stiffness and controlled attenuation parameters in the third trimester, which can be normal pregnancy physiology.
Upper endoscopy	Upper endoscopy is acceptable in pregnancy. Recommended in the second trimester.	Acceptable modality with consideration of the compatibility of sedation in lactation	Ensure informed consent with a discussion about fetal risks.
	Consideration of compatibility of sedation in pregnancy.		Ensure adequate oxygenation and haemodynamic stability during the procedure.
			Ensure left lateral decubitus position — to avoid IVC compression.

27. Hyperemesis Gravidarum (HG)

Condition	Signs/symptoms and implications	Action
HG • Nausea and vomiting in pregnancy begin in the first trimester • *Diagnosis of exclusion* • Prevalence: 69% • Recurrence rate: 54–83% **HG** refers to *severe* nausea and vomiting in pregnancy. *Defined by the presence of:* o >5% pre-pregnancy weight loss o Dehydration o Electrolyte imbalance *Incidence of HG*: 1.1% 75% of women with HG considered not getting pregnant again 15% had TOP due to HG Up to 27% considered TOP due to HG **Risk factors:** • Previous HG • Multiple/molar pregnancy • Family history • Genetics	• Symptoms begin between 4–7 weeks, peak at 9 weeks, subside by 20 weeks in 90% of patients. • 24% have persistent symptoms throughout pregnancy. • Nausea, vomiting — duration, onset. • Severity — whether the woman can retain orally. • Any weight loss? • Assess for dehydration. • Use the PUQE score to determine the severity. **Maternal risks:** • Fluid and electrolyte imbalance — low sodium/potassium/chloride/magnesium, metabolic hypochloraemic acidosis. • Starvation ketoacidosis. • Malnutrition. • Hepatic dysfunction. • Thiamine (vitamin B1) deficiency → can result in *Wernicke's encephalopathy*. They present with blurring of vision, confusion, memory problems and drowsiness. *Signs* include nystagmus, ophthalmoplegia, sixth nerve palsy and ataxia. IV dextrose-containing fluids can precipitate it. MRI scan is diagnostic. Treatment is with *thiamine*. There is complete remission in 29% and possible residual permanent impairment.	• Relieve nausea and vomiting. • Correct dehydration and electrolyte abnormalities. • Improve hydration and weight gain. • VTE prophylaxis for hospitalised patients. • Psycho-social support. • Folic acid supplementation. • Dietitian review. • Urinary ketones. • UFEME, urine culture to screen for UTI. • Monitor BP, HR, Weight and BMI. • Neurological examination. • Renal panel and electrolytes. • Hypocount to exclude DKA • For severe/refractory HG, consider LFTs (deranged in 15–50% of HG) and TFTs. • Ultrasound scan for dating/viability. • Rarely TOP may be considered in refractory HG with severe weight loss, depression and lack of family support. **Pharmacological management** (refer to Chapter 18: *Medications in Pregnancy and Lactation*) • IV fluids — normal saline with KCl/vitamin replacement. • Avoid dextrose-containing fluids — risk of Wernicke's encephalopathy if thiamine deficient. • Initiate **anti-emetics** in the following order: ***First line*:** 1. Diclectin® (pyridoxine/doxylamine). 2. Antihistamines, e.g., promethazine, cinnarizine, dimenhydrinate. 3. Phenothiazines, e.g., prochlorperazine (Stemetil®), chlorpromazine.

(Continued)

(*Continued*)

	• *Korsakoff psychosis* consists of a triad of retrograde amnesia, impaired learning ability and confabulation. The recovery rate is 50% and residual impairment is common. • *Vitamin B12 and B6 deficiency*: Anaemia, peripheral neuropathy. • Mallory–Weiss tear. • VTE. • *Psychosocial* — depression, anxiety, post-traumatic stress disorder (PTSD). **Fetal risks:** • IUGR. • Preterm birth. • Increase in risk of neurodevelopmental conditions/behavioural disorders.	***Second line:*** 1. Dopamine antagonists, e.g., metoclopramide — risk of extrapyramidal side effects. 2. Serotonin inhibitors, e.g., ondansetron — currently, the available data do not suggest that use in the first trimester is associated with an overall risk of fetal anomalies. Some small studies show a small risk of cleft palate and cardiac defects, but the absolute risk is small. The background risk for orofacial clefts is 11 per 10,000 pregnancies versus 14 per 10,000 pregnancies after ondansetron use in the first trimester. Avoid ondansetron in the first trimester, if possible. In KKH, we perform an ultrasound scan of the fetus at 15–16 weeks and a high-risk fetal anomaly scan at 20 weeks for maternal ondansetron use. ***Third line:*** 1. Steroids — use only in refractory HG, possible small increased risk of oral clefts in first trimester. ***Acid suppression therapy:*** 1. Antacids/famotidine. 2. Omeprazole. **Laxatives** if constipation.

28. Obstetric Cholestasis/Intrahepatic Cholestasis in Pregnancy (ICP)

Diagnosis of ICP is based on the peak bile acid (BA) concentration, the highest BA concentration recorded during a woman's pregnancy.

The upper limit of normal BA concentrations in pregnancy is 18 μmol/L.

Definitions (RCOG 2022 guideline on ICP):

1. Gestational pruritus = Maternal pruritus and peak BA concentration <19 μmol/L → women can develop ICP up to 15 weeks from the diagnosis of gestational pruritus.
2. *Mild* ICP = Maternal pruritus and peak BA concentration 19–39 μmol/L.
3. *Moderate* ICP = Maternal pruritus and peak BA concentration 40–99 μmol/L.
4. *Severe* ICP = Maternal pruritus and peak BA concentration ≥100 μmol/L.

Condition	Signs/symptoms and implications	Action
Obstetric Cholestasis (OC)/Intrahepatic Cholestasis in Pregnancy (ICP) – Most commonly in the third trimester, although it can be earlier. – More common in South American and Asian women. ***Diagnosis (RCOG 2022 guideline)*** – Pruritus in the absence of a primary skin condition with abnormal maternal BA concentrations. – Confirm the diagnosis of ICP in the postnatal period by measuring LFT and BA **at least 4 weeks post-delivery**, which should normalise and the itch resolves. – If the patient is unwell, other diagnoses should be suspected and repeat the LFT earlier. Refer to gastroenterologist if required **Risk factors/aetiology of OC** — likely multifactorial – Previous OC. – Genetics. ▪ Some women have mutations in the biliary transporters ABCB11 and ABCB4 or pathogenic mutations in other genes. They can have a 3–5-fold increase in gallstone pancreatitis, cirrhosis and biliary tract cancer. Hence, they will require long-term follow-up with a gastroenterologist. – Family history. – Oestrogens. **Recurrence rate:** Up to 90%	**Clinical features:** • Pruritus, typically of palms and soles — typically worse at night → BA concentrations do not correlate with itch severity • No rash • Nausea/anorexia • Jaundice — rare, <1%, usually mild • Dark urine/pale stools (steatorrhoea) • Abnormal LFTs ↑ Transaminases (<3-fold) — especially ALT (60%) ↑ Alkaline phosphatase more than the pregnancy range ↑ Serum bilirubin (25%) ↑ Serum BAs • Liver failure — *not typical* of ICP **Maternal risks:** • Sleep deprivation • Higher risk of pre-eclampsia/GDM • PTL (spontaneous/iatrogenic): higher risk for *moderate* and *severe* OC • IOL • CS • Vitamin K deficiency • PPH 2–22% — *no* increased risk of uncomplicated ICP • Gallstones • Increased risk of GDM, HLD	**Management of OC:** • *Multidisciplinary team care* — maternal–fetal specialist, anaesthetist and neonatologist. • Refer to a gastroenterologist if the woman develops ICP in the first or second trimester or persistence of itch/abnormal LFT/BA post-partum, at least 4 weeks. ***Investigations:*** • Routine use of other investigations to rule out differential diagnoses is no longer recommended. – Perform these investigations in women with an atypical presentation/uncertain diagnosis of ICP, e.g., severe transaminitis, early onset in the first or second trimester, rapidly worsening biochemical results, features of liver failure/acute infection or persistent post-partum. ➢ Ultrasound of the hepatobiliary system. ➢ Viral serology (Hep A, B, C, EBV and CMV). ➢ Autoimmune screen for chronic active hepatitis and biliary cirrhosis. • Patient education — especially fetal movement charting. • Serial growth scans — ultrasound and CTG *do not* predict or prevent stillbirth. • Routine OGTT screening at 24–28 weeks. • Repeat LFT and BAs 1 week after diagnosis and individualise the frequency of monitoring based on the severity. – <u>Mild ICP:</u> Weekly testing from 38 weeks. – <u>Moderate ICP:</u> Weekly testing from 35 weeks. – <u>Severe ICP:</u> MDT care. May need to expedite delivery. • Perform coagulation testing if indicated, e.g., in complicated ICP. ***Medications:*** • Topical emollients for pruritus (calamine lotion/aqueous cream with menthol). • Antihistamines, especially at night. • Ursodeoxycholic acid 250 mg BD or TDS. – In women with BA ≥40 μmol/L who are 34–36 weeks, ursodeoxycholic acid may have some benefit in reducing late preterm births.

Condition	Signs/symptoms and implications	Action
Bile acids (BA) interpretation: ***Singleton pregnancy*** – <u>*Mild* ICP</u> and no other risk factors: The risk of stillbirth (0.13%) is similar to the background risk. BA >40 μmol/L is associated with adverse pregnancy outcomes. – <u>*Moderate* ICP</u> and no other risk factors: Risk of stillbirth similar to background risk **until 38–39 weeks when risk increases.** – <u>*Severe* ICP</u>: The risk of stillbirth is (3.4%) significantly higher than the background risk. Presence of risk factors, e.g., pre-eclampsia/GDM/multiple pregnancy, appears to increase the risk of stillbirth. ***Multiple pregnancy*** – The risk of stillbirth is higher than a twin pregnancy without ICP.	**Fetal risks** • Preterm birth (25–60%) — mostly iatrogenic • Meconium-stained liquor: 25–45% (common in preterm OC) • Fetal distress (33%) • Intracranial haemorrhage • Stillbirth (SB)/IUD • Increased admission to NICU/special care nursery for respiratory distress syndrome (RDS) • Increased perinatal morbidity and mortality	• Consider maternal vitamin K only if there is reduced absorption of dietary fats (e.g., the woman has steatorrhoea) or abnormal prothrombin time. • **Timing of delivery (ICP with no other risk factors):** – <u>*Mild ICP:*</u> Deliver by 40 weeks of gestation. – <u>*Moderate ICP:*</u> Deliver at 38–39 weeks of gestation. – <u>*Severe ICP:*</u> Deliver at 35–36 weeks of gestation. • Continuous intrapartum CTG. • Active management of third stage. • The mode of delivery is dependent on obstetric indication. ***Postpartum*** • Repeat LFT/BA at least 4 weeks postpartum. If the LFT/BA remain elevated after 4–6 weeks — refer to a gastroenterologist to exclude underlying liver disorders. • Safe to breastfeed baby. • IM vitamin K for neonate. • <u>*Contraception:*</u> ICP itself does not affect the type of contraception/HRT. – Previously, it was thought that women with ICP may have an increased risk of cholestasis when using oestrogen-containing contraception, but this is unlikely for most women. Hence, oestrogen-containing contraception is *not a contraindication*. If itch recurs or abnormal LFT develop while on oestrogen-containing contraception, stop the oestrogen-containing contraception and advise other methods. – For women with ICP and previous cholestasis due to oestrogen-containing contraception, use non-hormonal/progestogen-only methods. • Risk of recurrence of ICP. Perform a baseline LFT and BA at booking visits for subsequent pregnancies.

29. Acute Fatty Liver of Pregnancy (AFLP)

Condition	Signs/symptoms and implications	Action
AFLP • Typically presents in the third trimester • ~20% present postnatally • Incidence: 1 in 7,000–15,000 pregnancies ***Risk factors:*** • Long-chain L-3 hydroxyacyl-CoA dehydrogenase deficiency (LCHAD) • First pregnancy • Low BMI • Pre-eclampsia • Male fetus • Multiple pregnancy ***Differential diagnosis:*** • Pre-eclampsia/HELLP syndrome • Acute viral hepatitis • OC ***Diagnosis via the Swansea criteria (≥6 of the criteria):*** – Nausea and vomiting – Abdominal pain – Polydipsia/polyuria – Confusion/encephalopathy – Renal impairment (creatinine >150 μmol/L) – Hypoglycaemia (<4 mmol/L) – Transaminitis (AST/ALT >42 IU/L) – Hyperbilirubinaemia (>14 mmol/L) – Hyperuricaemia (>340 mmol/L) – Coagulopathy (INR >1.3/PT >14 seconds/APTT >34 seconds) – Raised ammonia (>47 mmol/L) – Leukocytosis (>11 × 10^9/L) – Ascites or echogenic liver on ultrasound – Microvesicular steatosis on liver biopsy	**Symptoms:** – Abdominal pain – Nausea, vomiting – Malaise, anorexia – Fever – Headache – Jaundice – Polyuria – Polydipsia **Signs:** • Epigastric/right hypochondrial tenderness • Jaundice • HTN (in 70% of patients with AFLP) • Tachycardia • Late-onset pyrexia • Confusion • Hepatic flap • Hypoglycaemia (70% of cases) **Maternal risks:** <u>*Multisystem involvement*</u> • AKI • Encephalopathy • GI bleeding • Pancreatitis • Coagulopathy • Metabolic acidosis secondary to impaired clearance of serum lactate by damaged hepatocytes • Transient diabetes insipidus • Circulatory collapse • Persistent liver failure • Mortality (18%) **Fetal risks:** • Altered acid-base status • Neonatal mortality up to 85% — can reduce to 23% with prompt recognition and management	• Resuscitation and stabilisation • Involve HDU/ICU • *Multidisciplinary team care*: anaesthetist, gastroenterologist, MF specialist and neonatologist • Broad-spectrum IV antibiotics • Correct hypoglycaemia, coagulopathy ***Investigations:*** • FBC, UECr, PT/PTT, uric acid, serum bilirubin • LFT: Transaminitis (up to 3–10× of normal, raised ALP) • Hypocount • *Viral hepatitis screen*: ***Hepatitis A:*** Hep A IgM, IgG ***Hepatitis B:*** HBsAg (If HbsAg positive, do HBeAg, HBeAb, HBV-DNA) ***Hepatitis C:*** Anti-HCV antibodies ± **CMV:** CMV IgM and IgG ± **EBV**: EBV IgM and IgG ± **Autoimmune liver panel** US HBS • Expedite delivery • If fulminant hepatic failure or encephalopathy, the patient may need liver transplant. • Postnatal surveillance of LFT (derangement may continue for up to 1 week before recovery) • Recurrence risk of 25%

Renal Disorders in Pregnancy

30. Acute Kidney Injury (AKI) in Pregnancy

Condition	Signs/symptoms and implications	Action
AKI in pregnancy ***Definition*:** – Sudden loss of kidney function causing an accumulation of urea and other nitrogenous waste products, dysregulation of extracellular volume and electrolytes **Causes can be obstetric-related or non-obstetric related** ***Obstetric-related causes:*** **1. Early pregnancy** (<20 weeks) – Hyperemesis gravidarum – Acute tubular necrosis (ATN) from septic abortion **2. Late pregnancy** • Severe pre-eclampsia ± HELLP • Acute tubular necrosis (ATN) associated with haemorrhage • Rarer causes: o Haemolytic uraemic syndrome (HUS) o Thrombotic thrombocytopaenic purpura (TTP) o AFLP o Amniotic fluid embolism o Gravid uterus causing urinary tract obstruction ***Non-obstetric-related causes:*** – Acute pyelonephritis – Sepsis – Drugs, e.g., NSAID use – Glomerulonephritis/interstitial nephritis – Urinary tract obstruction	**Signs/symptoms:** – Oliguria – Hypovolemia – Hypertension/ hypotension – Shock – Sepsis – Proteinuria – Rising serum creatinine **Maternal risks:** • Pre-eclampsia • Placental abruption • PTL • CS • DIC • HDU/ICU admissions • Death • CKD, renal failure ± requiring dialysis/ renal transplant **Fetal risks:** • Miscarriage • Prematurity • IUGR • LBW • IUD • Perinatal morbidity/ mortality	**Management:** • *Multidisciplinary team care*: Maternal–fetal specialist, nephrologist, haematologist, intensivist, ID physician and neonatologist. • Admit to HDU/ICU if haemodynamically unstable. ***Investigations for AKI*:** ➢ FBC, serum UECr ➢ Serum LDH, serum bilirubin and reticulocyte count, haptoglobin (*to exclude haemolysis*) ➢ Urine FEME, culture, urine PCR ➢ Renal tract ultrasound ± Septic workup in sepsis ± Renal biopsy, immunological investigations • Supportive management • Treat the underlying cause • Monitor intake/output • Stop nephrotoxic drugs **Pre-renal causes** (volume depletion) → *volume resuscitation* (crystalloids/ colloids ± blood products) **Post-renal causes** → ureteral stents, percutaneous nephrostomy, or delivery, if indicated **Consider dialysis in refractory cases of:** A — (metabolic) acidosis E — electrolytes, e.g., hyperkalaemia I — intoxication O — (fluid) overload U — uraemia

31. Chronic Kidney Disease (CKD) in Pregnancy

Condition	Signs/symptoms and implications	Action
CKD in pregnancy • More difficult conception due to irregular menses/amenorrhoea • Even mild CKD has a higher risk of adverse maternal and fetal outcomes • Use serum creatinine instead of eGFR (eGFR is not validated in pregnancy) • High-risk pregnancy *Renal biopsy in pregnancy:* • Indicated if it is going to change management • Unable to diagnose through less invasive means • Accurate diagnosis is required to save the mother's life • Usually done <28 to 30 weeks of gestation Low threshold to start dialysis in pregnant patients. The risks of preterm delivery outweigh the risks of dialysis. *Indications for initiating dialysis in pregnancy:* • Urea >17 mmol/L • Serum creatinine 310–450 μmol/L • Glomerular filtration rate (GFR) <20 ml/min	**Maternal risks:** • Miscarriage • Pre-eclampsia • Anaemia • Blood transfusion risks • GDM • PTL/delivery • CS • Infection • CKD progression to end-stage renal failure • May need acute dialysis or other renal replacement therapy • Cardiovascular disease • Mental issues, e.g., depression • Mortality **Fetal risks:** • Prematurity • IUGR • LBW • Stillbirth • NICU admission • Neonatal mortality **Effect of pregnancy on dialysis:** • Worsens anaemia and increases the need for transfusion • Increased demand for dialysis • Increased heparin doses to prevent dialysis lines from being clotted	**Management:** *Multidisciplinary team care*: Maternal–fetal specialist, renal physician, neonatologist, dietician and pharmacist. Consider adjusting doses of medications that can be continued in pregnancy if indicated. **Pre-conception planning:** • Stop nephrotoxic/fetotoxic drugs, e.g., ACE inhibitors, ARBs, NSAIDs, statins, immunosuppressants, e.g., MTX, mycophenolate, cyclophosphamide. • Optimise control of comorbidities, e.g., diabetes, SLE, hypertension. • FBC, UECr, LFT, HbA1c (for DM). • Urine dipstick, urine PCR. • Routine antenatal vaccinations. • Genetic counselling for women with inheritable renal diseases. **Antenatal:** • Booking BMI. BP, weight, urinalysis every visit — aim for BP **≤135/85.** • Initiate dialysis if indicated. • Treat anaemia with iron supplements/erythropoietin stimulating agents (EPO). • Folate ± vitamin D supplements. • Early dating scan — assess gestational age (GA) accurately. • Fluid management is important. • Regular antenatal visits. • First trimester screening for aneuploidy. – First-trimester screening and maternal serum screening: Reduced clearance of β-hCG, PAPP-A unreliable in late CKD. There is an increased false positive. • Start LDA 150 mg ON from 11–14 weeks till 36 weeks of gestation to prevent pre-eclampsia (new KKH 2022 protocol). • Start calcium in calcium-deficient women. • Screening scan at 20 weeks — look for fetal anomalies (FA), e.g., polycystic kidneys. • OGTT at 24–28 weeks (or earlier if previous GDM, on steroids or calcineurin inhibitors). • Serial growth scans ± Doppler if IUGR.

Condition	Signs/symptoms and implications	Action
		• VTE prophylaxis — start LMWH if nephrotic-range proteinuria (urine PCR >300 mg/mmol or 3 g/day or ACR >250 mg/mmol) or sub-nephrotic range proteinuria with other risk factors. May need a renally adjusted dose depending on creatinine. **Delivery:** • Vaginal delivery is preferred (if there are no obstetric contraindications). • Continuous intrapartum CTG. • Avoid nephrotoxic drugs, e.g., NSAIDs. • Judicious fluid management. • I/O chart — to monitor fluid balance. • Aim delivery at term. May need earlier delivery <37 weeks if there are maternal/fetal indications. • *Consider earlier delivery if maternal/fetal indications*, e.g.: o Worsening renal function, especially if reaching dialysis threshold >34 weeks. o Refractory hypertension, pulmonary oedema, symptomatic hypoalbuminaemia. o Severe pre-eclampsia. o IUGR/NRFS. **Postnatal/long-term:** • Screen for depression. • Psychological/social support. • Safe to breastfeed. • Follow-up by renal physician. ***Contraception*:** • POP, Depo-Provera, progesterone subdermal implant, progesterone/copper intra-uterine device, sterilisation. Avoid oestrogen-containing contraception if the woman has cardiovascular risk factors. • ***Emergency contraception*:** Progesterone-only pill is safe, copper IUCD.

(Continued)

(Continued)

<table>
<tr>
<td>

Renal allograft recipients

<u>Obstetric outcomes</u>

<table>
<tr><th>Renal status</th><th>Successful outcome (%)</th><th>Long-term sequelae (%)</th></tr>
<tr><td>Serum creatinine <125 μmol/L</td><td>97</td><td>7</td></tr>
<tr><td>Serum creatinine >125 μmol/L</td><td>75</td><td>27</td></tr>
</table>

</td>
<td>

Maternal risks:

- Ectopic pregnancy (due to adhesions from previous surgery, peritoneal dialysis)
- Pre-eclampsia
- UTI
- GDM
- Preterm delivery
- Preterm premature rupture of membranes (PPROM)
- Opportunistic infections, e.g., rubella, CMV, toxoplasmosis, HSV, hepatitis B/C
- Acute graft rejection

Fetal risks:

- IUGR
- Prematurity
- Perinatal morbidity/mortality

Effects of pregnancy on renal transplant:

- If baseline creatinine is normal or <100 μmol/L: No adverse effects on long-term graft function or survival
- If an impaired renal function with creatinine >130 μmol/L: Graft survival will reduce
- The risk of renal graft deterioration is higher with baseline impaired renal function, hypertension or proteinuria

</td>
<td>

Management:

Multidisciplinary team care: Maternal–fetal specialist, renal physician, neonatologist, dietician and pharmacist.

Pre-pregnancy counselling:

- Renal transplant recipients — to wait until kidney function is stabilised before conception (usually >1 year) — *as graft function is stable and on stable levels of immunosuppressants, hence, minimising the risks to the fetus.*

<u>Can try to conceive when:</u>

- No transplant rejection within the last 1 year.
- Adequate and stable graft function.
- No/minimal proteinuria (<500 mg/24 hours).
- On stable maintenance doses of immunosuppressive drugs.
- No acute infections that may affect the fetus.
- Optimise control of comorbidities, e.g., HTN, DM.

Continue immunosuppressives at pre-pregnancy dosages

- Safe to continue prednisolone, azathioprine, ciclosporin, tacrolimus.
- Avoid MMF due to the risk of FA, first-trimester pregnancy loss.

- Screen for CMV, HIV, HSV, hepatitis B/C.
  - If CMV is negative, re-check titres every trimester.
- First-trimester screening for aneuploidy.
  - NIPT: False positive for gender.
- OGTT at 24–28 weeks.
- Manage hypertension — safe to continue methyldopa, labetalol, nifedipine.
- For preterm delivery, consider antenatal steroids and IV $MGSO_4$ for fetal neuroprotection ($MgSO_4$ dose needs to be adjusted based on renal function).
- Aim delivery at term if there are no maternal/fetal indications.
- Vaginal delivery is preferred. CS is reserved for obstetric indications.
- Allograft in the false pelvis does not obstruct fetal delivery. However, there is a 1–2% risk of injury to the kidney or transplanted ureter during a CS. Therefore, manage in conjunction with a transplant surgeon for elective/emergency caesarean. Consider a midline skin incision to avoid injury to the allograft. Use ultrasound pre-operatively to locate the allograft.

</td>
</tr>
</table>

32. Pregnancy in Women on Dialysis

Condition	Signs/symptoms and implications	Action
Pregnancy in women on dialysis: • More difficult conception due to irregular menstruation/ amenorrhoea ***Indications for dialysis in pregnancy:*** • Severe refractory nephropathy • Severe electrolyte imbalance • Volume overload — CCF • Pulmonary oedema refractory to diuretics • Bilateral renal cortical necrosis (oliguria >1 week) • Severe metabolic acidosis • Uraemia	**Maternal risks:** • Hypertension/pre-eclampsia, HELLP • Anaemia • Blood transfusion risks • Miscarriage • Preterm labour • Induced labour • CS • Infections/bacteraemia • Depression • May need permanent dialysis in the future ***Effects of dialysis on pregnancy:*** – <u>Pros:</u> Positive correlation with pregnancy outcomes, i.e., gestational age, birth weight and live birth rate. Improve BP control, reduce hypotension risk and improve maternal nutrition. – <u>Cons:</u> Miscarriage, IUD, pre-eclampsia, PTL, PPROM, polyhydramnios secondary to uraemia, placental abruption. – Risk of bleeding due to the use of heparin during dialysis. – Peritoneal dialysis-associated complications, e.g., peritonitis, limited exchange volume in pregnancy. – Aim for pre-dialysis urea <17 mmol/L. **Fetal risks:** • Prematurity • IUGR • LBW • Stillbirth • Perinatal morbidity and mortality	**Management:** • *Multidisciplinary team care*, e.g., maternal–fetal specialist, nephrologist, haematologist, intensivist, neonatologist, pharmacist and dietician. • Consider changing peritoneal dialysis → haemodialysis during pregnancy. • Increase duration + frequency of haemodialysis (≥20 hours/week) to improve pregnancy outcomes. • Optimise control of comorbidities, e.g., SLE or DM. • Booking BMI, BP and proteinuria at every visit — aim post-dialysis BP <140/90 mmHg and avoid intradialytic hypotension <120/70 mmHg. • Baseline renal function, urine PCR. • Dating ultrasound scan. • Folate supplementation. • Review all medications. • Start LDA 150 mg ON from 11–14 weeks till 36 weeks gestation to prevent pre-eclampsia (new KKH 2022 protocol). • Screen for anaemia and treat with iron supplements/EPO. • Measure calcineurin inhibitor levels — tacrolimus/cyclosporin. • Screen for hepatitis B and C virus, HSV, CMV, toxoplasmosis and rubella. • Assess VTE risk. • First-trimester screening for aneuploidy. – First-trimester screening and maternal serum screening: Reduced clearance of βHCG, PAPP-A unreliable in dialysis. There is an increased false positive result. – NIPT: Cell-free DNA may be partially cleared by haemodialysis. • Screening scan at 20 weeks of gestation. • Monitor FBC, UECr, uric acid and urine PCR regularly. • OGTT at 24–28 weeks (earlier if previous GDM, on steroids or calcineurin inhibitors). • Monthly urine culture — to screen for asymptomatic bacteriuria. • Serial growth scans ± Doppler if IUGR. • For preterm delivery, consider antenatal steroids and IV $MgSO_4$ for fetal neuroprotection. ($MgSO_4$ dose needs to be adjusted based on renal function). • Aim delivery at term >37 weeks if no maternal/fetal indications. • Vaginal delivery is preferred. CS is reserved for obstetric indications. • Continuous intrapartum CTG. • Safe to breastfeed. • Avoid oestrogen-containing contraceptives due to increased cardiovascular risks. • *Postnatal*: Monitor BP. Continue pre-pregnancy dialysis regime. • Screen for depression.

33. Urinary Tract Infections (UTIs) in Pregnancy (Asymptomatic Bacteriuria, Acute Cystitis and Acute Pyelonephritis)

It is a spectrum of diseases from asymptomatic bacteriuria → acute cystitis → acute pyelonephritis.

Proper management of bacteriuria and urinary tract infections is necessary for patient care and to reduce antibiotic resistance.

Risk factors:

- Urinary stasis/reflux (physiological changes in pregnancy)
- Glycosuria
- Sexual activity
- Previous UTI
- Concomitant urinary tract anomalies, e.g., duplex ureter/kidney, reflux nephropathy
- Renal calculi
- Neurogenic bladder (e.g., spina bifida)
- In-out/indwelling catheterization
- Maternal disease, e.g., DM, immunosuppressed state, e.g., HIV/sickle cell disease/SLE
- History of maternal renal conditions, e.g., chronic glomerulonephritis (GN), adult polycystic kidney disease, chronic pyelonephritis, renal transplantation → associated with acute pyelonephritis in pregnancy

Causative organisms:

- *Escherichia coli* (*E. Coli*) — 80–90% of infections; *Proteus mirabilis* and *Klebsiella pneumoniae.*
- Gram-positive cocci, e.g., *Staphylococcus saprophyticus*, Group B haemolytic Streptococci (GBS)*, *Staphylococcus aureus*, acid-fast mycobacterium.
- *Chlamydia trachomatis*; *Neisseria gonorrhoeae.*
- Non-bacterial organisms: Yeasts, e.g., *Candida.*

*Group B Streptococcus is strongly associated with PPROM and PTL and is a proven cause of neonatal sepsis.

	Asymptomatic bacteriuria (ASB)	Acute cystitis	Acute pyelonephritis (recurrence risk: 8–20%)
Definition and clinical manifestations	• Asymptomatic • Persistent colonization of the urinary tract by **≥10^5** colony-forming units (CFU)/ml • Mostly occurs in early pregnancy • Incidence: 2–10% in pregnancy	• Lower UTI • Bacteriuria ≥10^5 CFU/ml • *Symptoms* include dysuria, urgency, frequency, nocturia, haematuria, cloudy urine, suprapubic pain • No evidence of systemic illness, such as fever	• Upper UTI. • Bacteriuria ≥10^5 CFU/ml. • Cystitis and/or signs and symptoms of systemic illness, e g., flank/renal angle pain, pyrexia, chills, rigors, nausea and vomiting. • Incidence: 1–2% in pregnancy. • Common in second and third trimesters with a history of ASB/recurrent UTI/previous pyelonephritis.
Maternal and Fetal Risks	**Maternal risks:** • Symptomatic cystitis/pyelonephritis: If untreated in 40% of pregnant women • Pre-eclampsia • Anaemia • PPROM • PTL • Chorioamnionitis • Postpartum endometritis **Fetal risks:** • LBW • Prematurity • Mental retardation • Developmental delay • Perinatal mortality	**Maternal risks:** • Pre-eclampsia • Recurrent cystitis *No clear correlation has been established between acute cystitis during pregnancy and increased risk of LBW, preterm delivery, or pyelonephritis.*	**Maternal risks:** • Pyonephrosis • Perinephric abscess • ± Gram-negative bacteraemia • Septic shock, DIC • Renal impairment • Multiple organ failure • ARDS • Persistent/recurrent UTI* • Miscarriage • Pre-eclampsia • PTL/delivery • Anaemia • PPROM • Chorioamnionitis • Postpartum endometritis • Mortality **Fetal risks:** • NRFS • LBW • Prematurity • Developmental delay • Perinatal mortality

(Continued)

(*Continued*)

	Asymptomatic bacteriuria (ASB)	Acute cystitis	Acute pyelonephritis (recurrence risk: 8–20%)
Investigations	• Screen for ASB with mid-stream urine for culture and sensitivity (C&S) at booking • No need for repeat screening if first urine C&S is negative, unless the patient has risk factors for UTI • The specimen is considered contaminated if >20 squamous cells under microscopic HPF or ≥3 organisms identified in the urine culture — repeat the test. *N.B.: Urine dipstick has a lower sensitivity/specificity than urine C&S → hence, it is not recommended for ASB screening.*	• Send mid-stream urine for FEME, C&S	• Send mid-stream urine for FEME, C&S. • *Bloods*: FBC, CRP, UECr, blood cultures. • ± Serum lactate if the patient is septic. • *Ultrasound scan of kidney, ureter and bladder* (KUB) — to evaluate for causes or complications of pyelonephritis, e.g., abscess, calculi, renal tract malformations.
Management: Refer to local antibiogram for choice of antibiotics as antibiotic resistance differs between countries. **Avoid trimethoprim** in the <u>*first trimester*</u> in patients with folate deficiency or on folate antagonists **Avoid nitrofurantoin** in the <u>*third trimester*</u> and patients with G6PD deficiency — the risk of neonatal haemolysis. **In G6PD-deficient patients, to avoid:** • Sulphur drugs • Nitrofurantoin • Nalidixic acid	• Empirical oral antibiotics • Continue/change to culture-directed treatment when urine C&S results are out • Increase fluid intake • Repeat urine C&S at least 2 weeks after treatment for the test of cure. ***Screening and treatment of ASB reduce the risk of acute pyelonephritis in pregnancy*** **GBS bacteriuria:** • If GBS growth ≥10^5 CFU/ml on urine culture in current pregnancy → to start antibiotics (PO amoxicillin/cefalexin) when detected • Will also require intrapartum IV penicillin G (if not allergic) for vaginal delivery or if SROM occurs before planned CS (category 2 or 3 caesarean)	**Similar management to ASB:** • The duration of antibiotics is 5–7 days. • Consider starting antibiotic prophylaxis if ≥3 episodes of recurrent cystitis during pregnancy.	• Admit patient • I/O charting • IV hydration • Empirical broad-spectrum IV antibiotics till afebrile for ≥24–48 hours • Continue with culture-directed oral antibiotics to complete 10–14 days. • In severe cases, *MDT care* — involve an ID physician, microbiologist, pharmacist. • Analgesia (avoid NSAIDs) • Antipyretics • VTE prophylaxis (TEDS ± LMWH) — if reduced mobility/prolonged bed rest/hospitalisation • Assess for PTL. • Repeat urine C&S at least 2 weeks after treatment for the test of cure.

*For additional information on UTI/recurrent UTI, refer to Chapter 48: *Urogynaecology*.

34. History of Second-Trimester Fetal Loss

Risk factor	Implications	Action
History of second-trimester fetal loss – Check if the cause of fetal loss was found. ***Risk factors:*** – History of excisional biopsy of cervix, e.g., cone biopsy/LLETZ and if the depth of excision is >1 cm – Previous dilatation and curettage/ evacuation of uterus – Congenital Müllerian anomalies, e.g., bicornuate, septate, didelphys uterus – History of submucosal fibroids – Autoimmune diseases, e.g., SLE, APS – DM, HTN, thyroid disease – Infections, e.g., chorioamnionitis – Abdominal trauma – Fetal anomalies	**Maternal risks:** – Recurrence (dependent on aetiology) – PTL – PPROM – Depression/anxiety **Fetal risks:** – Extreme prematurity – Miscarriage/IUD	**Management:** – Treat the underlying cause of previous fetal loss, if identified. – *For the next pregnancy*: • Accurate dating ultrasound scan. • Folic acid supplements. • Screen for infections, e.g., lower genital tract infection (LGTI) via VP3 test, urine culture. • First-trimester aneuploidy screening. • Serial TVUS for cervical length from 16 to 24 weeks. If cervical length is ≤2.5 cm, <u>options for short cervix:</u> 1. Recommend ultrasound-indicated *cervical cerclage* (RCOG 2021). – Cervical cerclage after first-trimester aneuploidy screening between 12 and 16 weeks. – Counsel on cervical cerclage procedure and risks. – In women who have failed transvaginal cerclage, consider a transabdominal cerclage. – Not applicable to multiple pregnancy based on current literature. – Plan for cervical cerclage removal before labour, around 36+1 to 37+0 weeks or during elective CS. 2. *Medical* — progestogens, e.g., vaginal micronised progesterone 400 mg BD or Arabin pessary. – There is no evidence that progesterone or Arabin pessary is more or less effective than cerclage (RCOG). 3. *Conservative* – Screening scan at 20 weeks for fetal anomalies. – OGTT at 24–28 weeks. – Rest of management as per routine antenatal care.

35. Preterm Labour (PTL)

Risk factor	Implications	Action
PTL – Birth <37 completed weeks – Incidence: 10% (singleton) 50–60% (twins) **Risk factors:** – Previous PTL – Short cervix – Uterine anomalies – Assisted reproductive therapy – Multiple pregnancy – Past gynaecological conditions/ surgeries – Abdominal surgery in pregnancy – Current pregnancy complications, e.g., pre-eclampsia and DM – Antepartum haemorrhage — placenta praevia or abruption – Infections, e.g., chorioamnionitis, bacterial vaginosis – STIs – PPROM – Low or high BMI – Smoking, alcohol or substance abuse – Nutritional deficiencies – Extremes of age – Nulliparity – Short inter-pregnancy interval – Domestic violence – Stress – Maternal chronic medical conditions	**Maternal risks:** **Recurrence risk:** – 15–30% after 1 preterm birth – Up to 60% after 2 preterm births (UpToDate) – Malpresentation – CS: Technically difficult caesarean **Fetal risks:** – Prematurity risks – LBW – NICU admission (if NICU bed is unavailable — consider an *in utero* transfer if the woman is stable and delivery is not imminent) – Perinatal morbidity/mortality – HIE – Cerebral palsy – Long-term neurodevelopmental and learning disabilities	**Management:** – Booking BMI. – Record BP, urine protein every antenatal visit. – Folic acid supplementation. – Screen and treat infection — urine culture, VP3, GBS swab. – **Actim® Partus.** – Treat asymptomatic bacteriuria. – Start IV penicillin G (if there are no allergies) while awaiting the GBS swab result. – Consider "rescue" cerclage in a small select group of patients. – *Multidisciplinary team care*: Maternal–fetal specialist, neonatologist. – Consider serial cervical length monitoring via TVUS from 16 to 24 weeks if previous preterm birth <34 weeks. – *Offer tocolysis* (nifedipine) between 26 and 33+6 weeks if membranes are intact and in PTL. *Consider tocolysis* between 24+0 and 25+6 weeks (NICE Guidelines). – CTG monitoring. – Bed rest is not recommended — **ineffective** for PTL and increases VTE risk. – If preterm delivery is anticipated, administer antenatal steroids if delivery is <34 weeks and IV $MGSO_4$ for fetal neuroprotection if delivery is <32 weeks (RCOG <30 weeks) and there is a high risk of delivery within 24 hours. o Stop tocolysis 24 hours after steroid completion/when on IV $MGSO_4$. o Adjust $MgSO_4$ dose in women with renal impairment. – If short cervical length ≤2.5 cm — cervical cerclage or PV micronised progesterone until 34 weeks (reduces preterm birth by 20%). – Avoid vacuum delivery if <34+0 weeks. – Delayed cord clamping if no fetal distress. – If the woman remains stable, perform a growth scan (presentation, EFW, AFI and placental location).

36. Preterm Prelabour Rupture of Membranes (PPROM)

Risk factor	Implications	Action
PPROM – PPROM occurs from 24 to 36+6 weeks gestation and before the onset of labour – Up to 3% of pregnancies _Diagnosis:_ Maternal history _Sterile speculum exam:_ 1. Pool of liquor seen — confirm PPROM 2. If no amniotic fluid seen, use a. **Actim® PROM** (detects insulin-like growth factor-binding protein 1 (IGFBP-1)) **OR** b. **AmniSure®** (detects placental alpha microglobulin-1 (PAMG-1) test of vaginal fluid) _Risk factors for PPROM_ – Previous PPROM – Genital tract infection – Antepartum bleeding – Smoking – Polyhydramnios _Signs/symptoms of chorioamnionitis:_ _N.B.: May have subclinical chorioamnionitis, e.g., rising baseline fetal heart rate — difficulty in diagnosis._ • Abnormal vital signs — tachycardia (maternal/fetal), hypotension, fever • Abdomen: Abdominal pain, uterine tenderness • Foul-smelling vaginal discharge/pus • Uptrending FBC/CRP	**Maternal risks:** • PTL • Placental abruption • Chorioamnionitis • Risk of IOL, Caesarean and instrumental delivery • Postpartum fever, endometritis, sepsis • PPH, DIC • Severe pelvic infections • Subcutaneous wound infection • PTSD **Fetal risks:** • Pulmonary hypoplasia, limb contractures, Potter sequence (<23 weeks) • Cord prolapse • Cord compression → NRFS • Prematurity risks • Meconium-stained liquor • Preterm birth • Stillbirth • Increased neonatal morbidity–neonatal sepsis, extreme prematurity • Vertical transmission if maternal HIV positive • Increased NICU admissions • Cerebral palsy • Neonatal mortality	• _MDT_ — maternal–fetal specialist, neonatologist • Inpatient management until delivery • Avoid VE unless suspecting cord prolapse or if labour progression • Pad charting • Routine vitals monitoring • Monitor clinically for signs and symptoms of chorioamnionitis • Low vaginal swab (LVS) and VP3 to exclude GBS and other LGTI • UFEME, urine culture • FBC/CRP twice weekly/trend as necessary • KIV lactate if the patient is septic • TEDS, VTE prophylaxis • Ultrasound scan for presentation, AFI, placenta and estimated fetal weight, repeat as indicated • Start IV penicillin G until GBS result out or if GBS positive • PO erythromycin × 10 days/until the woman is in established labour (whichever is sooner) • Discuss expectant management till 37 weeks versus IOL at diagnosis ≥34 weeks * Deliver earlier if there is chorioamnionitis, NRFS, cord prolapse, placental abruption. • Neonatologist to standby for delivery • IV $MgSO_4$ for fetal neuroprotection if delivery imminent before 30–32 weeks or planned within 24 hours • Antenatal steroids will cause a rise in total white cell count within 24 hours of steroids → normalise within 3 days • To give antenatal steroids between 24 and 34+6 weeks' gestation • Tocolysis is _not_ recommended

(_Continued_)

(Continued)

• CTG abnormalities, e.g., fetal tachycardia, reduced baseline variability, lack of accelerations/cycling, rising baseline fetal heart rate **Delivery latency** from PPROM remains relatively constant at 8–10 days, from 24 to 28 weeks and then decreases to 5 days at 31 weeks. **Recurrence risk** (7%) — can consider cerclage if cervical length ≤25 mm to reduce risk in a subsequent pregnancy.	**Differential diagnosis:** – Appendicitis – UTI – Pyelonephritis – Pneumonia	**Post-delivery:** • Placenta swab for culture and histology • Neonatal — paired cord blood gases • Emotional support

37. Chorioamnionitis/Intra-Amniotic Infection

Risk factor	Symptoms/signs and implications	Action
Chorioamnionitis/intra-amniotic infection High clinical index of suspicion needed Risk factors: • History of leaking liquor • Prolonged labour • Multiple vaginal examinations • Meconium-stained liquor • History of STI • GBS carrier • Previous chorioamnionitis **Suspected** intraamniotic infection *Clinical criteria:* Maternal intrapartum fever and ≥1 of: Maternal leucocytosis, purulent cervical discharge, fetal tachycardia **Confirmed** intraamniotic infection *Criteria:* • Positive amniotic fluid test result (Gram stain, glucose level or culture results consistent with infection) • Placental histological evidence of infection or inflammation	• Abdominal pain • Foul-smelling vaginal discharge • Fever in labour (one temperature reading of ≥38°C or two consecutive readings 1 hour apart ≥37.5°C) • May have signs of septic shock: Tachycardia, hypotension • Tender uterus • Foul-smelling vaginal discharge/pus on speculum examination • CTG anomalies: Fetal tachycardia/fetal distress • Rising inflammatory markers **Maternal risks:** • Dysfunctional labour • Placenta abruption • Uterine atony with PPH • Wound infection • Endometritis, peritonitis, sepsis, septic thrombophlebitis, pelvic abscess • ARDS • Mortality **Fetal risks:** • Prematurity • Neonatal pneumonia, meningitis, sepsis • Long-term complications, e.g., bronchopulmonary dysplasia and cerebral palsy • Mortality	■ Resuscitation and stabilisation. ■ Start SEPSIS bundle within 1 hour of presentation. ■ Fluid resuscitation — initial rate of 20 ml/kg in pregnancy due to increased risk of pulmonary oedema in pregnancy. ■ Early re-course to vasopressors to achieve MAP >65 mmHg. ***Investigations:*** ■ CTG monitoring. ■ FBC, CRP, UECr, LFT, PT/PTT GXM. ■ Serum lactate. • Re-measure if initial lactate is >2 mmol/L. • Lactate >2 mmol/L should prompt critical care input. If lactate >4 mmol/L despite IV fluid resuscitation + vasopressor use, set a CVP line. • Aim CVP ≥8 mmHg and central venous oxygen saturation ($ScvO_2$) ≥70%. ■ Obtain cultures before giving antibiotics: • Blood cultures. • UFEME, urine culture. • Vaginal swab culture. ■ Placental swab culture and histology at delivery. ■ IV broad spectrum antibiotics based on the institution's protocol. KK Hospital: ■ ***If the patient is stable:*** IV ampicillin 2 g q6H, gentamicin 5–7 mg/kg q24H, metronidazole 500 mg q8H. ■ ***If the patient is in shock:*** IV ceftriaxone 2 g q24H, metronidazole 500 mg q8H. ■ ***If the patient is allergic to penicillin:*** IV clindamycin 900 mg q8H, gentamicin 5–7 mg/kg q24H. ■ If PTL, administer antenatal steroids and IV $MgSO_4$ if indicated. Do not delay delivery if there are maternal/fetal indications for immediate delivery. ■ CS is mainly for obstetric indication unless the woman is in DIC. ■ PPH prophylaxis and management. ■ Neonatal standby at delivery.

38. Thrombocytopenia in Pregnancy

Thrombocytopenia (~10% of all pregnancies)

- Spurious (EDTA-induced platelet aggregation) → send a citrate sample to exclude this.
- Repeat FBC and do a PBF to confirm thrombocytopenia and exclude the presence of red cell fragments (suggestive of microangiopathies).
- Do a serum vitamin B12 and folate levels.
- Perform autoimmune and viral screen as required.
- For diagnosis in the second trimester onwards: Perform a coagulation screen, check renal function, liver function and haemolysis screen to exclude pre-eclampsia/HELLP syndrome/haemolytic-uraemic syndrome (HUS).

Pregnancy-related causes	Non-pregnancy-related causes
Isolated thrombocytopenia • Gestational (75% — most common) — isolated thrombocytopenia *Thrombocytopenia with systemic or multi-organ involvement* • Pre-eclampsia/hypertension (20%)/HELLP syndrome (<1%) • DIC • AFLP (<1%)	*Isolated thrombocytopenia* • Autoimmune — immune thrombocytopenic purpura (ITP): 3–4% • Congenital — rare *Thrombocytopenia with systemic or multi-organ involvement* • Autoimmune — SLE, APS • Drug-induced (frusemide, NSAIDs, penicillins, quinidine, sulphonamides, ranitidine), heparin-induced thrombocytopenia (HIT), especially unfractionated heparin (UFH), *not LMWH* • Viral infections — HIV, EBV, CMV, dengue fever • Von-Willebrand type IIB disease • HUS/TTP • Marrow disease/hypersplenism/liver disease • Folate deficiency

Conditions ***treated*** by delivery of the fetus	Conditions ***not treated*** by delivery of the fetus
Pre-eclampsia	TTP
HELLP	Drug-induced thrombocytopenia
DIC secondary to an obstetric cause	DIC secondary to a non-obstetric cause
AFLP	Immune thrombocytopenia (ITP)

Condition	Implications	Action
Gestational thrombocytopenia (GT) – The most common cause of thrombocytopenia in pregnancy (70–80% cases) – **Diagnosis of exclusion** – Occurs in second half of pregnancy (most commonly detected during delivery) – Usually mild — PLT count: 100–150 × 10^9/L, tend to be >50 × 10^9/L – No personal history of thrombocytopenia – Bleeding time is normal unless the platelet count is <100 × 10^9/L	**Maternal risks:** – Limited labour analgesia options if platelet (PLT) <80 × 10^9/L – No epidural/spinal, to avoid NSAIDs – No association with maternal haemorrhage – Risk of recurrence in a subsequent pregnancy *(Women with previous GT have a 14-fold increased risk of recurrent GT (UpToDate)* **Fetal risks:** No fetal or neonatal thrombocytopenia	No need for specific investigations apart from monitoring platelet count. – Platelet count >100 × 10^9/L: 1–2 monthly monitoring. – Avoid NSAIDS and intramuscular (IM) injections. – Low-dose aspirin can be given unless there is a high risk of bleeding. Generally, a platelet count of >50 × 10^9/L is safe for aspirin use. ➔ Ensure that thrombocytopenia resolves spontaneously within 7 days to 6 weeks postpartum. ➔ If thrombocytopenia persists, consider other differential diagnoses of thrombocytopenia.
Immune thrombocytopenia (ITP) – 1–5 cases/10,000 pregnancies – 100 times less common than GT – The majority of cases occur in isolation – **Diagnosis of exclusion** – Rarely associated with SLE, HIV or drugs – Can occur anytime in pregnancy – Asymptomatic or presents with ecchymosis, petechiae, purpura, gum bleeding – May be present pre-pregnancy but sometimes diagnosed during pregnancy	**Maternal risks:** – Spontaneous bleeding if platelet count <20 × 10^9/L – Risk of internal bleeding if PLT count <10 × 10^9/L – Occasionally require splenectomy in second trimester – Epidural haematoma if PLT <80 × 10^9/L – Steroid side effects (if the woman is on steroids)	*Multidisciplinary team care* — involving the maternal–fetal specialist, neonatologist, haematologist and anaesthetist. *Monitor platelet counts:* monthly until the third trimester, then 2 weekly and weekly from term onwards. May require more frequent monitoring depending on the severity and rate of decline. **Refer to an anaesthetist at 32 weeks for assessment.** ***Platelets levels during pregnancy:*** – Antenatal period: >20–30 × 10^9/L if patient is asymptomatic – Delivery/procedure: >50 × 10^9/L – Epidural/spinal anaesthesia: >80 × 10^9/L ***Indications for treatment:*** – Treat if symptomatic – Platelet count <20 × 10^9/L – Treat if PLT count <50 × 10^9/L in late pregnancy, even if asymptomatic, to increase PLT count before delivery – Before invasive procedures, e.g., chorionic villus sampling

(Continued)

(*Continued*)

	Fetal risks: – Rarely causes fetal thrombocytopenia unless platelet count <50 × 10^9/L → 0.5–1.5% risk of intracranial haemorrhage (ICH) → may require cranial ultrasound (even if asymptomatic)	***Indications for platelet transfusion:*** **1. Therapeutic** — aim platelet >50 × 10^9/L if active bleeding (>100 × 10^9/L if CNS bleeding) **2. Prophylactic** *Epidural* — aim PLT count >80 × 10^9/L *Most major surgeries/procedures* — aim PLT count >50 × 10^9/L. If PLT count <10 × 10^9/L — to prevent spontaneous bleeding **Treatment options:** **1. Steroids** — start PO prednisolone 20–30 mg/day. Can decrease dose for maintenance dose. (Consider stress steroids intrapartum to reduce risk of adrenal suppresion — Refer to Chapter 64 for regime) **2. Intravenous immunoglobulin (IVIG) —** indicated for women resistant/intolerant to prednisolone. **3. Anti-D immunoglobulin** • Given as an IV bolus. • May increase platelet count in non-splenectomised rhesus-positive women. • Monitor for neonatal anaemia and jaundice. • Check the neonate for direct anti-globulin test positivity. **4. Splenectomy** Rarely, may need splenectomy in second trimester. Will need penicillin prophylaxis throughout pregnancy post-splenectomy. **5. *Others*,** e.g., IV methylprednisolone, azathioprine, cyclosporin. **The mode of delivery is based on obstetric indication.** **Aim PLT count >50 × 10^9/L before delivery,** preferably >80 × 10^9/L to allow epidural – Standby platelet if PLT count <50 × 10^9/L – Allow vaginal delivery if PLT count >30 × 10^9/L. – Allow operative vaginal/caesarean delivery if PLT count >50 × 10^9/L. – Safe for anticoagulation if PLT count is >50 × 10^9/L ***Other precautions for thrombocytopenia*:** – Avoid NSAIDs, aspirin. – Avoid IM injections. – Aim for atraumatic delivery → avoid ventose delivery, rotational forceps, scalp electrode, fetal blood sampling. **Neonate** Send cord blood to test for PLT count. Defer IM vitamin K injection until the platelet count is known.

Differential diagnosis of Gestational Thrombocytopenia (GT) versus Immune Thrombocytopenia (ITP)

Characteristic	GT	ITP
Onset during pregnancy	Mid-late second/third trimester. Frequency increases as term approaches.	Anytime in pregnancy
Evidence for alternative aetiology	No	No
Platelet count $\times 10^9$/L	>50* decreases as term approaches	Any <100
Thrombocytopenia before pregnancy	No	Possible
Neonatal thrombocytopenia	No	Possible†
Postpartum resolution	Yes	Possible

*Rare cases have been reported with platelet counts at term about 40–50 × 10^9/L.
†A total of 10% of infants have platelet counts of <50 × 10^9/L.

Clinical and Laboratory Features of Microangiopathies of Pregnancy

Feature	Pre-eclampsia	HELLP	AFLP	aHUS	TTP	C-APS	SLE
Peak time of onset	**Third trimester**	**Third trimester**	**Third trimester**	**Post-partum**	**Anytime, second/third trimester/postpartum**	**Anytime**	**Anytime**
Hypertension	+++	+++	+	++	No	+/−	++
Proteinuria	+++	++	+/−	+++	+/−	+	+++
Nausea/vomiting	+	+	++	+/−	+/−	+/−	+/−
Abdominal pain	+/−	++	++	+/−	+/−	+/−	+/−
Jaundice	+/−	+/−	++	+/−	+/−	+/−	+/−
Neurological symptoms	+	+	+	+/−	++	++	+
Thrombocytopenia	+/−	+++	+	+++	+++	+	+
Haemolysis	+/−	+++	+	+++	+++	+/−	+
Raised bilirubin	+/−	+++	+++	+++	++–	+/−	+/−
Renal impairment	+/−	+	++	+++	+	++	++
DIC	+/−	++	+++	+/−	No	+/−	+/−
Hypoglycaemia	+/−	+/−	+++	+/−	+/−	+/−	+/−
Elevated ammonia	+/−	+/−	+	+/−	+/−	+/−	+/−
Elevated transaminases	+	+++	+++	+/−	+/−	+/−	+
Management	Deliver fetus	Deliver fetus; blood transfusion	Deliver fetus; correct metabolic abnormalities	Supportive treatment	Plasmapheresis	Aspirin; LMWH	Aspirin ± LMWH ± hydroxychloroquine/other immunosuppressants

C-APS, catastrophic antiphospholipid syndrome; aHUS, atypical haemolytic uraemic syndrome.
+/− rare or absent (0–20% of cases), + fairly common (20–50% of cases), ++ common (50–80% of cases), +++ very common or constant feature (80–100% of cases).

39. Previous Caesarean Sections (CS) (≥2)

Risk factor	Implications	Action
Previous CS (≥2) We *do not* conduct VBAC for ≥2 previous CSs in KKH. Risk increases with the number of previous CSs, especially those with ≥4 previous CSs (critical number for most major complications). Review the type of uterine scar and previous complications to assess the risk of uterine rupture and determine the timing of CS.	**Maternal risks:** • Scar ectopic • Placenta accreta spectrum (PAS) • Placenta abruption • Uterine dehiscence/rupture • PPH • Blood transfusion risks • Difficult CS and prolonged operating time due to adhesions and increased risk of visceral injury — bladder, ureter, bowel and difficult delivery of the fetus • Hysterectomy • VTE • Maternal morbidity/mortality **Long-term maternal risks:** • Chronic pelvic pain • Numbness/pain at skin incision • Hernia **Fetal risks:** • Prematurity (spontaneous/iatrogenic) • Birth injuries • Respiratory distress syndrome • NICU admission • Fetal death • Perinatal morbidity/mortality	**Management:** – Early booking scan to *exclude scar ectopic pregnancy* and accurate pregnancy dating. – *MDT care* — involve experienced obstetricians, anaesthetist, and surgical assistants. – Optimise haemoglobin level. – Folate supplementation. – Aneuploidy screening. – Screening scan at 20 weeks to exclude fetal anomalies (FA) and placenta praevia. • If anterior lower placenta, to suspect PAS. – Repeat US scan at 32–34 weeks to monitor placenta and fetal growth. – Consider an MRI scan if PAS is suspected. – If preterm delivery is anticipated, administer antenatal steroids if delivery is <34 weeks and IV $MGSO_4$ for fetal neuroprotection if delivery is 30 to 32 weeks. – Plan for elective CS at term by an experienced obstetrician, anaesthetist and assistants. To offer sterilisation. – If PAS, may need uterine artery embolisation (UAE) or hysterectomy. – For PAS, standby blood and blood products. – Consider cell salvage. – VTE — pharmacological thromboprophylaxis once bleeding risk is low. ***Contraception:*** – Postpartum sterilisation or male vasectomy if the patient has completed family. – LARC.

40. Advanced Maternal Age (≥35 Years Old) at Expected Date of Delivery (EDD)

Risk factor	Implications	Action
Advanced maternal age (AMA) ≥35 years at EDD **VAMA —** very advanced maternal age ≥45 years at EDD	**Maternal risks:** • Miscarriage • Ectopic pregnancy • Multiple pregnancy • Molar pregnancy • Assisted reproductive technology (ART) pregnancy • Pre-eclampsia/hypertension • GDM/DM • Placenta praevia/abruption • PTL • Instrumental delivery/CS • Postnatal depression • Breastfeeding issues • VTE risk • Other chronic medical conditions, e.g., cardiac disease/IHD • Maternal mortality **Fetal risks:** • Chromosomal anomalies • Fetal anomalies, especially cardiac defects • Prematurity • IUGR/LBW • Stillbirth • Perinatal morbidity/mortality • Autism spectrum disorder	**Management:** – Accurate dating scan. – Folic acid in the first trimester. – Booking BMI, urine for protein and glucose and at every visit. – Start LDA 150 mg ON from 11–14 weeks till 36 weeks of gestation to prevent pre-eclampsia (KKH 2022 protocol). If another moderate risk factor for pre-eclampsia is present. – Aneuploidy screening — refer to Chapter 25: *Prenatal Screening for Chromosomal Defects and Invasive Diagnostic Tests.* – First-trimester screen (done between 11 and 13+6 weeks). – NIPT (done after 10 weeks gestation). – Screening scan at 20 weeks for fetal anomalies. – OGTT at 24–28 weeks. – Serial growth scans. – If preterm delivery is anticipated, administer antenatal steroids if delivery <34/52 and IV $MgSO_4$ for fetal neuroprotection if delivery occurs <30–32 weeks. – If uncomplicated pregnancy, aim for delivery at 39–40 weeks due to an increased risk of stillbirth. – Postnatal support. – Screen for postnatal depression. – VTE prophylaxis if indicated. **Contraception:** – Age alone is *not* a contraindication for any form of contraception. – **Caution** with combined oral contraceptives and IM Depo-Provera >40 years — recommend to stop by 50 years old. – For smokers, recommend stopping COC pills after 35 years old.

41. Teenage/Adolescent Pregnancy

Risk factor	Implications	Action
Teenage/adolescent pregnancy Refers to women <20 years who are pregnant (WHO). Pregnancy may be unplanned. Patients often have *inadequate* antenatal care — there is a risk of booking late or defaulting their appointments. In Singapore, sex under 16 years of age is considered statutory rape. Therefore, make a police report if the patient is <16 years old at the time of sexual intercourse.	**Maternal risks:** – Anaemia – Pre-eclampsia, eclampsia – STI – PTL – PPROM – Chorioamnionitis – Obstructed labour – Instrumental delivery – CS – PPH – Domestic violence – Financial and social issues – Depression/anxiety – Postnatal endometritis – Systemic infections – Mortality **Fetal risks:** – Fetal anomalies (FA) — CNS, gastroschisis – Prematurity – LBW – NICU admissions – Perinatal mortality	**Management:** – Record booking BMI – Record BP, urine protein every visit – *Multidisciplinary team care* — medical social worker, mental wellness, ± psychiatrist – STI screening – Iron, folic acid supplementation – Postnatal support groups – Effective contraception, e.g., COCP/LARC/IUCD

42. Grand Multiparity (Parity ≥5)

Risk factor	Implications	Action
Grand multiparity – Parity ≥5 – Increased parity is usually associated with reduced inter-pregnancy intervals and older maternal age at delivery. – If deliveries were via CS → refer to the section *Previous CS* (≥2) in this chapter	**Maternal risks:** – Anaemia – Placenta praevia/abruption – DM, hypertension – Cord prolapse – Meconium-stained liquor – Malpresentation – Uterine rupture – IUD – PPH – Maternal mortality – *Long-term risks:* Pelvic organ prolapse, diastasis recti **Fetal risks:** – Macrosomia – Prematurity – Low Apgar scores – Perinatal mortality	**Management:** – Booking BMI + maternal age – Folic acid and iron supplementation – Record BP, urine protein/glucose at every antenatal visit – Aneuploidy screening – Screening scan at 20 weeks – DM screening at 24–28 weeks – Serial growth scans – Close intrapartum monitoring – Judicious oxytocin use – CTG monitoring – Monitor for labour/shoulder dystocia – PPH prophylaxis – Effective contraception counselling is important. – Discuss options, e.g., LARC, postpartum sterilisation (patient), vasectomy (partner)

43. Obesity in Pregnancy (BMI ≥30)

Risk factor	Implications	Action
Maternal obesity Recommended weight gain for singleton pregnancy: 5–9 kg (IOM guidelines) ***Risk factors for high BMI*** – Dietary indiscretion – Low physical activity – Genetics – Childhood obesity – Psychological/psychiatric disorders – Medications, e.g., anti-psychotics, anti-depressants, steroids, anti-epileptic medications	**<u>Maternal risks:</u>** **1. Antenatal** – Miscarriage – Multiple pregnancy – Gestational HTN/pre-eclampsia – GDM – PTL – Vitamin D deficiency – Inaccurate scans due to maternal habitus – Inaccurate clinical assessment of presentation/fetal growth – Post-term **2. Intrapartum** – Difficult venous access – Difficult CTG monitoring – Labour/shoulder dystocia – Instrumental delivery – Higher chance of CS and difficult CSs – Anaesthetic complications **3. Postpartum** – PPH – Wound dehiscence/infection – Infectious morbidity – VTE – Postnatal depression – Mortality **4. Long-term risks** – Cardiovascular disease – Obstructive sleep apnoea – DM – Metabolic syndrome **<u>Fetal risks</u>** – Fetal anomalies (FAs), e.g., NTD, cardiac defects – Macrosomia – Birth injuries – IUD/neonatal death – **Long-term**: Obesity, cardio-metabolic morbidity, asthma, DM	**Management:** • Document booking BMI • Check BP + urine protein/glucose during every antenatal visit • *Multidisciplinary team care* • Refer to a dietician • Moderate amount of exercise • Avoid dieting during pregnancy • Folic acid and vitamin D supplementation • Consider low-dose aspirin (LDA) for pre-eclampsia prophylaxis if another moderate risk factor for pre-eclampsia is present • Fetal aneuploidy screening is affected by high BMI, e.g., inaccurate NIPT due to lower fetal fraction detected. • Screening scan at 20 weeks • Experienced sonographer required for ultrasound scans • DM screening (OGTT) at 24–28 weeks • Anaesthetic review at 32 weeks • Regular fetal growth scans • Consider using a fetal scalp electrode if poor recording is seen on external CTG • Special equipment/operative bed to accommodate maternal weight at delivery • Anticipate shoulder dystocia if vaginal delivery • Experienced surgeon/assistants for CS • *<u>VTE prophylaxis:</u>* TEDS, calf compressors, LMWH (weight-adjusted), early ambulation • SpO_2 monitoring, especially after anaesthesia • Encourage breastfeeding (helps with weight loss) • *Contraception* — consider LARC • Postnatal depression screening Postnatally — lifestyle modifications (diet, exercise), consider bariatric surgery if BMI >40 or BMI >35 with co-morbidities

44. Low Body Mass Index (BMI) in Pregnancy (BMI <18.5)

Risk factor	Implications	Action
Low BMI in pregnancy Recommended weight gain for singleton pregnancy = 12.5–18 kg (IOM guidelines) ***Risk factors for low BMI*** – High physical activity – Chronic illness – Genetics – Psychological/psychiatric disorders, e.g., eating disorders – Malabsorptive disorders – Malnutrition – Medications – Stress	**Maternal risks:** • Miscarriage • Anaemia • Vitamin deficiencies • Osteoporosis *These women may have menstrual disturbances, subfertility before pregnancy.* **Fetal risks:** • Prematurity • IUGR • LBW • Stillbirth • Death	**Management:** • Folic acid supplementation in first trimester • Refer to a dietician • Screening for eating disorders • Screen for alcohol use • Consider organic causes, e.g., hyperthyroidism, coeliac disease/malabsorption disorders • Adjust medications according to weight, e.g., paracetamol, LMWH — enoxaparin or clexane • Serial growth scans

45. Alcohol Consumption in Pregnancy

Risk factor	Implications	Action
Alcohol use in pregnancy *"There is no known safe amount of alcohol use during pregnancy or when trying to conceive."* ***Risk factors for alcohol use:*** – Psychiatric disorders – Substance abuse – Social issues, e.g., stress, financial problems, relationship issues, peer pressure – Family history	**Maternal risks:** – Miscarriage – PTL – Stillbirth – Nutritional deficiencies – <u>Long-term health issues:</u> Cirrhosis, pancreatitis, liver/breast cancer, osteoporosis – Psychiatric disorders – Death **Fetal risks:** – Prematurity – IUGR – LBW – Fetal alcohol syndrome (FAS) – Childhood learning/behavioural/physical/mental problems	– Screen all pregnant women for concurrent smoking and substance abuse – Consider STI screen – Folic acid supplementation – Dating scan – *<u>Multidisciplinary team care</u>* — social worker, mental wellness/psychiatrist, maternal–fetal specialist, neonatologist – Abstain from alcohol – Refer to an alcohol cessation programme – Join support groups – Screening scan at 20 weeks – Serial growth scans – Refer to neonatology for the possibility of neonatal withdrawal/screening for FAS – Avoid breastfeeding if ongoing alcohol use postnatally

46. Cigarette Smoking in Pregnancy

Risk factor	Implications	Action
Cigarette smoking in pregnancy *N.B.: Smoking is the only environmental exposure known to* <u>*reduce*</u> *the risk of pre-eclampsia consistently.* – Quitting smoking at any stage of pregnancy is associated with improved pregnancy outcomes. If women quit before 15 weeks, they are at *no greater* risk of adverse pregnancy outcomes than non-smokers. – ~50% re-start smoking 2 months postnatally.	**Maternal risks:** – Miscarriage – Ectopic pregnancy – PTL – PPROM – IUGR – Placental abruption/praevia – Stillbirth – <u>*Chronic issues:*</u> Lung disease, e.g., bronchitis, asthma, lung cancer, hypertension, DM, cardiovascular disease **Fetal risks:** – Fetal anomalies (FA): Cleft lip/palate, cardiac defects – Prematurity – LBW – Sudden infant death syndrome (SIDS) – Withdrawal symptoms in the baby – <u>*Chronic issues:*</u> Atopy, ear/chest infections, asthma, behavioural problems, e.g., ADHD, poor school performance, childhood obesity	– Screen all pregnant women for concurrent alcohol and substance abuse. – Folic acid supplementation. – <u>*Multidisciplinary team care:*</u> Social worker, mental wellness/psychiatrist, maternal–fetal specialist and neonatologist. – Abstain from smoking + avoid second-hand smoke. – Refer to a smoking cessation programme. – Join support groups. – Nicotine replacement therapy is safe in pregnancy. – In women ≥35 years old who smoke, avoid oestrogen-containing contraception (FSRH guidelines). – Counsel on the long-term implications of cigarette smoking on general health.

47. Venous Thromboembolism (VTE) Prophylaxis in Pregnancy

Condition	Risk factor	Management
VTE thromboprophylaxis in pregnancy – It consists of DVT and pulmonary embolism (PE). – The risk of thrombosis is 5–10 times higher in pregnancy due to the: ▪ Increase in clotting factors. ▪ Compression of the gravid uterus on pelvic veins. ▪ Pelvic vascular endothelial injury at delivery. – Pulmonary embolism is the leading cause of direct maternal deaths worldwide. – In a Hong Kong study, the VTE incidence was 1.88/1,000 deliveries. In total, 75% of cases occurred postpartum and following caesarean section. There is a higher prevalence of congenital thrombophilia, such as anti-thrombin III, protein C and S deficiencies in Asian women, whereas in the West, factor V Leiden and prothrombin gene mutations are more prevalent.	**VTE assessment:** – All women should undergo a documented assessment of risk factors for VTE in early pregnancy. – Risk assessment for VTE should be repeated for any antenatal admission to the hospital, inter-current problems and in the immediate postpartum period. – Thromboprophylaxis should be individualised according to the patient's risk factors (risk stratification). – Although there is no clear evidence from high-quality studies, consensus-derived clinical practice guidelines can be based on indirect evidence to guide clinical management. Refer to Table 11.1: *Risk Factors for VTE (Adapted From SCOG Consensus Statement 2021)*	Multidisciplinary team care involving the maternal–fetal medicine specialist, haematologist, anaesthetist and pharmacist. Women at high risk of VTE in pregnancy, such as previous VTE, should be offered pre-pregnancy counselling and a prospective management plan for thromboprophylaxis in pregnancy. <u>Investigations:</u> – Diagnostic tests for thrombophilia should not be performed during pregnancy. – Protein S levels may be falsely low due to complement binding. – A previous history of isolated low protein C/S or antithrombin level is not diagnostic of thrombophilia; should be repeated when the patient is not pregnant. <u>Mechanical VTE thromboprophylaxis during the antenatal period:</u> – Mechanical thromboprophylaxis includes the use of graduated compression stockings (GCS) — with a pressure of 14–15 mmHg at the calf and intermittent pneumatic compression (IPC) devices that work by reducing venous stasis. – IPC and/or GCS should be considered if hospitalised, especially if >3 days. – Patients at high risk of VTE but have contraindications to pharmacological thromboprophylaxis should be considered for mechanical thromboprophylaxis. However, data supporting this in the antenatal population are limited. <u>Pharmacological VTE thromboprophylaxis:</u> 1. <u>LMWH</u> – Drug of choice. – Based on maternal weight (either weight at booking or the most recent weight). – Monitoring PLT counts after initiating LMWH is only necessary if the woman has had prior exposure to UFH. – Monitoring of anti-Xa levels is not required. – Women with a history of VTE associated with high-risk thrombophilia (e.g., protein S or C deficiency, anti-thrombin deficiency) or APS should be considered for higher doses of LMWH (50–100% of therapeutic dose) antenatally and for 6 weeks postpartum or until return to oral anticoagulation therapy.

(Continued)

(Continued)

– DVT can lead to post-thrombotic syndrome and chronic venous ulcers.
– Therefore, thromboprophylaxis for VTE in pregnancy should be prioritised as VTE is largely preventable with appropriate measures.

– These women should be co-managed with a haematologist.
– Suggested doses for antenatal and postnatal LMWH thromboprophylaxis for all other women are shown in the chart below:

Weight (kg)	Enoxaparin (clexane)	Dalteparin	Nadroparin (fraxiparine)
<50	20 mg daily	2,500 units daily	
50–90	40 mg daily	5,000 units daily	0.3 ml daily (2,850 units)
91–130	60 mg daily	7,500 units daily	
131–170	80 mg daily (or 40 mg BD)	10,000 units daily	
>170	0.6 mg/kg/day	75 units/kg/day	

These doses are recommended doses for women with normal renal function. Patients with renal impairment may require dose adjustment of the LMWH.

<u>Contraindications or to use with caution in:</u>

✓ Known bleeding disorder
✓ Active bleeding
✓ Thrombocytopenia <75 × 10^9/L
✓ Acute stroke within the past 4 weeks
✓ Severe liver or renal disease
✓ Uncontrolled hypertension >200/120

2. <u>Unfractionated testing (UFH)</u>

– Has a shorter half-life than LMWH.
– The interval between the prophylactic dose of UFH and regional anaesthesia is 4 hours.
– Higher risk of HIT and 2% risk of heparin-associated osteoporosis.
– If used after a CS, need to monitor PLT count every 2–3 days from day 4 to 14 post-surgery or till UFH is stopped.

3. <u>Warfarin</u>

– Use only if heparin is unsuitable.
– Can be converted from LMWH to warfarin postpartum, usually 5–7 days post-delivery for women who need long-term anticoagulation.

Condition	Risk factor	Management
		4. Others, e.g., danaparoid or fondaparinux Their use is only after consultation with a haematologist and is usually reserved for women intolerant of heparin compounds. **Intrapartum management:** – Women receiving antenatal LMWH should be advised to stop LMWH if they have any vaginal bleeding or signs and symptoms of labour. – Regional analgesia should be avoided until at least 12 hours after the last dose of prophylactic LMWH or 24 hours after therapeutic LMWH. – LMWH should not be given until 4 hours after spinal anaesthesia or after removing the epidural catheter. – The epidural catheter should not be removed within 12 hours of the prophylactic dose of LMWH. – If there are no contraindications to anticoagulation, the first thromboprophylaxis dose of LMWH should be given 4–6 hours after delivery, considering the risk of PPH – Intermitting pneumatic compression or GCS may be offered as alternatives if the postpartum bleeding risk is high and the woman is deemed unsuitable for early LMWH after delivery. **For caesarean deliveries:** – Patients at high risk of VTE and undergoing CS should be prescribed a combination of LMWH and GCS and/or IPC. – If there are contraindications to LMWH, GCS and/or IPC should be prescribed. This is based on evidence extrapolated from studies on the non-pregnant population. – The use of knee-length GCS is recommended over thigh-length GCS as the former is associated with a higher adherence rate and a lower risk of adverse effects such as skin breaks.

(*Continued*)

		Postpartum management – Start anticoagulation if the bleeding risk is low. Balance risks of thrombosis with the risk of bleeding and consult the haematologist. – All women requiring antenatal LMWH will require at least 6 weeks of prophylactic postnatal LMWH. – If the total score is >2 postnatally, consider thromboprophylaxis with LMWH for at least 7 days. If these risk factors persist beyond 7 days, consider extended thromboprophylaxis. – If the total score is >3, consider extended thromboprophylaxis with LMWH for up to 6 weeks. – If the patient is re-admitted within the puerperium period, consider LMWH thromboprophylaxis. – If pharmacological thromboprophylaxis is not suitable, consider mechanical thromboprophylaxis as an alternative. – LMWH and warfarin are safe for breastfeeding.

Table 11.1 Risk Factors for VTE (Adapted From SCOG Consensus Statement 2021)

	Tick	Score
VTE history		
Previous unprovoked VTE and oestrogen-related VTE		4
Previous non-oestrogen-provoked VTE		3
Family history of unprovoked or oestrogen-related VTE in a first-degree relative		1
Inherited thrombophilia		
Known high-risk thrombophilia: Antithrombin deficiency		4
Known high-risk thrombophilia: Protein S deficiency Protein C deficiency Homozygous factor V Leiden mutation Homozygous prothrombin gene mutation Compound heterozygote (factor V Leiden/prothrombin gene mutation)		3
Known low-risk thrombophilia (no VTE): Heterozygous prothrombin gene mutation Heterozygous factor V Leiden mutation Persistent antiphospholipid antibodies (ACL antibodies, LAC, $\beta 2$ glycoprotein 1 antibodies) without any clinical features of APS		1[a]
Existing risk factors		
Medical co-morbidities, e.g., cancer, HF, active systemic lupus erythematous, inflammatory polyarthropathy or active IBD Type 1 DM with nephropathy Sickle cell disease Current intravenous drug user		3
Obesity		
BMI 30–39.9		1
BMI >40		2
Parity >3		1
Smoker		1
Age >35 years (postnatal assessment only)		1
Obstetric risk factors		
Pre-eclampsia in current pregnancy		1
ART/IVF (antenatal assessment only)		1
Multiple pregnancy		1
Elective CS		1
Emergency CS		2

Table 11.1 (*Continued*)

	Tick	Score
Prolonged labour (>24 hours)		1
PPH (>1 L or transfusion required)		1
Preterm birth <37+0 weeks in current pregnancy		1
Stillbirth in current pregnancy		1
Transient risk factors		
Any major surgical procedure in pregnancy or puerperium (excluding CS)		3
Hyperemesis gravidarum (defined by PUQE score)		3
OHSS (first trimester only)		4
Current systemic infection		1
Immobility		1
Dehydration		1

[a] *If the known low-risk thrombophilia is in a woman with a family history of VTE in a first-degree relative, postpartum thromboprophylaxis should be continued for 6 weeks.*

Venous Thromboembolism (VTE) in Pregnancy

Condition	Symptoms and signs	Management
VTE in pregnancy: – Most women have symptoms. – 15–25% will develop pulmonary embolism (PE) if DVT is not treated. – PE in pregnancy can result in mortality in 15% of these women. – Left-sided DVT: right-sided DVT: 9:1 due to the venous stasis being more significant on the left.	**Symptoms:** – Leg swelling/pain – Lower abdominal pain – Buttock/back pain (seen in iliac vein thrombosis) – Chest pain – SOB – Haemoptysis – Pleuritic chest pain – Fever **Signs:** – Haemodynamic instability – Maternal collapse – Pyrexia – Tachycardia – Tachypnoea – Raised jugular venous pressure – Loud S2 – Right ventricular heave – Calf tenderness – Lower limb swelling – *ECG changes*: sinus tachycardia, S1Q3T3	*Multidisciplinary team care* involving the maternal–fetal medicine specialist, haematologist, anaesthetist and pharmacist. ***Investigations*** *If DVT is suspected:* **1. Compression duplex ultrasound (CUS)** of the lower limbs for DVT. ± **Iliac vein duplex Doppler ultrasound if** iliac vein DVT is suspected. – Consider starting anticoagulation first if there is high clinical suspicion and the bleeding risk is low. Stop if CUS is negative. – If initial CUS is negative, but there is high clinical suspicion, perform serial CUS on days 3 and 7. *If pulmonary embolism (PE) is suspected:* **1. CXR with abdominal shield.** **2. Perform CUS if there is suspected DVT with PE.** – If CUS is positive, there is no need to investigate for PE. If CUS is negative, proceed with the other investigations for PE. **3. CT pulmonary angiogram (CTPA) for PE.** – *Modality of choice*: Lower fetal radiation dose than a V/Q scan, can exclude other causes of the symptoms. – Fetal radiation exposure is 0.5 mGy. Fetal radiation exposure <1 mGy is similar to the dose received annually from natural background radiation and is considered to pose a negligible risk. **4. Ventilation/perfusion — V/Q scan for PE.** – There is a slightly increased risk of childhood cancer, but it is associated with a lower risk of maternal breast cancer than CTPA. – Fetal radiation exposure is 0.1 mGy. – Consider V/Q as first line for young women, especially if there is a family history of breast cancer or if the patient has had a previous CT chest. – May be used in women with a normal CTPA but persistently high clinical suspicion of PE. **5. Baseline — FBC, UECr, LFT, PT/PTT, T&S.** **Do not** perform D-dimer in pregnancy. Thrombophilia screen before starting treatment is *not* recommended.

(*Continued*)

(Continued)

Treatment of VTE

Mechanical methods for DVT:

Encourage early ambulation.

✓ Reduces acute DVT — associated pain.

✓ Does not result in worsening of the DVT nor increase the risk of pulmonary embolism.

- GCS/compression therapy can be used to reduce the pain and oedema associated with DVT.
- However, its role in reducing the risk of the post-thrombotic syndrome is unclear.

Pharmacological treatment:

Anticoagulation should continue throughout pregnancy until 6 weeks postpartum and for a minimum of 3 months.

6. LMWH.

– Preferred due to greater ease of administration, lower risk of HIT and osteoporosis.

– LMWH doses are shown in the chart below:

Weight (kg)	Enoxaparin (clexane)	Dalteparin	Tinzaparin
<50	40 mg BD	5,000 units BD	175 unit/kg once daily
50–69	60 mg BD	6,000 units BD	
70–89	80 mg BD	8,000 units BD	
90–109	100 mg BD	10,000 units BD	
110–125	120 mg BD	12,000 units BD	
>125	Discuss with haematologist		

These doses are recommended doses for women with normal renal function. Patients with renal impairment may require dose adjustment of the LMWH.

Monitor anti-Xa levels in the following patients:

- Weight <50 kg or >90 kg.
- Recurrent VTE despite therapeutic anticoagulation.
- Renal impairment (eGFR <30 ml/min).
- Non-compliance to LMWH.

Monitor PLT count if:

Previous LMWH or UFH exposure in the last 100 days: Check PLT count 24 hours after LMWH initiation.

Condition	Symptoms and signs	Management
		7. Warfarin — avoid unless exceptional circumstances in consultation with a haematologist. **8. Direct oral anticoagulants (DOACs)** — not recommended. ***Use of IVC filter:*** Consider in women with recent proximal DVT where anticoagulation is absolutely contraindicated due to high bleeding risk OR recurrent VTE despite being on anticoagulation. Remove the IVC filter as soon as it is safe to be on anticoagulation. **For life-threatening or massive VTE with haemodynamic instability:** – *Multidisciplinary team care*, including the vascular surgeon and intensivist. – Systemic thrombolytic therapy may be required. – Intravenous UFH is the preferred anticoagulant. **Intrapartum management:** – Mode of delivery is based on obstetric indication. Consider a planned date for delivery for ease of managing anticoagulation in the peripartum period. – Women receiving antenatal LMWH should be advised to stop LMWH if they have any vaginal bleeding or signs and symptoms of labour. – Regional analgesia should be avoided until at least 24 hours after therapeutic LMWH. – Some women may need UFH during labour if the risk of thrombosis is very high. – LMWH should not be given until 4 hours after spinal anaesthesia or after removing the epidural catheter. – The epidural catheter should not be removed within 12–24 hours of the therapeutic dose of LMWH. – If there are no contraindications to anticoagulation and the risk of bleeding is low, the first prophylactic dose of LMWH should be given 4–6 hours after delivery, followed by a therapeutic dose within 24 hours post-delivery. **Postpartum management:** – LMWH and warfarin are safe for breastfeeding. – Offer option of either LMWH or warfarin. If the woman is not breastfeeding, they can be offered DOACs as an alternative. – If the woman chooses warfarin, continue bridging clexane until INR is between 2 and 3 and warfarin should only be started 5–7 days post-delivery.

48. Intrauterine Death (IUD) and Stillbirth

Definitions:

Definitions vary across the world.

(a) *RCOG guideline*:
- IUD is defined as *in utero* death that occurred ≥24 weeks of pregnancy.
- Stillbirth is defined as a newborn delivered with no signs of life ≥24 weeks of pregnancy.

(b) The WHO defines stillbirth as a newborn delivered with no signs of life ≥28 weeks of pregnancy or a birth weight of ≥1,000 g.

The WHO's international classification of diseases (ICD) *10th Revision 2008* defines stillbirth as a fetus delivered with no signs of life with a birth weight of ≥500 g or ≥22 weeks of pregnancy or crown-to-heel length of ≥25 cm.

(c) The *United States National Centre for Health Statistics* defines stillbirth as the death or loss of a fetus at ≥20 weeks of gestation and before or during birth.

(d) In Singapore, the Ministry of Health (MOH) defines stillbirth as the demise of the fetus that has reached the gestational age of fetal viability, which is 24 weeks of pregnancy, based on local data and MOH's review.

Condition	Signs and symptoms	Management
Intrauterine death (IUD) ■ Occurs in ~1 in 160–200 babies ***Risk factors:*** ■ Nulliparity ■ Non-Hispanic black women ■ Advanced maternal age ■ Obesity ■ Maternal medical conditions: Pre-existing diabetes, chronic hypertension, thrombophilias ■ Smoking/alcohol/recreational drug use ■ Assisted reproductive technology (ART) pregnancies ■ Multiple pregnancy ■ Previous history of IUD/stillbirth ***Aetiologies:*** ■ Unexplained (~50%) ■ Fetal growth restriction ■ Maternal conditions, e.g., pre-eclampsia, placental abruption ■ Fetal abnormalities ■ Genetic abnormalities ■ Intrauterine infections/chorioamnionitis ■ Hydrops fetalis ■ Fetomaternal haemorrhage (FMH)	■ Decreased/absent fetal movements. *There is a possibility of passive fetal movements after IUD.* ■ Abdominal pain/vaginal bleeding/discharge. ***Diagnosis:*** ■ Ultrasound scan of the fetus: Absent fetal heart activity. <u>*Other findings:*</u> ■ Spalding sign — overlapping skull bones. ■ Fetal skull oedema. ■ Fetal hydrops. ■ Maceration resulting in unrecognisable fetal mass. ■ Intrafetal gas (within the heart, vessels and joints). ***Examination:*** ■ Assess maternal status — ensure that she is haemodynamically stable. Check vitals: Temperature, BP, heart rate, oxygen saturation. ■ Abdominal examination: Tense and woody hard uterus. ■ Speculum/vaginal examination. ***Investigations:*** No cause is found in 50% of IUD.	■ If the woman is alone, offer to call her partner/family. Break bad news. ■ Investigate the cause of IUD. ■ Assess for complications, e.g., coagulopathy. ■ Intravenous (IV) access. ■ Start IV broad-spectrum antibiotics if sepsis is suspected. ■ Anti-D immunoglobulin as soon as possible for rhesus-negative women. – Perform an urgent Kleihauer test. The anti-D dose may have to be adjusted based on the result. ■ ***Timing of delivery:*** >85% of women with IUD will go into labour spontaneously within 3 weeks. – Advise for immediate delivery if there are maternal indications, e.g., chorioamnionitis, sepsis, severe pre-eclampsia, active bleeding or ruptured membranes. – If the woman is well with intact membranes with no indication for immediate delivery, advise her that they are unlikely to have complications if they delay for a short period. However, with prolonged delay, they may develop complications and anxiety. – If the woman delays labour for >48 hours, do a coagulation screen to rule out DIC twice weekly. ■ ***Mode of delivery*** – Vaginal delivery is recommended in the absence of contraindications. Contraindications to vaginal delivery include placenta praevia or previous classical CS. – IOL protocol varies according to the institution. – Discuss the pros and cons of IOL for women with previous CS. ***KKH's IUD protocol 2021*** 1. **For women with an unscarred uterus:** ➢ **24 to 26+6 weeks of gestation:** vaginal (PV) misoprostol 100 mcg 4 hourly × 5 doses. If undelivered, rest for 8 hours, then consider an increased dose of 200 mcg 4 hourly × 5 doses.

(Continued)

(*Continued*)

Aetiologies: ▪ Placental abnormalities, e.g., velamentous cord insertion ▪ Umbilical cord anomalies or accidents	***Maternal investigations:*** *Blood tests* ▪ To rule out pre-eclampsia: Full blood count, renal panel, LFT. ▪ Coagulation screen: PT/APTT, fibrinogen. ▪ Antibody screen. Group and cross match. ▪ CRP. ▪ Septic workup if sepsis is suspected: Urine FEME, urine culture, blood culture, serum lactate. ▪ Kleihauer–Betke test. ▪ HbA1c and random serum glucose level: To rule out DM. ▪ TFT. ▪ Serum BA if obstetric cholestasis is suspected. ▪ Serology for infections: Syphilis, parvovirus, CMV, toxoplasmosis, rubella ± herpes simplex virus. ± Thrombophilia screen (if there is evidence of IUGR or placental disease). ± Anti-Ro/La antibodies (if there is fetal hydrops, endomyocardial fibro-elastosis or AV node calcification at postmortem examination of the fetus). ± Alloimmune anti-platelet antibody (if there is fetal ICH). ± Parental karyotype(s).	➢ **27–35+6 weeks of gestation:** PV misoprostol 50 mcg 4 hourly × 5 doses. If undelivered, rest for 8 hours and consider an increased dose of 100 mcg 4 hourly × 5 doses. ➢ **≥36 weeks of gestation:** As per the usual obstetric IOL protocol by using prostaglandin E2 (prostin) followed by artificial rupture of membranes (ARM) and oxytocin. ➢ If still undelivered, consult a maternal–fetal medicine specialist. 2. **For women with a <u>scarred uterus</u>.** ▪ **<u>For women ≤2 lower segment CS (LSCS)</u>:** ➢ **24–35+6 weeks of gestation:** Discuss the pros and cons of IOL. For women with one LSCS, IOL with prostaglandins is generally safe but not without risks. For women with two LSCS, the risk of uterine rupture from IOL with prostaglandins is slightly higher than in women with one LSCS. However, medical management is still preferred to avoid the increased risks and morbidity associated with repeat CS for future pregnancies. PV misoprostol 50 mcg 4 hourly × 5 doses. If still undelivered, consult a maternal–fetal medicine specialist. ➢ **≥36 weeks of gestation:** Discuss the pros and cons of IOL. Consider IOL with ARM and a short trial of oxytocin. ▪ **<u>For women >2 LSCS:</u>** The safety of IOL is unknown. Consider CS due to the <u>risk of uterine rupture</u> and maternal morbidity. ▪ Allow the woman/couple to have contact with the baby if they are keen. ▪ Offer them to keep artefacts of remembrance. ***Post-delivery*** ▪ Provide adequate privacy. Manage in a Gynaecological ward instead of an obstetrics ward. – Some women may choose to donate their breast milk. ▪ Allow the patient/family to take photos ▪ Check with the patient if she is claiming the fetus ▪ Refer to a medical social worker for grief counselling ± mental wellness/psychiatrist. ▪ VTE prophylaxis.

Condition	Signs and symptoms	Management
	Others: ■ Vaginal swab for infections. ■ Placental histology. ■ Placental swab if an infection is suspected. ***Fetal investigations:*** ■ Inform the neonatologist to conduct a general examination of the fetus: Any dysmorphic features, measure the weight, length and head circumference. ■ Fetal tissues for karyotype and chromosome microarray (CMA): Deep fetal skin/fetal cartilage. ■ Postmortem examination of the fetus — if the family is uncomfortable with a full autopsy, they can consider a partial autopsy or gross examination with imaging, e.g., X-rays.	■ Suppress lactation with dopamine agonists. (if patient is agreeable) ➢ ***First line:*** PO cabergoline: 1 mg STAT (if lactation is not established) or 0.25 mg BD for 2 days (if lactation has been established). It is contraindicated in pre-eclampsia, postpartum hypertension or a family history of VTE. ➢ ***Second line:*** PO bromocriptine 2.5 mg BD for 14 days. There is a possibility of rebound galactorrhoea. ■ Discuss fertility and contraception. ***At the postnatal follow-up appointment*** ■ Assess the woman's physical and mental well-being. Debrief the couple. ■ Review results of investigations. ■ Explain recurrence risk and any interventions to reduce the risk of subsequent fetal loss. *There is an increased risk of recurrence of IUD following a previous IUD. Recurrence risks have been reported to range from 2- to 10-fold, depending on the cause. For unexplained IUD, there is no consensus regarding recurrence risk.* ■ Healthy lifestyle and dietary advice. ■ The couple can conceive when they are physically and mentally ready. ■ Counselling for future pregnancies. An interpregnancy interval of less than 6 months is not associated with an adverse pregnancy outcome in the next pregnancy. A woman may delay future pregnancy until she feels she has reached closure and psychological stability after the stillbirth. The typical interval is 6 to 12 months. ***For subsequent pregnancy*** ■ Regular antenatal follow-up. ■ Screen for GDM. ■ If there is a history of a small-for-gestational-age fetus, do serial growth scans. ■ Discuss IOL: take into account the gestational age of the IUD, previous intrapartum history and safety of IOL. ■ Monitor for postpartum depression.

CHAPTER 12

Multiple Pregnancy

Multiple pregnancy is the presence of more than one fetus in the abdomen of a pregnant woman. According to their number, they could be categorised into twins (most common), triplet, quadruplet, etc.

Incidence of Multiple Pregnancy

According to Hellin's law [$1{:}80^{(n-1)}$] this rule applies to *spontaneous multiple pregnancy*. The incidence of twins is 1:80, for triplet $1{:}(80)^2$, for quadruplet $1{:}(80)^3$ etc. *Multiple pregnancy* is one of the greatest perinatal challenges. Changing demographics and fertility practices have resulted in the global epidemic of multiple pregnancy, substantially inflating the perinatal disease burden for clinicians, parents and society.

Twins

Twins account for 3% of all live births. They can be either:

- *Monozygotic (MZ)* (synonyms: identical, uniovular) arising from the fertilisation of a single ovum or
- *Dizygotic (DZ)* (synonyms: fraternal, binovular) due to fertilisation of two separate ova.

MZ twins account for one-third of twins, with a worldwide incidence of 1 in 250.

DZ twins have a varied rate depending on maternal age, parity, race, family history, geographical location, use of ovulation induction, and other assisted reproductive techniques (ART).

Zygosity refers to the genetic makeup of the twin pregnancy, and **chorionicity** indicates the placental composition. **Chorionicity** is determined by the mechanism of twinning and, in MZ twins, by the timing of embryo division.

DZ twins: Each blastocyst generates its own chorionic and amniotic sacs. Hence, they always have **dichorionic diamniotic (DCDA)** placentation.

MZ twins: The pregnancy is created by the spontaneous cleavage of one fertilised ovum. Thus, the type of placentation that develops is determined by the **timing of this cleavage (refer to Table 12.1)**.

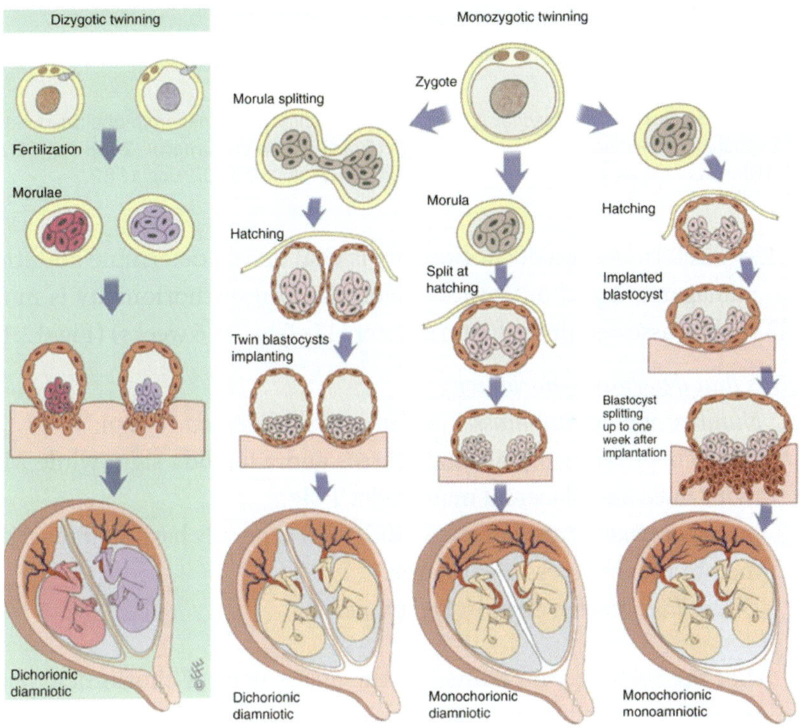

Source: McNamara HC, Kane SC, Craig JM, Short RV, Umstad MP. A review of the mechanisms and evidence for typical and atypical twinning. *Am J Obstet Gynecol* 2016; 214(2): 172–191. doi:10.1016/j.ajog.2015.10.930.

Table 12.1 Type of Placentation in Monozygotic (MZ) Twin Pregnancy

Timing of cleavage of fertilised ovum	Resulting placentation	% of MZ twins
<72 hours	Dichorionic diamniotic (DCDA)	25–30
Days 4–7	Monochorionic diamniotic (MCDA)	70–75
Days 8–12	Monochorionic monoamniotic (MCMA)	1–2
>Day 13	Conjoined twins	Very rare

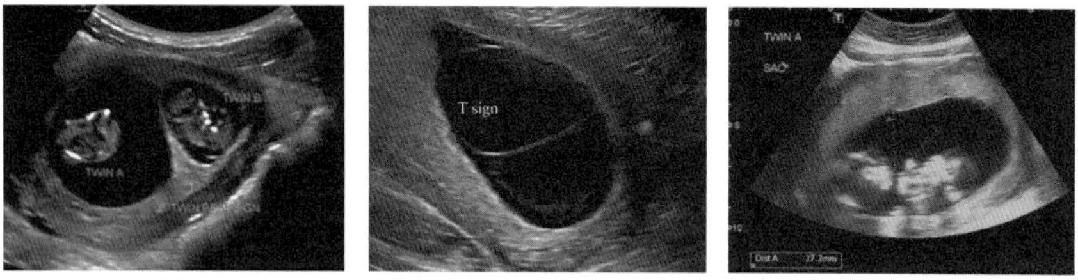

(a) (b) (c)

Fig. 12.1 (a) DCDA twins with twin peak sign ("lambda sign"). (b) MCDA twins with "T sign." (c) MCMA twins.

Source: Khalil A, Rodgers M, Baschat A, *et al*. ISUOG Practice Guidelines: role of ultrasound in twin pregnancy [published correction appears in *Ultrasound Obstet Gynecol*. 2018 Jul; 52(1): 140]. *Ultrasound Obstet Gynecol* 2016; 47(2): 247–263. doi:10.1002/uog.15821.

Early determination of chorionicity is vital to help determine obstetric risks, management and outcomes. Determination of chorionicity is most reliable when assessed in the first trimester (11+0 to 13+6 weeks) (Fig. 12.1).

<u>*Factors that determine chorionicity:*</u>

1. *Number of placental masses and presence of lambda /T sign*:
   DC twins have two placental masses and a lambda sign, while MC twins have one placental mass and a T sign.
2. *Inter-twin membrane thickness*: MC twins generally have an inter-twin membrane thickness of <1.8 mm.
3. *Discordant gender*: Seen in DC twins.

After the early second trimester, the assessment of chorionicity and amnionicity becomes less accurate. It is done by determining the number of placentas and the gender of fetuses. Cases of *indeterminate chorionicity* are followed as MC twins for their antenatal care.

Risks of Multiple Pregnancy

A twin pregnancy is a high-risk pregnancy accounting for about 6.3% of stillbirths and 12.7% of neonatal deaths. Almost every obstetric complication, except for **macrosomia** and **post-term gestation**, is more common with multiple pregnancy. In general, the risk rises in proportion to the number of fetuses.

MC twins are at higher risk of adverse outcomes than DC twins. MC twins have higher rates of fetal anomalies, preterm delivery, lower birth weight, intrauterine death (IUD) and neonatal deaths.

Maternal Risks of Multiple Pregnancy

During pregnancy	During labour	During puerperium
Hyperemesis gravidarum Increased mechanical symptoms of pregnancy Gastro-oesophageal reflux Mechanical distress such as palpitations, dyspnoea, varicosities and haemorrhoids Anaemia Hypertensive disorders (25%)/gestational diabetes mellitus (2–3 times) Antepartum haemorrhage (APH) — Placenta praevia or abruption Polyhydramnios (10%) Preterm labour Premature pre-labour rupture of membranes (PPROM) Malpresentations Acute fatty liver and peripartum cardiomyopathy — rare Neonatal intensive care unit (NICU) admission Maternal death — very rare	Pre-labour rupture of the membranes (PROM) Cord prolapse Incoordinate uterine contractions Labour dystocia Operative interventions Placental abruption after delivery of first baby Postpartum haemorrhage (PPH)	Subinvolution of uterus Infection Postpartum haemorrhage Lactation failure Perinatal mental health disorders, e.g., depression

Table 12.2 Fetal Risks of Singleton Versus Twin Pregnancy

	Singleton (%)	Dichorionic (DC) (%)	Monochorionic (MC) (%)
Miscarriage at 11–23 weeks	1	2	10
Perinatal death	0.5	1.5	3
Intrauterine growth restriction (IUGR)	5	20	30
Preterm delivery <32 weeks	1	5	10
Major birth defects	0.5	1	4

Antenatal Management

- Check BP, maternal weight, urine protein and glucose at each visit.
- Optimise maternal nutrition and weight gain: the recommended caloric intake for normal BMI women with twins is 40–45 kcal/kg daily (an additional 300 kcal/day).
- Women should be given iron, folate and calcium supplements.
- Ultrasound scan at 11–13+6 weeks (CRL 45–84 mm).
- Scan for viability, dating, chorionicity and nuchal translucency (NT).
- Offer aneuploidy screening at 11–13+6 weeks.
- Start low-dose aspirin (LDA) at 150 mg ON from 11 to 14 weeks till 36 weeks of gestation for pre-eclampsia prophylaxis (new KKH protocol 2022) if an additional moderate risk factor for PE is present (NICE).
- Fetal abnormality scan at 19–22 weeks.
- OGTT at 24–28 weeks to screen for GDM.
- Fetal growth scans: MC twins two weekly from 16 weeks, DC twins four weekly from 16 weeks.

First-trimester aneuploidy screening — Refer to Chapter 25: *Prenatal Screening for Chromosomal Defects and Invasive Diagnostic Tests.*

The risk of Down syndrome for MC twins is the same as that for singleton, but for DC twins, this risk is doubled as each fetus has its risk.

Test of choice: Combined first trimester screening (cFTS) at 11–13+6 weeks with a combined risk for the pregnancy in MC twins and an individual risk per baby for DC twins.

Non-invasive prenatal testing (NIPT) or cell-free DNA (cfDNA) — can be challenging in twin pregnancy due to a higher failure rate. Serum screening and NIPT should **not** be performed on triplets and higher-order multiple pregnancy.

In situations such as co-twin demise/vanishing twin where the performance of serum screening and NIPT is uncertain, a NT and nasal bone ultrasound scan can be performed instead.

Chorionic villus sampling (CVS) and amniocentesis are possible invasive diagnostic options performed in a maternal–fetal medicine unit. The risk of miscarriage is about 1%.

Screening for Fetal Anomalies (FA)

The frequency of fetal anomalies in DC twins is comparable to that of singleton pregnancies (2–4%). However, fetal anomalies are more frequent in MC gestations, up to 10%, including neural tube and heart defects. In addition, in MC twins, abnormal vascular connections predispose to limb reduction defects and bowel atresia.

Most MC twins appear to be almost identical. However, there are MC twins who may be genetically and phenotypically dissimilar. Possible mechanisms may include unequal allocation of blastomeres between the two embryos, disrupted embryonic migration, somatic mosaicism or chimerism and variations in penetrance producing phenotypic discrepancy.

Complications of Multiple Pregnancy

IUD of One Twin

- Up to 21% of twins are complicated by either miscarriage or the loss of one twin in the early stages. The risk of "vanishing twin" is higher with advanced maternal age, MC gestation, higher-order multiples and early dating ultrasound scan.
- The first-trimester loss of a twin is common, usually without any consequences. It does not appear to impair the development of the surviving twin. Therefore, no increased surveillance is necessary in pregnancy.
- Loss of a co-twin in the second or third trimester carries risks of preterm delivery, neurological sequelae or death to the remaining fetus (Table 12.3). It may result in the phenomenon known as fetus papyraceous.
- After the death of a co-twin, damage to MC twins is caused by acute haemodynamic changes around the time of death, with the survivor

Table 12.3 Impact of Single Fetal Death in Multiple Pregnancy

	Preterm birth (%)	*In utero* death (%)	Neurological sequelae (%)
DC twin	50	1	4
MC twin	68	15	26

essentially exsanguinating into the circulation of the dying twin. Resultant transient or persistent hypotension and low perfusion lead to ischaemic organ damage, notably but not exclusively to the brain.

- These patients should be counselled on the prognosis for the surviving twin.
- MRI of the fetal brain is advised in MC pregnancy 4 weeks after a co-twin demise.

Twins with a discordant fetal anomaly

- In nearly 85% of cases, the anomaly is confined to one fetus and the co-twin is normal (Fig. 12.2).
- <u>*Management options*</u>
  (1) Expectant management of both fetuses.
  (2) Termination of the entire pregnancy.
  (3) Selective termination of the abnormal fetus.
- *Selective termination of a single fetus in multiple pregnancy*:
  The approach is determined by chorionicity.
  In DC twins, intracardiac injection of potassium chloride (KCl) is the method of choice.

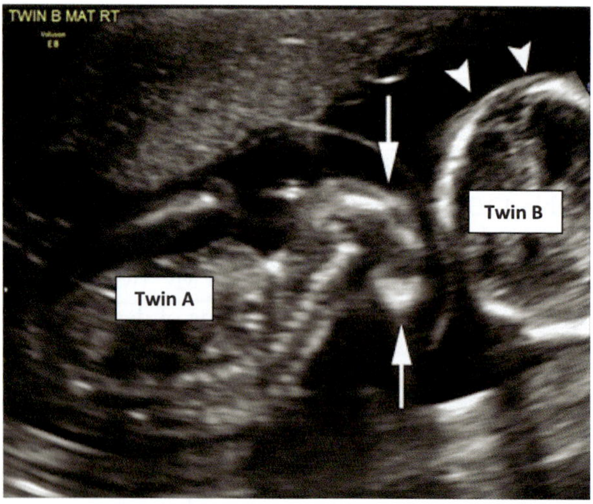

Fig. 12.2 *Twins with a discordant anomaly*: twin A with anencephaly, twin B — normal.

In MC twins, selective termination is far more challenging. Ablation of the umbilical cord of the abnormal fetus is needed to avoid acute haemodynamic change.
It is performed by bipolar cord coagulation or radiofrequency ablation.

IUGR

- Increased risk of IUGR with 20% in DC and 30% in MC twins. Fetal weight discordance is estimated using ≥2 biometric parameters at each scan from 20 weeks.
- Criteria for diagnosis of IUGR in twins (Delphi criteria):
  - Estimated fetal weight (EFW) <3rd percentile of one fetus OR
  - At least two of the following four criteria:
    1. EFW <10th percentile for one twin
    2. Abdominal circumference <10th percentile for one twin
    3. Weight discordance ≥25% [Formula = (EFW larger twin weight – EFW smaller twin weight)/(EFW larger twin weight) × 100]
    4. Umbilical artery pulsatility index (UAPI) >95th percentile for the smaller twin
- Referral to a tertiary centre should be made if IUGR is diagnosed.
- Surveillance of IUGR twins include monitoring the fetal Dopplers (umbilical artery, middle cerebral artery and ductus venosus) and liquor volume.
- These twins should be managed by a maternal–fetal medicine specialist (dedicated multiple pregnancy clinic) to optimise the outcome for both twins.

Complications Unique to Monochorionic Twin Pregnancy

1 Twin–Twin Transfusion Syndrome (TTTS) (Figure 12.3)

Occurs in 10–15% of MCDA pregnancies. TTTS is characterised by an imbalance of fetal blood flow through communicating vessels across a shared placenta, which leads to *under-perfusion* of the *donor* twin and *over-perfusion* of the *recipient*. It results in *hypovolaemia and oligohydramnios in the donor twin* and *overload and polyhydramnios in the recipient twin*. TTTS usually presents after 16 weeks of gestation and rarely after 26 weeks.

Quintero introduced the ultrasound staging of TTTS to describe a progression from early (stage I) to late (stage IV) disease (refer to Table 12.4). However, the progression of TTTS is unpredictable and may not happen in a chronological pattern. Untreated TTTS may result in a perinatal loss of 70–90%.

Table 12.4 The Quintero Classification System

Stage	Classification
I	Discrepancy in amniotic fluid volume with oligohydramnios of a maximum vertical pocket (MVP <2 cm) in one sac and polyhydramnios in the other sac (MVP >8 cm). The bladder of the donor twin is visible and Doppler studies are normal.
II	The bladder of the donor twin is not visible, but Doppler studies are normal.
III	Abnormal Doppler studies in either donor or recipient twin, characterised by reversed end-diastolic flow (EDF) in the umbilical artery, reversed flow in the ductus venosus (DV) or pulsatile umbilical venous velocities.
IV	The presence of hydrops in one or both twins.
V	Death of one or both twins.

Management of TTTS

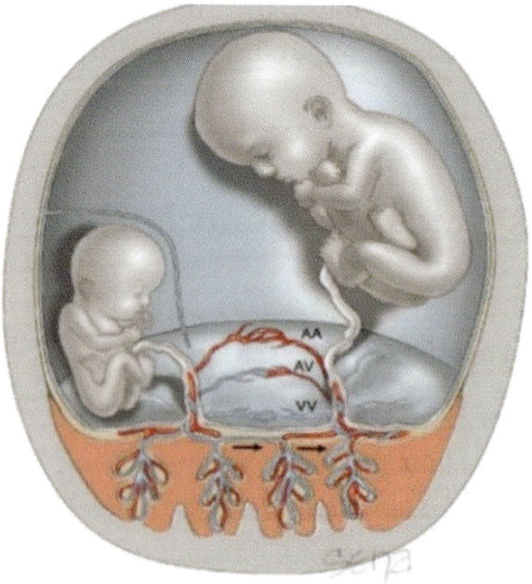

Fig. 12.3: Twin-twin transfusion syndrome (TTTS).

<u>*Treatment options for TTTS*</u>

1. *Selective fetoscopic laser photocoagulation of intertwin vascular anastomoses*. Treatment of choice **up to 26 weeks**. Complications include PPROM, preterm labour, TTTS recurrence, development of twin anaemia — polycythaemia sequence (TAPS) and fetal death.
2. *Cord occlusion* may be appropriate if there is severe hydrops in the recipient or evidence of cerebral damage in either twin.
3. *Serial amnioreduction, with or without septostomy*, favourably changes intra-amniotic pressure and placental intravascular pressure, allowing re-distribution of placental blood flow and normalisation of amniotic fluid volume in each sac. This can be done at **26–28 weeks**.
4. *Selective reduction of one twin* (via radiofrequency ablation or cord coagulation).
5. *Immediate delivery* may be considered **beyond 28 weeks** based on each institution's NICU gestational age-dependent survival.
6. Some women may request *termination of pregnancy* for severe TTTS — the option of abortion should also be discussed (if before 24 weeks — the legal limit for abortion in Singapore).

<u>*Management post-TTTS treatment*</u>

- Close follow-up with MF specialist.
- Regular ultrasound scan of the fetuses: viability, EFW, fetal Dopplers — UAPI, MCA PSV, DVP.
- Delivery timing is usually between 34+0 and 36+6 weeks, with antenatal steroids cover.
- Consider earlier delivery of the surviving twin(s) if there are any concerns.

2 Twin Anaemia Polycythaemia Sequence (TAPS)

- TAPS is a form of TTTS where there is fetal anaemia in the donor twin and polycythaemia in the recipient twin without significant amniotic fluid discordance. This is due to small artery-vein anastomoses allowing slow transfusion of blood from the donor to the recipient twin.
- TAPS is seen in 13% of TTTS post-laser-ablation and 2% of uncomplicated MCDA twins.
- <u>Prenatal diagnosis</u>: The MCA PSV in the donor twin is >1.5 MoM while the recipient twin is <1.5 MoM.

- *Postnatal diagnosis:* Difference in haemoglobin between the twins of >8.0 g/dL and a reticulocyte count ratio of >1.7.
- *Management options for TAPS*
  - Expectant
  - Intrauterine blood transfusion (IUT)
  - Selective fetocide
  - Fetoscopic laser surgery
  - Delivery

3 Twin Reversed Arterial Perfusion (TRAP)

- Rare complication unique to MC placentation.
  Occurs in 1% of MC twins.
- It occurs when, with an apparent lack of well-formed cardiac structure, an acardiac twin is abnormally perfused by a structurally normal co-twin ("pump twin") via a single superficial artery-to-artery anastomosis.
- With conservative management, intrauterine death of the pump twin occurs in 25%, polyhydramnios in 50% and preterm birth in 80% of cases.
- The pump twin survival rate with **no** intervention is 60%.
- *Conservative management* should be contemplated in cases of TRAP sequence where there is an abdominal circumference ratio of <50% with no evidence of compromise of the pump twin.
- *Management of TRAP*: *In utero* interventions performed under ultrasound or fetoscopic guidance are bipolar cord occlusion or intrafetal laser ablation.

4 Selective Growth Restriction (sGR)

- Defined as ≥20% difference in EFW between the twins
  % EFW discrepancy = (EFW of larger twin — EFW of smaller twin)/ EFW of larger twin × 100%
- sGR is found in 10–15% of MC twins without TTTS and 50% of MC twins with TTTS
- **Three types of SGR:**
  Type I: Growth discrepancy with positive diastolic velocities in both fetal umbilical arteries
  - Favourable outcome with >90% perinatal survival

- Aim for delivery between 34 and 36 weeks in case of satisfactory growth and normal Dopplers

Type II: Growth discordance with absent or reversed end-diastolic velocities (AREDV) in one or both fetuses
- Up to ~30% risk of intrauterine death of growth-restricted twin and/or preterm delivery
- Aim for delivery at 32 weeks unless there is abnormal growth velocity or worsening Dopplers

Type III: Growth discordance with cyclical umbilical artery diastolic waveforms (positive followed by absent, then reversed end-diastolic flow in a cyclical pattern over several minutes [intermittent AREDV: iAREDV])
- 10–20% risk of unexpected fetal death of the smaller twin and 10–20% risk of neurological injury in the larger twin
- Aim for delivery at 32 weeks unless there is abnormal growth velocity or worsening Dopplers

o Earlier delivery if there is an abnormal DV waveform or abnormal CTG

Management Options of SGR

- Cord coagulation for selective fetocide
- Laser coagulation of placental anastomoses
- Delivery

MCMA Twins

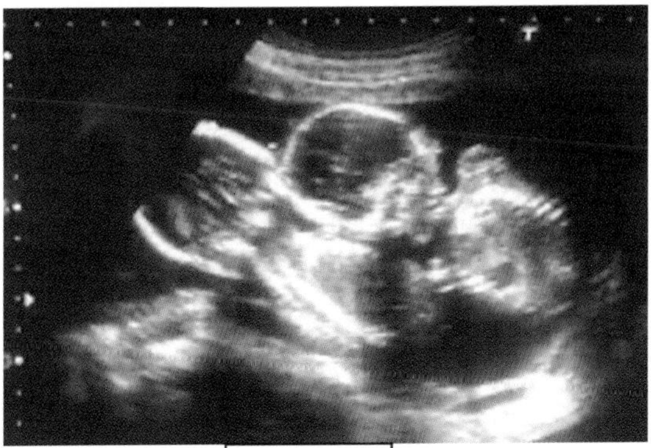

MCMA Twins

- Occurs in 1–2% of monochorionic twin pregnancies.
- Ultrasound shows a single placenta and two freely moving fetuses with no inter-twin membrane.
- Among all types of twins, MCMA are associated with the highest perinatal loss rate ~30–60% in most series due to umbilical cord accidents and prematurity, along with higher rates of fetal anomaly (20–25%) and growth restriction.
- Despite the shared placenta, chronic TTTS appears less common (5%).
- Elective delivery at 32 weeks of gestation following antenatal steroids is usually advocated.

Conjoined Twins

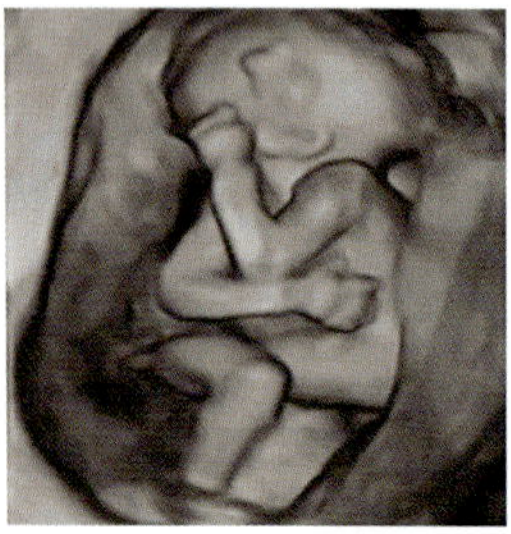

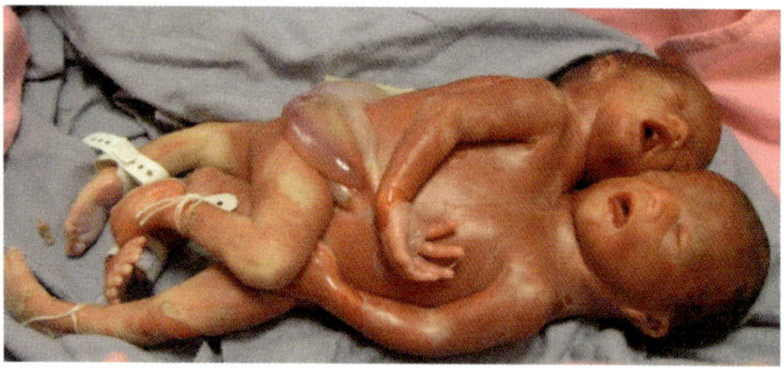

- Incomplete division of the embryo may result in conjoined twins.
- The classification depends on the anatomical areas joined.
- Conjoined thorax (thoracopagus) is the commonest, whereas conjoined thorax and abdomen (thoraco-omphalopagus) and conjoined pelvis and head (ischiopagus and craniopagus) are much less common.
- Prenatal diagnosis of conjoined twins is now well-reported.
- 20% of parents opted for abortion and 10% of fetuses may die *in utero*.
- Overall individual survival rate was about 25%.
- Conjoined twins are usually delivered by elective caesarean section.
- Vaginal deliveries, labour dystocia and uterine rupture have been reported.

Table 12.5 Management of Twin Pregnancy

Summary of management of twins	
DC twins	**MC twins**
Multidisciplinary team BP and urinalysis at every visit Ultrasound scan at 11–13+6 weeks: (a) viability, (b) chorionicity, (c) NT: aneuploidy screen Aneuploid screening, i.e., cFTS at 11–13+6 weeks Structural abnormality scan: 19–22 weeks Serial fetal growth scans every 4 weeks Discussion of woman's needs relating to twins <u>*34–36 weeks:*</u> Discussion of the timing, mode of delivery and intrapartum care Elective delivery at 37–38 weeks gestation if uncomplicated Postnatal advice and support — to include breastfeeding and contraception	Multidisciplinary team BP and urinalysis at every visit Ultrasound scan at 11–13+6 weeks: (a) viability, (b) chorionicity, (c) NT: aneuploidy screen/TTTS Aneuploid screening, i.e., cFTS at 11–13+6 weeks Scan surveillance for TTTS and discordant growth every 2 weeks from 16 weeks onwards Structural abnormality scan at 19–22 weeks (including fetal echocardiography) Discussion of woman's needs relating to twins <u>*32–34 weeks:*</u> Discussion of the timing, mode of delivery, intrapartum care and caesarean section Elective delivery at 36–37 weeks gestation if uncomplicated Postnatal advice and support — to include breastfeeding and contraception

Triplets

Incidence is about 1 in 6000–8000 births for spontaneous triplet pregnancy.

Table 12.6 Type of Triplets

Types	Monochorionic Triamniotic (MCTA)	Dichorionic Triamniotic (DCTA)	Trichorionic Triamniotic (TCTA)
Type of Triplets	A single fertilised egg splits into three	Two sperms fertilising two eggs, and one of the two fertilised eggs split into two	Three sperms fertilising three eggs. Three different placenta and amniotic sacs

Table 12.7 Complications of Singleton Versus Triplets

	Singleton	Triplets
Spontaneous reduction	20%	50%
Aneuploidy	Age-related risk	Three times age-related risk
Hyperemesis gravidarum	Common	More common
Premature rupture of membranes	2%	15–30%
Mean gestation at delivery	38 weeks	32 weeks
Birth weight	<2,500 g: 5% <1,500 g: 1.1%	<2,500 g: 95% <1,500 g: 35%
Pre-eclampsia	5%	20–50%
Anaemia	25%	50%
PPH	0.5%	10–35%

Considerations for the Mode and Timing of Delivery in Multiple Pregnancy (Table 12.5)

- The nadir of perinatal mortality for twin and triplet pregnancies occurs at about 38 and 35 completed weeks of gestation, respectively.
- NICE guidance recommends delivery at 37–38 weeks for uncomplicated DCDA twins and 36–37 weeks for uncomplicated MCDA twins.
- Consider antenatal steroids for planned preterm births as per RCOG guidelines.
- The use of prostaglandins for induction and oxytocin for induction/augmentation of labour is acceptable alternatives to elective caesarean delivery.
- Mode of delivery should consider gestational age, fetal presentations, EFW and the experience/skill of the obstetrician. A trial of labour is appropriate when both twins are in cephalic presentation. For MCMA, a caesarean section is required.
- Mode of delivery should be individualised for cephalic/non-cephalic twins and caesarean delivery is recommended if the presenting twin is non-cephalic.
- Follow-up studies indicate that twins may be disadvantaged in subsequent physical growth and intellectual achievement.
- The management of twins is challenging due to the wide range of perinatal, neonatal, neurodevelopmental and parenting problems.

CHAPTER 13

Hydrops Fetalis

Definition: Abnormal fluid accumulation in ≥2 fetal compartments — ascites, pleural effusion, pericardial effusion, skin oedema (>5 mm). It may be associated with polyhydramnios, placental oedema, hepatosplenomegaly and anaemia.

Incidence: 3–24 per 10,000 live births.

Pathophysiology — exact pathophysiology is unclear.

Possible causes:

- Obstructed lymphatic drainage
- Increased vascular permeability
- High central venous pressure/intravascular hydrostatic pressure
- Low osmotic pressure

Usually, it is incidentally diagnosed during antenatal ultrasound scans. If polyhydramnios is present, symptoms may include abdominal distension/bloating, sudden rapid weight gain, shortness of breath, orthopnoea or pedal oedema. Women may also present with a uterus that is larger than dates, or decreased fetal movements.

Causes of Hydrops Fetalis

Divided into *immune* versus *non-immune*

In developed countries, >90% of hydrops are due to non-immune causes.

a. **Immune hydrops (<10%):** Iso-immunisation:
   - o Formation of maternal antibodies to red cell antigens, including Rhesus (Rh), ABO, Duffy and Kell, which cross into fetal circulation, causing haemolysis and anaemia.
   - o Mainly due to Rh isoimmunisation.

b. **Non-immune hydrops (>90%):** *Hydrops* without *maternal circulating red cell antibodies.*

Possible causes:

Cardiovascular (20–35%)

- **Structural** (aortic stenosis, hypoplastic left heart, Ebstein anomaly)
- **Non-structural**
  - Arrhythmias: *tachyarrhythmias* (supraventricular tachycardia) Atrial flutter, *bradyarrhythmias* (complete heart block)
  - Tumours/vascular abnormalities
  - Infections
  - Cardiomyopathy

Chromosomal (10%)

- Trisomies (Down or Edward syndrome)
- Turner syndrome
- Triploidy
- Single gene disorders, e.g., skeletal dysplasia, G6PD deficiency

Haematological (5–12%)

- Haemoglobinopathies, e.g., alpha thalassaemia (Bart)
- Fetal haemorrhage (intracranial/intraventricular, feto-maternal haemorrhage (FMH), twin-to-twin transfusion syndrome)
- Disorders of red blood cell metabolism (G6PD deficiency, pyruvate kinase deficiency)
- Disorders of RBC production (congenital dyserythropoietic anaemia, Diamond–Blackfan syndrome, Fanconi anaemia)
- Disorders of RBC membrane (hereditary spherocytosis/elliptocytosis)
- Leukaemias

Infections (5–7%): Parvovirus B19, cytomegalovirus (CMV), syphilis, herpes simplex virus (HSV), toxoplasmosis, hepatitis B, adenovirus, listeria monocytogenes, coxsackievirus type B, ureaplasma urealyticum.

Thoracic (5%): Congenital diaphragmatic hernia (CDH), congenital pulmonary airway malformation (CPAM), congenital hydrothorax, chylothorax.

Urinary (2–3%) — congenital nephrosis, Prune Belly syndrome, urinary ascites due to ruptured bladder/renal collecting system.

Gastrointestinal — volvulus, meconium peritonitis, biliary atresia, malrotation of intestines.

Lymphatic dysplasia (5–6%).

Metabolic (1.3%): Inborn errors of metabolism (glycogen storage disease type IV, lysosomal storage diseases), fetal hypo or hyperthyroidism.

Extra-thoracic tumours: Sacrococcygeal teratoma, lymphangiomas, haemangiomas.

Twin-to-twin transfusion syndrome (4.1%).

Placental/cord: Chorioangiomas, angiomyxoma of cord.

Maternal diseases — diabetes mellitus, hyperthyroidism.

Idiopathic (19.8%).

Maternal Risks of Hydrops

Pre-eclampsia-like "mirror syndrome" (also known as Ballantynes syndrome):

Generalised maternal oedema, often with pulmonary involvement and hypertension — "mirrors" the oedema of the hydropic fetus and placenta.

Placental abruption
Preterm delivery
Prolonged hospitalisation
Caesarean section
Risk of dystocia during delivery and birth trauma
Retained placenta and postpartum haemorrhage
Emotional distress with anxiety

Fetal or Neonatal Risks of Hydrops

Miscarriage
Intrauterine death (IUD)
Perinatal/early neonatal death
Admission to the neonatal intensive care unit (NICU)
Risks of prematurity, e.g., intraventricular haemorrhage, retinopathy of prematurity

Respiratory distress syndrome, necrotising enterocolitis
Cognitive defects and neurodevelopmental delay

Evaluation of Hydrops Fetalis

History: to identify possible causes of hydrops fetalis
Consanguinity

Current pregnancy: Rh status, fetal anomaly (FA) scan, history of infections in pregnancy, contact history

Past obstetric history: Previous pregnancy with FA or pregnancy loss, e.g., IUD/neonatal or infant death

Past medical history: Autoimmune conditions, thalassaemia

Family history: Developmental delay, FA, genetic conditions, fetal loss or neonatal death. Enquire about symptoms of mirror syndrome

Examination
Vitals, BP, weight, urine dipstick for proteinuria
Heart/lungs: pulmonary oedema
Abdomen: distension, uterus larger than dates
Pedal oedema

Investigations for Hydrops Fetalis

Ultrasound Scans

- *Detailed FA scan:* Presentation, amniotic fluid index (AFI), estimated fetal weight (EFW), placental and cord abnormalities, fetal anomalies, placenta, ultrasound features of maternal–fetal infection (e.g., ventriculomegaly, microcephaly, echogenic bowel), fetal echocardiography, assessment for fetal arrhythmias, Doppler studies for umbilical artery, ductus venosus, middle cerebral artery (MCA)
- *Doppler scan* of MCA PSV in all hydropic fetuses >16 weeks for fetal anaemia — **MCA PSV >1.5 MoM** indicates fetal anaemia
- If fetal anaemia is suspected, consider cordocentesis/FBS (fetal blood sampling)

Blood Tests

- *Maternal blood group and antibody status*
- *Antibody screen with indirect Coomb's test* — to determine if immune or non-immune cause
- *Thalassaemia tests*: alpha-globin genotyping for α-thalassaemia, haemoglobin electrophoresis for β-thalassaemia
- *Paternal and fetal genotyping if maternal antibodies present* — non-invasive prenatal testing or invasive testing [via chorionic villus sampling (CVS) or amniocentesis] may be performed for the Rh status of the fetus (refer to Chapter 24: *Approach to Management of Red Cell Antibodies in Pregnancy*)
- *Kleihauer–Betke test* for FMH
- *Test for maternal–fetal infections*: CMV, toxoplasmosis, parvovirus, rubella, syphilis

Invasive Testing — CVS/Amniocentesis/Cordocentesis

- Genetic testing [e.g., fetal karyotype, chromosomal microarray analysis (CMA), Bart haemoglobin].
- Fetal genotyping for Rh status of the fetus.
- Studies for fetal infection (e.g., CMV/toxoplasma PCR).
- A sample of amniotic fluid may be frozen for further testing in future.
- *Cordocentesis*: For fetal full blood count (FBC), direct Coomb's test, blood group, Rh status, Hb electrophoresis. Also used for intrauterine transfusion (IUT).

Other Tests

- All cases of *unexplained fetal hydrops* should be referred to the geneticist for detailed postnatal evaluation and counselling.
- *Post-delivery*, echocardiogram, FBC, thyroid function test and metabolic panel may be performed for the neonate.
- Post-mortem examination of the fetus/placenta, molecular and genetic studies are recommended for all cases of fetal/neonatal death or termination of pregnancy.
- Amniotic fluid and/or fetal cells should be stored for future genetic testing.

Management of Hydrops Fetalis

- *Multidisciplinary team management* (maternal–fetal specialist, sonographer, geneticist, paediatric cardiologist/surgeon, pharmacist, medical social worker, neonatologist) at a tertiary centre with a fetal-medicine unit that can perform fetal procedures.
- *Key management strategies:*
  - Identify cases caused by disorders that may be treated *in utero*
  - Deliver the fetus when the benefits of prolonging pregnancy are outweighed by the risks of IUD or risk of maternal deterioration
- Treatment is dependent on the cause and whether the aetiology may be determined
- Parents need to be involved in shared decision-making should they choose to continue with the pregnancy

Antenatal Care

- Monitor BP and perform urine dipstick to assess for pre-eclampsia-like "mirror syndrome".
- If the diagnosis of hydrops was made before 24 weeks of gestation and a poor prognosis was expected, e.g., chromosomal abnormality, discuss the option of termination of pregnancy.
- Need to exclude structural cardiac abnormalities and chromosomal disorders before performing intra-uterine interventions, as these conditions are **not** amenable to *in utero* treatments.

Intrauterine Interventions are Available for Certain Fetal Conditions

- *IUT for fetal anaemia.*
  - If fetal anaemia is diagnosed before 34 weeks, IUT may be performed.
  - Blood used for IUT should be ABO compatible with the neonate and mother, RhD negative (or RhD identical with fetus), K negative, negative for the corresponding antigen to which the woman has an antibody and cross-match compatible with the woman's blood sample.

    - Blood should also be <5 days old (to ensure low supernatant potassium levels), CMV negative, irradiated and with plasma removed to increase the haematocrit to 70–85%.
  - Thoracocentesis/pleuroamniotic shunt insertion for fetal pleural effusion.
  - Fetal procedures (laser vessel or radiofrequency ablation/fetal surgery).
    - Some teratomas can be resected via *in utero* surgery.
- Anti-arrhythmic drugs such as digoxin, sotalol, flecainide and amiodarone are used to treat fetal SVT.
- Anti-thyroid medications can be used to treat fetal thyrotoxicosis.
- Cardiotocography (CTG) as appropriate.

Intrapartum Care

- Delivery at a tertiary centre with level 3 neonatal care facilities.
- Delivery is usually recommended by 34 weeks after completion of antenatal steroids. Delivery should not be beyond 37–38 weeks in the absence of known lethal anomaly, maternal or fetal deterioration, or other indications for earlier delivery.
- If the patient decides on comfort care for the fetus due to poor prognosis, e.g., Edward syndrome, vaginal delivery is preferred.
- If the patient decides on active management and neonatal resuscitation for the fetus, there should be continuous CTG monitoring and a low threshold for caesarean section for non-reassuring fetal status (NFRS).
- Ultrasound-guided percutaneous aspiration of large ascites/pleural effusion before delivery may reduce the risk of dystocia and aid in neonatal resuscitation.
- *Ex utero* intrapartum therapy (EXIT) procedure may be performed at caesarean delivery for fetuses with congenital cardiac and thoracic anomalies.

Postnatal Care

- Admission to the NICU.

- Initial resuscitation of neonate — the majority will require endotracheal intubation due to respiratory depression.
- Identification and treatment of the underlying cause of hydrops.
- Thoracocentesis, paracentesis and cardiocentesis may be performed for neonatal pleural effusion, ascites and pericardial effusion, respectively.
- Neonatal blood transfusion for severe anaemia.
- Severe tachyarrhythmias may be corrected with cardioversion, anti-arrhythmic drugs and pacing.
- Emotional support for the woman and her family.

Prognosis of Hydrops Fetalis

Prognosis depends on the underlying aetiology, available fetal therapies to resolve hydrops and gestational age at delivery. If associated with chromosomal/structural abnormalities or genetic metabolic disorders, the prognosis is usually poorer — this could help parents decide whether to continue the pregnancy. Other factors affecting prognosis include gestational age at diagnosis, time of delivery, amount of fetal oedema and if intrauterine interventions are possible.

Despite aggressive treatment and advances in fetal diagnosis and therapy, the survival rate is still low. Surviving infants commonly suffer from neurodevelopmental and cognitive defects. The recurrence rate is highest in women whose infants have genetic disorders (e.g., autosomal dominant/recessive conditions) or Rh incompatibility.

CHAPTER 14

Fetal Growth Restriction (FGR)/ Intrauterine Growth Restriction (IUGR)

Fetal growth restriction (FGR) refers to a fetus with slow or static growth *in utero*, which implies a failure of a fetus to achieve its endorsed growth potential. FGR, intrauterine growth restriction (IUGR) and small for gestational age (SGA) are often used interchangeably.

Definition

- **FGR is diagnosed when the sonographic estimated fetal weight (EFW) or abdominal circumference (AC) is <10th percentile for gestational age on a standardised population growth curve.**
- **Severe FGR is defined as EFW or AC <3rd percentile.**
- <u>Early-onset FGR</u> is FGR that occurs <32+0 weeks of gestation.
- <u>Late-onset FGR</u> is FGR that occurs from 32+0 weeks of gestation.

FGR complicates about 4–8% of pregnancies. It is the primary cause of stillbirth in 6.6% of cases and an associated cause in 19%. Both screening and diagnosis of FGR rely on accurate dating by an early ultrasound (preferably first trimester) and are based on ultrasound biometry.

Aetiology

- Most fetuses with an EFW of <10th percentile (up to 70%) are constitutionally small and not at risk of adverse perinatal outcomes.
- The remaining 30% are *pathological FGR*, and these fetuses (and neonates) are most at risk.
- If a fetus is >10th percentile on a population growth curve but has fallen in its growth trajectory by two quartiles, it is still at risk of poor

perinatal outcomes secondary to not meeting its individualised growth potential.

The **causes of FGR** can be divided into 3 basic categories (refer to Table 14.1):

1) Maternal factors
2) Fetal factors
3) Placental factors

Although the pathophysiology of each factor is different, **maternal factors** (e.g., chronic hypertension) and **placental factors** may have a common final pathway of decreased placental perfusion and transfer of nutrients across the placenta to the fetus. **Fetal factors** include conditions in which growth is reduced secondary to genetic, chromosomal, structural malformations or infectious causes.

Table 14.1 Aetiology of FGR/IUGR

Maternal factors	Fetal factors	Placental factors
• Age/race/parity • Low BMI/small stature • Maternal history of SGA • Low socio-economic status/malnutrition • Smoking (13%)/alcohol/ substance abuse • Uteroplacental insufficiency (70%) • Pre-existing hypertension/pre-eclampsia • Pre-existing type 1/ type 2 DM • Thrombophilia-antiphospholipid syndrome (APS) • Autoimmune disorders • Chronic renal disease • Drugs: antiepileptics, corticosteroids	• Chromosomal and genetic defects (4–25%) • Fetal infections (5–10%), e.g., CMV, toxoplasmosis, rubella, malaria, herpes HSV, HIV, varicella, syphilis • Structural anomalies (1–2%): congenital heart disease, gastroschisis • Inborn error of metabolism • Multiple pregnancy (3%)	• Chronic placental abruption • Placental mosaicism • Abnormal placentation-circumvallate placenta, single umbilical artery (SUA), velamentous or marginal cord insertion • Placental tumour — chorioangioma • Abnormal analytes on serum screening

Table 14.2 Complications of FGR/IUGR

Mother	Need for close antenatal surveillance Increased risk of pre-eclampsia: FGR may precede the onset of pre-eclampsia in 50% of cases Increased risk of caesarean section, as high as 90% of cases Increased risk of post-traumatic stress disorder (PTSD), anxiety/depression Risks related to co-morbidities or other pregnancy complications 20% recurrence risk of FGR
Fetus	Associated with fetal anomaly Oligohydramnios Non-reassuring fetal heart testing (NRFS), birth asphyxia Meconium aspiration syndrome Severe prematurity *In utero* demise/stillbirth: 5-fold increased risk of stillbirth beyond 37 weeks
Neonate	Iatrogenic or spontaneous preterm birth and its consequences Increased NICU admissions/need for intubation Low birth weight Low Apgar score Hypoglycaemia/electrolyte disturbances/acidosis Hyperviscosity syndrome Hypoxic-ischaemic encephalopathy (HIE) Seizures, death
Infant and child	Impaired neurodevelopmental delay, cerebral palsy, lower intelligence quotient, mental retardation, speech/reading disabilities, attention and learning deficits, poor academic achievement and short stature
Adult	Hypertension, coronary artery disease, stroke, diabetes, obesity, social and financial problems

Complications of FGR can occur *in utero* and later in life (Table 14.2).

Classification of FGR

- FGR is classified into two phenotypes: when the onset is either early or late in gestation, its association with pre-eclampsia, and the natural history of fetal deterioration (Table 14.3).
- Present evidence suggests that FGR is defined by the existence of placental insufficiency. Placental insufficiency in <u>*early FGR*</u> is

Table 14.3 Classification of FGR

Early-onset FGR (rare)	Late-onset FGR (common)
Definition: AC/EFW <3rd centile or absent end diastolic flow in the umbilical artery (UA) or 1. AC/EFW <10th centile combined with 2. Pulsatility index (PI) in the uterine artery (UtA) >95th percentile and/or 3. PI in the UA >95th percentile	**Definition:** AC/EFW <3rd centile or At least 2 out of 3 of following 1. AC/EFW <10th centile 2. Crossing centiles of >2 quartiles on growth centiles 3. Cerebroplacental ratio (CPR) <5th centile
Causes: Severe placental insufficiency, chronic hypoxia (rule out genetic causes) **Association with early pre-eclampsia** in 70% **Dopplers:** UA Doppler largely affected. Doppler cascade changes are usually seen **Natural history:** If left unchecked, deterioration to uncompensated hypoxia-mortality before term **Difficult to manage —** severe prematurity versus intrauterine death (IUD) **Perinatal mortality and morbidity:** High	**Causes:** Mild placental insufficiency Association with pre-eclampsia: 15% **Dopplers:** Abnormal CPR. Ductus venosus (DV) changes. Doppler cascade changes are usually not seen **Natural history:** Lacks chronological changes. Acute deterioration may happen before or during labour **Undiagnosed late FGR:** Large share of term stillbirths **Easy to manage:** Deliver **Perinatal mortality and morbidity:** Low Stillbirth risk is high in undiagnosed cases

associated with histological signs of abnormal early implantation. Late FGR is probably a mild form of abnormal placental implantation in early pregnancy or superimposed placental damage occurring during the second half of pregnancy.

- Both phenotypes of growth restriction are associated with poor long-term neurodevelopmental, cardiovascular and metabolic outcomes secondary to chronic exposure to an adverse intrauterine environment resulting in adverse fetal programming.

Diagnosis of FGR/IUGR

- All women should be assessed for risk factors for a growth-restricted fetus at the booking visit.

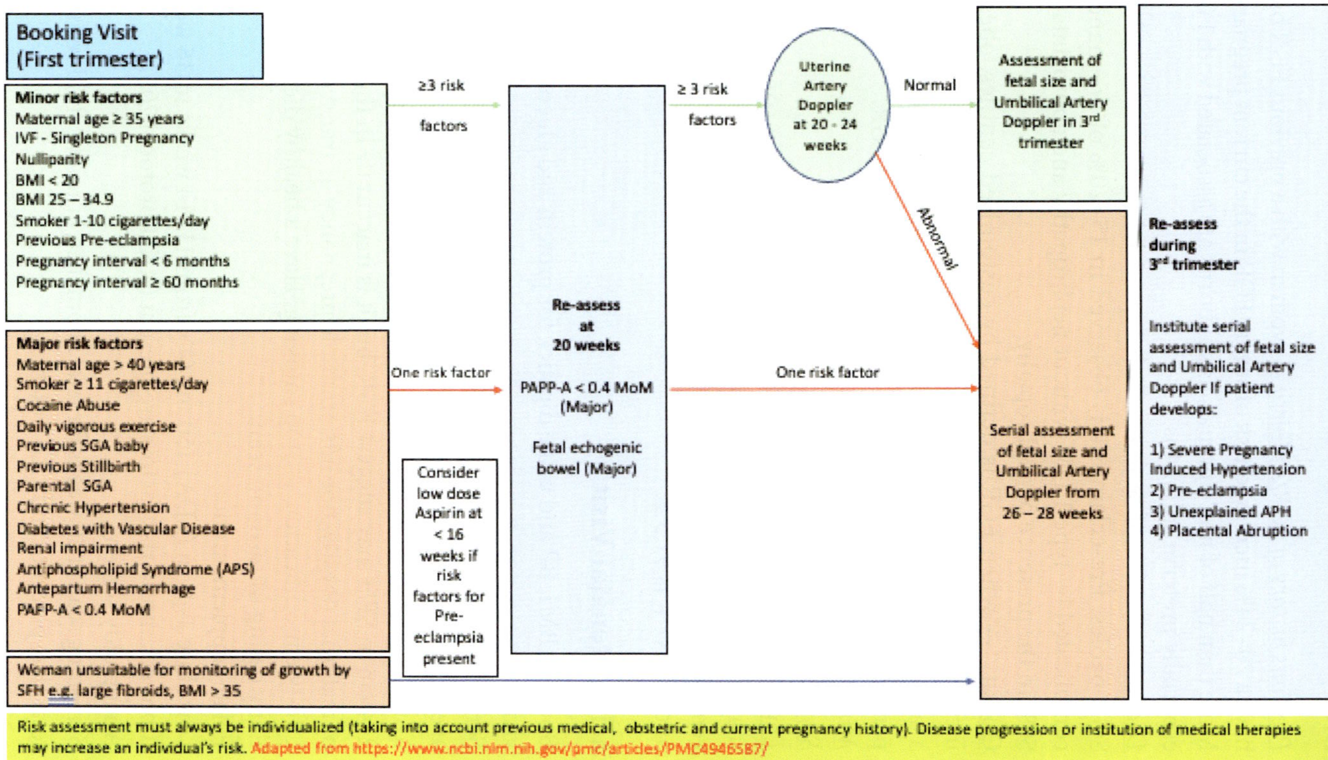
Booking Visit
(First trimester)
Minor risk factors
Maternal age ≥ 35 years
IVF - Singleton Pregnancy
Nulliparity
BMI < 20
BMI 25 – 34.9
Smoker 1-10 cigarettes/day
Previous Pre-eclampsia
Pregnancy interval < 6 months
Pregnancy interval ≥ 60 months
Major risk factors
Maternal age > 40 years
Smoker ≥ 11 cigarettes/day
Cocaine Abuse
Daily vigorous exercise
Previous SGA baby
Previous Stillbirth
Parental SGA
Chronic Hypertension
Diabetes with Vascular Disease
Renal impairment
Antiphospholipid Syndrome (APS)
Antepartum Hemorrhage
PAFP-A < 0.4 MoM
Woman unsuitable for monitoring of growth by SFH e.g. large fibroids, BMI > 35
≥3 risk factors
One risk factor
Consider low dose Aspirin at < 16 weeks if risk factors for Pre-eclampsia present
Re-assess at 20 weeks
PAPP-A < 0.4 MoM (Major)
Fetal echogenic bowel (Major)
≥ 3 risk factors
One risk factor
Uterine Artery Doppler at 20 - 24 weeks
Normal
Abnormal
Assessment of fetal size and Umbilical Artery Doppler in 3rd trimester
Serial assessment of fetal size and Umbilical Artery Doppler from 26 – 28 weeks
Re-assess during 3rd trimester
Institute serial assessment of fetal size and Umbilical Artery Doppler If patient develops:
1) Severe Pregnancy Induced Hypertension
2) Pre-eclampsia
3) Unexplained APH
4) Placental Abruption
Risk assessment must always be individualized (taking into account previous medical, obstetric and current pregnancy history). Disease progression or institution of medical therapies may increase an individual's risk. Adapted from https://www.ncbi.nlm.nih.gov/pmc/articles/PMC4946587/

History

- *Previous history of FGR/stillbirth* — women with a previous FGR baby have a 20–24% increased risk of severe FGR in the current pregnancy. More than half of non-anomalous stillborns are associated with FGR, especially preterm stillbirths.
- *Diabetes* — 15% of women with type 2 DM are found to have SGA babies. Pre-eclampsia is observed in 15–20% of pregnancies complicated by type 1 DM without nephropathy and approximately 50% in the presence of nephropathy.
- Obesity — when FGR is defined by customised centiles, obesity increases the risk of FGR by 50%. Such relative smallness is pathological: a large population-based study reported that in obese women, higher perinatal mortality is associated with higher rates of FGR.
- *Multiple pregnancy*
- *Smoking*
- *Low PAPP-A* — low PAPP-A <0.415 MoM should be considered a major risk factor for delivery of a SGA neonate. When PAPP-A is <5th centile, the sensitivity of detecting FGR is 10.4%, the PPV is 18.7%, and the NPV is 91.3%.

At Each Antenatal Visit

- Booking BMI, BP and urine dipstick for protein and glucose at every visit.
- Serial measurement of symphysis fundal height (SFH) is recommended at each antenatal visit from 24 weeks, as this improves the prediction of a SGA neonate. In addition, it is inexpensive and easy to use. A lag of 2–4 cm in SFH may suggest FGR, but it is inaccurate in the presence of maternal obesity, fibroids, multiple pregnancy or transverse lie.
- Lifestyle modification — stop smoking. Have a healthy diet.
- Early dating ultrasound scan.
- Folate supplementation.
- Low-dose aspirin (LDA) 150 mg ON from 11–14 weeks to 36 weeks if pre-eclampsia risk factors are present (KKH protocol 2022).
- Aneuploidy screen.
- Screening scan at 20 weeks for fetal anomalies, amniotic fluid volume, fetal size, placenta and UtA notching.

- **When the risk of FGR is high, ultrasound should be the primary modality to screen for fetal growth abnormalities** by assessing fetal biometry, Dopplers and amniotic fluid.
- *Normal growth* is defined by measurements of the head (biparietal diameter, head circumference), abdominal circumference (AC) and femur length (FL) within normal ranges for gestational age plotted on population-specific growth charts.
- A decrease in the umbilical venous flow and reduction in fetal cardiac output leads to the downregulation of the glucose-insulin-IgF growth axis and decreased glycogen storage in the liver before the clinical onset of FGR. Reduction in liver size results in a fall in the AC before the EFW falls below the 10th centile.
- *Serial measurements at 2 to 3 weekly intervals* are needed to define normality and abnormality.
- Both fetal growth decline and the rate of decline in late pregnancy are important considerations. It is the rate of growth that is more important than the absolute value at a given time. It is reassuring if the fetus is in lower centiles but continues the growth within those centiles. However, if growth is slow, this is a cause for concern.

Management for FGR/IUGR

- MDT care with MF specialist, neonatologist, geneticist, etc.

Investigations for FGR/IUGR

- The first step is to confirm the gestational age by checking the dating scan to ensure that the fetus is truly small.
- *Review risk factors:* check medical history and BP. If abnormal BP, exclude pre-eclampsia.
- In addition, any substance abuse should be discussed. Advise cessation.
- Evaluation of fetal anatomy, placenta and amniotic fluid by ultrasound scan.
- Assessment of the UA by Doppler (refer to Chapter 26: *Ultrasonography and Fetal Doppler in Obstetrics*).
- *Infection workup:* Maternal serum IgG and IgM for CMV and toxoplasmosis. Rubella immunity should be ascertained.

- *Screen for anti-phospholipid syndrome*: Lupus anticoagulant, anti-cardiolipin (ACL) IgM and IgG, anti-$\beta 2$ glycoprotein. Perform if obstetric history suggestive of Anti-Phospholipid syndrome, e.g. previous unexplained intrauterine death, severe preterm pre-eclampsia or recurrent miscarriage.
- *Amniocentesis* to rule out aneuploidy [karyotype + chromosomal microarray (CMA)] and infection (PCR for CMV, toxoplasmosis).
- Maternal urine albumin.
- Maternal workup for pre-eclampsia should be performed if indicated.
- Maternal placental growth factor (PlGF) level — low circulating PlGF <100 pg/ml distinguishes the healthy small-for-gestational age fetus from the fetus with placenta-mediated FGR that is at risk of stillbirth and asphyxia-related morbidity. These patients need close surveillance during pregnancy and labour.

The clinician should discuss possible complications and prognosis, including planned antenatal surveillance, pregnancy termination option, delivery thresholds and timing of antenatal steroids. The prognosis of FGR depends largely upon the underlying aetiology. Aneuploidy, fetal anomalies and intrauterine infection are associated with a worse prognosis. Once these factors have been excluded, gestational age at delivery is one of the best predictors of perinatal outcomes.

Follow-Up of FGR — Aims of Antepartum Surveillance

Maximise intrauterine stay for the fetus
Optimise timing of delivery
Minimise stillbirths/neonatal morbidity and mortality

Doppler Changes in FGR/IUGR

Doppler velocimetry is the cornerstone of the management and follow-up of FGR (refer to Chapter 26: *Ultrasonography and Fetal Doppler in Obstetrics*).

Stage	Doppler changes	Comments
Initial stage	Placental vascular dysfunction $\rightarrow$ Increased impedance in UA	Impaired fetal growth
Diagnosis of FGR	A decrease in UA end-diastolic flow (EDF) with elevated resistance indices — high PI	Associated with abnormalities in 30% of fetal vessels
As condition worsens	With the increase in placental vascular resistance $\rightarrow$ UA absent EDF and then reversed EDF	60–70% of fetal villous vessels are abnormal. $\geq$50% of fetuses will be hypoxaemic and have higher incidences of preterm birth, intrauterine death, neonatal morbidity/mortality and neurodevelopmental impairments.
	Fetal middle cerebral artery (MCA) impedance decreases $\rightarrow$ decrease in MCA PI This results in a decreasing CPR Low amniotic fluid index (AFI)	The growth-restricted fetus re-organises its blood flow, shunting blood from visceral, i.e., less essential organs, to vital organs like the brain and heart. In FGR fetuses, MCA PI is a surrogate marker of hypoxia, particularly valuable for identifying and predicting adverse outcomes among late-onset FGR. *Late FGRs* with abnormal MCA PI have poorer neuro-behavioural competence at birth and at 2 years.
	Abnormal venous Doppler: Decreased or reversed a-wave in DV	DV Doppler is the strongest single Doppler parameter to predict the *short-term risk* of fetal death in early-onset FGR. DV flow waveforms become abnormal only in advanced stages of fetal compromise. **Abnormal DV Doppler occurred in up to 70% of FGR cases 7 days to 24 hours before CTG abnormalities.** Overall, the sensitivity for perinatal death is 40–70%.
Fetal deterioration	Pulsatile flow in umbilical vein and DV <u>*CTG changes*</u>: Decreased variability, non-reassuring fetal status (NRFS)	

Surveillance for FGR/IUGR

FGR is probably among the obstetrical entities with the greatest variation in clinical practice. There is no therapy currently available which can reverse FGR. The only intervention possible in most cases is *delivery*. The main consideration is appropriate timing, balancing the risk of iatrogenic prematurity and continued exposure to an unfavourable intrauterine environment.

- Timing and delivery of the FGR fetus should be individualised, based on gestational age, the severity of FGR, Doppler velocimetry, growth/ Doppler and CTG findings. Gestational age is the most important determinant of survival until about 30–32 weeks.
- If preterm delivery is anticipated within 24 hours, administer antenatal steroids if delivery is <34 weeks (up to 34+6 weeks — RCOG) and IV $MgSO_4$ for fetal neuroprotection if delivery is <32 weeks in KKH (Offer IV $MgSO_4$ from 24+0 to 29+6 weeks and consider from 30 to 33+6 weeks — RCOG).

  RCOG green top guidelines (2013)
  - **If UA Dopplers are normal.** Perform growth + Dopplers two weekly. Perform MCA Doppler if >32 weeks.
  - **If UA Doppler is abnormal but EDF is positive:** Perform Dopplers twice weekly.
  - **If UA is absent/reversed EDF:** Perform Dopplers daily.
  - **Timing of delivery**
    - *In preterm FGR fetus with absent/reversed EDF <32 weeks:*
      - DV Doppler is normal → deliver no later than 32 weeks
      - DV Doppler becomes abnormal/UV pulsations appear → Deliver provided fetus is considered viable and after antenatal steroids completed
    - *FGR fetus with normal UA Dopplers and MCA Doppler:* Deliver if static growth over 3 weeks or offer delivery at 37 weeks with the involvement of a senior obstetrician
    - *FGR fetus with normal UA Doppler but abnormal MCA Doppler:* Deliver no later than 37 weeks

Gratacos *et al.* (2014) proposed a protocol that integrates the best available evidence that can help reduce clinical practice variation for abnormal fetal Dopplers.

Stage-Based Classification and Management of FGR

Stage	Pathophysiological correlation	Criteria (any of)	Monitoring*	GA/mode of delivery
I	*Mild* placental insufficiency-low risk of fetal deterioration before term	EFW <3rd centile CPR <5th centile UA PI >95th centile MCA PI <5th centile UtA PI >95%	Weekly	37 weeks IOL with a cervical balloon High risk of intrapartum fetal distress
II	*Severe* placental insufficiency-risk of abnormal neurodevelopment	UA AEDV	Bi-weekly	34 weeks Elective CS
III	*Advanced* fetal deterioration-higher risk of stillbirth	UA REDV DV-PI >95%	1–2 days	30 weeks CS
IV	*High-suspicion* of fetal acidosis and fetal death	DV reverse 'a' flow, CTG: FHR decelerations	12 hours	26 weeks with antenatal steroids** CS

All Doppler signs described above should be confirmed at least twice, ideally at least 12 hours apart.
GA, gestational age; IOL, induction or labour; CS, caesarean section.
*Recommended intervals in the **absence** of severe pre-eclampsia.
If FGR is accompanied by pre-eclampsia, strict fetal monitoring is warranted regardless of the FGR stage.
**Lower GA threshold is recommended according to current literature reporting at least 50% intact survival. The threshold could be tailored according to parents' wishes or adjusted according to local statistics of intact survival.

Mode of Delivery

There is insufficient evidence to assess the mode of delivery associated with the best outcomes for a FGR fetus. Therefore, a trial of labour for a vertex FGR fetus can only be attempted if fetal monitoring is reassuring.

RCOG Green Top Guidelines 2013

- *If normal UA Doppler or abnormal UA Doppler but positive EDF* → Offer induction of labour. There is an increased risk of caesarean section.

- *<u>If absent/reversed EDF</u>* → Recommend caesarean section.

Inform the neonatal team to standby for delivery. Send paired cord blood gases.

The placenta should be sent for histology after the delivery of a FGR fetus.

Recurrence Risk of FGR/IUGR

Recurrence risk is linked mainly to the underlying aetiology in the affected pregnancy. With a prior FGR baby, the risk of FGR in a subsequent singleton pregnancy is about 20–24%. Recurrence of FGR in cases associated with aneuploidy is low, but the risk of aneuploidy in subsequent pregnancies is higher than the risk of maternal age. When FGR is due to infection from a viral source, recurrence risk is low, as the patient would have attained immunity.

CHAPTER 15

Infections in Pregnancy

List of Infections in Pregnancy

Bacterial Vaginosis
Candidiasis
Trichomoniasis
} Refer to Chapter 49: *Vaginal Discharge and Recurrent Vulvo-Vaginal Candidiasis*

Chlamydia trachomatis and *Neisseria gonorrhoeae* — Refer to Chapter 51: *Sexually Transmitted Infections (STI)*

1. COVID-19 (SARS-CoV-2)
2. Cytomegalovirus (CMV)
3. Dengue
4. Genital Warts (Condyloma Acuminata)
5. Group B Streptococcus (GBS) Infection
6. Hand–Foot–Mouth Disease (HFMD)
7. Hepatitis B virus (HBV) Infection
8. Hepatitis C virus (HCV) Infection
9. Hepatitis E virus (HEV) Infection
10. Herpes Simplex Virus (HSV) Infection
11. H1N1 Influenza Infection
12. Human Immunodeficiency Virus (HIV) Infection
13. Listeriosis (*Listeria* Infection)
14. Malaria
15. Parvovirus B19 ("Fifth Disease")
16. Rubella ("German Measles")
17. Shingles/Herpes Zoster-Varicella-Zoster Virus, (VZV) Infection
18. Syphilis (*Treponema pallidum*)
19. Toxoplasmosis
20. Tuberculosis (TB)
21. Varicella/Chickenpox-Varicella-Zoster Virus (VZV) Infection
22. Zika Virus Infection

Antenatal Screening for Infection in KKH

Do's	Don'ts
Hepatitis B: Hepatitis B surface antigen (HbsAg) Human immunodeficiency virus (*HIV*): HIV antibody *Rubella*: Rubella IgG to assess immunity *Syphilis*: Treponemal chemiluminescent microparticle immunoassay (CMIA) *Urine analysis (UFEME) and culture* for asymptomatic bacteriuria Group B *Streptococcus (GBS) screening* ±Chlamydia/gonorrhoea (urine PCR) — *if STI risk factors present, e.g., age <25 years, history of STI*	Asymptomatic bacterial vaginosis Cytomegalovirus (CMV) Toxoplasmosis Hepatitis C — *if hepatitis C risk factors present, e.g., patient has HIV, history of intravenous drug abuse*

History

Date and time of exposure
Time of onset of symptoms
History of previous vaccination or infection
Current gestation of pregnancy

Examination

Temperature, pulse rate and blood pressure
Maternal well-being
Stigmata of infection

Investigations

Confirm maternal infection by testing for pathogen-specific IgG/IgM or viral polymerase chain reaction (PCR)

Management

Refer to infectious disease specialist and maternal–fetal specialist

Diagnose fetal infection — Definitive testing is by PCR via invasive testing. Amniotic fluid PCR analysis will <u>not</u> be positive until 6–8 weeks after the

maternal infection. Fetal urination is not well established until 18–20 weeks of gestation.
Ultrasound (US) surveillance of the fetus
Therapeutic options — depending on the type of infection

Limitations

Fetal infection does **not** necessarily mean that the fetus will be infected by the pathogen.

Risks of transmission and fetal damage depend on the pathogen and gestation at infection.

Invasive techniques may cause maternal–fetal transmission and infect a non-infected fetus.

Infections Associated with ***Perinatal*** Infections	Infections Associated with ***In utero*** Infections	Infections Not Associated with ***In utero*** or ***Perinatal*** Infections
Hepatitis B Hepatitis C HIV Herpes simplex (type 1/2) GBS	CMV Toxoplasmosis Rubella Parvovirus Varicella Syphilis Listeriosis Zika virus	COVID 19 (Severe Acute Respiratory Syndrome Coronavirus, SARS-CoV-2) Dengue

1. COVID-19 (SARS-CoV-2)

Maternal Risks

Pregnant women do not seem more susceptible to infection but are at an increased risk of developing complications.
Higher rates of Anxiety and Depression due to the COVID pandemic.

Fetal Risks

2–3-fold increased risk of preterm labour, 2-fold risk of IUD/stillbirth, increased risk of fetal distress during labour and caesarean section
No increased risk of congenital anomalies
Vertical transmission is rare

Management

Multidisciplinary team care. Infection control measures and donning of personal protective equipment (PPE).

Supportive treatment.

VTE thromboprophylaxis, including prophylactic LMWH, unless delivery is expected to happen within 12 hours or there is a risk of bleeding.

Continuous CTG monitoring in labour.

Chest X-ray with abdominal shielding is safe and essential if the woman is unwell.

Watch for signs of deterioration: increased oxygen requirements, respiratory rate ≥25/minutes, oliguria, acute kidney injury, drowsiness.

Therapy for ill pregnant women includes corticosteroids, tocilizumab, remdesivir.

The mode of delivery is based on obstetric indications.

Entonox can be safely offered.

Epidural or spinal anaesthesia is *not* contraindicated.

Vaccination

mRNA vaccines are safe for pregnant and breastfeeding women. It has been shown to effectively reduce the severity of infection, hospitalisation and ICU stay.

The adverse side effects of the vaccines are similar to those of the non-pregnant population.

Current data have shown that antibodies are transmitted via the placenta to the fetus and are also detected in breast milk. However, the nature and extent of protection for these babies remain uncertain. Long-term studies will be required to determine the effect of these vaccines.

The mRNA vaccines can be taken at any gestational age in pregnancy and during breastfeeding.

The mRNA vaccines do **not** affect fertility. Therefore, couples should be vaccinated before conceiving and do **not** need to defer their plans to start a family.

2. Cytomegalovirus (CMV)

Incidence

The most common viral cause of congenital infections — 3 to 4/1000 live births. The second most common cause of mental retardation after Down syndrome.

2% seroconvert during pregnancy. 70–90% of women of childbearing age have antibodies to CMV, with the highest seroprevalence in regions such as Southeast Asia and Africa.

Maternal Symptoms

1. **Primary infection** (most common).
2. **Non-primary infection** is either due to reactivation of prior infection or due to reinfection with a different viral strain.

Asymptomatic or flu-like illness.

Fetal Risks

The most common cause of congenital sensorineural hearing loss (SNHL)

30–40% risk of congenital infection for *primary* maternal infection

1–2% risk for *non-primary* infections

Risk of transmission increases with the trimester but the severity of fetal infection decreases.

US abnormalities appear at least ≥12 weeks after maternal infection.

a) ***Cranial findings***, e.g., ventriculomegaly, intracranial calcifications, periventricular cysts.
b) ***Extracranial findings***, e.g., hepatosplenomegaly, cardiomegaly, hydrops.
c) ***Placenta/amniotic fluid* abnormalities,** e.g., placentomegaly, placental calcifications, poly/oligohydramnios.

Miscarriage, stillbirth
Intrauterine growth restriction (IUGR)
Microcephaly, learning disability, seizures
Thrombocytopenia, jaundice, haemolytic anaemia
Chorioretinitis, micro-ophthalmia, cataract, optic atrophy

The main prognostic indicator for symptomatic fetal infection is fetal cerebral abnormality. Consider performing a fetal cranial US scan and/or MRI brain.

	Risk of CMV Transmission (%)	Risk of Severe Symptoms at Birth
Preconception	0–10	Negligible
Periconception	25–45	70%
First trimester	25–45	20%
Second trimester	45	5%
Third trimester	47–78	Negligible

If both scans are normal, there is a low risk of infant disability. However, this is **not** indicative of hearing outcomes. There is still a risk of SNHL.

CMV-infected Fetus	Definition	Prognosis
Asymptomatic fetus	• No US abnormalities • Normal cerebral MRI and normal biological parameters, fetal platelet count	• **Generally good** • Residual risk of SNHL
Mild or moderately symptomatic fetus	• Isolated biological abnormalities on full blood count (FBC) with no brain US abnormality OR • Isolated US abnormality	• Uncertain prognosis • Further follow-up with US or MRI • Discuss the option of termination of pregnancy (TOP)
Severely symptomatic fetus	• Severe cerebral US abnormality with thrombocytopenia	• **Poor prognosis** • Counsel on TOP

Diagnosis

Usually investigated after findings of an abnormal US scan or IUGR.

Maternal CMV-specific IgG and IgM antibodies but IgM persist for 4–7 months.

CMV IgG avidity test can help distinguish primary CMV infection from reactivated infection.

Low avidity (<30%) — **Primary CMV infection** within the past 3 months.

High avidity (>60%) — **Past CMV infection** >3 months ago or secondary infection.

Amniocentesis to detect CMV DNA PCR in amniotic fluid but should be delayed for 8 weeks after maternal seropositivity and after 18–20 weeks of gestation to allow for the accumulation of CMV in fetal urine. Non-primary infection is a difficult diagnosis. It needs CMV PCR of amniotic fluid for confirmation.

Interpretation of CMV IgG and IgM Serology in Pregnancy

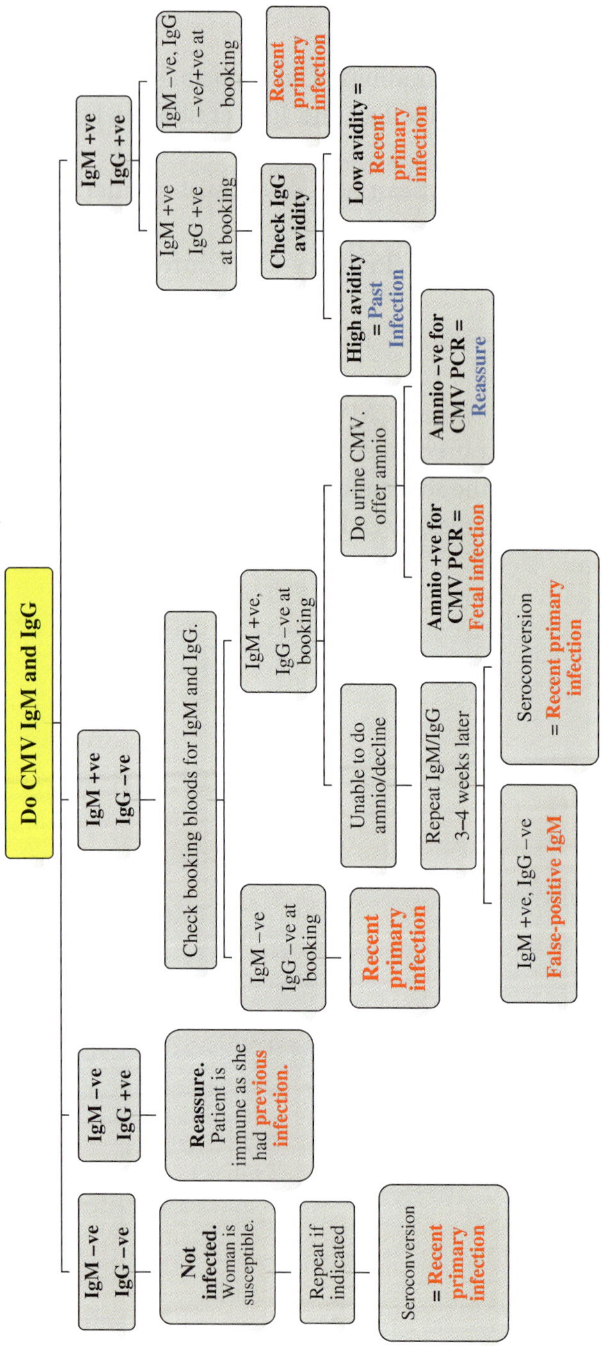

Management

Symptomatic relief for maternal symptoms. If CMV is detected in amniotic fluid, assume that the fetus is infected. Consider TOP if the primary infection is diagnosed in the first trimester. Take serial fetal US scans every 2–4 weeks for fetal abnormalities. Maternal antiviral treatment is currently *not* recommended routinely but should only be given in the context of research due to a lack of randomised controlled trials. However, high-dose valaciclovir has shown promising results as it increases the proportion of asymptomatic neonates.

Maternal CMV-specific hyperimmune globulin therapy (HIG) has not been shown to be effective in preventing congenital infection. Congenital CMV should be confirmed at birth, even if the fetal diagnosis is made by invasive sampling. Test the neonate's urine sample or saliva swab for CMV PCR immediately after birth or within 3 weeks of birth. Neonatal treatment with ganciclovir or valganciclovir for neonates with symptomatic congenital CMV and central nervous system (CNS) signs at birth.

Prevention

Hygiene and behavioural modifications: Avoid sharing utensils/food/drinks/ with young children, not kissing children on the lips and hand-washing after contact with their urine/saliva. No licensed vaccine is currently available for CMV.

3. Dengue

Maternal Risks

Acute fever, headache, retro-orbital pain, severe muscle and joint pains
Fine petechial rash
Dengue haemorrhagic fever
Dengue shock syndrome

Clinical confusion can occur with haemolysis, elevated liver enzymes and low platelets (HELLP) syndrome as they have a similar clinical presentation.

Pregnancy does not predispose to more severe disease.
Higher risk of adverse maternal outcomes with severe dengue, e.g., postpartum haemorrhage if there is marked thrombocytopenia.
Mortality.

Fetal Risks

There are conflicting data on dengue in pregnancy and adverse outcomes such as preterm delivery and low-birth weight.

Not shown to be associated with a higher risk of fetal anomalies.

If maternal infection occurs near delivery, infants might develop congenital dengue infection — fever, thrombocytopenia and hepatomegaly.

Management

Dengue should be considered as a differential diagnosis for pregnant patients with fever and no obvious localising signs and symptoms.

Supportive treatment with fever reduction measures
Inpatient management for pregnant patients
Careful maintenance of fluid and electrolyte balance
Trending of FBC if thrombocytopenic and liver function test (LFT) if transaminitis is present

Prevention

Avoid travel to dengue-endemic areas.

Mosquito bite-preventive measures should be advised, including using an effective insect repellent containing 50% DEET. Other alternatives, if 50% DEET is not tolerated, are para-menthane-diol, IR3535, picaridin or oil of lemon eucalyptus.

4. Genital Warts (Condyloma Acuminata)

Maternal Risks

Genital warts can proliferate and become friable during pregnancy.
Growth can be rapid and extensive during pregnancy.
Complete resolution of warts during pregnancy is seldom achieved.

Fetal Risks

Very small risk of warts on the larynx, mucosa or conjunctiva in infants and children. The most severe but rare condition is juvenile-onset respiratory papillomatosis (*JRP*). The route of transmission, whether transplacental, perinatal or postnatal, has *not* been established.

Caesarean section is indicated only for obstetric indications, if genital warts obstruct the pelvic outlet or if vaginal delivery would result in excessive bleeding or cause dystocia. It has *not* been shown to prevent human papillomavirus (HPV) transmission or JRP.

Management

Imiquimod, sinecatechins, podophyllin, podophyllotoxin, interferon, fluorouracil and podofilox should **NOT** be used during pregnancy.

Cryotherapy with liquid nitrogen, electro-cautery and laser treatment can be considered.

Trichloroacetic acid can be used. It is not absorbed into the system and has no known fetal effects.

5. Group B Streptococcus (GBS) Infection

Incidence

The most common cause of severe infection in newborns.

Overall mortality in early-onset GBS disease (presents within 7 days of birth) is up to 19% in preterm and 2% in term babies.
The prevalence of colonisation in pregnant women is 10–40%.
The risk of transmission to neonates is 50% among colonised women.

Universal screening is practised by most obstetricians in Singapore and involves a swab from the vagina and anorectum between 35 and 37 weeks of gestation or 3–5 weeks before the anticipated date of delivery.

- If the woman has a known penicillin allergy, request for clindamycin susceptibility for routine antenatal vaginal GBS screen (KKH protocol).

Treatment

No evidence that antepartum antibiotics reduce the GBS carriage rate or affect the outcome.

Treatment for GBS bacteriuria detected antenatally is recommended for any symptomatic women or if $\geq 10^5$ CFU/ml. These women will also need intrapartum antibiotics.

Offer treatment to women identified to be at risk of having an infected infant with intrapartum antibiotic prophylaxis.

No evidence that intrapartum vaginal cleaning will reduce the risk of neonatal GBS infection.

Indications for Intrapartum GBS Prophylaxis

1. GBS disease in a previous baby
2. GBS incidentally detected in the vagina or urine (GBS bacteriuria) at any time during the current pregnancy
3. Unknown GBS status at the onset of labour AND any of the following:
    a. Preterm labour <37 weeks of gestation
    b. Amniotic membrane rupture ≥18 hours
    c. Maternal pyrexia ≥38°C

When GBS Prophylaxis Is NOT Indicated

1. GBS colonisation/GBS bacteriuria in a previous pregnancy (unless there is an indication in the current pregnancy)
2. Negative GBS screening in the late gestation of the current pregnancy
3. Caesarean delivery before labour onset in women with intact amniotic membranes

Intrapartum Management

KKH regime:

- Intravenous 5 MU Pen G stat and intravenous 2.5 MU Pen G 4 hourly OR IV ampicillin 2 g stat then 1 g 4 hourly
- If penicillin allergy is suspected, but the reaction is *non-anaphylactic/ severe*: IV cefazolin 2 g stat then 1 g cefazolin 8 hourly

- If penicillin allergy is present and GBS is sensitive to clindamycin: IV clindamycin 900 mg 8 hourly
- If severe penicillin allergy is present and GBS is resistant to clindamycin: IV vancomycin 25–30 mg/kg/dose (max 2 g) once, then 15 mg/kg/dose (max 1 g) 12 hourly

Aim to complete at least 4 hours of intravenous antibiotics before delivery to be considered adequate neonatal GBS prophylaxis. In women with preterm premature rupture of membranes (PPROM), stop GBS prophylaxis if the GBS screen is negative or after 48 hours if the woman is not in labour.

Neonatal Management

Neonatologist to review baby after delivery.

Consider treatment if intrapartum antibiotics were *not* given or if the first dose is <4 hours before delivery.
Observe for at least 12 hours in high-risk groups.
Treat if the baby develops signs and symptoms of infection.

6. Hand-Foot-Mouth Disease (HFMD)

Symptoms

Blister-like or pimple-like rash on hands, feet, buttocks, mouth ulcers and fever.

Some may get sore throat, runny nose, vomiting and diarrhoea.

Fetal Risks

Normally, no risk to the fetus, but there have been very rare cases of miscarriage and stillbirth in infected pregnant women. Infection in the newborn can occur if pregnant women acquire infection close to delivery. Most infected newborns have mild infections but, in rare cases, may have severe morbidities such as overwhelming sepsis, multi-organ failure and mortality.

Prevention

Ensure good hygiene. Wash hands immediately after contact with an infected child, handling diaper changes or before handling food. Wear a mask when in close contact with children suffering from runny nose and cough.

7. Hepatitis B Virus (HBV) Infection

Incidence

3–4% of the population in Singapore are hepatitis B carriers.

Fetal Risks

No congenital syndrome.

Neonatal hepatitis — high mortality.

90% become chronic carriers if vertically infected.

Chronic carriers have a 25% risk of dying from cirrhosis ± hepatocellular carcinoma (the incubation period is 20–30 years).

5% occur due to transplacental transmission.

95% occur during delivery.

For women who are both hepatitis B surface antigen (HbsAg) and Hepatitis B e antigen (HbeAg) positive, the vertical transmission risk is 90%.

For women who are HbsAg-positive but HbeAg-negative, the vertical transmission risk is 2–10%.

Vertical transmission risk is higher in women with a higher viral load.

Management

Counsel, screen and vaccinate the partner, children and family.

Refer to a gastroenterologist for management, risk assessment and determine the need for antenatal antiviral therapy.

Record in notes and notify carers. Notify the Ministry of Health (MOH).

If HbsAg is positive, do HbeAg, HBV DNA viral load, LFT and coagulation panel. These should be done before 24 weeks of gestation.

Refer to the gastroenterologist for management and further workup, such as an ultrasound of the hepatobiliary system. Antiviral treatment is safe in pregnancy and is indicated in women with active HBV infection, cirrhosis or high viral load (>200,000 IU/ml, equivalent to >5.3 log 10 IU/ml). Tenofovir disoproxil is the preferred antiviral for treating hepatitis B in pregnancy.

Prevention of Neonatal Infection

Universal infection control measures during invasive procedures.

Immunisation is 85–95% effective for preventing HBV infection and subsequent development into a chronic carrier. Give hepatitis B immune globulin (HBIg) to the neonate within 12 hours of delivery. Singapore adopts a universal hepatitis B immunoglobulin policy. Therefore, all infants of HBsAg-positive mothers receive HBIg, irrespective of maternal HbeAg status.

First dose of HBV vaccine within 12 hours of birth
Second dose at 1 month, third dose at 6 months
Test for HbsAg and HbsAb at 9–12 months

8. Hepatitis C Virus (HCV) Infection

High-Risk Groups

Current or past intravenous (IV) drug users.

Diagnosis and Management

Anti-HCV positive — a positive hepatitis C antibody test implies a persistent infection. Check HCV PCR. Counsel and screen partner, children and family. Record in notes and notify carers. Notify MOH. Refer to a gastroenterologist for management and workup. Universal infection control measures during invasive procedures.

Maternal Risks

Increased risk of obstetric cholestasis (OC), which may occur earlier in pregnancy.

Pregnancy itself does not worsen the condition.

Interferon and ribavirin treatment are **not** recommended during pregnancy.

Fetal Risks

5% risk of vertical transmission unless the mother is co-infected with HIV (20%).

HCV RNA status negative, no reported transmission.

Babies of infected mothers need testing for HCV RNA at 6 and 12 months of age.

Breastfeeding is *not* contraindicated.

Vaccine — Not available.

9. Hepatitis E Virus (HEV) Infection

Transmission

Water-borne infection with faecal-oral transmission.

Maternal Risks

Usually, a self-limiting infection, but pregnancy is associated with a 6-fold increase in maternal mortality. Especially in the third trimester with hepatic encephalopathy, 15–20% fulminant hepatic failure and 5% mortality.

Treatment — Supportive treatment. Refer to a gastroenterologist for management. Notify MOH.

10. Herpes Simplex Virus (HSV) Infection

Incidence

Genital herpes lesions are usually caused by HSV type 2 virus
Increasing incidence of HSV type 1 amongst young adults
HSV1 is *not* protective against HSV2

Transmission Risk

40% transmission risk if vaginal delivery occurs with active primary infection from 28 weeks onwards or within 6 weeks of delivery. <3% transmission risk if: the primary infection occurred before 28 weeks of gestation or delivery was after 6 weeks of infection or in recurrent infection.

Maternal Risks

75% will have at least one recurrent infection
Infection is *not* more severe in pregnancy
The risk of neonatal herpes is low

Fetal Risks

1. **Neonatal herpes**
   30% will have localised disease in the skin, eyes or mouth, while the rest will be localised CNS or disseminated infection with multi-organ involvement.
   With *localised* CNS disease, 70% have neurological morbidity and 6% mortality.
   With *disseminated* disease, 17% have neurological morbidity and 30% mortality.
   Requires early recognition and treatment with acyclovir.

2. **Congenital herpes (rare)**
   There are case reports where the skin, eyes and CNS are affected.
   There may be fetal growth restriction or intrauterine death (IUD).

Current Practice

Diagnose with viral HSV PCR — offer HSV 1 and HSV 2 IgG serology to confirm if it is primary or recurrent genital herpes. Screen for other STIs. Treatment with acyclovir is associated with reduced severity of symptoms and duration of viral shedding.

Acyclovir is safe in pregnancy and has *not* been associated with fetal anomalies. It can also be used in breastfeeding women. Start oral acyclovir 400 mg TDS for 5 days and supportive treatment such as analgesia and topical lignocaine gel.

Most recurrent herpes is self-limiting and resolves within 7–10 days without antiviral treatment.

Start *suppressive therapy from 36 weeks* with either oral acyclovir 400 mg TDS daily or valacyclovir 500 mg BD daily to reduce recurrence at term and asymptomatic viral shedding.

Start earlier from 32 weeks for women with HIV.

A caesarean section is recommended for all women presenting with first episode of genital herpes at the time of labour or within 6 weeks of the expected date of delivery.

Routine caesarean section is *not* recommended for women with *recurrent* genital herpes infection.

11. H1N1 Influenza Infection

Maternal Risks

Pregnant women are at increased risk of developing complications. Four-fold increase in the risk of being hospitalised for complications compared to the non-pregnant population. Risk is highest in the third trimester. Women with asthma, morbid obesity, chronic obstructive pulmonary disease (COPD), diabetes mellitus (DM) and heart disease appear to have a higher risk of severe disease.

Effect on Pregnancy

It is associated with preterm delivery, especially in women admitted to ICU. Vertical transmission has *not* been reported.

Criteria for Hospital Referral

Signs of respiratory distress, oxygen saturation <94% in room air, dehydration, shock, sepsis, altered consciousness level or seizures.

Risk Factors for ICU Admission

Dyspnoea, tachypnoea (respiratory rate >30/min)
Supplementary oxygen requirement
Pneumonia
Tachycardia
Altered consciousness level

Antiviral Therapy

Most effective if given within 48 hours of the onset of symptoms. Inhaled zanamivir may be a good choice as there is no systemic absorption. Oseltamivir (Tamiflu) is an alternative.

Vaccination

Inactivated H1N1 virus.
Antibody response in pregnant women is as effective as in non-pregnant women.
Side effects: Pain at the injection site, myalgia, Guillain-Barre syndrome (rare).
Influenza vaccines are safe to be given in all trimesters of pregnancy.

12. Human Immunodeficiency Virus (HIV) Infection

Incidence — very low in Singapore.

Transmission Risk

Without treatment, mother-to-child transmission (MTCT) is 15–25%. It can be reduced to <1% with anti-retroviral therapy (mother and neonate). Mode of delivery is dependent on viral load. Breastfeeding is contraindicated.

Maternal risks — Pregnancy does *not* affect the prognosis and progression of HIV.

Fetal risks — Risk of miscarriage, preterm delivery, low birthweight in advanced maternal disease.

Management

A multidisciplinary team including an obstetrician, infectious disease specialist and neonatologist. Screen partner and children. Notify MOH. Universal precautions. At booking, check hepatitis B, C, syphilis, LFT, CD 4 count, HIV viral load and viral resistance test. Screen for genitourinary infections.

High-dose folic acid 5 mg daily. Prophylaxis against *Pneumocystis carinii* pneumonia is dependent on the CD4 count.

Advise all women to continue combined anti-retroviral therapy (cART) if they were on them preconception. If not, they should start cART by 24 weeks gestation to achieve an undetectable viral load of <50 copies/ml before delivery. Planned vaginal delivery is possible in women taking highly active anti-retroviral therapy (HAART) with a viral load of <50 copies/ml.

Delivery by elective caesarean section at 38–39 weeks in

(a) Women taking HAART with a viral load of ≥400 copies/ml.
For 50–399 copies/mL, consider a caesarean section.

(b) Women taking zidovudine monotherapy

- All pregnant women with HIV and hepatitis C should be on cART, regardless of CD4 count or HIV viral load.
- Vaginal delivery is possible for women receiving effective cART for HIV, regardless of HCV viral load.

Neonatal Management

Early cord clamping.
Early bathing of the neonate.
Anti-retroviral therapy within 4 hours of birth for 4 weeks.
Avoid breastfeeding.
HIV PCR test should be performed during the first 48 hours of life, 6 weeks and 12 weeks.
A confirmatory HIV antibody test should be done at 18–24 months of age.

13. Listeriosis (*Listeria* Infection)

Infections occur via food-borne transmission.

Prevention

Do not eat unpasteurised dairy products, soft-ripened cheese and pate.

Maternal Symptoms

Asymptomatic OR

Flu-like symptoms

Usually, a mild illness but can cause severe acute respiratory distress syndrome (ARDS).

More common in third trimester

Need a high index of clinical suspicion

Positive *Listeria monocytogenes* in blood, placenta, liquor or neonatal cultures

Meconium stained liquor

Maternal/Fetal Risks

Miscarriage, intrauterine death, premature labour.
Congenital listeriosis is a cause of hydrops fetalis.
Perinatal listeriosis.

Treatment

High-dose ampicillin/amoxycillin and gentamicin.
Co-trimoxazole can be used with high-dose folic acid for those with penicillin allergy.
Early aggressive treatment may allow the continuation of pregnancy with a good outcome.

14. Malaria

Maternal Risks

Pregnant women are twice as likely to be bitten by mosquitoes (*Anopheles* mosquito), to contract and die from malaria than non-pregnant women.

Fetal Risks

Miscarriage, preterm birth, stillbirth, IUGR, fetal anaemia.

Prevention in Pregnancy

Do not travel to a malaria-endemic country unless essential.
If travel is unavoidable, advise women to seek guidance from the centre with expertise in risk and avoidance strategies.

"ABCD" of malaria prevention

- o **Awareness** of risk — transmission risk, rainy or dry season, drug-resistant strains, rural or urban travel, length of stay.
- o **Bite prevention** — risk period dawn to dusk, skin repellents containing 50% DEET, knock-down mosquito sprays, insecticide-treated bed nets, clothing and room protection.
- o **Chemoprophylaxis** — no malaria prophylaxis is 100% protective. *Mefloquine* is the drug of choice. An *alternative* is chloroquine plus

proguanil but *not* efficacious in areas with resistance. Atovaquone plus proguanil can be considered, but there is *insufficient safety data*, and an infectious disease specialist should be consulted.

- **Diagnosis and treatment** must be prompt — suspect if flu-like illness and temperature >38°C when travelling or upon returning home for up to 1 year or more.

Safety of Malaria Drugs in Pregnancy

Mefloquine — safe in the second and third trimesters.

Its use in the first trimester may be justified if the risk of acquiring *Plasmodium falciparum* is high.

- Contraindicated in depression, epilepsy, hypersensitivity to quinine or mefloquine.

Atovaquone and proguanil — use if resistant to mefloquine or chloroquine.

Doxycycline — contraindicated as it affects fetal bone growth and teeth discolouration.

Primaquine — contraindicated as it causes haemolysis.

Chloroquine — contraindicated due to widespread drug resistance.

Symptoms

Fever, headache, myalgia, nausea, vomiting, diarrhoea, cough, jaundice, pyrexia, splenomegaly, respiratory distress.

Diagnosis

Blood film and Malaria rapid antigen test.

Management

Start anti-malarials immediately according to the species and severity of the disease

Multidisciplinary team care

Notify MOH

Watch for complications: coma (cerebral malaria), hyperpyrexia, convulsions, acute pulmonary oedema, hypoglycaemia, coagulopathy, venous thromboembolism (VTE)

15. Parvovirus B19 ("Fifth Disease")

Incidence

1% of susceptible adults are infected each year.
1 in 400 pregnancies.
The annual seroconversion rate among susceptible primary school employees is 5%, and hospital staff is 2%.

Maternal Presentation

Asymptomatic (30–40%) OR

Flu-like illness, arthralgia, rash (erythematous infectiosum), slapped cheek appearance.

Once the rash appears, viraemia has resolved.

60–75% of adults are immune.

Fetal Risks

Transplacental transmission rate — 30%.

No evidence of an increased risk of congenital anomalies.

Fetal anaemia can result in cardiac failure and hydrops fetalis.

If there is no hydrops, there is a 6% risk of perinatal death but a negligible risk of neurodevelopmental anomalies.

There is a 4–13% risk of fetal hydrops, which occurs about 3 weeks after the primary maternal infection.

Once hydrops occurs, there is a 50% risk of intrauterine death, 30% perinatal death and 10% neurodevelopmental anomalies. Spontaneous resolution can occur between 1 and 7 weeks.

No congenital syndrome.

Diagnosis

Maternal B19 specific IgM — detectable 3 days after the onset of symptoms and may persist for up to 6 months. Parvovirus B19 IgG is detectable by the 7th day of illness and persists for life. Conveys lasting immunity to infection. Elevated maternal serum αFP may be a marker for fetal parvovirus B19 infection. Invasive testing is only done when there are signs of fetal anaemia or hydrops. Fetal parvovirus B19 DNA by PCR is required via amniocentesis or fetal cord blood.

Interpretation of Parvovirus IgG and IgM Serology in Pregnancy

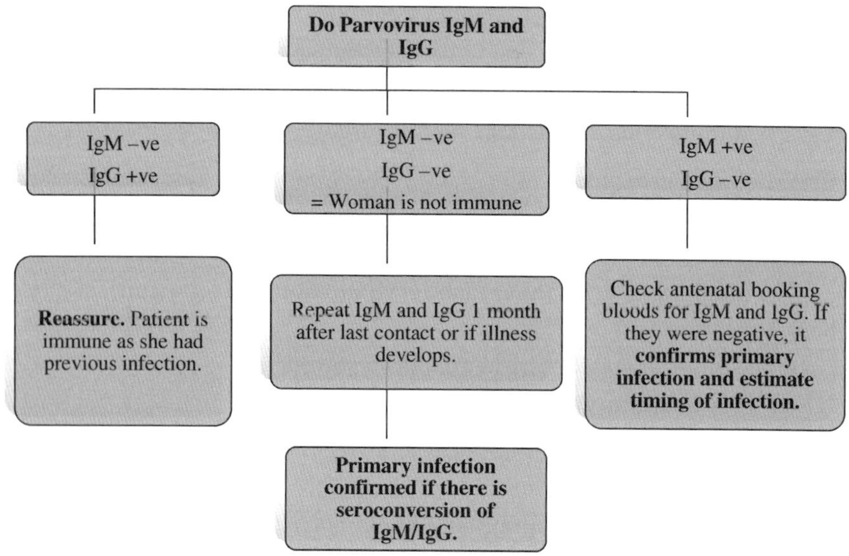

Management

a) If parvovirus IgG is positive — reassure the patient.
b) If IgG is negative, check serum IgM and IgG 1 month after contact.
c) If IgG and IgM are negative, the patient is susceptible but not infected.

Reassure the patient and follow up on any future contact.

If IgM is positive — refer to a tertiary centre. Multidisciplinary team care involving MF specialist and neonatologist.

Serial US scans: Start 4 weeks after infection/seroconversion and 1–2 weekly for up to 12 weeks (monitor MCA-PSV for fetal anaemia, MCA-PSV >1.5 MoM). Look for signs of fetal hydrops, e.g., skin oedema, ascites, cardiomegaly, pericardial effusion.

Fetal blood sampling and intrauterine blood transfusion. This results in the resolution of hydrops in 55%, usually within 6 weeks of transfusion. The common site is the placental insertion of the umbilical cord. Another site: the intrahepatic umbilical veins.

The fetus may need earlier delivery depending on the gestation.

16. Rubella ("German Measles")

Incidence

1–2% of women of childbearing age are thought to be susceptible.

Maternal Presentation

Asymptomatic OR

Mild symptoms, e.g., malaise, cold-like symptoms
Maculopapular rash
Arthralgia
Infectious from 7 days before until 7 days after onset of rash

Incubation period: 14–21 days

Fetal Risks

The risk of transmission decreases and the severity of infection decreases with gestation

***First 12 weeks*:** 90% risk of fetal infection, 97% risk of congenital anomalies

***12–16 weeks*:** 55% risk of fetal infection, 20% risk of congenital anomalies

***After 16 weeks*:** 45% risk of fetal infection, minimal risk of deafness between 16 and 20 weeks and a very small risk of congenital anomalies

Congenital rubella syndrome (***classic triad*:** *cardiac defects, cataracts, hearing loss*)

Eyes: cataract, retinopathy, glaucoma, micro-ophthalmia

Heart: patent ductus arteriosus (PDA), pulmonary stenosis (PS), coarctation of aorta, ventricular septal defect (VSD), atrial septal defect (ASD)

Ear: bilateral and progressive hearing loss

IUGR, oligohydramnios
Neonatal hepatosplenomegaly, purpura, jaundice, meningoencephalitis, thrombocytopenia

Diagnosis

Rubella-specific IgM antibodies peak at 10 days and present for 4–8 weeks.
IgG is present 1 week after the onset of the rash.
Use avidity test if indicated to distinguish between recent and past infection.
- Detect rubella DNA PCR in amniotic fluid.

Management

If infected in the first trimester, offer TOP.
Fetal growth scans.
Fetal echocardiography.

Prevention

Vaccination programme (15-year protection — 98%).

Check rubella IgG (immunity) before pregnancy; 2% of those vaccinated are non-immune.

If seronegative, advise MMR vaccination before pregnancy or after delivery. To avoid pregnancy for 28 days afer MMR vaccine.

Maternal reinfection in immune women has been reported, but the fetal risk is <5%.

Vaccine — live attenuated vaccine (MMR). Avoid pregnancy for 4 weeks after MMR vaccination.

MMR is contraindicated in pregnancy due to its theoretical risk.

No adverse outcomes or congenital defects are linked to inadvertent MMR vaccines. TOP should *not* be recommended solely on the theoretical risk of rubella embryopathy.

Interpretation of Rubella IgG and IgM Serology in Pregnancy

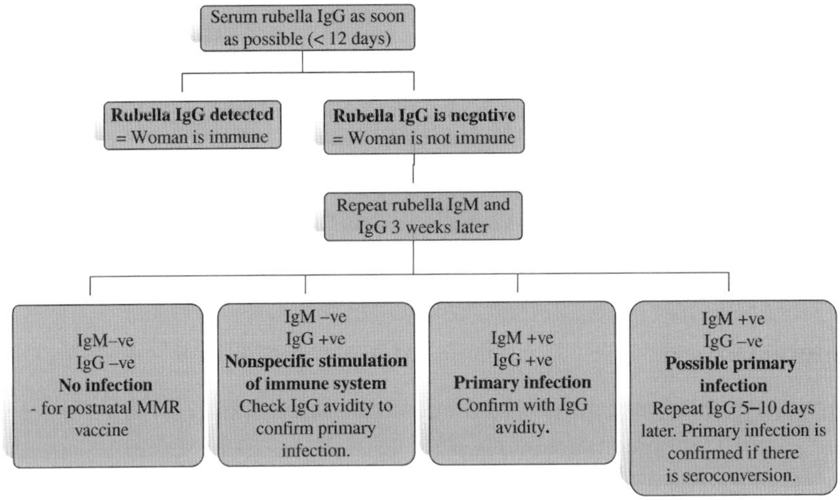

17. Shingles/Herpes Zoster-Varicella-Zoster Virus, (VZV) Infection

Mode of Transmission

Shingles, also known as herpes zoster, only occurs if a person previously had chickenpox because both conditions are caused by the same virus, Varicella-Zoster virus (VZV).

If a person is not immune to chickenpox, it is possible to be infected by someone with shingles.

However, the risk is low, particularly if the area of the rash is covered, e.g., by clothing or a dressing.

In shingles, the virus is passed by direct contact with the rash. Therefore, the risk is higher if the rash is widespread or on an exposed part of the body, such as the face.

Fetal Risks

Does not appear to have any fetal sequelae.

Management

Symptomatic treatment for pain.

Avoid contact with other pregnant women in case they are not immune to VZV.

Keep the rash covered until the last blister has scabbed.

18. Syphilis (*Treponema pallidum*)

Incidence

Active syphilis is usually detected by routine screening.

5 in 10,000 pregnancies.

Maternal Symptoms

Asymptomatic or positive serology at routine antenatal screening.

Primary infection

- Single painless ulcer (chancre) or regional lymphadenopathy.
- Heals spontaneously over 3–8 weeks.

Secondary infection

- Rash, fever, sore throat, weight loss, malaise.
- Resolves in 1–3 months; can enter the latent phase.

Fetal Risks

Transplacental infection occurs at any gestation.

Risk increases as gestation increases and with the stage of syphilis.

- **Transmission risk** — up to 100% risk if primary syphilis, 40% if *early* latent syphilis, 10% if *late* latent syphilis.
- IUGR, low birth weight, ascites, hydrops, hepatosplenomegaly, intrahepatic calcifications, 25% preterm birth, 30–40% intrauterine death.

- *30% congenital syphilis* — jaundice, pink nasal discharge ("bloody snuffles"), rash, skeletal anomalies, Hutchinson's triad (Hutchinson's teeth, interstitial keratitis, eighth cranial nerve deafness), mulberry molars, clutton joints (painless knee arthritis), saddle nose and anterior mid-tibia bowing ("sabre shins").

Management

Treat with penicillin G — cures maternal and fetal infection but will *not* reverse established fetal damage. If there is penicillin allergy/intolerance, refer to an allergist.

Consider desensitisation.

Watch for Jarisch–Herxheimer reaction as it occurs in up to 45% of pregnant women.

Symptoms occur within the first 24 hours of treatment, e.g., fever, rigours, rash and uterine contractions.

It is self-limiting and treatment is supportive.

- Screen for other STI.
- Refer to an STI physician. Perform contact tracing. Notify MOH.

Treatment of Syphilis in Pregnancy

	Primary/Secondary/ Latent Infection <2 years	Latent Infection >2 years/ Unknown Duration
First or second trimester	IM benzathine penicillin G 2.4 MU × 1 dose	IM benzathine penicillin G 2.4 MU weekly × 3 doses
Third trimester	IM benzathine penicillin G 2.4 MU weekly × 2 doses	

19. Toxoplasmosis

Incidence

2 per 1,000 pregnancies.
90% of women of childbearing age are susceptible.

Maternal Presentation

Asymptomatic OR

Non-specific febrile illness

Transmission to Fetus

The risk of infection *increases* with gestational age.

15% in first trimester, 30–40% in second trimester, >60% in third trimester

The severity of infection *decreases* with gestational age:

60% in the first trimester, 25% in the second trimester, 9% in the third trimester

The highest risk of having an affected fetus is between *15 and 30 weeks.*

Fetal Risks

The classic triad of intracerebral calcification, hydrocephalus, chorioretinitis (uncommon).

Spontaneous first-trimester miscarriage

IUGR, microcephaly, learning disability

Hepatosplenomegaly

10% of infected neonates will be symptomatic at birth, but if infected, up to 90% will develop neurological or ophthalmic problems later.

All infected babies must be treated at birth.

Maternal Diagnosis

Toxoplasmosis-specific IgG/IgM antibodies.
IgM appears within 2 weeks of exposure and can persist for 18 months.
IgG appears 2 weeks after exposure and is lifelong.
Immunity is lifelong unless the woman becomes immunocompromised.
IgG avidity test can be done to determine when infection likely occurred.
High avidity is associated with primary infection >4–5 months ago.

Fetal Diagnosis

Amniocentesis from 18 weeks to detect the presence of *Toxoplasma gondii* DNA in amniotic fluid.

May need to repeat amniocentesis as the presence of toxoplasmosis in amniotic fluid may take up to 6 weeks after maternal seroconversion, and fetal diuresis is only fully established from 18 to 20 weeks.

No accurate method to predict the severity of fetal disease.

Treatment

Spiramycin therapy for infected mothers results in a 60% reduction in the risk of fetal infection. Initiate within 3 weeks of maternal infection.

A combination of daily pyrimethamine, sulfadiazine and weekly folinic acid is more effective than spiramycin alone in preventing vertical transmission. Sulfadiazine is **contraindicated** in G6PD carriers as it causes haemolysis.

Treat fetal infection with **pyrimethamine, sulphadiazine and folinic acid** throughout pregnancy and the infant for the first year of life.

Serial US scans throughout pregnancy. Consider *MRI fetal brain* to detect subtle brain anomalies. If fetal studies are normal, there is a 30% risk of long-term sequelae, especially chorioretinitis and vision loss.

Prevention

Source: Undercooked or cured meat with Toxoplasma tissue cysts. The cat is the host.
Wash hands before handling food.
Thorough washing of fruits and vegetables, including ready-prepared salads, before eating.
Thorough cooking of raw meats and ready-prepared chilled meats.
Wear gloves and thoroughly wash hands after handling soil and gardening.
Avoid cat faeces in cat litter or soil.

20. Tuberculosis (TB)

Incidence

More likely in areas with a higher incidence of tuberculosis.

TB infection should be suspected in women who come from endemic areas and ethnic minorities with non-specific symptoms.

Maternal Symptoms

Fever, cough, shortness of breath.
Weight loss, night sweats, malaise.

Maternal Risks

The outcome of TB infection is *not* affected by pregnancy. Delayed or untreated infection can result in increased maternal morbidity.

Fetal Risks

Increased risk of preterm labour and IUGR. Congenital TB is very rare — primary hepatic complex and caseating granulomas in infants

Investigations

Tuberculin skin testing (TST/Mantoux test) is safe in pregnancy and the result is not affected by pregnancy.
Blood test — interferon-gamma release assays (IGRA).
After a positive TST/IGRA, evaluate for active TB. Look for symptoms and signs.
Do a chest X-ray (radiation <0.01 mGy) with an abdominal shield — safe in pregnancy.
If CXR is suggestive of TB, send off 3 sputum samples for acid-fast bacilli (AFB) smears and cultures and one sputum specimen for mycobacterium TB nucleic acid amplification testing (NAAT).

Treatment

Multidisciplinary team care including an infectious disease specialist, maternal–fetal specialist and neonatologist. Isoniazid, rifampicin, pyridoxine (reduces the risk of isoniazid-induced neuropathy) and ethambutol can be used in pregnancy.

Patients are non-infectious 2 weeks after initiation of TB treatment. Breastfeeding can be continued for women with latent TB on treatment or after 2 weeks of treatment for active TB. Breastfeeding is *contraindicated* in untreated TB or women with active TB that have *not* completed 2 weeks of TB treatment.

21. Varicella/Chickenpox-Varicella-Zoster Virus (VZV) Infection

Incidence

Primary chickenpox infection occurs in 3 in 1,000 pregnancies. 90% of the adult population is immune.

Maternal Risks

Severe disease in adults, particularly in pregnancy.
Severity increases with increasing gestational age.
Complications include pneumonia, hepatitis and encephalitis.

Women at greater risk of pneumonia are those who smoke, have COPD, are immunocompromised, have an extensive or haemorrhagic rash or are in the later half of pregnancy.

Fetal Risks

Fetal varicella syndrome (FVS) — 1% risk if <28 weeks, very rare between 20 and 28 weeks and does not occur if >28 weeks of gestation. Risk is lowest in early pregnancy — 0.5% in the first trimester and **highest from 13 to 20 weeks**. Defects do not occur at the time of initial infection but are secondary to a herpes zoster type reactivation *in utero*: Skin loss and scarring, usually unilateral and segmented hypoplasia of limbs, rudimentary digits, mental retardation with cortical and cerebellar atrophy, microcephaly, microophthalmia, chorioretinitis and cataracts, bladder and bowel sphincter dysfunction.

Diagnosis

Clinical diagnosis if a rash is present.
If there is a history of past infection, reassure the patient. Check maternal VZV IgG to confirm immunity.
If there is significant contact (face-to-face for 5 minutes or in the same room for ≥15 minutes), test IgG status.
Detection of VZV DNA in amniotic fluid does **not** imply fetal varicella syndrome; thus, amniocentesis is **not** recommended.

Management of Suspected Exposure to Varicella in Pregnancy

If IgG is positive, reassure the patient.

If IgG is negative, recommend VZIG as soon as possible. Effective within 10 days of contact.

The patient is potentially infectious from 8 to 28 days after VZIG administration.

The patient should be advised to notify a doctor if a rash develops after VZIG administration.

Check for seroconversion (VZV IgM) 3 weeks after exposure.

Management of Varicella in Pregnancy

Avoid contact with susceptible individuals (other pregnant women and neonates) until the lesions have crusted over.

Symptomatic treatment and hygiene to prevent secondary bacterial infection.

Oral acyclovir if the woman presents within 24 hours of the onset of the rash (800 mg 5 times per day for 7 days). Oral acyclovir is safe in pregnancy and reduces the duration of fever and symptoms.

Refer to the hospital if the patient develops: chest or neurological symptoms, haemorrhagic rash or bleeding, or a dense rash with or without mucosal lesions.

Can breastfeed if the woman is well. Express milk from the affected breast until lesions have crusted over, if there are active lesions close to the nipple.

Neonatal Varicella

The severity of the infection depends on the timing of the maternal infection. It is greatest if maternal infection occurs within 4 weeks of pregnancy, especially 1 week before and 1 week after delivery. Up to 50% will be infected, and 25% will develop clinical varicella. Mortality is up to 30% of cases. Varicella-zoster immune globulin (VZIG) is recommended if the mother develops chickenpox 7 days before or after delivery. Neonatal infection should be treated with acyclovir following a discussion with the neonatologist.

Vaccination

Two doses 4–8 weeks apart (s/c 0.5 ml varilrix or s/c 0.5 ml varivax) live attenuated vaccine.

Safe for breastfeeding. Should be considered pre-pregnancy or postpartum in women who are found to be seronegative for varicella.

Avoid pregnancy for 4 weeks after the last vaccine dose. Avoid contact with other susceptible pregnant women should a post-vaccination rash occur. Inadvertent exposure to the varicella vaccine in pregnancy has **not** been associated with fetal varicella syndrome or an increase in fetal anomalies. No need to recommend TOP.

22. Zika Virus Infection

Epidemiology

Transmitted by aedes mosquito or sexual contact.

Maternal Symptoms

Up to 80% of infected women have minimal or no symptoms.
Rash, fever.
Arthralgia, conjunctivitis.

Fetal Risks

Congenital Zika Syndrome (CZS):

Microcephaly.
Craniofacial disproportion, neurological symptoms.
Intracerebral calcifications.
Unclear if the risk is related to gestational age.
It may be independent of the presence/absence of maternal symptoms.
Limited knowledge of prognosis for CZS.

Management

Routinely ask pregnant women about their travel history.

Investigate for Zika if:

- ✓ Suggestive symptoms AND
- ✓ History of recent travel to a high or moderate Zika-affected area OR
- ✓ Sexual contact with a person returning from an affected area

Send serum and urine for Zika real-time reverse transcriptase PCR (RT-PCR).

An antibody test can be done if >1 week has passed since the onset of symptoms.

Serology tests have a false-positive risk due to cross-reactivity with other viruses, e.g., dengue.

Multidisciplinary team care. Refer to a maternal–fetal specialist, neonatologist.

Amniocentesis to test for Zika by RT-PCR should only be done after 20 weeks of gestation.

Serial US scans of the fetus.

Consider MRI fetal brain.

Discuss the option of TOP if <24 weeks of gestation.

The legal limit for abortion in Singapore is 24 weeks.

Prevention

No vaccines are available.

Women should avoid conceiving while travelling to an area with a risk of Zika virus transmission.

Both men and women returning from Zika-affected areas should practise safe sex/abstinence for:

- ✓ 3 months after returning from Zika-affected areas/last possible Zika virus exposure, if both partners have travelled together.
- ✓ 3 months after returning from Zika-affected areas/last possible Zika virus exposure, if only the male partner has travelled.
- ✓ 2 months after returning from Zika-affected areas/last possible Zika virus exposure, if only the female partner has travelled.

The last possible Zika virus exposure is either the date of leaving an area with a risk of Zika virus transmission or the date on which the last unprotected sexual contact with a potentially infectious partner took place, whichever is later.

After a Zika infection, a woman should avoid conceiving for 2 months following recovery from the infection.

CHAPTER 16

Skin Disorders in Pregnancy

Categories of Skin Conditions in Pregnancy

Hormone-related

There is an increase in pigmentation due to increased oestrogen, progesterone and melanocyte-stimulating hormone.

Common skin changes include:

- Linea nigra.
- Striae gravidarum (stretch marks).
- Hyperpigmentation such as around the nipple, areola and genitalia. **Melasma** refers to the light-brown to grey-brown macules or patches on the face. They are typically found on the cheeks and forehead.
- Hair, nail and vascular changes.

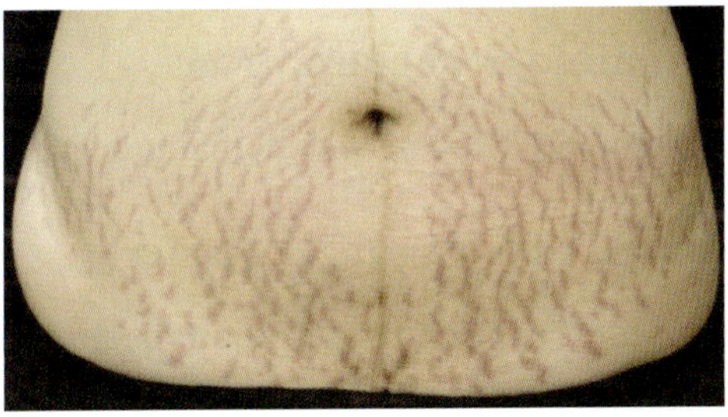

Striae gravidarum

Pre-Existing Dermatological Conditions

Atopic dermatitis, psoriasis, fungal infections, cutaneous tumours.

Pregnancy-Specific

Dermatoses specific to pregnancy are:

Most common

- Polymorphic eruption of pregnancy (PEP), previously known as pruritic urticarial papules and plaques of pregnancy (PUPPP)
- Atopic eruption of pregnancy (AEP)

Less common

- Obstetric cholestasis (OC)/intrahepatic cholestasis of pregnancy (ICP)
- Pemphigoid (herpes) gestationis
- Pustular psoriasis in pregnancy (PPP), previously known as impetigo herpetiformis
  - Most skin conditions resolve postpartum and only require symptomatic treatment.
  - Specific treatments are required for ICP, impetigo herpetiformis and pemphigoid gestationis.
  - Antepartum surveillance is mandatory for ICP, pemphigoid gestationis and impetigo herpetiformis, as these conditions can have adverse effects on the fetus, e.g., intrauterine growth restriction (IUGR), preterm delivery and stillbirth.

Coincident Dermatological Conditions

Acne, rosacea, erythema multiforme, erythema nodosum.

Skin Manifestations of Systemic Disorders

Dermatological symptoms can be manifestations of an underlying systemic illness.

- *Infections*
  - Bacterial, e.g., *Streptococcus*
  - Viral, e.g., human immunodeficiency virus (HIV)
  - Mycobacterial, e.g., tuberculosis (TB)
- *Autoimmune disorders*, e.g., systemic lupus erythematosus (SLE), rheumatoid arthritis

- *Endocrine disorders*, e.g., diabetes mellitus (DM)
- *Malignancy*, e.g., lymphoma, leukaemia

Drug Eruptions

Drug eruption is an adverse cutaneous reaction to a medication. It can range from a mild rash to severe cutaneous adverse reactions (SCARs). **SCARs** encompass acute generalised exanthematous pustulosis (AGEP), Steven–Johnsons syndrome (SJS)/toxic epidermal necrolysis (TEN) and drug reaction with eosinophilia and systemic symptoms (DRESS).

Pregnancy-Specific Skin Disorders

Evaluation

A. *History*
- Dermatological symptoms, e.g., rash, pruritus, itch, blisters
- Location, duration and time course of symptoms
- Exacerbating/relieving factors
- Any previous or current treatment
- Contact history
- Drug history
- Past medical/surgical history
- Family history
- Obstetric history

B. *Physical examination*
- Vitals, body mass index (BMI)
- Distribution and morphology of the skin lesions

C. *Investigations*
- <u>*Blood tests*</u>, e.g., liver function test, bile acids, if suspicious of OC
- <u>*Skin biopsy*</u> — indicated if the diagnosis is unclear or to confirm pemphigoid gestationis or pustular psoriasis in pregnancy (PPP)

Types of Pregnancy-Specific Dermatoses

Condition	Clinical Feature	Rash Presentation	Pregnancy Risk	Treatment
1. **Polymorphic eruption of pregnancy (PEP)** (previously known as PUPPP) 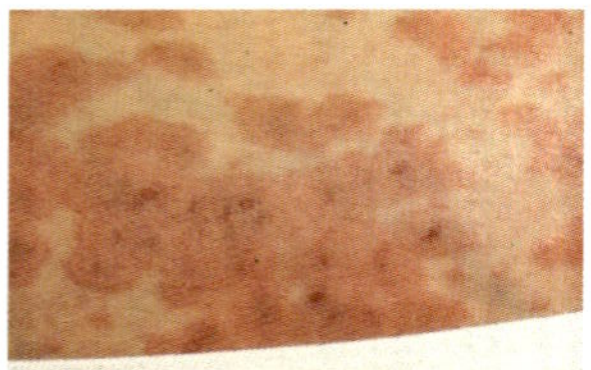	▪ Most common dermatosis associated with pregnancy. ▪ Mainly occurs in the first pregnancy ▪ Usually presents during third trimester to 1 week postpartum ▪ The condition may worsen immediately postpartum but resolves after a few weeks	▪ Intensely pruritic, erythematous papules, plaques or wheals ▪ Vesicles may rarely be seen ▪ **No** blisters ▪ Rash first appears on the abdomen, often along striae and spreads to involve the extremities ▪ Umbilical-sparing ▪ Face and scalp are usually *not* affected ▪ Palms and soles are usually *not* affected	▪ No identified maternal or fetal adverse effects	▪ Oral antihistamines (chlorpheniramine 4 mg ON). ▪ Topical corticosteroids (e.g., betamethasone valerate cream 0.1%) ▪ Topical anti-pruritic creams (e.g., suu balm cream, menthol 1% in aqueous cream) ▪ Systemic corticosteroids may be required for severely affected patients ▪ Resolves rapidly after pregnancy ▪ Recurrence is very rare. If it does recur, it is usually mild.
2. Atopic eruption of pregnancy (AEP) 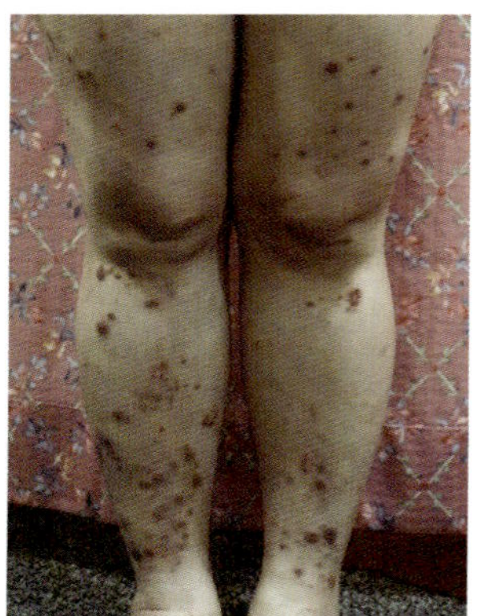	▪ Can present during any trimester but most commonly during the second trimester ▪ There is often a personal or family history of atopy ▪ 80% of women experience it for the first time in their life or after a long period of remission ▪ 20% will be an exacerbation of pre-existing atopy	▪ Pruritic, erythematous, scaly, excoriated papules and nodules on the extensor surfaces of the extremities ▪ No urticarial or vesicles **2 Types:** ▪ <u>*E-type*</u>: Eczematous changes affecting typical atopic sites, e.g., flexural surfaces, face and neck ▪ <u>*P-type*</u>: Mainly on limbs and trunk, prurigo nodules on arms and shins	▪ No identified maternal or fetal adverse effects ▪ The child may have a higher risk of developing atopic skin conditions	▪ Topical moisturisers 2–3 times daily ▪ Low-potency topical corticosteroids (e.g., betamethasone valerate cream 0.025%) to the thinner areas ▪ Mid- to high-potency topical corticosteroids (e.g., betamethasone valerate cream 0.1% or mometasone furoate cream 0.1%) to the trunk and limbs (e.g., neck, groin, flexures) ▪ Oral antihistamines ▪ Phototherapy, e.g., narrow-band ultraviolet light (UVB), may be required in more severe cases ▪ It can recur in subsequent pregnancies

3. **Pemphigoid gestationis** (previously known as herpes gestationis) 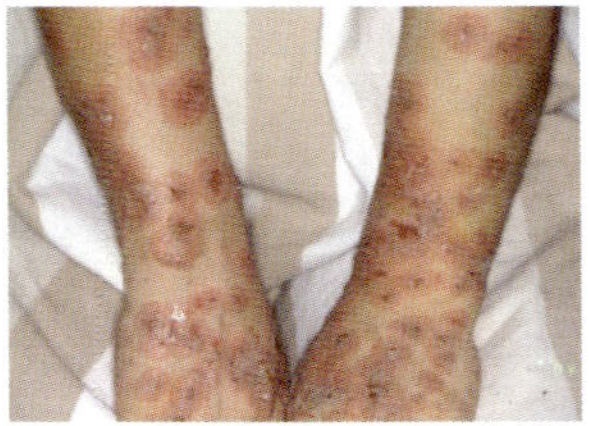	▪ Rare but severe autoimmune condition ▪ May have a genetic predisposition — associated with HLA-DR3/HLA-DR4 ▪ Associated with other autoimmune conditions, e.g., Graves' disease, type 1 DM ▪ Usually, onset is in the second/third trimester ▪ Postpartum onset (20%)	▪ Involves the umbilicus — initial periumbilical lesions (90%) may generalise ▪ Palms and soles are commonly involved ▪ Mucosal sparing ▪ Pruritic papules, plaques, and vesicles evolve into generalised vesicles or **bullae** ▪ The face and scalp are usually *not* affected	*Risks to fetus*: ▪ Newborns may develop similar urticarial, vesicular, or bullous lesions due to the maternal transfer of antibodies (10%) ▪ Usually mild and resolves within days to weeks ▪ Associated with – Low birth weight – Preterm delivery – Stillbirth	▪ Diagnosed by skin biopsy and direct immunofluorescence (DIF) – *Skin biopsy* shows sub-epidermal blistering with eosinophils – *DIF* from peri-lesional skin is positive – *IIF*-indirect immunofluorescence from serum may be positive (30–100%) <u>*Treatment of pemphigoid gestationis*</u> ▪ High-risk pregnancy Multidisciplinary (MDT) care ▪ Oral antihistamines ▪ Topical corticosteroids for mild cases. ▪ Systemic corticosteroids (oral) ▪ Topical or systemic immunosuppressants for severe cases (cyclosporin or tacrolimus) ▪ Serial growth scans for the fetus ▪ Avoid combined oral contraceptive pills (COCPs) postpartum, as they may cause flare-ups ▪ Recurs in subsequent pregnancy: Maybe earlier onset and increase in severity ▪ Recurs with COC pills and menstruation

(Continued)

(*Continued*)

Condition	Clinical Feature	Rash Presentation	Pregnancy Risk	Treatment
4. **Pustular psoriasis in pregnancy (PPP)** (previously known as impetigo herpetiformis) 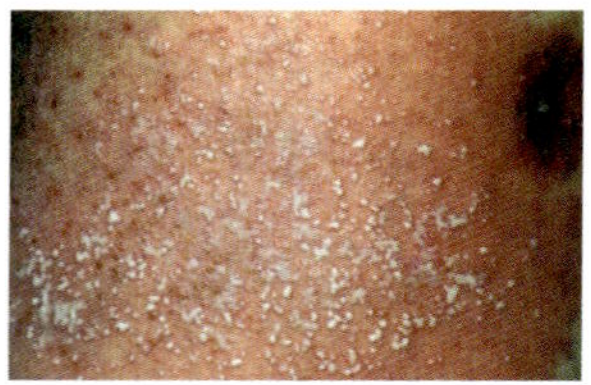 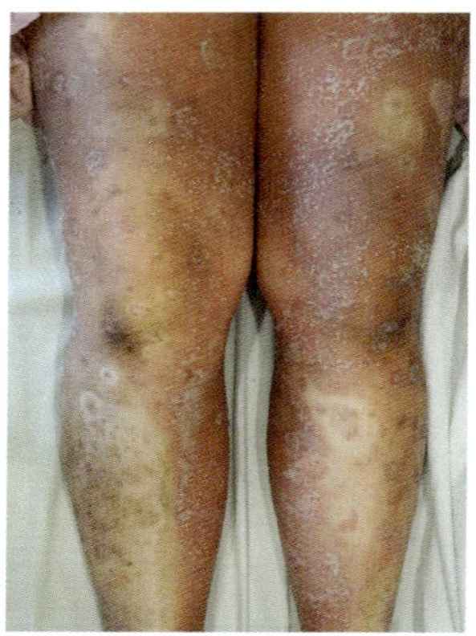	▪ Very rare variant of generalised PPP ▪ Patients may or may not have a history of psoriasis before the pregnancy ▪ Usually begins in the second or third trimester	▪ Face, hands and feet are *not* affected ▪ Usually *no* pruritus ▪ Round, arched or polycyclic patches covered with small painful pustules on an erythematous base that coalesce to form superficial sheets of pus ▪ Most commonly appears on thighs and groin in major flexures ▪ The rash may coalesce and spread to the trunk and extremities ▪ Can have systemic symptoms such as fever, malaise, vomiting and diarrhoea	▪ Reports of increased fetal morbidity ▪ Severe and extensive forms can be associated with: – Miscarriage – IUGR – Low birthweight – Stillbirth	▪ Diagnosed by skin biopsy – Presence of spongiform pustules, neutrophils, psoriasiform hyperplasia and parakeratosis **<u>Treatment of PPP</u>** ▪ High-risk pregnancy. MDT care ▪ Topical moisturisers ▪ Topical corticosteroids *<u>For more severe cases:</u>* ▪ Systemic corticosteroids ▪ Oral immunosuppressives (e.g., cyclosporin) ▪ Biologics (infliximab) ▪ Serial growth scans ▪ May recur in subsequent pregnancies: maybe earlier onset and more severe
5. **Obstetric cholestasis/ Intrahepatic cholestasis of pregnancy (OC/ICP)**	*For OC* — Refer to Chapter 11: *Medical Disorders in Pregnancy* Pruritus present but no rash			

CHAPTER 17

Depression in Pregnancy and Postnatal Psychiatric Disorders

Depression in Pregnancy

Depression affects about 1 in 10 pregnant and postpartum women.

Women with major depression who discontinue anti-depressants have an increased risk of relapse during pregnancy, hence the need for specialist care planning.

Recognition of symptoms of depression is important:
*(cardinal symptoms of depression***)

- Low mood/irritability**
- Loss of interest/pleasure**
- Poor sleep
- Poor appetite
- Low energy/fatigue
- Agitation or retardation
- Excessive self-blame
- Negative thinking
- Feelings of hopelessness
- Suicidal/infanticidal impulses

Look out for comorbid anxiety symptoms:

- Excessive worrying
- Palpitations
- Giddiness
- Nausea
- Breathlessness
- Muscle cramps

- Abdominal pain
- Tremors
- Panic attacks

Look out for comorbid obsessional compulsive or intrusive symptoms:
- Preoccupation with cleanliness
- Excessive cleaning
- Fear of contamination
- Intrusive morbid thoughts

Look out for psychotic symptoms:
- Hallucinations
- Delusions
- Irrational/bizarre beliefs

Screening for Antenatal/Postnatal Depression (PND)

A. Use the Edinburgh Postnatal Depression Scale (EPDS)
- Antenatal depression — cut-off score of 15
- PND — cut-off score of 13

B. Whooley questions

Two questions can be effectively used to identify possible depression:

1. "During the past month, have you often been bothered by feeling down, depressed or hopeless?"
2. "During the past month, have you often been bothered by having little interest or pleasure in doing things?"

A "**yes**" answer to either one or both questions is suggestive of depression, and the patient can be offered help with the question: "Is this something you feel you need or want help with?"

Screening also includes identifying those at greater risk of adverse outcomes, especially maternal suicide. It is strongly recommended that specialist psychiatric care be arranged for pregnant or postpartum women with the following:

- Past or present severe mental illness, including schizophrenia, bipolar disorder, psychosis in the postnatal period and severe depression.

- Previous treatment by a psychiatrist/specialist mental health team, including inpatient care (NB: *If the patient is currently seeing a psychiatrist, please check if that psychiatrist is aware of the patient's pregnancy — the patient can choose to continue with her preferred care provider).*
- A family history of perinatal mental illness.

Antenatal Depression is associated with:

a) Poor antenatal compliance/nutrition
b) Poor maternal fetal attachment
c) Higher risk of low birth weight babies
d) Higher risk of preterm delivery
e) Substance abuse as a means of self-medication

If untreated, antenatal depression progresses into the postpartum period in up to 50% of cases.

Management of Antenatal Depression

- **Refer to a psychiatrist and medical social worker (MSW)**

The main goals of treatment are:

1. Maintaining euthymic mood in the mother throughout pregnancy.
2. Preventing postpartum depression.

Treatment options:

1. **Psychological therapies supportive counselling** — consider as an initial treatment for mild to moderate symptoms of anxiety disorders before pharmacotherapy is considered.
   - Cognitive behavioural therapy (CBT)
   - Psychotherapy
   - Support and education
2. **Medications** — refer to Table 17.1: List of Psychotropic Medications.
   - General information regarding psychotropic medications in pregnancy and the postpartum period (NICE 2020 guidelines).
     - Small increased risk of postpartum haemorrhage with selective serotonin reuptake inhibitor (SSRI) and serotonin and norepinephrine reuptake inhibitors (SNRI) anti-depressants when used in the month before delivery.

Table 17.1 List of Psychotropic Medications

Medication	Dose	Comments
(a) Selective serotonin reuptake inhibitors (SSRI)		
Sertraline (zoloft)	PO 50 mg daily (max 200 mg daily)	May be taken in the daytime/night-time, depending on the patient's preference — most patients feel sedated and calm; starting dose can be 25 mg (half tab) with a gradual increase if well tolerated. Concern with worsening suicidal ideation and risk of septal defects. If used during the third trimester, there are risks of persistent pulmonary hypertension of the neonate and neonatal adaptation syndrome.
Fluoxetine (prozac)	PO 20 mg OM (max 60 mg daily)	Best studied SSRI in pregnancy for safety and efficacy — most evidence is available regarding its adverse effects in pregnancy. Has a long half-life and active metabolite.
Escitalopram (lexapro)	PO 10–20 mg daily	Start with 5 mg (half tab) first; can be helpful for those with obsessive-compulsive symptoms. Concern with worsening suicidal ideation and risk of septal defects. If used during the third trimester, there are risks of persistent pulmonary hypertension of the neonate and neonatal adaptation syndrome.
Paroxetine (paxil)	PO 20 mg OM	Controversy regarding its safety in pregnancy due to the risk of cardiac defects — *not* the first line SSRI in pregnancy. Need to perform fetal echocardiography during pregnancy.
(b) Serotonin and norepinephrine reuptake inhibitors (SNRI)		
Venlafaxine	PO 37.5–75 mg/day	Possible small risk of birth defects, e.g., cardiac, neural tube defects, cleft lip/palate, gastroschisis and hypospadias.
(c) Tricyclic antidepressants (TCA)		
Dothiepin	PO 25 mg ON (max 75 mg ON)	Concern with cardiotoxicity in overdose, family members to monitor the patient closely. Can be sedating with initial use; start low and titrate gradually. Possible adverse effects include constipation and dry mouth. May be used in second trimester for moderate-severe depression. Should be tapered off in the last trimester if depression is less severe.
Imipramine	Max 25 mg daily	More experience with its use, but poor side effect profile, e.g., constipation and dry mouth.
Amitriptyline	PO 10 mg ON (max 25 mg daily)	

Medication	Dose	Comments
(d) Typical/first generation antipsychotics		
Haloperidol	PO 500 mcg BD (max 2–10 mg daily)	For short-term management of severe anxiety. It may be used throughout pregnancy.
Trifluoperazine (phenothiazines)	PO 2–4 mg in divided doses	
(e) Atypical/second generation antipsychotics		
Olanzapine	PO 5–10 mg daily (max 20 mg daily)	Risk of maternal metabolic syndrome. Monitor maternal weight and screen for gestational diabetes mellitus (GDM).
Quetiapine	PO 25 mg BD (max 600 mg daily in 2–3 divided doses)	
Risperidone	PO 4–6 mg daily (max 16 mg daily)	
Aripriprazole	PO 10–30 mg daily	

- Risks of fetal cardiac abnormalities and persistent pulmonary hypertension in the newborn.
- Risk of discontinuation symptoms in the woman and neonatal adaptation syndrome in the baby with most tricyclic anti-depressants (TCAs), SSRIs and SNRIs, especially paroxetine and venlafaxine.

- The potential risks of drugs include major fetal malformations (during first-trimester exposure), neonatal toxicity (during third-trimester exposure) and long-term neurobehavioural effects.
- *Types*:
    - TCAs have been widely used throughout second-trimester pregnancies without apparent detriment to fetuses and are preferred in pregnancy.
    - *SSRI anti-depressants* also generally have a good safety profile in the second trimester. However, there are concerns about the risks of septal defects and spontaneous abortion with exposure during the first trimester and the risk of persistent pulmonary hypertension of the neonate with late trimester exposure.
- Management strategy includes using a minimal effective dose in divided doses to minimise peak levels and, therefore, fetal exposure.
- The use of anti-depressants should be gradually tapered off in the last 1 month to minimise neonatal withdrawal symptoms.
- If the pregnant mother is severely depressed and requires continued dosing, neonatal standby should be arranged peripartum.

  Psychotropic drugs to avoid unless there are no better alternatives:
    - *Lithium* — the risk of Ebstein anomaly in the fetus.
    - *Sodium valproate* — 10% risk of major congenital malformations, e.g., neural tube defects, cardiac defects, cleft palate and a 20–40% risk of poor neurodevelopmental outcomes.
        - Use effective contraception while on sodium valproate.
        - It should not be used in women of childbearing potential unless there are no other suitable or effective alternatives.
        - Switch to a safer option when the patient is trying to conceive.

3. For **insomnia in pregnancy**, can consider prescribing promethazine theoclate 25 mg ON (avomine).

Postnatal Depression (PND)

Definition

- Refers to a major depressive episode following childbirth (in some studies, it might also include milder forms of depression, otherwise known as a minor depressive episode).
- Typical onset is during the first 8 weeks but can arise during the first 6 months after delivery.
- It may resolve within several months if the woman is not treated but can persist beyond the first year postpartum.
- Depressive symptoms include depressed mood, loss of interest, poor sleep, loss of weight and appetite, tiredness or fatigue, poor concentration, excessive self-blame, negative thinking, and feelings of hopelessness or suicide.
- PND can be easily screened by asking two questions on low mood and loss of interest in the past month, with a positive screen being a "yes" to either question.
- With early intervention, PND is highly treatable.

PND is associated with:

a) Early cessation of breastfeeding
b) Marital strain
c) Impaired mother–infant bonding
d) Decreased maternal sensitivity — *impaired mother–child interactions can affect the infant's cognitive and emotional development.*
e) Maternal self-harm/suicide
f) Infanticide

Management of Postnatal Depression

Refer to a psychiatrist and medical social worker (MSW)

- Psychological therapies and supportive counselling are readily acceptable and effective for mothers.
- It is important to note that medication safety in breastfeeding should be considered.
- Switching anti-depressant medications is *not* advisable if the condition is stable.

- New mothers need not discontinue breastfeeding even if they initiate anti-depressants.
- *Common anti-depressants used:* escitalopram (PO 10 mg/day), sertraline (PO 50 mg/day) and venlafaxine (PO 75 mg/day).
- Fluoxetine is linked to irritability, sleep disturbance and poor feeding in some infants exposed to it in breast milk. However, there is little evidence of adverse effects with most medications.
- Aim for the lowest minimum effective dose if the mother is breastfeeding.
- *Common anti-depressants used in non-breastfeeding mothers:* fluoxetine (PO 20–40 mg/day), sertraline (PO 50–100 mg/day), escitalopram (PO 10–20 mg/day) and venlafaxine (PO 37.5–75 mg/day).
- There is good clinical experience with using dothiepin, a TCA (PO 25–75 mg/day in divided dosing) for nursing mothers, with no adverse effects in nursing infants.

Postnatal Mental Conditions

(a) Postnatal Blues

- Postnatal blues ("baby blues") is common following childbirth and occurs in 50–80% of women.
- Characterised by mood lability, tearfulness and lacking confidence in caring for the newborn.
- Usually peaks on the fourth to fifth postnatal day and resolves by 1–2 weeks after delivery.
- Postnatal blues is self-limiting and mild and is not considered a disorder.

Management of Postnatal Blues

- Reassurance
- Encourage support from her partner, family and friends to cope with the newborn.
- Improves with sleep and rest
- **Refer to a psychiatrist** for evaluation if mood disturbance persists for more than 2 weeks.

(b) Postnatal Depression (PND)

Refer to the previous section on postnatal depression.

(c) Postnatal Psychosis

- It is rare and occurs in 1–2 per 1,000 births.
- Is a medical emergency with a risk of self-harm (suicide) and infanticide.
- Usually occurs within the first month after delivery.
- Symptoms include affective (emotional) lability, agitation, confusion, hallucinations or delusions.
- *Risk factors*
  - If the patient has a history of postpartum psychosis, the recurrence risk is 25–50%.
  - If the patient has a history of bipolar disorder, the risk of postnatal psychosis is 25–40%.
  - If the patient has a history of bipolar disorder and a family history of postpartum psychosis, the risk is 50%.
  - Family history of bipolar disorder.
  - First pregnancy.

Management of Postnatal Psychosis

- Urgent referral to a psychiatrist and medical social worker (MSW).
- Requires close acute-phase outpatient management with case management or inpatient management if there are concerns with a risk of self-harm/suicide or infanticide, and if the family is unable to manage the patient.
- Treatment depends on presenting symptoms: start the woman on mood stabilisers (lithium/valproic acid/carbamazepine), anti-depressants, antipsychotic medications and benzodiazepines as indicated.
- Women on lithium need to stop breastfeeding as it is secreted into the breastmilk and can cause neonatal toxicity.
- For severe cases, electroconvulsive therapy (ECT) may be required. ECT is well-tolerated and rapidly effective.

CHAPTER 18

Medications in Pregnancy and Lactation

This chapter intends to share some common medications used extensively in pregnancy. Before considering any recommendations in this chapter, healthcare professionals are advised to check for the latest guidance and carefully weigh the evidence, or lack thereof, before use.

All pregnant women will encounter the use of medications during pregnancy. However, not all medicines are safe to take during pregnancy. In addition, there are concerns that some medicines could be potential teratogens that may cause birth defects, pregnancy loss, prematurity, infant death or developmental disabilities. Thus, the use of medications in pregnancy requires careful assessment of the evidence available to balance the risks of fetal exposure against the potential benefits of maternal treatment.

Teratogenic Mechanisms Associated With Medication Use

A teratogenic medication can cause abnormalities in the form or function of a developing fetus. It is important to note, however, that the response is highly individualised and influenced by multiple factors such as the following:

a) Genetic susceptibility

The genetic make-up of the mother and fetus can affect the susceptibility to teratogenic agents; for example, a fetal methylenetetrahydrofolate reductase

(MTHFR) gene defect and inadequate maternal folate intake may increase the risk of neural tube defects (NTDs).

b) Dose and duration of exposure

Most medications have a threshold dose, i.e., the lowest dose of a drug that may cause birth defects. For exposures below the threshold dose, the risks of birth defects are *not* higher than those in non-exposed controls.

Certain medications may be more harmful when the exposure is prolonged, whereas some may be harmful even when given as a single dose if the dose exceeds the threshold.

c) Route of exposure

Topical medications generally have lower absorption than systemic exposure from oral or injectable drugs; for example, ketoconazole cream applied to the skin is considered safe, but *oral* ketoconazole may *not* be.

However, *not* all topical medications are recommended in pregnancy.

d) Timing of exposure

The exposure of a developing fetus to a teratogenic medication at different gestational stages causes different patterns and types of malformation. The embryo is most vulnerable during organogenesis in the first trimester (refer to the figure on the critical period of development of various organs in the fetus).

e) Concurrent exposure or illness during pregnancy

Exposure to infectious agents or untreated/uncontrolled maternal illnesses, e.g., toxoplasmosis, herpes simplex, syphilis, diabetes mellitus or autoimmune disorders, may cause complications in the fetus.

Critical Period of Development of Various Organs in the Fetus

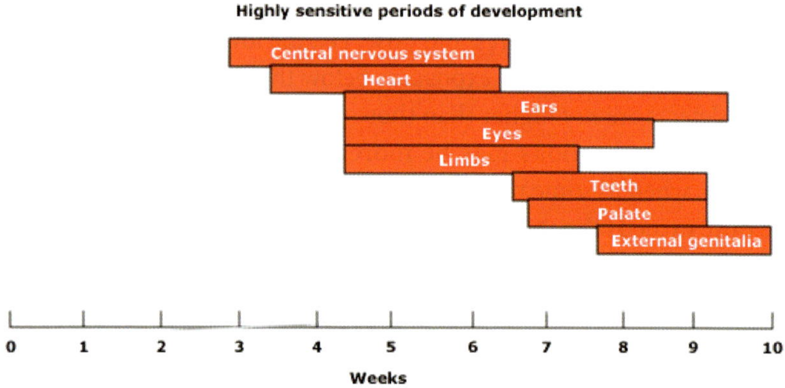

Adapted from: Unborn Patient: Prenatal Diagnosis and Treatment. Harrison, Golbus, Filly (eds). Philadelphia, Saunders, 1990. p. 44.

List of Medications That Require Special Precautions Before or During Pregnancy

The medication list we have compiled serves only as a rough guide for reference. It is relatively comprehensive but not exhaustive. The information given is accurate at publication based on the current literature.

When using drugs during pregnancy for a specific medical condition, always remember to balance the benefits against the risks and prescribe after shared decision-making with the patient. In addition, it is important to counsel women that there is a 2–4% background risk of fetal anomaly (FA) in the general population.

If in doubt, please consult the drug information pharmacist, general practitioner, obstetrician or maternal–fetal specialist for advice or clarification.

Medication	Remarks	When to Avoid
Cardiovascular		
Angiotensin-converting-enzyme inhibitors (ACEi), e.g., enalapril, lisinopril **Angiotensin receptor blockers (ARBs),** e.g., losartan, valsartan	Fetal hypotension results in fetal kidney hypoperfusion, anuria, oligohydramnios, limb contractures and pulmonary hypoplasia. It can cause renal tubular aplasia, cranial bone hypoplasia, intrauterine growth restriction (IUGR), prematurity, patent ductus arteriosus (PDA) and neonatal death. Possible association with increased risk of cardiac (e.g., atrial/ventricular septal defects) and neurological abnormalities (e.g., microcephaly) with first-trimester use.	Avoid in all trimesters of pregnancy. If the patient gets pregnant while on ACEi/ARBs, switch to safe alternatives immediately, e.g., labetalol/nifedipine.
Statins (e.g., simvastatin, atorvastatin)	Affect cholesterol biosynthesis. No consistent association with birth defects. Possible skeletal malformation. Linked to increased miscarriage, preterm labour (PTL) and low birth weight.	Stop at least 3 months before conception. For women with familial hypercholesterolaemia (FH): stop at least 1 month before conception. Avoid routine use during pregnancy (FDA). Caution: May consider continuing statins in high-risk patients (e.g. homozygous FH, history of AMI, CVA or established cardiovascular disease). Consult the cardiologist/ neurologist. Avoid breastfeeding while on statins.
Diuretics	Cause intravascular depletion, possibly causing IUGR and oligohydramnios.	Avoid in pregnancy. They may be used to treat pulmonary oedema, cardiac failure or idiopathic intracranial hypertension.
Beta blockers, e.g., propranolol	Can cause IUGR, fetal and neonatal bradycardia, hypoglycaemia and respiratory depression.	Use for short term if indicated.
Analgesics		
NSAIDs May adversely affect platelet and renal function. Can exacerbate asthma in about 10% of asthmatics. Can also cause gastric ulcers and bleeding.	May cause premature closure of fetal ductus arteriosus and oligohydramnios. Can be associated with persistent pulmonary hypertension in the newborn and renal problems in the neonate.	Avoid NSAIDS after 30 weeks of gestation. The US Food and Drug Administration (FDA) recommends avoiding NSAIDS after 20 weeks of gestation. It is safe to prescribe low-dose aspirin 150 mg ON for pre-eclampsia prophylaxis from 11–14 weeks to 36 weeks of gestation in women with risk factors for pre-eclampsia.

(Continued)

(*Continued*)

Medication	Remarks	When to Avoid
Opioids, e.g., morphine, fentanyl, remifentanil	Limited data available do *not* indicate teratogenic risks. Maternal sedation, constipation, urinary retention, nausea, vomiting and dependence if chronic use. Opioid use near delivery can cause maternal and neonatal respiratory depression and neonatal hypothermia. Withdrawal symptoms in the neonate (neonatal abstinence syndrome).	Short-term use with the lowest effective dose is recommended. Close monitoring of respiratory depression in the woman and neonate is needed.
Pethidine or meperidine for labour pain relief	*Maternal* sedation, nausea, vomiting, drowsiness, delayed gastric emptying. Usually given with an anti-emetic (metoclopramide). *Fetus*: reduced baseline fetal heart rate variability on CTG (maximum duration 60 minutes). *Neonate*: respiratory depression (the baby is likely to be affected if delivery happens within 1–4 hours of pethidine use) and neurobehavioural changes.	Do not use pethidine if delivery is expected within the next 4 hours of use. *Antidote*: Naloxone. Close monitoring of the neonate is needed.
Anti-emetics		
Ondansetron	*No* increased risk of stillbirth, PTL or small for gestational age (SGA). Currently, the available data do not suggest that use in the first trimester is associated with an overall risk of fetal anomalies (FA). Some small studies show a small risk of cleft palate and cardiac defects, but the absolute risk is small. The background risk for orofacial clefts is 11 per 10,000 pregnancies versus 14 per 10,000 pregnancies after use in the first trimester.	Avoid in the first trimester of pregnancy unless needed as the second-line treatment for hyperemesis gravidarum. In KKH, we perform an ultrasound scan of the fetus at 15–16 weeks and a high-risk FA scan at 20 weeks for maternal ondansetron use.
Skin/hair medications		
Retinoids or vitamin A derivatives: oral isotretinoin	Miscarriages and retinoic acid embryopathy: abnormalities of the central nervous system (CNS) (e.g., microcephaly), face, eyes, ears (e.g., abnormally formed or absent external ear) and skull, cardiovascular anomalies and thymus gland aplasia.	Avoid for at least one to three months before conception (the washout period of the drug is at least 35 days).
Acitretin		Avoid pregnancy four weeks before treatment, during treatment and for at least three years after stopping treatment.

(*Continued*)

Medication	Remarks	When to Avoid
Minoxidil	Promotes fetal hair growth and hirsutism in newborns.	Avoid in the first trimester.
Anti-depressants		
Lithium	*First trimester:* can cause cardiac defects, most commonly Ebstein anomaly of the tricuspid valve. *Second and third trimesters:* can lead to lithium toxicity and neonatal complications.	Avoid in pregnancy unless the benefits outweigh the risks. Consult a psychiatrist.
Selective serotonin reuptake inhibitors (SSRIs), e.g., paroxetine	Most studies indicate that SSRIs are *not* major teratogens. Some small studies show an increased risk of cardiac defects and postpartum haemorrhage with paroxetine. **SSRIs**: little or no increased risk of miscarriage, prematurity, low-birth-weight babies and perinatal death. Can cause neonatal serotonin syndrome, neonatal adaptation syndrome (withdrawal) and persistent pulmonary hypertension in the newborn.	Use as advised by a perinatal psychiatrist.
Psychotropic drugs: teratogenic risks from highest to lowest: sodium valproate, carbamazepine, lithium, lamotrigine, anti-psychotics, anti-depressants		
Anti-psychotics		
Typical antipsychotics or first-generation anti-psychotics	The risk of birth defects is *not* increased. Chronic use in the third trimester can cause neonatal toxicity and withdrawal syndrome.	Use if the benefits outweigh the risks, as recommended by the perinatal psychiatrist.
Atypical anti-psychotics or second-generation antipsychotics	The risk of birth defects is *not* increased, except possibly slightly increased risk with risperidone. Increase maternal obesity and gestational diabetes mellitus (GDM) with atypical anti-psychotics Chronic use in the third trimester can cause neonatal toxicity and withdrawal syndrome.	Use if the benefits outweigh the risks, as recommended by the perinatal psychiatrist.
Benzodiazepines		
Diazepam **Temazepam** **Alprazolam**	Best evidence: *no* increased risk of birth defects. Antenatal exposure is associated with miscarriage and preterm	Use only if the benefits outweigh the risks; use the lowest effective dose for the shortest duration possible.

(*Continued*)

(*Continued*)

Medication	Remarks	When to Avoid
Advised to use drugs with a short half-life, e.g., lorazepam, for short-term treatment of severe anxiety, insomnia and agitation	delivery (PTD), caesarean delivery and the neonate needing ventilatory support. Chronic use in the third trimester can cause neonatal toxicity and neonatal withdrawal syndrome, which occurs more in preterm infants.	Avoid use in the first and third trimesters and during lactation.
Anti-epileptic drugs (AEDs)		
Among the AEDs, lamotrigine and levetiracetam are safer to use in pregnancy. They do not increase the risk of physical birth abnormalities compared to the general population.		
Sodium valproate Used as a mood stabiliser and for epilepsy The highest risk of major FA: ~10% The background risk of FA in the general population: 2–4%	Can cause **fetal valproate syndrome**: NTD, oral clefts, midfacial hypoplasia, cardiovascular and urogenital abnormalities, hypospadias, polydactyly, craniosynostosis and microcephaly. It can also cause infant liver toxicity, IUGR and intrapartum fetal distress. It has a 30–40% risk of adverse neurodevelopmental outcomes, including lower IQ, autistic spectrum disorder, autism, behavioural problems and attention-deficit hyperactivity disorder (ADHD). The absolute risk of causing NTDs when valproic acid is used between the 17th and 30th days of fertilisation is 1–2%.	It should *not* be used in women of childbearing potential unless other AEDs are ineffective or not tolerated, as advised by a neurologist. Effective contraception is essential in women on sodium valproate. Start folic acid 5 mg when trying to conceive until at least the end of the first trimester.
Phenytoin Risk of FA: 6%	Can cause **fetal hydantoin syndrome**: abnormal head and face development, orofacial clefts, cardiac (ventricular septal defect) and urogenital defects, possible IUGR and adverse neurodevelopmental outcomes and intellectual disability.	Risk is highest 18–60 days post-conception. Take if the benefits outweigh the risks for epilepsy control in pregnancy, as recommended by the neurologist. Folic acid 5 mg daily.
Phenobarbitone Risk of FA: 6–7% Dose-dependent risk for major FA	<u>*First trimester*</u>: Birth defects: cardiac, orofacial and urogenital defects. <u>*Third trimester*</u>: Respiratory depression and neonatal withdrawal symptoms up to 14 days, IUGR and possible adverse neurodevelopmental outcomes.	Use in the first and third trimesters is associated with risks. Take if the benefits outweigh the risks for epilepsy control in pregnancy, as recommended by the neurologist. Folic acid 5 mg daily. Consider vitamin K supplements in the woman and neonate.

(Continued)

Medication	Remarks	When to Avoid
Carbamazepine Risk of FA: 4–5%	Increased risk of craniofacial defects (e.g., cleft palate, facial dysmorphology), NTD, and cardiovascular, genitourinary, brain and skeletal defects.	Take if the benefits outweigh the risks for epilepsy control in pregnancy, as recommended by the neurologist. Folic acid 5 mg daily.
Topiramate Risk of FA: 4–5% Dose-dependent risk for major FA	Oral clefts. IUGR.	Take if the benefits outweigh the risks for epilepsy control in pregnancy, as recommended by the neurologist. Folic acid 5 mg daily.
Trimethadione/ paramethadione	Facial dysmorphology, V-shaped eyebrows, low-set ears, high-arched palate, CNS defects and severe neurodevelopmental delay.	Take if the benefits outweigh the risks for epilepsy control in pregnancy, as recommended by the neurologist. Folic acid 5 mg daily.
Anti-coagulants		
Warfarin Vitamin K antagonist	**Fetal warfarin embryopathy** (5–10%). Nasal hypoplasia, skeletal abnormalities including short limbs and digits (brachydactyly) and stippled epiphysis, ocular abnormality and IUGR. Late pregnancy exposure can cause CNS malformations because of intracranial bleeding.	Avoid in the first trimester, especially in weeks 6–12.
Anti-thyroid drugs		
Propylthiouracil (PTU)	2–3% reported malformations: primarily face and neck cysts (minor birth defects) and urinary tract abnormalities (in males).	Consult an endocrinologist. It can be used in pregnancy. Dose <150 mg/day is *unlikely* to cause problems in the fetus. Risk of maternal hepatotoxicity with PTU exposure.
Carbimazole (converted *in vivo* to methimazole) It can cause agranulocytosis. Safe for breastfeeding.	2–4% reported malformations: *Most frequently reported:* congenital aplasia cutis and craniofacial malformations (choanal atresia, facial dysmorphism). *Other anomalies* include omphalocele, oesophageal atresia, patent vitello-intestinal duct, omphalomesenteric duct anomaly and VSD.	Consult an endocrinologist. Dose <15 mg/day is *unlikely* to cause problems in the fetus. Avoid in the first trimester, especially from weeks 6 to 10, for newly diagnosed women. Use PTU instead. It can be used in pregnancy if the patient conceives while on it. For such a case, we may *not* need to switch to PTU to avoid the potential risk of suboptimal thyroid control during the switching process and avoid exposure to 2 different anti-thyroid drugs.

(Continued)

(*Continued*)

Medication	Remarks	When to Avoid
Radioactive iodine Sodium iodide — 131 Fetal thyroid tissue is present by 10–12 weeks	*No* increased risk of birth defects. Destroys fetal thyroid, thus causing fetal hypothyroidism, mental retardation, cretinism and malignancy.	*Contraindicated* in pregnancy and breastfeeding: to confirm with a negative pregnancy test 48 hours before radioactive iodine treatment. Avoid conception for at least 6–12 months after treatment.
Antibiotics		
Chloramphenicol	Can cause bone marrow suppression, grey baby syndrome.	The grey baby syndrome begins 2–9 days after starting chloramphenicol treatment.
Aminoglycosides, e.g., streptomycin	Can cause fetal nephrotoxicity and ototoxicity.	Use if benefits outweigh risks; usually use gentamicin.
Trimethoprim	Interferes with folic acid metabolism → increased risk of NTD, cardiovascular defects and possibly oral clefts.	Avoid in the first trimester.
Nitrofurantoin	Possible haemolytic anaemia and neonatal jaundice.	Avoid in the third trimester.
Sulphonamides	Interferes with folic acid metabolism: risk of NTD. Can cause haemolysis in the third trimester → neonatal jaundice.	Avoid in the first and third trimesters. Avoid breastfeeding in premature or G6PD-deficient babies if on sulphonamides.
Tetracyclines e.g., doxycycline, minocycline, tetracycline	Can cause tooth and bone discolouration. High doses can suppress skeletal bone growth and cause teeth enamel hypoplasia.	Avoid in the second and third trimesters.
Quinolones	*Conflicting literature* on safety in humans. Animal studies show increased birth defects and carcinogenesis. Can cause renal, cardiac and CNS toxicity, impaired cartilage/limb development.	Avoid during pregnancy.
Macrolides, e.g., azithromycin, clarithromycin, erythromycin	Increased cardiac and genital defects.	*First trimester*: birth defects. *All trimesters*: genital defects.
Augmentin	Increased risk of necrotising enterocolitis (NEC) in neonates.	*Avoid* in preterm premature rupture of membranes (PPROM).
Metronidazole	Some clinicians avoid use in the first trimester as it crosses the placenta and has the potential for teratogenicity. However, meta-analysis has *not* found any	Caution in the first trimester (*conflicting data*). *CDC/BASHH*: *Safe to use* metronidazole in pregnancy, including the first trimester.

(*Continued*)

Medication	Remarks	When to Avoid
	relationship between exposure during the first trimester and congenital anomalies. An additional concern is that the drug is mutagenic in bacteria and carcinogenic in mice, but there is no evidence of harm in humans.	
Anti-fungal		
Azoles, e.g., fluconazole	A high dose (>400 mg/day) can cause miscarriages, craniosynostosis, mid-facial hypoplasia, and musculoskeletal, cardiac and eye defects.	Avoid in the first trimester. USE *topical* antifungals in pregnancy instead.
Anti-tuberculosis drugs		
Para-amino salicylic acid	Hypospadias, limb and ear defects	Avoid in the first and possibly in the second trimester.
Hormones		
Androgens **Androgen-derived progestins**, e.g., norethisterone, norethindrone **Danazol**	Can cause virilisation in female fetuses: <u>*First trimester:*</u> labioscrotal fusion <u>*Second and third trimesters:*</u> clitoral hypertrophy may cause ambiguous genitalia. Norethisterone is associated with hypospadias in male fetuses. Exposure after 8–10 weeks may be associated with clitoral enlargement in ~1% of female infants. The risk is increased with higher doses, e.g., 15 mg/day.	Avoid in pregnancy. The critical period is between 8 and 12 weeks.
Tamoxifen SERM (selective oestrogen receptor modulator)	*Animal studies and case reports*: *In utero* exposure may cause fetal harm/birth defects. Some defects are similar to those caused by DES.	Use is *contraindicated in* pregnancy. Good effective contraception is essential if on tamoxifen. The washout period is 2–3 months. **Differing data:** avoid for two to six months before conception (for RCOG, avoid for three months).
Misoprostol Prostaglandin E1	Induces uterine contractions and abortion. May cause skull defects, cranial nerve palsies, facial malformations, limb reduction defects and Möbius syndrome.	Avoid in pregnancy.

(*Continued*)

(*Continued*)

Medication	Remarks	When to Avoid
Glucocorticoids, e.g., **prednisolone**: <10% of the maternal dose reaches fetal circulation. **Betamethasone or dexamethasone**: 88% of the maternal dose reaches fetal circulation.	*Inconsistent data*: high doses may be associated with a cleft palate risk. Steroid use in pregnancy may increase the risk of PROM, IUGR, GDM, pregnancy-induced hypertension, infection and osteoporosis.	Avoid in the first trimester if possible unless for the treatment of refractory hyperemesis gravidarum. Consider the use of stress steroids in women on long-term or high doses of steroids at delivery. High-dose steroid use in pregnancy can cause neonatal adrenal suppression.
Spironolactone (anti-androgen)	Risk of feminisation of a male fetus.	The critical period is between 8 and 12 weeks.
Chemotherapy		
Anti-metabolites methotrexate (MTX)/ aminopterin Folic acid antagonist	Miscarriages. Can cause *methotrexate embryopathy or fetal aminopterin–methotrexate syndrome* (IUGR, microcephaly, meningomyelocele, decreased ossification of the calvarium, hypoplastic supraorbital ridges, small low-set ears, micrognathia, limb defects and mental retardation).	Avoid in pregnancy. Folic acid 5 mg daily when planning to conceive and throughout pregnancy. <u>Most critical period:</u> 18–60 days post-conception. Avoid conception for three months after stopping MTX. Advised effective contraception for women and men while on therapy.
Alkylating agent, e.g., cyclophosphamide Risk of primary ovarian insufficiency (POI)	Miscarriage, *birth defects* (malformations of the eye, skeleton and limbs, omphalocele, absent digits, cleft palate, a single coronary artery, IUGR and fetal bone marrow suppression) when used later in pregnancy.	Avoid use during pregnancy. <u>First trimester:</u> for birth defects and <u>Second and third trimesters:</u> for IUGR and pancytopenia. For a planned pregnancy, avoid conception for at least three months after stopping treatment.
Thalidomide	*Multiple defects in the following systems*: limbs (e.g., amelia, phocomelia), craniofacial, major organs (lungs, cardiovascular, gastrointestinal, genitourinary) and inguinal hernia. Neonatal mortality at or shortly after birth has been reported in about 40% of pregnancies.	Avoid use during pregnancy. <u>Most critical period:</u> 22–36 days post-conception. Effective contraception is recommended for men and women during therapy (including dosing interruptions) and for four weeks after the last dose.
Anti-rheumatic/immunosuppressives (disease-modifying anti-rheumatic drugs)		
Mycophenolate mofetil (MMF)	Miscarriage (45–49%), congenital malformations (23–27%), e.g., facial malformations (cleft lip/palate), eye and ear abnormalities (e.g., abnormally formed or absent external ear), distal limbs, cardiac, congenital diaphragmatic hernia (CDH), oesophagus, skeletal, kidney and NTD.	Avoid use during pregnancy. Avoid conception for six weeks after stopping treatment in women taking MMF. Sexually active male patients and/or their female partners should use effective contraception during the treatment of the male patient and for at least 90 days after the last dose.

(Continued)

Medication	Remarks	When to Avoid
Methotrexate	Refer to the earlier section on MTX and cyclophosphamide. Avoid use during pregnancy.	
Cyclophosphamide		
Aminosalicylates (sulphasalazine, mesalazine)	Relatively safe drug if taken with folate supplements. *Not* associated with birth defects, miscarriage, IUGR, stillbirth or PTD. Does *not* appear to increase the risk of NNJ or kernicterus.	Safe to use during pregnancy. Folic acid 5 mg daily. Can breastfeed term infants — stop if the infant has bloody diarrhoea. Avoid breastfeeding in premature or G6PD-deficient babies if taking sulphasalazine.
Leflunomide	Reports of birth defects in animals. Limited human data on safety.	Avoid conception for at least two years after stopping the treatment or use cholestyramine to enhance drug clearance to undetectable serum levels (<0.02 mg/L).
Tumour necrosis factor-alpha inhibitors **Anti-TNF (biologics),** e.g., infliximab, etanercept, adalimumab, certolizumab	*No* evidence of teratogenicity. *No* increased risk of miscarriage, PTD, stillbirth, IUGR or infections. Placental transfer of drugs begins at 14 weeks and increases towards delivery, with maximum transfer in the last four weeks of pregnancy.	Can use in pregnancy if the benefits outweigh the risks. **Avoid in the late second or third trimester.** *General guide*: To stop biologics at 22–24 weeks of gestation (to discuss with a medical specialist). *Infliximab*: stop at 21–22 weeks. *Etanercept* can be given until 32 weeks and, if needed, throughout pregnancy. *Adalimumab*: stop at 30–32 weeks. *Certolizumab* can be continued till delivery. **Avoid live vaccines, e.g., BCG, for infants for at least 6 to 12 months, ideally until 12 months after birth.**
Rituximab CD20-directed cytolytic antibody	Risk of infant B cell depletion. Limited human data on safety in pregnancy.	Avoid use during pregnancy. Stop for 12 months before conception.
Osteoporosis		
Bisphosphonates	Limited data in pregnancy. Theoretical risk of fetal harm, e.g., skeletal.	Avoid use during pregnancy. Stop for three months before conception. No need to terminate the pregnancy if there is inadvertent exposure. Need to monitor growth, skeletal development and neonatal calcium levels.
Live vaccines		
MMR/BCG, rotavirus/ varicella, herpes zoster, yellow fever, smallpox	Refer to Chapter 3: *Vaccination in Pregnancy*.	

Removal of FDA pregnancy letter categories

The health regulatory agency in Singapore does not assign pregnancy categories; hence, the US FDA letter categories were widely used. These letter categories by the FDA — A, B, C, D and X — have since been removed and replaced by the "pregnancy and lactation labelling rule" **(PLLR)**. The former system is often viewed as confusing and overly simplistic, and is misinterpreted as a grading system on medication risks. Thus, the content and format of the information presented in the prescription medication labelling under the PLLR are more comprehensive. The information is presented in the following subcategories: the pregnancy exposure registry, risk summary, clinical considerations and data. This aims to assist healthcare providers in assessing benefits versus risks and facilitate counselling of pregnant and breastfeeding mothers who need to take medication, allowing them to make informed and educated decisions.

Commonly Prescribed Medications During Pregnancy

Healthcare providers need to assess the benefits and risks of each medication before prescribing any medicine during pregnancy. The data on the safety of medications in pregnancy are usually collected from registries, case studies, case reports or animal studies.

In this section, we share some of the commonly used medications in certain conditions in pregnancy that have been recognised as safe to be used at the time of writing. The dose in a pregnant adult is the same as in a non-pregnant adult unless otherwise specified.

Analgesics

Medications	Comments
Paracetamol	Remains the safest choice in pregnancy. (**Dose** 500 mg — 1 g QDS.) Do not exceed eight tablets/day or two tablets/dose.
Paracetamol/ orphenadrine (Anarex®)	Commonly used as a muscle relaxant in non-pregnant adults. There is limited information on the safety of the component orphenadrine in pregnancy. Not recommended to use.

(*Continued*)

Medications	Comments
NSAIDs	Avoid NSAIDS >30 weeks of gestation (US FDA: avoid NSAIDS >20 weeks). May be considered for severe pain at the lowest effective dose and shortest duration possible (only if there are no suitable alternatives) It is safe to continue low-dose aspirin 150 mg every night (ON) for pre-eclampsia prophylaxis till 36 weeks in women with risk factors (KKH protocol 2022).**
Codeine (also available as a combination product with paracetamol, Panadeine®)	Codeine should be avoided in the first and third trimesters. Potential small increased risk of congenital birth defects associated with opioid use in the first trimester. Risk of neonatal withdrawal syndrome in the third trimester due to prolonged or chronic use of opioids during pregnancy. Codeine should be administered only if the potential maternal benefit outweighs the fetal risk, at the lowest effective dose and the shortest duration possible. To use for a maximum duration of 7 days. ***Maximum dose:*** Panadeine 2 tablets QDS (64 mg/day) Procodin 10 ml TDS (54 mg/day) Codeine phosphate 30–60 mg/day
Tramadol (also available as a combination product with paracetamol, Ultracet®)	Tramadol is a synthetic, centrally acting, analgesic analogue of codeine: refer to information on *codeine*. Short-term and occasional use only if no other suitable alternatives are available. **Dose:** 50–100 mg QDS.

Supplements in Pregnancy

Medications	Comments
Folic acid/folate	Folic acid decreases the risk of NTDs. All females planning a pregnancy should start folic acid before conception and continue during the first trimester. The recommended dietary allowance (RDA) in pregnancy is 400–800 μg/day, but higher doses are required in females at high risk of NTDs. In KKH, we routinely give all pregnant women folic acid 5 mg daily.

(*Continued*)

(*Continued*)

Medications	Comments
Iron	Iron is necessary for fetal brain and placental development; there are increased maternal iron requirements during pregnancy because of the expanding blood volume of the mother. The RDA for elemental iron in pregnancy is 27 mg/day, which is contained in most antenatal supplements. **Iron-deficiency anaemia (IDA)** is associated with adverse pregnancy outcomes such as low birth weight and preterm birth and, hence, should be treated in pregnancy. Refer to Chapter 11: *Anaemia in Pregnancy.* Oral supplementation is effective and usually preferred; however, parenteral iron therapy may be considered (from the second trimester onwards) if there is a poor response or if rapid iron replacement is required.
Calcium and vitamin D	Calcium and vitamin D are required for fetal skeletal development. Vitamin D potentially regulates many other cellular functions as well. The RDA for elemental calcium in pregnancy is 1,000–1,200 mg/day, depending on age. Women may increase their calcium intake through increased dietary consumption of calcium-rich food. Conversely, those with low dietary calcium intake may benefit from additional calcium supplementation. International guidelines recommend vitamin D3 up to 4000 IU/day in pregnancy and lactation or 100 μg maximum. Women at increased risk of vitamin D deficiency may require additional vitamin D supplementation of 1,000–2,000 IU/day.
Docosahexaenoic acid (DHA)	DHA is necessary for the normal development of the fetal brain and retina. The recommended intake of DHA is 200–300 mg/day. Seafood consumption (including fish) during pregnancy can help achieve the DHA intake goal; however, pregnant women should choose fish that are low in mercury and other contaminants. DHA supplements are also available.
Magnesium	**Dose:** 250 mg (elemental) tablets Recommended for leg cramps in pregnancy

Components of Commonly Prescribed Antenatal Vitamins

Medication	Comments
Ganilia®	**Dose:** 2 tablets daily — contains DHA and eicosapentaenoic acid (EPA), which are long-chain omega-3 fatty acids. *Contents of 1 capsule*: Vitamin A 950 IU, vitamin B1 1.05 mg, vitamin B2 1.05 mg, vitamin B5 3 mg, vitamin B6 1.3 mg, vitamin B12 1.56 μg, vitamin C 63.9 mg, vitamin D 100 IU, vitamin E 2.2 IU, iron 14.25 mg, iodine 57 μg, folic acid 400 μg, calcium (elemental) 76 mg, DHA 150 mg, EPA 30 mg, niacinamide 8.35 mg.
Natal Care Plus®	Helps support the fetus' brain and eye development. **Dose:** 1–2 capsules daily. DHA 102 mg, EPA 27 mg, arachidonic acid 18 mg, oleic acid 70 mg, D-alpha-tocopherol 4 mg. Suitable for all trimesters; recommended from 12 weeks onwards.
NeuroGain S®	Helps support the fetus' brain and eye development. **Dose:** 1 tablet OM. DHA 383 mg, EPA 23 mg. DHA-rich edible with added vitamin E as an antioxidant in a soft vegetable capsule. Suitable for all trimesters; recommended from 12 weeks onwards.
New Obimin®	**Dose:** 1 tablet OM. *Contents of 1 tablet*: vitamin A 3,000 USP units, vitamin D 400 USP units, vitamin C 100 mg, vitamin B1 10 mg, vitamin B2 2.5 mg, vitamin B6 15 mg, vitamin B12 4 μg, niacinamide 20 mg, calcium pantothenate 7.5 mg, folic acid 1 mg, iron 30 mg, calcium 35 mg, copper 100 μg, iodine 100 μg. To be taken before food for better absorption.
Prenaforte®	**Dose:** 1 tablet OM. *Contents of 1 tablet*: vitamin A 4,000 IU, vitamin B1 1.5 mg, vitamin B2 1.7 mg, vitamin B5 8.33 mg, vitamin B6 2.6 mg, vitamin B12 4 μg, vitamin C 100 mg, vitamin D 400 IU, vitamin E 11 IU, iron 27 mg, iodine 150 mcg, folic acid 800 μg, calcium (elemental) 100 mg, copper 2 mg, phosphorus 40 mg, selenium 20 μg, zinc oxide 25 mg.

Gastrointestinal Disorders

Medications	Comments
Acid-suppressing agents	**Antacids (e.g., magnesium carbonate mixture).** Generally, when prescribed at the usual recommended doses, most antacids containing aluminium, magnesium, calcium and simethicone may be used to treat heartburn or gastroesophageal reflux in pregnant women. Higher doses of aluminium-containing antacids should be *avoided* because of concerns over neurotoxicity. Simethicone is physiologically inert and not absorbed systemically; it is used as an antiflatulent and relieves bloating. **Dose:** antacid 1–2 tablets TDS, magnesium carbonate 10 mls TDS. **Histamine H2-receptor antagonists (H2RAs), e.g., famotidine.** To date, there are *no* known teratogenic effects with the use of H2RA; hence, it can be used safely throughout pregnancy. **Dose:** Famotidine — oral (PO) 20–40 mg daily or twice a day (BD), Ranitidine — PO 150 mg BD or IV 50 mg q8 hourly. **Proton-pump inhibitors (PPIs)** Evidence suggests low risk in pregnancy with good short-term use safety profiles. There is limited data for the newer PPI agents such as dexlansoprazole, esomeprazole and rabeprazole. Most of the data on safety in pregnancy are based on the first available PPI, i.e., omeprazole. **Dose:** PO/IV omeprazole 20 mg BD or 40 mg OM.
Anti-diarrhoeal agents	For **acute diarrhoea** in pregnant women, adequate hydration should be maintained. **Oral rehydration salts** may be used. **Probiotics can be given, e.g., lacteol fort 1–2 sachets TDS.** Activated charcoal may be considered, mainly for diarrhoea and poisoning due to foods and drugs. It is not absorbed systemically. **Dose:** two tablets of charcoal (500 mg) TDS. If an antimotility agent is required for more severe symptoms or decreasing the frequency of stools, loperamide or lomotil (atropine sulphate 25 μg, diphenoxylate HCl 2.5 mg) is an option. **Dose:** PO loperamide 2–4 mg TDS, PO lomotil 1–2 tablets TDS.
Laxatives	The initial treatment of constipation in pregnancy is similar to that in non-pregnant adults, i.e., non-pharmacological options such as increasing dietary fibre and fluid intake, and moderate exercise should be considered. **Bulk-forming laxatives** (e.g., ispaghula husk/psyllium) are safe in pregnancy as they are not absorbed from the gastrointestinal tract. However, these agents may take a few days to work and, therefore, are ineffective in improving acute symptoms and should not be used for faecal impaction. **Dose:** fybogel 1 sachet OM. Takes up to 48 hours to see the effects.

(*Continued*)

Medications	Comments
	Lactulose and polyethylene glycol (PEG) are **osmotic laxatives** that are poorly absorbed systemically and are commonly used in pregnancy. **PEG** is the preferred choice in pregnancy based on several sources. It does not cause any significant fluid or electrolyte imbalance. **Lactulose (semi-synthetic disaccharide)** should be used with caution in patients with diabetes mellitus and those requiring a low galactose diet. **Dose:** lactulose 10–20 ml BD. **Stimulant laxatives** are more effective in relieving constipation, but regular or chronic use *should be* avoided (e.g., bisacodyl, sennosides, senna). The use of stimulant laxatives may cause abdominal pain or cramping. If suppositories are required for faecal impaction/loading, **bisacodyl or glycerine suppositories** can be safely used. **Dose:** 5–10 mg once (rectal). **Dose for senna:** 1–2 tablets daily or BD. There are *no published studies* on the use of phosphate enemas during pregnancy; hence, these should be used with caution.

Nausea and Vomiting

Medications	Comments
Doxylamine **10 mg/** pyridoxine **10 mg combination** (Diclectin®)	If available, doxylamine (antihistamine)/pyridoxine (vitamin B6) is recommended as first-line pharmacotherapy to manage nausea and vomiting in pregnancy. May cause drowsiness. **Dose:** 2 tablets ON → can increase to 1 tablet every morning (OM), 1 tablet mid-afternoon and 2 tablets ON for severe nausea and vomiting.
Promethazine theoclate/ dimenhydrinate/ diphenhydramine	Antihistamines are used as an anti-emetic in pregnancy. These are preferred to metoclopramide because of their lower risk of extrapyramidal side effects. May cause drowsiness. **Dose:** PO/IV promethazine 25 mg TDS.
Metoclopramide	Dopamine agonists can be an adjunct treatment when symptoms persist following initial pharmacologic therapy. Because of the increased risk of extrapyramidal side effects (including oculogyric crisis), it should be used as the second-line therapy and its use should be minimised to 5 days. May cause drowsiness. Concurrent use of metoclopramide and prochlorperazine may increase the risk of extrapyramidal side effects (e.g., tardive dyskinesia) or rarely neuroleptic malignant syndrome (a life-threatening reaction, including high fever, confusion, rigid muscles and symptoms of autonomic nervous system instability). **Dose:** PO/IV metoclopramide 10 mg TDS.

(*Continued*)

(*Continued*)

Medications	Comments
Prochlorperazine	Phenothiazine derivative **can be used as the first-line therapy.** Concurrent use of metoclopramide and prochlorperazine may increase the risk of extrapyramidal side effects or rarely neuroleptic malignant syndrome (a life-threatening reaction, including high fever, confusion, rigid muscles, and symptoms of autonomic nervous system instability.) **Dose:** PO 5–10 mg 6–8 hourly, IV 12.5 mg 8 hourly.
Pyridoxine (vitamin B_6)	Pyridoxine monotherapy may be associated with improvement in mild nausea and vomiting symptoms. However, the combination of doxylamine/pyridoxine is more effective. **Doses** range from PO 10 to 25 mg TDS–QDS, although a commonly prescribed dose in KKH is 50 mg once daily to improve compliance.
Ondansetron	Ondansetron may be considered for treating severe or refractory nausea and vomiting in pregnancy when preferred agents have failed. **Refer to the earlier section on ondansetron risks in pregnancy.** **Dose:** PO 4–8 mg 6–8 hourly, IV 8 mg over 15 minutes 12 hourly.
Thiamine (vitamin B_1)	Women with prolonged, severe vomiting risk dehydration and a rare maternal complication, Wernicke encephalopathy. Intravenous hydration and vitamins should be administered, and thiamine should be administered before dextrose infusion to prevent Wernicke encephalopathy. **Dose (KKH regimen 2022):** *For first 3 days of admission*: IV intermittent thiamine 100 mg OM (diluted in 100 ml of 0.9% normal saline and run over 30 min) + IV hydration. If a dextrose-containing drip is indicated, it can be given after the first dose of thiamine. *If the patient has persistent vomiting after 3 days*: May continue IV thiamine, up to a total of 3–5 days of treatment. • IV vitamin cocktail daily (i.e., 2 ml of vitamin B complex and 500 mg of vitamin C to 500 ml of IV hydration) to 1 pint of IV hydration regardless of the intended volume of total hydration per day. • Dextrose-containing drip can still be given since thiamine is considered replenished.

Cough and Cold

Cough and cold medications often exist as a combination product; thus, careful consideration of the individual components is required.

Medications	Comments
Antihistamines	Chlorphenlramine (first-generation antihistamine) is usually the antihistamine of choice during pregnancy because of its long history of use with good safety data. However, it causes drowsiness. **Dose:** PO 4 mg TDS. When a non-sedating antihistamine is preferred, cetirizine or loratadine (second-generation antihistamines) is an acceptable alternative, preferably from the second trimester. **Dose:** PO cetirizine 10 mg OM, PO loratadine 10 mg OM.
Cough suppressants	Promethazine HCl and dextromethorphan preparations are safe to be used in pregnancy. **Dose:** dextromethorphan 10 ml TDS. Codeine-containing cough preparations should be avoided, especially in the first and third trimesters. The lowest effective dose should be used for the shortest duration if necessary. **Dose:** PO procodin 10 ml TDS, maximum duration of 7 days. Refer to information on *codeine*.
Cough expectorants	Diphenhydramine (with ammonium chloride) and guaifenesin preparations may be used for productive (phlegmy) cough. **Dose:** PO diphenhydramine 10 ml TDS.
Mucolytics	Acetylcysteine and bromhexine may be used in pregnancy. **Dose:** PO acetylcysteine 600 mg daily/200 mg BD or TDS, PO bromhexine 1 tablet TDS
Nasal preparations	Isotonic or hypertonic sodium chloride nasal preparations are suitable for rhinitis in pregnancy. Oxymetazoline may be considered if acute relief of severe nasal congestion is needed, but for short-term use only. There is a risk of rebound congestion with prolonged use. **Dose:** oxymetazoline, 0.05% nasal drops, 1 drop TDS PRN. Decongestants containing phenylephrine or pseudoephedrine may be associated with an increased risk of congenital anomalies (e.g., gastroschisis, small intestinal atresia) in the first trimester, possibly because of vasoconstrictive effects; their use is **not** recommended in pregnancy.

Anti-Asthmatics

During pregnancy, asthma should be well controlled to prevent maternal and fetal complications such as pre-eclampsia, preterm birth, fetal growth restriction and neonatal hypoxia. The principles of pharmacologic therapy for asthma during pregnancy are similar to those for non-pregnant patients, as the risks of uncontrolled asthma are greater than any possible adverse effects of conventional asthma medications.

In general, medications used to treat asthma are safe in pregnancy and pregnant women need to continue their medications during pregnancy to ensure good asthma control.

Medications	Comments
Short-acting β_2 agonists (e.g., salbutamol, inhaler or nebulising solution)	Short-acting β_2 agonists should be used as usual for acute asthma exacerbations in pregnancy.
Long-acting β_2 agonists (e.g., salmeterol, formoterol)	Long-acting β_2 agonists should be used together with an inhaled corticosteroid (ICS), usually as a combination product. There are more data on salmeterol (with ICS) in pregnancy. However, the patient should be on the same asthma medication as before pregnancy if her condition is well controlled.
ICS (Inhaled corticosteroids) (e.g., budesonide, beclomethasone, fluticasone, ciclesonide)	ICS should be used as usual for anti-inflammatory and maintenance treatment in pregnancy. The lowest dose that maintains asthma control should be used. There are more data on budesonide, beclomethasone and fluticasone in pregnancy. However, the patient should be on the same asthma medication as before pregnancy if her condition is well controlled.
Systemic steroids	Systemic steroids should be used as usual to treat asthma exacerbations and severe asthma if indicated during pregnancy. Prednisolone is the oral steroid of choice in pregnancy as it is extensively metabolised by placental enzymes, so only a small amount reaches the fetus. **Dose:** 10–20 mg daily, maximum of 60 mg daily. Hydrocortisone may be used for parenteral administration.
Montelukast	There are limited data on the use of montelukast in pregnancy, but available data have *not* demonstrated an increased risk of teratogenic effects. Montelukast should *not* be withheld during pregnancy when clinically indicated.
Theophylline	Theophylline may be used in pregnancy to maintain asthma control, but monitoring of levels is recommended because of pregnancy-induced physiologic changes.

Common Skin Conditions in Pregnancy (Eczema/Acne)

Eczema

Medications	Comments
Emollients/moisturisers (e.g., aqueous cream, soft white paraffin ointment)	Skin hydration is a key component of the overall management of eczema, including in pregnant women. Emollients are safe for use in pregnancy.
Topical corticosteroids	Topical corticosteroids may be used in pregnancy to treat eczema when the use of emollients alone is insufficient. ▪ These should *not* be used on extensive areas, in large amounts or for prolonged periods in pregnant women. ▪ It is recommended that lower potency (mild to moderate) topical corticosteroids are used in pregnancy rather than the potent ones. ▪ *If absolutely necessary*, the potent or very potent preparations should be used for the shortest duration possible, in very small amounts. ▪ Limited data suggest that prolonged use of potent topical corticosteroids

Types and Dosages of Topical Creams

Medication	Dose	Comments
Betamethasone cream (0.025%)	Once daily or when necessary	Topical use. Apply thinly.
Calamine lotion	When necessary	Topical use
Chlorhexidine 1% cream	Once daily or when necessary	Antiseptic cream
Combiderm/Triderm® (Betamethasone 0.05%/ Clotrimazole 1%/ Gentamicin 0.1% cream)	Once daily or when necessary	Allergy and inflammatory dermatitis, dermatomycosis
Hydrocortisone cream 1%	Once daily or when necessary	Topical use. Apply thinly.
Miconazole 2% cream	Contains miconazole	Antifungal cream. Apply thinly.
Miconazole 2%, hydrocortiscone 1%	Once daily or when necessary	
Neoderm® (neomycin/ hydrocortisone) cream	Once daily or when necessary	Corticosteroid cream with an anti-infective agent
Travocort® cream (Isoconazole, diflucortolone valerate)	Once daily or when necessary	Broad-spectrum antifungal with a steroid additive. Apply thinly.

(*Continued*)

(*Continued*)

Medications	Comments
Topical corticosteroids	may be associated with lower birth weight, although the risk is likely low. ▪ Topical corticosteroids should be applied with caution to areas with high percutaneous absorption (e.g., face, armpits, skin folds, vulva) or broken skin. ▪ Infected eczema areas may be treated with a combination product of topical corticosteroids and antimicrobials such as fusidic acid.
Antihistamines	Chlorpheniramine (first-generation antihistamine) is usually the antihistamine of choice during pregnancy because of its long history of use with good safety data; however, it causes drowsiness. When a non-sedating antihistamine is preferred, cetirizine or loratadine (second-generation antihistamines) is an acceptable alternative, preferably from the second trimester onwards.

Acne

Treatment of acne in pregnant women requires consideration of the severity of the acne and the safety of the medications in pregnancy.

Common acne therapies contraindicated in pregnant women include oral retinoids (isotretinoin), tetracyclines (doxycycline, minocycline) and hormonal medications.

Topical retinoids such as adapalene are also *not* recommended in pregnancy.

Refer to the section: *List of Medications That Require Special Precautions Before or During Pregnancy* for isotretinoin and tetracyclines.

Medications	Comments
Topical antibiotics and acne agents	Topical clindamycin and erythromycin are available as both individual and fixed-combination products; combining antibiotic therapy with benzoyl peroxide decreases the development of antibiotic resistance and improves treatment efficacy. These can be used safely during pregnancy. Topical azelaic acid can also be used during pregnancy; additionally, this is useful in patients with acne and post-inflammatory hyperpigmentation as it induces hypopigmentation in darker skin. Topical salicylic acid is also unlikely to pose a risk to the fetus.
Oral antibiotics	Erythromycin can be used as a second-line treatment or for more severe acne in pregnancy. Cephalexin is also safe for use in pregnancy.

GDM and Diabetes Medications

GDM is a condition in which carbohydrate intolerance develops during pregnancy. Women with GDM have a higher risk of developing pre-eclampsia, undergoing caesarean delivery and developing diabetes (mainly type 2) later on. There are also significant fetal risks, such as macrosomia, neonatal hypoglycaemia and neonatal respiratory distress syndrome (RDS).

GDM may be adequately controlled with lifestyle changes, mainly dietary modifications and exercise. However, pharmacologic treatment is recommended when these interventions alone cannot achieve target glucose levels.

Medications	Comments
Insulin	Insulin is a naturally occurring polypeptide hormone; it is the preferred treatment for diabetes in pregnancy. None of the currently available human insulin preparations have been demonstrated to cross the placenta.
Biguanide: Metformin	Metformin is associated with a lower risk of neonatal hypoglycaemia and less maternal weight gain than that with insulin, but it crosses the placenta. Data have shown no increase in the risk of fetal abnormalities or neonatal adverse outcomes. Short-time data on metformin in pregnancy has been reassuring. Metformin may be considered in pregnant women who decline insulin therapy, are unable to administer or cannot afford insulin. About 40% of women taking metformin will require additional insulin therapy.
Sulphonylureas	Sulphonylureas, particularly short-acting sulphonylureas such as glipizide, are known to cross the placenta and have been associated with increased neonatal hypoglycaemia. Glibenclamide (also known as glyburide) is a long-acting sulphonylurea that can be used in pregnancy. Data have shown no increase in the risk of FA. However, compared to insulin, it results in higher birth weight and a higher risk of neonatal hypoglycaemia. About 20% of women taking glibenclamide will require additional insulin therapy.
Other oral and non-insulin injectable anti-diabetic agents	*Not* recommended at this point because of the lack of safety and long-term data on pregnancy.

Hypertension in Pregnancy

Hypertensive agents such as ACEi (e.g., enalapril) or ARBs (e.g., losartan) are *contraindicated* during pregnancy. In addition, certain beta-blockers, such as atenolol, are also *not* recommended in pregnancy because of the risk of fetal growth restriction and low birth weight.

In general, only agents mentioned in the table below are used to manage hypertension in pregnancy.

Medications	Comments
Labetalol	Labetalol is a non-selective β-blocker (β_1 and β_2) with α_1-blocking activity. It is the first-line treatment option for hypertension in pregnancy. It has potential *bronchoconstriction effects*; hence, it should be *avoided* in women with *asthma*, chronic obstructive lung disease, pre-existing myocardial disease, heart failure, bradycardia and greater than first-degree heart block. Intravenous labetalol is recommended for use in the management of acute onset, severe hypertension in pregnant women. **Dose:** PO 100–400 mg BD/TDS, maximum 2,400 mg/day.
Nifedipine	Nifedipine is a calcium channel blocker. The long-acting or extended-release formulation is one of the preferred anti-hypertensives for managing hypertension in pregnancy. **Dose:** PO 30–60 mg OM, maximum dose of 120 mg/day. The short-acting or immediate-release formulation may be used for the management of acute-onset, severe hypertension in pregnant women, but it should *not* be used for chronic management as it can cause rapid fluctuations in blood pressure (BP). **Dose:** PO 10 mg STAT.
Methyldopa	Methyldopa is a central α-agonist. Available data show that use during pregnancy does *not* cause fetal harm, but it may not be as effective as other medications and higher dosages are limited by the side effects, e.g., sedation, depression and dizziness. Methyldopa should be *avoided* in the *postnatal period* because it has been associated with *depression*. **Dose:** 125–500 mg BD-QDS, maximum 3 g/day.
Hydralazine	Hydralazine is a vasodilator. The intravenous form is typically used for acute onset, severe hypertension with pre-eclampsia or eclampsia in pregnant women but has a slower onset of action than intravenous labetalol. Common limiting side effects, particularly with higher doses, include reflex tachycardia, maternal hypotension, headaches, palpitations, flushing, anxiety, tremor, vomiting, epigastric pain and fluid retention. **Dose:** IV 5 bolus over 20 minutes, up to three doses. Start IV infusion at 5 mg/hour — can increase infusion up to a maximum of 10 mg/hour [ACOG 2020].
Diuretics, i.e., hydrochlorothiazide, furosemide	They are *not* prescribed as monotherapy but may be considered to treat oedema with pathological causes. There is a theoretical concern that diuretics may cause intravascular volume depletion, leading to IUGR or oligohydramnios.

Thyroid Disease in Pregnancy

Hyperthyroidism

The medications used for treating hyperthyroidism are thioamides such as carbimazole (or its active form, methimazole) and PTU. The choice of medication mainly depends on the pregnancy trimester and response to prior therapy. The goal of treatment is to maintain the serum-free T4 concentration in the normal range, using the lowest possible dose. *Radioactive iodine* is *contraindicated* in pregnancy because of the risks associated with fetal irradiation.

Medications	Comments
Carbimazole	Refer to the section: *List of Medications That Require Special Precautions Before or During Pregnancy.* **Dose:** – **Initial:** PO 15–40 mg daily. – **Maintenance**: PO 20–40 mg TDS/QDS.
Propylthiouracil (PTU)	Refer to the section: *List of Medications That Require Special Precautions Before or During Pregnancy.* **Dose:** – **Initial:** PO 200–400 mg daily. – **Maintenance:** PO 50–150 mg daily.
Propranolol	Refer to the section: *List of Medications That Require Special Precautions Before or During Pregnancy.* **Dose:** PO 10–40 mg TDS–QDS. The intravenous form may also be used to control tachycardia in managing thyroid storm or thyrotoxic heart failure in pregnancy.
Iodine	Intravenous sodium iodide, oral potassium iodide or Lugol's iodine may be used to manage thyroid storm or thyrotoxic heart failure in pregnancy.

Hypothyroidism

Pregnant women with overt hypothyroidism should be treated with adequate thyroid hormone replacement to minimise the risk of adverse outcomes. However, liothyronine (T_3) is *not* preferred as it does not provide the fetus with sufficient concentrations of T_4 required for the developing fetal brain.

Medications	Comments
Levothyroxine (T_4)	Levothyroxine is the preferred treatment for maternal hypothyroidism. It is compatible throughout pregnancy. The dose may need to be uptitrated because of an increased demand for T_4 requirement in pregnancy, likely related to the increased oestrogen production. ACOG states that an anticipatory 25% dose increase can be considered for women receiving treatment for known hypothyroidism at presentation to prenatal care. It is recommended to use the same brand/formulation as switching between different products may result in variations in dose and TSH values. If formulations are changed, close monitoring of TSH is recommended.
Liothyronine (T_3)	Liothyronine does *not* increase the risk of teratogenic or adverse effects following use in pregnancy. However, maternal supplementation with liothyronine does *not* provide the fetus with sufficient concentrations of T_4 required for the developing fetal brain; hence, it is *not* the preferred treatment for maternal hypothyroidism.

Common Gynaecological Infections in Pregnancy

Bacterial Vaginosis

Medications	Comments
Clindamycin	Clindamycin may be used safely throughout pregnancy. Some clinicians prefer clindamycin to metronidazole in the first trimester; refer to *metronidazole* safety in pregnancy (stated below). The recommended dose is PO clindamycin 300 mg BD for 7 days. Intravaginal clindamycin 2% cream may also be considered (not available in Singapore).
Metronidazole	There are conflicting reports on the safety of metronidazole in pregnancy because of concerns of carcinogenicity in some animal species; most of the published data suggest that metronidazole does *not* represent any significant risk of teratogenicity. The Centers for Disease Control and Prevention (CDC) recommends the twice-daily dose for non-pregnant and pregnant women in all trimesters, as symptomatic bacterial vaginosis has been associated with adverse pregnancy outcomes. The recommended dose is PO metronidazole 400 mg BD for 7 days (because of the availability of the 200-mg-strength tablet in our institution). Intravaginal metronidazole 0.75% gel may also be considered (not available in Singapore).

Vulvovaginal Candidiasis

Medications	Comments
Vaginal azoles	Intravaginal azole therapies are the treatment of choice for pregnant women. *The common therapies used are the following*: **a) Clotrimazole pessary** o PV 100 mg ON for 6 days o PV 200 mg ON for 3 days o PV 500 mg once **b) Isoconazole pessary** o PV 600 mg ON as a single dose
Fluconazole	A single dose of PO 150 mg fluconazole may be associated with spontaneous abortion and congenital abnormalities in the first trimester. Oral fluconazole should be used only after considering benefits versus risks (e.g., failed topical therapy).

Urinary Tract Infections (Uncomplicated, Lower UTI — Cystitis)

Initial management is often empiric, followed by tailored therapy for the susceptibility pattern of the isolated organism once urine culture results return.

Medications	Comments
Amoxicillin Co-amoxiclav (Augmentin®) Cephalexin Fosfomycin	These antibiotics are safe during pregnancy. One study reported an association between co-amoxiclav and NEC when the antibiotic combination was used near preterm birth/near term. Avoid augmentin in women with PPROM. Plain amoxicillin is safe in pregnancy. **Dose:** cephalexin 500 mg TDS × 1 week.
Nitrofurantoin	Nitrofurantoin may be used in the first and second trimesters. It is ***contraindicated*** at term (38–42 weeks of gestation), during labour and delivery or when the onset of labour is imminent because of the possibility of haemolytic anaemia in the newborn.
Trimethoprim or trimethoprim/sulphamethoxazole (commonly known as Bactrim®, Septra®)	Trimethoprim is generally ***avoided*** in the first trimester because it is a folic acid antagonist; refer to the section: *List of Medications That Require Special Precautions Before or During Pregnancy*. Because of theoretical concerns that sulphonamides cross the placenta and may increase the risk of kernicterus in the newborn, trimethoprim/sulphamethoxazole is avoided in the third trimester (from 32 weeks onwards).

Anti-D Immunoglobulin (Ig) in Pregnancy

Anti-D Ig (commonly known as Rhogam®/HyperRHO®) should be administered to non-sensitised **rhesus (Rh)-negative** pregnant women with rhesus-incompatible fetuses for the following indications: routine antenatal and postnatal anti-D prophylaxis and following any potentially sensitising events in pregnancy.

Anti-D Ig should be administered as soon as possible and within 72 hours of the potentially sensitising event. However, if not given, there may still be some protection if anti-D Ig is given up to 10 days after the sensitising event.

Anti-D Ig: 1,500 international units (IU) = 300 mcg.

Definition of Potentially Sensitising Events

1. For pregnancies <12 weeks + miscarriage/threatened miscarriage: Give anti-D Ig if there is heavy or repeated vaginal bleeding or bleeding associated with abdominal pain.
2. Termination of pregnancy (medical/surgical)
3. Molar pregnancy
4. Ectopic pregnancy
5. Miscarriage/threatened miscarriage >12 weeks
6. Chorionic villus sampling (CVS)/amniocentesis/cordocentesis
7. *In utero* therapeutic procedures, e.g., transfusion, surgery, insertion of shunts or laser surgery
8. Abdominal trauma sufficient to cause a fetomaternal haemorrhage
9. Antepartum haemorrhage
10. Intrauterine death (IUD)/stillbirth
11. External cephalic version (ECV)
12. Delivery (normal vaginal delivery/instrumental delivery/caesarean section)
13. Intraoperative cell salvage

Indications	Comments
Routine antenatal anti-D prophylaxis (RAADP)	There are 2 possible regimes: – 1-dose regime of 1,500 IU at around 28–30 weeks of pregnancy or – 2-dose regime of 500 IU each at 28 and 34 weeks of pregnancy. *Single-dose regimes* are preferred as they are logistically simpler and usually more cost-effective, potentially leading to improved compliance. A second dose is recommended for the single-dose regime if delivery does *not* occur within 12 weeks of administration. RAADP should be administered regardless of and in addition to any previous anti-D Ig given for a potentially sensitising event earlier in the same pregnancy. The half-life of anti-D Ig is approximately three weeks.
Postpartum prophylaxis	If the infant is confirmed to be Rh D-positive, all Rh D-negative women who are *not* known to be sensitised should receive anti-D Ig within 72 hours of delivery. 1,500 IU provides sufficient antibodies to prevent Rh sensitisation if the volume of the fetal Rh D-positive red blood cells (RBCs) exposure is ≤15 ml. Quantitative testing (such as the Kleihauer test) can be performed to determine if there is exposure to >15 ml of fetal Rh D-positive RBCs. If so, additional anti-D doses are required. Postpartum prophylaxis, if indicated, should be administered regardless of previous RAADP or any previous anti-D Ig given for a potentially sensitising event earlier in the same pregnancy.
Potentially sensitising events in pregnancy of <12 weeks	Anti-D prophylaxis (minimum dose 250 IU*) should be administered within 72 hours of the potentially sensitising event. Anti-D prophylaxis is **not required** for spontaneous complete miscarriage without uterine instrumentation or mild, painless vaginal bleeding. A test for feto-maternal haemorrhage (FMH) is **not** required.
Potentially sensitising events in pregnancy of 12 to <20 weeks	Anti-D prophylaxis (a minimum dose of 250 IU*) should be administered within 72 hours of the potentially sensitising event. A test for FMH is *not* required. In Rh D-negative women with continual uterine bleeding between 12 and 20 weeks of gestation, at least 250 IU* anti-D Ig should be given at a minimum of six weekly intervals.
Potentially sensitising events in pregnancy of ≥20 weeks	Anti-D prophylaxis (a minimum dose of 500 IU*) should be administered within 72 hours of the potentially sensitising event, regardless of whether RAADP has been administered at 28–30 weeks. FMH test is required, and additional doses may be necessary if the volume of FMH exceeds what is covered. With persistent vaginal bleeding, additional anti-D Ig may be required and may need to be given at more frequent intervals. Each new sensitising event should be managed with an appropriate additional dose of anti-D Ig regardless of the timing or dose of anti-D Ig administered for a previous event, including RAADP.

*In KKH, a standard anti-D dose of 1,500 IU (=300 mcg) is administered for these sensitising events as it is the only formulation available here.

Threatened Miscarriage

The 2 most used progesterone forms in pregnancy in KKH are **dydrogesterone** (sold under the brand name **Duphaston**) and **micronised progesterone** (also commonly known as **Utrogestan®**).

In the UK, the dose and progesterone used in women with a viable intrauterine pregnancy and who have a previous miscarriage but are currently having vaginal bleeding are vaginal micronised progesterone 400 mg BD till 16 weeks of gestation (NICE 2021).

Medications	Comments
Dydrogesterone (commonly known as Duphaston®)	Dydrogesterone is a synthetic progesterone that is safe in pregnancy. **The common doses used are:** a. *Threatened miscarriage* – PO 40 mg stat, then 10 mg TDS for two weeks or until symptoms remit. – Administration of PO 10 mg BD (with or without a loading dose) has also demonstrated efficacy. b. *Recurrent miscarriage* – PO 10 mg BD may be taken until week 20 of pregnancy.
Micronised progesterone (commonly known as Utrogestan®)	Utrogestan® is a natural progesterone in micronised form. **The common doses used are:** a. *Threatened miscarriage* – PO/PV 200–400 mg daily/BD until week 16 of pregnancy or symptoms remit. b. *Women with a short cervix and a history of preterm birth* – PV 200 mg ON from 16 weeks to at least 34 weeks of pregnancy (NICE guidelines).
Medroxyprogesterone, norethisterone	Medroxyprogesterone and norethisterone are synthetic forms of progesterone that are *contraindicated* in pregnancy; refer to the section: *List of Medications That Require Special Precautions Before or During Pregnancy.*

Lactation Promotion

Evidence for oral galactagogues (drugs or natural therapies) is generally limited.

Medications	Comments
Domperidone	Domperidone is used off-label as a galactagogue to increase breast milk supply. There is no established dosing; the common dose used is PO 10 mg TDS (maximum 30 mg/day). Higher doses are not recommended because of concerns over cardiac arrhythmias and sudden cardiac death. Avoid concurrent use with metoclopramide.
Fenugreek	There are mixed results on fenugreek's effect as a galactagogue; the evidence is mostly anecdotal. There is no established dosing; typical doses are one to three capsules BD/TDS (maximum nine capsules/day). Maple syrup odour in urine and sweat may be noticed.

Lactation Suppression

Medications	Comments
Cabergoline	There are 2 regimes available: a. <u>Inhibition of lactation</u> *(first day postpartum)* – The recommended dose is PO 1 mg stat. – This effectively inhibits milk secretion, breast engorgement and pain in 70–90% of women. b. <u>Suppression of established lactation</u> – The recommended dose is PO 0.25 mg BD for 2 days. – This is effective in 85% of women. – This dosage regimen has been demonstrated to be better tolerated than the single-dose regimen in this group of women having a lower rate of side effects, particularly in avoiding postural hypotension. The effect of cabergoline is usually irreversible, although in some cases, mothers may recover their milk supply following heavy pumping. Milk production for subsequent pregnancies will not be affected. It is **not** recommended to continue breastfeeding once cabergoline is administered.
Bromocriptine	Bromocriptine is an ergot-derived dopamine agonist, like cabergoline. However, it is **not** recommended for use to suppress lactation because of the increased risk of maternal stroke, seizures, cardiovascular disorders, death and possibly psychosis.

Antenatal Steroids — Benefits of Antenatal Steroids

1. Antenatal steroids given within 7 days before PTD have been shown to reduce RDS, perinatal and neonatal death. They are most effective in reducing RDS if delivery occurs between 24 hours and 7 days of administration of the second dose of steroids.
2. Some evidence shows that antenatal steroids reduce intraventricular haemorrhage (IVH) and developmental delay in childhood.
3. They reduce neonatal death when the first dose is given within 48 hours before birth.
4. There are still benefits if the first dose is given within 24 hours before birth.

Antenatal Steroids — Either Dexamethasone or Betamethasone

Dexamethasone	Betamethasone
– Intramuscular (IM) injection of 24 mg dexamethasone phosphate → either 12 mg 24 hours apart for 2 doses or 6 mg 12 hours apart for four doses. – In KKH, we give two doses of IM dexamethasone 12 mg 12 hours apart.	– IM betamethasone sodium phosphate/acetate mix or betamethasone sodium phosphate: two doses of 12 mg 24 hours apart.
– Compared to betamethasone, dexamethasone is more effective in reducing the risk of IVH. – Cheaper.	– Compared to dexamethasone, betamethasone is more effective in reducing the risk of RDS and may reduce the risk of chorioamnionitis.

When to Give Antenatal Steroids?

Things to assess

1. Singleton or multiple pregnancies (e.g., twins, triplets).
2. Gestational age of the fetus.
3. Indication.
4. Presence of sepsis
   - Weigh the benefits of steroids for the fetus against the risk of exacerbating maternal sepsis.
   - There is no evidence to suggest that a single course of steroids increases infection or antibiotic use, but caution should be exercised.

Delivery of the fetus/fetuses should *not* be delayed to await completion of antenatal steroids if there is maternal/fetal indication to expedite delivery, e.g., chorioamnionitis or non-reassuring fetal status.

Gestational age	Indication	Pros and Cons of Antenatal Steroids
Singleton		
22+0 to <24+0 weeks	Imminent PTD: decision for steroids should be after MDT counselling (including the maternal–fetal specialist and neonatologist) and if the woman has decided on *active resuscitation* for the neonate.	**Pros:** 1. Highly likely to reduce perinatal mortality, neonatal death and neonatal respiratory distress. 2. Likely to reduce IVH and childhood developmental delay. The above benefits are most likely seen if birth occurs 24–48 hours after starting treatment. If the birth occurs within 7 days of starting treatment, a reduction in respiratory morbidity but *not* IVH or mortality is seen. **Cons:** 1. Can affect maternal glucose tolerance for up to 5 days after steroid administration. For women with diabetes, hypocount monitoring with an insulin sliding scale is needed. 2. Likely to reduce birth weight if birth occurs >7 days after steroids are taken. 3. Likely no benefits if birth occurs >7 days after starting steroids. 4. May increase psychiatric and behavioural diagnoses if delivery occurs at term.
24+0 to 34+6 weeks	Imminent PTD: because of spontaneous PTL/ preterm pre-labour rupture of membranes (PPROM)/planned PTD. → **Offer antenatal steroids**	
35+0 to 36+6 weeks	Imminent PTD: because of spontaneous PTL/ PPROM/planned PTD. → **Consider antenatal steroids. Discuss the pros and cons of steroids.**	**Pros:** 1. Likely to reduce respiratory support. **Cons:** 2. Can affect maternal glucose tolerance for up to 5 days after administration. For women with diabetes, hypocount monitoring with an insulin sliding scale is needed. 3. Likely to increase neonatal hypoglycaemia. 4. May increase psychiatric and behavioural diagnoses if delivery occurs at term. Benefits seem unlikely if birth is >7 days after starting treatment, although there is a lack of studies on women at this gestational age.
≥37+0 to 38+6 weeks	Planned LSCS at ≥37+0 to 38+6 weeks. **No indication for steroids** for planned LSCS ≥39+0 weeks.	Discuss with the woman and family the pros and cons of steroids. The risk of respiratory morbidity at term is low, ~5%, and is usually transient. The risk decreases with advancing gestational age. **Pros:** 1. May reduce admission to the neonatal intensive care unit (NICU) for respiratory morbidity. **Cons:** 2. Can affect maternal glucose tolerance for up to 5 days after steroid administration. For women with DM, hypocount monitoring with an insulin sliding scale is needed. 3. Uncertain evidence regarding any reduction in RDS, transient tachypnoea of the newborn (TTNB) or NICU admission. 4. Increased risk of neonatal hypoglycaemia and possible developmental delay. 5. May reduce educational attainment in school.

Multiple Pregnancies

- Less evidence regarding the pros and cons in multiple pregnancies than in a singleton pregnancy.
- RCOG's recommendations are similar to those for a singleton pregnancy.
- **Offer** antenatal steroids for imminent PTD (because of either spontaneous PTL, PPROM or iatrogenic PTD) from 24+0 to 34+6 weeks.
- **Consider** antenatal steroids for imminent PTD from 35+0 to 36+6 weeks.

Repeat Course(s) of Antenatal Steroids

- Consult a maternal–fetal specialist and a neonatologist.
- Limited evidence to recommend repeat courses of steroids.
- If treatment was done >7 days ago, a repeat course might reduce the need for respiratory support, but it can result in lower birth weight (mean difference of 80 g), head circumference, length and neonatal BP. There is also no reduction in severe morbidity or long-term benefits with repeat courses.
- The maximum number of courses should *not* exceed three.

Low-Dose Aspirin for Pre-Eclampsia Prophylaxis

For risk factors for pre-eclampsia prophylaxis, refer to Chapter 1: *Pre-Conception Preparation.*

Since 2022, for pre-eclampsia prophylaxis in KKH, we have been using this regime as *per the ASPRE trial*: **start aspirin 150 mg ON from 11 to 14 weeks of gestation until 36 weeks of gestation.**

CHAPTER 19

Approach to Postnatal Problems

Maternal Physiological Changes in the Postpartum Period

The **postpartum period**, also known as the "fourth trimester", is defined as **the first six weeks of the postpartum period**. During this time, maternal physiological changes related to pregnancy return to the non-pregnant state.

a) Weight change

About 50% of gestational weight gain is lost in the first six weeks after delivery, with a slower rate of loss through the first six months after childbirth.

In total, 25% of women retain >5 kg of their pregnancy weight one year after delivery.

The target weight loss after delivery should be 1–2 kg per month.

Excessive exercise should be avoided as this can lead to a decrease in breast milk production.

b) Abdomen

The abdominal skin may remain lax postpartum.

Striae may fade from red to silvery or white, but are permanent.

Most of the abdominal wall will regain its normal tone over several weeks. However, in some women, diastasis of the rectus abdominis muscle may persist. It can cause long-term abdominal discomfort and affect cosmesis. Treatment with conservative measures includes physiotherapy, postnatal exercise or wearing an abdominal binder. Surgical treatment is reserved for those in which conservative measures have failed or the discomfort is severe.

c) Hair

Postpartum hair loss (telogen effluvium) is commonly noted one to five months after delivery. This is usually self-limiting, with the restoration of normal hair patterns 6–15 months after delivery.

d) ***Venous thromboembolism*** *(VTE) risk* — refer to Chapter 11: *Medical Disorders in Pregnancy*

Pregnant women are at a higher risk of developing VTE (four to six times) than non-pregnant women, and the risk is higher in the postnatal period.

Low-risk pregnant women should be advised on adequate hydration, ambulation and wearing compression stockings to reduce VTE risk. Consider prophylactic low-molecular-weight heparin (LMWH) for high-risk women. Pregnant women on long-distance travel for more than four hours should be warned of the increased VTE risk. They should be adequately hydrated, take regular walks around the plane, perform in-seat exercises and wear compression stockings.

Refer to a haematologist if deep vein thrombosis (DVT) is suspected with unilateral calf swelling and tenderness; perform a Doppler ultrasound (**US**) of the affected limb and consider starting LMWH.

Immediate Postnatal Follow-Up

Investigations to Review

Rhesus-negative women: If the baby is rhesus-positive, administer Rhogam (anti-D antibodies) within 72 hours after delivery.

Rubella IgG negative (i.e., non-immune): Offer measles, mumps and rubella (MMR) vaccination if the patient agrees.

i. Fetal rubella infection can cause hearing loss, blindness and fetal anomalies.
ii. In adults, rubella infection is usually mild, with low-grade fever, sore throat, headache and a rash.
iii. The MMR vaccine offers both maternal and fetal protection. In addition, it is safe for breastfeeding mothers.
iv. However, as it is a live vaccine, it is unsafe during pregnancy. Women should avoid pregnancy for 28 days after the MMR vaccine.

Gestational diabetes mellitus (GDM): Perform a two-point 75-g oral glucose tolerance test (OGTT) six weeks after childbirth (KKH protocol).

Anaemia: If maternal haemoglobin (Hb) is <10 g/dl or there is significant blood loss during delivery, check Hb postnatally. Consider packed cell transfusion (PCT) if the Hb is <8 g/dl. Consider intravenous (IV) ferric carboxymaltose if Hb is <10 g/dl, and oral iron can be restarted 5 to 7 days after IV iron and continued for three months to maintain iron stores.

Thrombocytopenia: Assess the cause; if it is related to pregnancy, e.g., gestational thrombocytopenia or haemolysis, elevated liver enzymes and low platelets (HELLP) syndrome, it is expected to resolve postpartum (usually normalises in six weeks).

If thrombocytopenia is due to disseminated intravascular coagulation (DIC), it should improve with the treatment of the underlying cause of DIC.

Thrombocytopenia caused by a condition unrelated to pregnancy, such as an inherited platelet disorder or immune thrombocytopenic purpura (ITP), will persist after delivery. Therefore, these women should be followed up by a haematologist.

Others: Review any other abnormal results during the antenatal period and follow up accordingly.

Contraception

Ovulation can occur as early as 25 days post-delivery (the average time to ovulation is 45–94 days); refer to Chapter 52: *Contraception for Postpartum Women*.

Outpatient Postnatal Follow-Up and Assessment

a) Women with uncomplicated vaginal deliveries are usually reviewed at 6 weeks.
b) Consider an earlier postnatal follow-up before 6 weeks if there were any complications.
c) Women with pre-existing medical conditions (e.g., hypertension, diabetes, thyroid disorders, renal disease, obesity and mood disorders) should continue to follow up with the relevant specialists or general practitioners (GPs) for ongoing care.

d) *During the postnatal follow-up*:

Enquire about the general well-being of the mother and child.

i. Assess for pain, lochia, urinary and bowel symptoms, abnormal vaginal discharge, fever and breastfeeding issues.
ii. Assess if the infant is growing well.
iii. Assess the psychological and emotional state of the mother, looking for signs of postnatal blues, depression or psychosis. Consider screening women with the Edinburgh Postnatal Depression Scale (EPDS) cut offscore of ≥13 for postnatal depression.
iv. Advise on the importance of good perineal hygiene, including daily showering of the perineum, frequent changing of sanitary pads, hand washing before and after, and pelvic floor exercises (PFEs).
v. Ensure the uterus is involuted.
vi. Assess the healing of the perineum (if the patient underwent vaginal delivery) or surgical/incision wound (if the patient underwent a caesarean section).
vii. Assess any complications post obstetric anal sphincter injury (OASIS), i.e., third- or fourth-degree tears, such as urinary or flatus/faecal incontinence. Multidisciplinary team care involving the colorectal surgeon may be required for fourth-degree tears or complex OASIS. In total, 60–80% of women may be symptomatic 12 months after delivery and OASIS repair.

Encourage and support breastfeeding.

Discuss contraception.

Perform cervical cancer screening, if not up-to-date: PAP smear for women 25–29 years old, human papillomavirus (HPV) testing for women ≥30 years old.

Take a mammogram if not up-to-date (for women ≥40 years old).

Ensure vaccinations are up-to-date (e.g., MMR, influenza, hepatitis B, COVID-19).

e) Debrief couples on adverse antenatal or perinatal events and discuss the implications on future pregnancies.

f) Patients with antenatal or postnatal complications, e.g., preterm birth, stillbirth or neonatal death, should have their laboratory or histology investigations reviewed. In addition, they should be counselled on recurrent risks (if any) and future pregnancy planning.

g) *Future pregnancy counselling*:

The ideal inter-pregnancy interval is 18–24 months. However, a shorter inter-pregnancy interval may be considered, given the reduced fertility with advanced maternal age.

Ask for an early booking visit with appropriate investigations, e.g., screening for infection in patients with previous preterm premature rupture of membranes (PPROM) or preterm labour and relevant prenatal genetic testing, if appropriate.

Advise on preconception folic acid (ideally to start 3 months before conception).

Women with risk factors for pre-eclampsia should be advised to start low-dose aspirin (LDA). Prescribe 150 mg every night from 11 to 14 weeks in the subsequent pregnancy until 36 weeks of gestation (KKH protocol 2022).

Advise the mode of delivery for future pregnancies.

Women with OASIS should be counselled on the recurrence risk (5–7%) and implications on future pregnancies. If the woman is symptomatic or has an abnormal endoanal ultrasound (US) (≥30°) or abnormal manometry (incremental squeeze pressure <20 mmHg), she should be advised on elective caesarean section. After a third-degree tear, asymptomatic women have a 20% risk of developing bowel symptoms following vaginal delivery.

Postnatal Issues

Pain (Wound/Uterus) — Identify cause and treat accordingly

Give analgesics

i. *Paracetamol and NSAIDs* are safe for breastfeeding.
ii. *Tramadol*: Use with caution — lowest dose (50 mg TDS) for the shortest duration. Monitor the infant for increased sleepiness, difficulty feeding, breathing difficulties or limpness.
   Prescribe metoclopramide 10 mg TDS to reduce the risk of nausea.
iii. *Lignocaine gel*, sitz bath, cooling pack (for vulva oedema) and doughnut pillows can be used to relieve pressure on the perineum.

Bleeding — Postpartum Haemorrhage (PPH) (Primary or Secondary)

Ensure the patient is haemodynamically stable, and check the haemoglobin level. Treat cause (the 4 Ts).

i. *Tone* (most common): Uterine atony.
ii. *Trauma*: Lacerations, haematomas, uterine inversion or rupture.
iii. *Tissue*: Retained placental tissue, invasive placenta.
iv. *Thrombin*: Coagulopathies.

Escalate early if the patient is unstable. Will need multidisciplinary care involving an anaesthetist, maternal–fetal specialist, haematologist, interventional radiologist, etc.

Puerperal Infection/Sepsis

Puerperal sepsis is an important cause of maternal death. It is ranked the third cause of maternal mortality by MMBRACE-UK 2019–2021 (1.12/100,000 maternities).

Puerperal sepsis is defined as sepsis developing after birth up to 6 weeks postnatally (includes non-genital tract infections).

i. ***Sepsis:*** Infection plus systemic manifestations of infection.
ii. ***Severe sepsis:*** Sepsis plus sepsis-induced organ dysfunction or tissue hypoperfusion (serum lactate ≥4 mmol/L).
iii. ***Septic shock:*** Persistence of hypoperfusion despite adequate fluid replacement therapy.

The physiological changes of pregnancy and the puerperium can obscure the signs and symptoms of sepsis in the obstetric population, warranting a high level of suspicion.

Early detection, accurate diagnosis and aggressive treatment are necessary to prevent morbidity and mortality.

Abdominal pain, fever (>38°C) and tachycardia (>90 bpm) are indications for IV antibiotics and senior clinician review.

The most common site of sepsis in the puerperium is the genital tract, particularly the uterus, resulting in endometritis.

Any widespread rash should suggest early toxic shock syndrome, especially if conjunctival hyperaemia or suffusion is present.

NSAIDs should be avoided for pain relief in sepsis as they may impede the ability of polymorphs to fight group A *streptococcus* (GAS) infection.

***Recommendations of the Surviving Sepsis Resuscitation Care Bundle*:**

i. Obtain blood cultures before antibiotic administration.
ii. Administer broad-spectrum antibiotics within 1 hour of recognition of severe sepsis. A combination of either piperacillin/tazobactam or a carbapenem plus clindamycin provides one of the broadest coverage of treatment for severe sepsis.
iii. Measure serum lactate.
iv. If hypotension or serum lactate >4 mmol/L: Deliver an initial minimum of 20 ml/kg of crystalloid/equivalent (RCOG recommendations). Apply vasopressors for hypotension not responding to initial fluid resuscitation to maintain MAP >65 mmHg.
v. In the event of persistent hypotension despite fluid resuscitation (septic shock) or serum lactate ≥4 mmol/L: Achieve a central venous pressure of ≥8 mmHg, a central venous oxygen saturation of ≥70% or a mixed venous oxygen saturation of ≥65%.

Causes of Puerperal Infection or Sepsis

Causes	Risk factors	Recommendations/Remarks
1. **Endometritis**	Group B *streptococcus* (GBS) colonisation/bacterial vaginosis Maternal diabetes mellitus Obesity Chorioamnionitis Prolonged labour or rupture of membranes A large amount of meconium in amniotic fluid Multiple vaginal examinations (VEs) Poor hand hygiene Operative vaginal delivery **Caesarean section** Manual removal of placenta Retained products of conception Poor perineal hygiene <u>Others:</u> Chronic medical disease Immunosuppression IV drug abuse	**Antibiotic prophylaxis during caesarean section:** IV cefazolin 2 g if <120 kg, 3 g if ≥120 kg and no allergies. *Alternative*: IV clindamycin 900 mg once. **Intrapartum antibiotic prophylaxis for maternal GBS colonisation:** IV penicillin G 5 MU once, then 2.5 MU Q4h till delivery. *Investigations*: FBC, renal panel, CRP, vaginal swab culture, urine and blood cultures, US pelvis. ***Early postpartum endometritis*** (first 48 hours, usually after caesarean section): IV ceftriaxone 2 g Q24h + IV metronidazole 500 mg Q8h. ***Late postpartum endometritis*** (48 hours to 6 weeks, usually after vaginal delivery): IV augmentin 1.2 g Q8h + IV gentamicin 5–7 mg/kg Q24h. Refer to a microbiologist or infectious disease (ID) physician if needed.

(Continued)

Causes	Risk factors	Recommendations/Remarks
2. **Urinary tract infection (UTI)** (Refer to Chapter 48: *Urogynaecology*.)	Indwelling catheter Epidural anaesthesia Urethral trauma Urinary tract anomalies	Early ambulation. Remove the catheter once the patient is ambulating or earlier if a catheter-associated urinary tract infection (CAUTI) is suspected. Obtain urine culture before initiating antibiotics. Differentiate between lower UTI (cystitis) and upper UTI (pyelonephritis).
3. **Skin and soft-tissue infection** *Sites of infection* i. IV cannula ii. Caesarean wound iii. Episiotomy wound	Prolonged IV cannula insertion Wound haematoma Diabetes mellitus Immunosuppression GAS (refer to point 8 in this table)	Remove the IV cannula as soon as no longer needed or if there is a suspected infection. Obtain swab cultures if a discharge is present. Empiric treatment of post-surgical wound infection with IV augmentin 1.2 g Q8h for ≥2–3 days, then switch to PO augmentin if clinically improving. If a patient is stable, she can be treated outpatient with oral augmentin. ***Necrotising skin and soft tissue infection:*** ***Necrotising fasciitis*** (IV penicillin G 4 MU + IV ceftazidime 2 g Q8h + IV clindamycin 900 mg Q8h). ***Fournier's gangrene*** (involves mainly perineum of the retroperitoneal region) (IV piperacillin/tazocin 4.5 g Q6h + IV clindamycin 900 mg Q8h). ***Streptococcal toxic shock syndrome (TSS)*** (IV penicillin G 4 MU + IV clindamycin 900 mg Q8h). These are **medical emergencies** and require prompt resuscitation, antibiotic administration and surgical debridement. Consider imaging (CT scan) if needed. Intensive care support is often required. Refer to an ID physician and a general surgeon. Continue IV antibiotics for ≥7 days.
4. **Mastitis** (refer to Chapter 20: *Lactation*)	Breast engorgement Cracked nipples Blocked ducts	Exclude breast abscess (refer to a breast surgeon if an abscess is present). Continue to express breastmilk (as stasis of breastmilk will predispose to infection). Symptom relief with cold cabbage and analgesics. PO cloxacillin or augmentin for 7–10 days. Refer to a lactation consultant.

(Continued)

(*Continued*)

Causes	Risk factors	Recommendations/Remarks
5. **Pneumonia**	Aspiration pneumonia from GA (Mendelson syndrome) Prolonged bed rest Smoking Unvaccinated status	Early ambulation and chest physiotherapy to reduce the risk of atelectasis. Sputum culture, COVID-19 testing. An arterial blood gas (ABG) test and a chest X-ray to determine the severity. Empiric antibiotic selection varies on the basis of the severity of illness, the likelihood of infection with drug-resistant pathogens and patient drug allergy. Refer to a respiratory medicine physician or an ID physician.
6. **Gastroenteritis**	Antibiotic-induced *Clostridium difficile* infection Other pathogens include *Salmonella* and *Campylobacter*	Appropriate use of antibiotics (to reduce the risk of antibiotic resistance). Ingestion of unpasteurised milk products raises the possibility of infection with *Salmonella*, *Campylobacter* or *Listeria*. <u>*Investigations:*</u> FBC, renal panel, stool culture, and ova, cysts and parasite (OCP) exam. Most cases of acute diarrhoea are caused by viruses and are self-limiting. Fluid replacement is the most important therapy in diarrhoeal illness. Empiric antibiotic therapy is <u>*not*</u> routinely recommended, but can be considered for those with suspected invasive bacterial infection (bloody or mucoid stools) or host factors that increase the risk of complications (e.g., immunocompromised). Antimotility agents (e.g., loperamide) should be used with caution as they may prolong the illness. Refer to a gastroenterologist or an ID physician if symptoms are severe/atypical/persistent.
7. **Spinal abscess** ***Classical triad:*** 1. Back pain 2. Fever 3. Neurological deficits	Regional anaesthesia Most commonly caused by *Staphylococcus aureus*	Inadvertent *rare* complication. Early diagnosis and prompt treatment are essential as prolonged neural compression can cause permanent spinal cord or cauda equina damage. Obtain blood cultures and send the aspirate or surgical specimens of the abscess contents for cultures. Imaging via a spine MRI with gadolinium contrast. Empiric treatment with IV vancomycin 15–20 mg/kg Q8-12h + IV ceftriaxone 2 g Q12h. Inform the anaesthetist. May need to refer to a neurosurgeon or an interventional radiologist for surgical decompression or CT-guided needle aspiration.

(Continued)

Causes	Risk factors	Recommendations/Remarks
8. **Invasive GAS infection** Up to 30% of the people are asymptomatic carriers — in the throat or skin.	URTI GAS infection Contact with young children during pregnancy Prolonged rupture of membranes Operative vaginal delivery	Consider a throat swab if the patient has a sore throat. Empiric antibiotics with IV penicillin G 4 MU Q4h + IV clindamycin 900 mg Q8h. Consider IV immunoglobulin (IVIg) for patients with streptococcal TSS.
9. **VTE** Refer to Chapter 11: *Medical Disorders in Pregnancy*.	Caesarean section Prolonged immobilisation Advanced maternal age Obesity Smoking Personal/family history of VTE Thrombophilia	Confirm diagnosis: Doppler US or computed tomography pulmonary angiogram (CTPA). Refer to a haematologist. Therapeutic anticoagulation with LMWH.

Antimicrobials (Choices and Limitations)

Antibiotic	Remarks
1. **Amoxycillin–clavulanic acid**	Does not cover MRSA, *Pseudomonas* or extended-spectrum beta-lactamase (ESBL)-producing organisms.
2. **Metronidazole**	Only covers anaerobes. Caution in breastfeeding.
3. **Clindamycin**	Covers most streptococci and staphylococci, including many MRSA, and switches off exotoxin production, significantly decreasing mortality. It also covers anaerobes. Not renally excreted or nephrotoxic. Risk of *C. difficile* infection.
4. **Piperacillin/tazobactam**	Covers most organisms except MRSA. Does not cover ESBL producers. Not renally excreted or nephrotoxic.
5. **Gentamicin** (as a single dose of 3–5 mg/kg)	Covers MRSA, Gram-negative bacilli and some Gram-positive bacteria (but not GAS or GBS) Poses no problem in normal renal function, but if doses are to be given regularly, serum gentamicin levels must be monitored. Dose adjustment is necessary in renal impairment.

Breast Issues — Refer to Chapter 20: Lactation

Insufficient milk supply: Identify cause and treat accordingly (the most common cause is inadequate sucking and emptying of the breast). Advise frequent and regular breastfeeding, always preceding complementary feed with breastfeeding, starting each feed on an alternate breast and ensuring adequate nutrition and hydration.

i. ***Galactagogues*:**
***Fenugreek*:** Herbal galactagogue.
Dose: Two capsules TDS (one capsule contains 600 mg).
***Domperidone*:** Dopamine D_2 receptor antagonist, which stimulates the release of prolactin. Dose: 10 mg TDS for up to 2 weeks. Avoid use in those with a history of cardiac arrhythmias (*common side effects*: dry mouth, dizziness, nausea, gastrointestinal symptoms and fatigue). In addition, metoclopramide should *not* be given concurrently with domperidone as they belong to the same class of medication.

Plugged duct: Encourage warm moist compress to the affected area 3–5 minutes before feeding to encourage milk flow.

Breast engorgement: Cold cabbage and analgesics; continue the regular expression of breast milk.

Mastitis: Gentle massage, antipyretics, fluids, antibiotics (PO cloxacillin or augmentin for 7–10 days). These antibiotics are safe for breastfeeding, and regular expression of breast milk should be continued.

Breast abscess: Symptoms similar to those of mastitis, but tender fluctuant palpable mass on examination. Start empiric antibiotics and refer to a breast surgeon for fine-needle aspiration or incision and drainage (I&D).

Nipple soreness/cracked nipples: This is usually due to poor positioning or latch-on. Advise correct positioning and attachment. Purified lanolin cream may be applied to promote healing.

Refer to a lactation consultant for any breastfeeding issues.

Wound Issues — Check Episiotomy/Caesarean Wound, Foul-Smelling Discharge/Ensure Normal Lochia

Lochia typically lasts four to six weeks after delivery. In the first few days after delivery, it is reddish-brown. It then becomes pinkish and watery for two to three weeks before turning yellowish-white.

In *non-lactating women*, menses usually resume in six to eight weeks.

Women who *exclusively breastfeed* may not have menses for that duration (can last ≥1 year after delivery).

Refer to O&G for signs of wound infection, breakdown or endometritis.

Refer to O&G for secondary PPH.

Urinary Symptoms: Urinary Retention/Urinary Tract Infection/Incontinence

- ***Urinary retention***: refer to Chapter 48: *Urogynaecology*

  Undetected and inadequately treated acute retention of urine (ARU) may result in temporary neurogenic detrusor dysfunction. This may lead to prolonged bladder overactivity and voiding dysfunction. In addition, it can cause incontinence and recurrent UTIs in the long-term. Therefore, early recognition and appropriate treatment of urinary retention are important to reduce the risk of long-term sequelae.

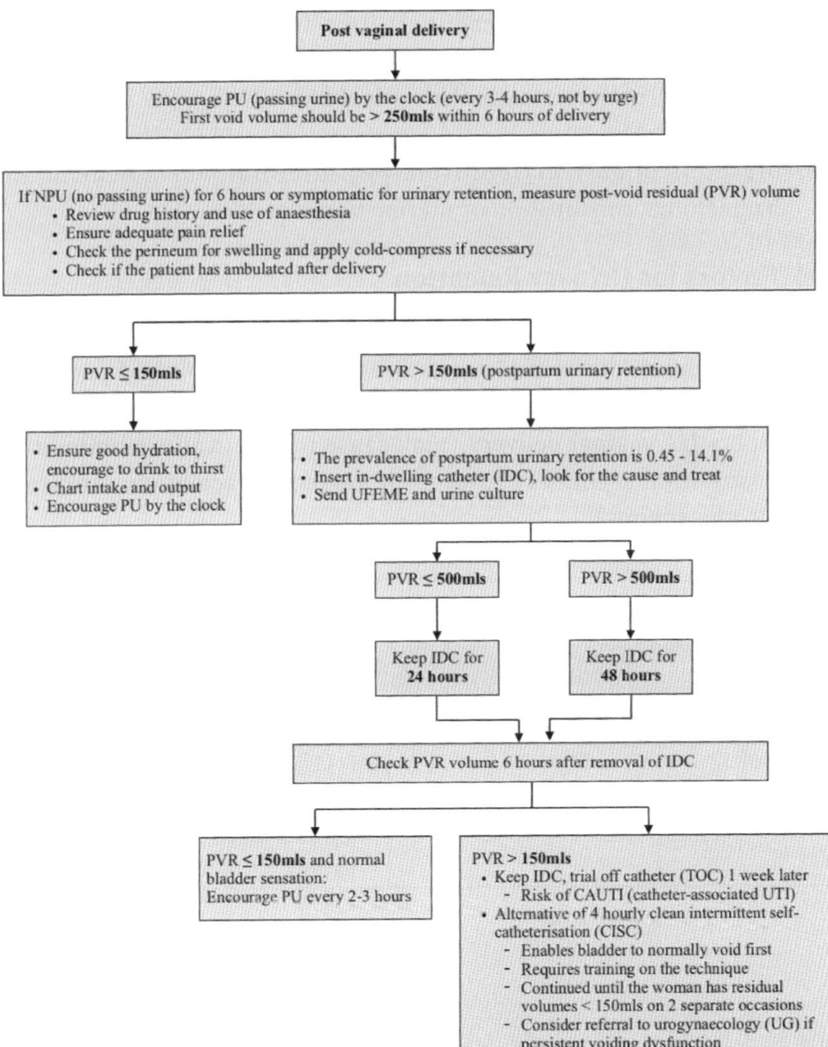

Common Causes of Postpartum Urinary Retention

1) ***Neurologic***
   a) Drugs with anti-cholinergic activity (e.g., anti-psychotics, anti-depressants and opioids such as morphine in epidural anaesthesia).
   b) Neuraxial analgesia (epidural/spinal). Conduction anaesthesia (epidural, spinal, combined spinal/epidural) blocks the sensory and motor nerve impulses of the sacral spinal cord, which suppresses the micturition reflex, decreases detrusor contractions and increases bladder capacity. Post caesarean section under spinal anaesthesia, bladder sensation may take ≥10 hours to return.
   c) Compromised bladder innervation from prolonged labour or fundal pressure.
2) ***Pain:*** UTI or from vaginal/perineal laceration with inadequate analgesia.
3) ***Mechanical obstruction:*** from peri-urethral, vulva oedema or haematoma, constipation or uterine fibroids.

Risk Factors for Urinary Retention

1) History of recurrent UTI or pre-existing voiding difficulties.
2) Long labour (due to prolonged pressure on the pelvic and pudendal nerves).
3) Operative vaginal delivery (may cause mechanical urethral outlet obstruction secondary to perineal oedema, haematoma or direct bladder trauma).
4) Extensive vaginal and perineal lacerations.
5) Immobility.

Measurement of PVR Volume	In/out Catheterisation	Bladder Scan
Advantages	Diagnostic and therapeutic	Non-invasive
Disadvantages	Risk of infection, haematuria, urethral injury, pain	Risk of overestimation due to the measurement of blood in the uterus. The risk of inaccurate estimation is higher in obese women because of habitus.

Lower UTI symptoms (e.g., dysuria, urgency, hesitancy, frequency, nocturia): Urine FEME and culture and treat with empiric antibiotics.

Urinary incontinence: Advise on PFE — refer for physiotherapy.
Refer to a urogynaecologist if incontinence persists after >3 months despite PFE.

Bowel Symptoms — Constipation/Haemorrhoids/Per-Rectal (PR) Bleeding

Ensure adequate hydration.
Iron supplements can aggravate constipation and cause dark stools (which may be mistaken for PR bleeding).
Anusol (Proctosedyl) cream/suppository, Daflon, Lactulose, Dulcolax, Agarol.
Refer to a colorectal surgeon for thrombosed piles/PR bleeding.

Postnatal Blues/Depression/Psychosis

Refer to Chapter 17: *Depression in Pregnancy and Postnatal Psychiatric Disorders.*

Risk factors: Prior history of postpartum depression or psychosis, personal or family history of mood disorder or antenatal depression.
Refer to a psychiatrist if symptoms persist for more than two weeks or if depressive symptoms or psychotic symptoms/risk of harm to self (i.e., have suicidal thoughts) or baby are noticed. Screen for postnatal depression with the EPDS. A score of ≥13 is used to identify postnatal women who are more likely to be suffering from depressive illness.

CHAPTER 20

Lactation

Introduction

The World Health Organization (WHO) recommends that infants be breastfeed for the first six months for optimal health and development and thereafter be fed other foods. Breastfeeding can be continued for two years and beyond as desired.

Benefits of Breastfeeding

Benefits for Infant

- Boosts the immune system.
- Early skin-to-skin contact between mothers and neonates may reduce infant crying and increase blood glucose levels.
- Decreases the incidence and severity of infection, gastroenteritis, diarrhoea, gastro-oesophageal reflux, respiratory tract infections, necrotising enterocolitis in preterm infants, otitis media and urinary tract infections.
- Decreases the incidence of late-onset sepsis in preterm infants.
- Decreases the risk of sudden infant death syndrome (SIDS) and infant mortality.
- Infants with a family history of allergies who exclusively breastfeed have a significantly lower incidence of atopic disease.
- Lowers the risk of obesity, diabetes mellitus, inflammatory bowel disease and dental caries.
- May lead to slightly better cognitive development.

Benefits for Mother

- Early skin-to-skin contact with neonates helps establish lactation and promotes ongoing breastfeeding.
- Reduces the risk of postpartum haemorrhage.
- More rapid postpartum weight loss.
- Premenopausal breast cancer is lower in women who have previously breastfeed.
- 20% decrease in the risk of developing ovarian cancer.
- Lower risk of endometrial cancer.
- Lower risk of hypertension and type 2 diabetes mellitus.
- The protective effects increase with a longer duration of breastfeeding.
- Economic benefit in terms of cost.

Contraindications of Breastfeeding

- Maternal HIV infection.
- Mother infected with human T-cell lymphotropic virus type I or type II.
- Mother with suspected or confirmed Ebola infection.
- Mother with active Monkeypox lesions (CDC).
- Mother who is undergoing treatment for cancer.
- Mother who is a drug abuser, e.g., using cocaine or phencyclidine.
- Baby with classic galactosemia (i.e., not Duarte variant).

Temporarily Cannot Breastfeed NOR Feed Expressed Breastmilk

- Mother with untreated brucellosis.
- Mother has active herpes simplex virus (HSV) infection with breast lesions (they can breastfeed from the unaffected breast but cover the contralateral breast lesions completely to avoid transmission).

Temporarily Cannot Breastfeed BUT Can Feed Expressed Breastmilk

Mother with active and untreated tuberculosis.

Antenatal Preparation

Breastfeeding education should be initiated as part of antenatal care.

Physician recommendations on breastfeeding often positively impact the woman's decision to breastfeed.

A breast examination should be performed to determine any structural problem or concern.

If the woman's nipples are inverted or non-protractile, reassure her and refer her to a lactation consultant for further advice. A niplette may be used from the second trimester for inverted nipples (Fig. 20.1).

The breasts start to produce colostrum between 12 and 18 weeks of pregnancy. Hence, some women may experience leaking from their nipples as early as 14 weeks but most commonly during the last few weeks of pregnancy and after delivery.

Refer to a breast surgeon if there is

- unilateral nipple discharge
- bloody nipple discharge
- nipple discharge associated with a breast mass/skin lesion
- new/rapidly growing breast mass

For women where the production of breastmilk may be difficult post-delivery or if the baby is anticipated to have difficulties with breastfeeding, antenatal breastmilk expression (aBME) from 36 to 37 weeks of gestation may be advised if there are no antenatal complications. For instance, women with diabetes during pregnancy may have difficulty in breastmilk production, and their newborns are at increased risk of hypoglycaemia and need to be feed early and frequently. Antenatal breastmilk expression from 36 weeks of gestation has not been shown to cause harm in women with diabetes during pregnancy and with low-risk pregnancies. The benefit of aBME is that it can improve lactation, decrease the chance of the newborn requiring infant formula and promote successful breastfeeding. The woman can express milk as often as three to four times a day for about 5 minutes, best by expressing by hand and should immediately stop expressing once they have contractions.

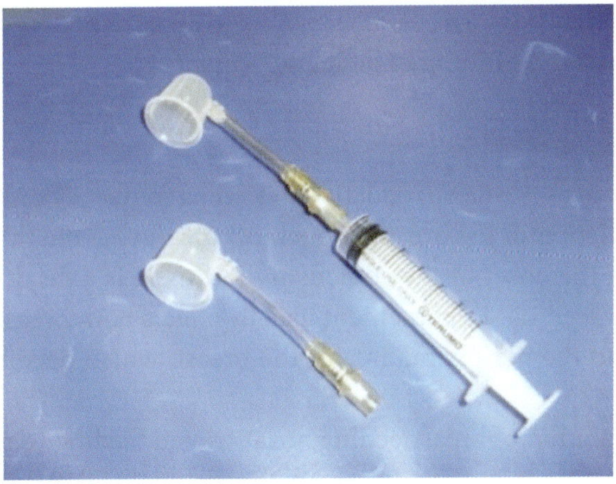

Fig. 20.1 Niplette.

Management of Breastfeeding Problems

Latching Difficulties

The newborn should take a large amount of the breast into their mouth, with more of the areola and the nipple pointing towards the soft palate. The mother should initially hold her breast during the attachment and draw the baby to the breast for a good latch.

Different feeding positions, such as the football hold or modified cradle hold, can be used by women encountering difficulties to facilitate latching onto the breast.

Women with inverted nipples often encounter difficulties latching their babies to the breast. Therefore, the use of a niplette as a non-surgical correction of inverted nipples may be recommended from the second trimester (Figure 20.1).

Sore Nipples

Sore nipples are usually the result of poor positioning or latch-on. Correct positioning/attachment is the key to preventing sore nipples. Hind milk treatment or purified lanolin cream may be applied to promote healing.

A breast shell may be worn between feeding to protect the sore nipples from rubbing against the clothing to facilitate healing.

Breast Engorgement

Engorgement occurs when a reduction in feeding frequency causes excessive milk accumulation in the breast. It often occurs during the first week after delivery with the onset of the copious milk if there is a delay in initiating or infrequent feeding. Engorgement usually affects both breasts, involving the areola and the peripheral area of the breast, which become full, hard and tender.

Early initiation of breastfeeding, unrestricted feeding (day and night) and ensuring proper latching for effective emptying will prevent or reduce the severity of breast engorgement. However, if engorgement is not relieved, milk production will be affected.

***Treatment of breast engorgement*:**

1. Massage the breast, nipple and areola area to clear any blockage to enhance milk flow.
2. Allow the baby to breastfeed frequently round the clock, as the baby's suckling is the most effective mechanism for the removal of milk.
3. *Apply a cold pack* or cold cabbage leaves on the breast in between feeding to help reduce swelling, warmth and pain.
4. *Avoid* warm compress as there will be increased vascular heat, which may aggravate the swelling if the ducts are blocked.
5. Administer analgesics to reduce the pain.

Plugged Ducts

A plugged duct is a localised blockage of milk resulting from milk stasis. It usually presents as a painful palpable lump with well-defined margins. It may be caused by inadequate drainage in one breast area or by tight or restrictive clothing.

Plugged ducts can develop into mastitis if not treated adequately. Massage of the breast is an effective way to help dislodge the blocked milk. Antibiotics are *not* indicated for plugged ducts unless there is mastitis.

Milk Blister

A milk blister is a whitish, tender area often found at the tip of the nipple. It seals the nipple pore, preventing the duct system from draining and causing milk buildup. An effective treatment is to break the epithelial tissue using a sterile needle. A breast massage should be done to clear the milk buildup. Breastfeeding should be continued to clear the blocked milk ducts.

Candidiasis

Symptoms often present as sharp shooting pain in the breast and soreness of the nipple. Treatment of candidiasis involves treating both the mother and infant simultaneously. The infant should be treated with oral nystatin. Treat the mother with either nystatin, miconazole or ketoconazole cream applied to the nipple after each feed. For persistent candidiasis, oral fluconazole (Diflucan) may be prescribed for the mother. In addition, the mother should boil and wash pacifiers, teats, teethers, breast pump parts, bras or reusable breast pads daily, as the spores are heat resistant.

Mastitis

It is a clinical diagnosis.

Definition: A unilateral bacterial infection of the breast. A common causative organism is *Staphylococcus aureus.*

***Management of mastitis*:**

1. Breast massage and clearing of plugged ducts, if present.
2. Application of a cold pack on the affected area to reduce swelling.
3. Increased fluids and bed rest.
4. Prescribe anti-pyretics.
5. Antibiotic therapy (augmentin or cloxacillin) for 7–10 days.
6. If allergic to penicillin, prescribe trimethoprim-sulfamethoxazole (Bactrim), erythromycin or clindamycin.
7. Continue with breastfeeding.

Breast Abscess

Antibiotic treatment is necessary. A breast surgeon may perform fine needle aspiration or incision and drainage (I&D) of the breast abscess. The mother can continue breastfeeding on the unaffected breast. She can hand-express or pump the milk from the affected breast to prevent breast engorgement and maintain the milk supply.

Increasing Milk Supply

Ensure a good latch so that there is effective milk removal by the baby.
Increase the frequency of breastfeeding.
Use breast compression during feeding to help increase the intake of milk by the baby.
Express milk after a feed to increase milk supply.

Pharmacological Methods to Increase Milk Supply

1. ***Metoclopramide (MAXOLON)***

Metoclopramide increases prolactin and thus improves the milk supply.
Effective for the initiation and maintenance of lactation.

Dose: PO 10 mg TDS for 7–14 days

Side effects: Fatigue, irritability, depression and extrapyramidal side effects, which may include tremors, bradykinesia (slow movements) and other dystonic reactions.

2. ***Domperidone*** — used commonly in our hospital.

Do not use it concurrently with metoclopramide.
Increases prolactin levels and improves milk supply.
Effective for the initiation and maintenance of lactation.
May take a week before the effect is seen and two to four weeks to achieve the maximum effect.

Recommended dose: PO 10 mg TDS — not to exceed 30 mg per day because of possible cardiac events.

Side effects: Headache (most common), abdominal pain, dry mouth and problem sleeping. Very rarely, restlessness and muscle spasms.

3. ***Fenugreek (a herbal supplement): Fenugreek capsules*** — used commonly in our hospital.

Fenugreek (the herb commonly used in cooking curry) has been used traditionally to increase milk supply. When used in moderation, Fenugreek is considered safe for breastfeeding mothers and is listed as GRAS (generally recognised as safe) by the US FDA. However, an excessive amount of Fenugreek may cause diarrhoea in the mother.

Fenugreek tea can be taken four times a day by adding three teaspoons of fenugreek seeds into a glass of hot water to improve milk supply. ***Fenugreek capsules*** are available from health food outlets and pharmacies. Two capsules QDS or three capsules TDS can be taken to improve milk supply.

Maintaining Milk Supply

Regular breastfeeding usually will ensure an adequate milk supply.

Milk supply increases with the baby's demand. Therefore, mothers need to understand that substituting or delaying breastfeeding may reduce milk supply because of a reduction in the stimulation of milk production. This is dependent on the infant's sucking and removal of milk from the breast.

Frequent feeding: 8–10 feeds a day are expected during the initial four to eight weeks after birth.

Separation of mother and infant should be avoided whenever possible. However, during separation, regular three hourly pumping of the breasts should be sufficient to maintain the milk supply. The expressed milk can be stored and given to the baby later.

Expressed milk can be safely stored for up to 4 hours at room temperature, 48 hours in the fridge (at 4°C), 3–6 months in the freezer (at –5 to –15°C) and 6–12 months in a deep freezer (at –20°C).

Avoid excessive accumulation of milk in the breasts, as this can affect milk supply.

Lactation Suppression

***Indications for lactation suppression*:**

1) Maternal anatomical abnormalities, e.g., hypoplastic breasts
2) Maternal breast infections or tumours

3) Maternal systemic illness, e.g., HIV or active or untreated tuberculosis
4) Maternal use of medications *not* safe for breastfeeding
5) Infant anatomical abnormalities that inhibit sucking
6) Death of the infant or stillbirth or infant adoption
7) Mother is too ill to breastfeed — in cases of severe obstetric morbidity
8) Maternal preference *not* to breastfeed

Methods for lactation suppression:

1. ***Non-pharmacological:***

Firm, supportive bra; cold compress with cold cabbage leaves; do not stimulate the breasts or nipples; limit the amount of milk removal; use nursing pads for milk leakage and do not limit fluid intake.

2. ***Pharmacological:***
   - *Analgesics* — paracetamol or NSAIDs, e.g., ibuprofen.
   - *Dopamine agonists* to reduce prolactin levels are commonly used in KKH.

     If breastfeeding **has not** been initiated, give cabergoline (Dostinex) 1 mg stat.

     If breastfeeding **has** been initiated, give cabergoline (Dostinex) 0.25 mg BD for two days.

     It may take days to weeks before the milk stops completely.
   - Consult a lactation consultant if there are problems with lactation suppression.

Breastfeeding after Breast Augmentation

If breasts have been surgically enlarged with silicone or saline implants, the nipples may vary in sensitivity.

Breastfeeding success depends on the type of surgery, but most approaches are compatible with breastfeeding.

If the surgery was for underdeveloped (hypoplastic) breasts, there might be trouble producing enough milk and a breast pump might be required after each nursing session to stimulate milk production.

Milk Bank

The Temasek Foundation Community Milk Bank Programme, run by the KKH Human Milk Bank, is a non-profit initiative to provide pasteurised donor human milk (PDHM) to hospitalised premature and sick infants and non-hospitalised infants who meet the eligibility criteria.

Who are eligible for PDHM?

- Preterm babies <35 weeks of gestation.
- Sick babies (>35 weeks of gestation) and children <1 year old admitted to NICU, children's ICU/step-down unit/high dependency with qualifying medical conditions, e.g., congenital heart disease, gastrointestinal disease or brain injury.
- Compassionate reasons:
  - Infants for whom their own mother's milk is contraindicated because of illness or medications (e.g., maternal HIV and maternal chemotherapy).
  - Infants who do not have access to their own mother's milk (e.g., adopted babies and deceased mothers).

CHAPTER 21

Frequently Asked Questions (FAQs) on Pregnancy

Air Travel in Pregnancy

Generally, occasional air travel is safe if the woman has a healthy pregnancy. However, the woman should be advised not to travel if the pregnancy is high-risk or has complications.

Contraindications to Air Travel in Pregnancy

- Increased risk of preterm labour (PTL)
- Severe anaemia
- Recent vaginal bleeding/antepartum haemorrhage (APH)
- Placenta praevia/placenta accreta spectrum (PAS)
- Long bone fracture
- Recent sickle cell crisis
- Recent major surgery
- Severe respiratory or cardiac problems
- Multiple pregnancies

Risks of Air Travel in Pregnancy

Air travel does not increase the risk of miscarriage. It does not induce PTL or preterm premature rupture of membranes (PPROM). However, any pregnant woman has a background risk of first-trimester miscarriage and PTL of 20% and 10%, respectively.

- There may be an increased risk of discomfort in pregnancy due to oedema, nasal congestion or nausea/vomiting.
- Long-distance travel (>4 hours) carries a small risk of venous thromboembolism (VTE).

For the fetus, the exposure to cosmic radiation is negligible. Passing through airport security scanners and metal detectors is not known to pose any risks to the mother or fetus. The National Council on Radiation Protection and Measurements and the International Commission on Radiological Protection recommend a maximum annual radiation exposure of 1 millisievert (mSv) for the general population and 1 mSv for a 40-week pregnancy (not exceeding 0.5 mSv in any month). However, the radiation may exceed the limit for aircrew or frequent air travellers, and they should be informed of the risk.

When to Travel?

The second trimester is generally the safest time to fly, as the incidence of obstetric emergencies is the lowest. Most airlines allow pregnant women with *singleton* pregnancies to fly *up to 36 weeks* of gestation. However, women pregnant with *twins* may be allowed to fly *up to 32 weeks* of gestation. Do check with the individual airlines regarding their policy on air travel for pregnant women, as it may vary by destination and carrier.

Precautions During Travel

- Bring along your medical records.
- Find out about the healthcare facilities at the destination.
- Have travel insurance.
- Check vaccination requirements and safety of travel destination.
- Avoid travelling to malaria-endemic areas.
- Practise food and hand hygiene.
- Wear seat belts continuously while seated; the seat belt should be below the abdomen (baby bump) and low on the pelvis.
- *Recommendations to reduce risks of deep vein thrombosis (DVT) during air travel*:
  - Regular walks around the plane every 30 minutes.
  - Periodic leg exercises.
  - Avoid restrictive clothing. Wear comfortable shoes.
  - Hydration at frequent intervals.
  - Limit caffeine/fizzy drinks and avoid alcohol.
  - Consider bringing anti-emetic medications on board.

- Use graduated elastic compression stockings (if the duration of air travel is >4 hours).
- LMWH (heparin) in women with additional risk factors for DVT.

Carrying Heavy Things During Pregnancy

It is common to hear that lifting heavy things during pregnancy is unsafe. However, the risk of injury is usually directed at the mother and not the baby. The increase in the level of hormones during pregnancy causes the ligaments to soften, which leads to joints that may be less stable. The pregnant woman's centre of gravity shifts, putting more stress on her back. These two factors make the woman more susceptible to injury when lifting heavy things.

Clothing in Pregnancy

If the pregnant woman is comfortable in her clothing, not too restrictive or tight, it will not impede the growth of the fetus. Likewise, exposing the belly has no known adverse effects on the fetus.

Dental Health Concerns in Pregnancy

Good dental hygiene is essential in pregnancy. Therefore, the pregnant woman should continue to visit the dentist regularly for routine care, at least every six months, as this is safe during pregnancy.

Periodontal Disease (Gum Disease)

Pregnancy increases the risk of developing gingivitis and periodontitis. **Gingivitis** is an inflammation of the gingiva (gums). As a result, the gingiva becomes erythematous and swollen and loses its normal shape. Bleeding also occurs easily, such as during tooth brushing (Fig. 21.1).

Periodontitis is a more severe form of gingivitis, involving the destruction of the supporting bone structure surrounding the teeth, resulting in mobility and, eventually, loss of the affected teeth.

The increased susceptibility is due to increased oestrogen and progesterone levels during pregnancy. An increase in gingivitis frequently

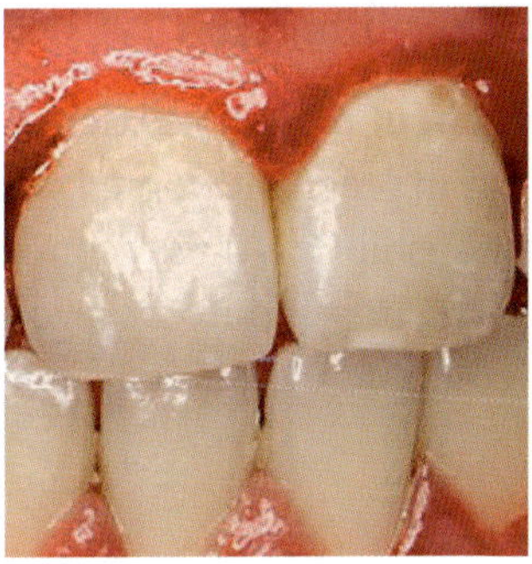

Fig. 21.1 Gingivitis.

appears between the second and eighth months of pregnancy. Studies have shown **a correlation between periodontal disease and an increased risk of PTL.**

Management

Good oral hygiene: Brush teeth after each meal, floss at least once a day and use an anti-plaque mouth rinse.

Caries (Dental Decay)

Morning sickness and general malaise in the first trimester can result in poor oral health, increasing the patient's susceptibility to caries. In addition, food cravings during pregnancy may result in higher or more frequent sugar intake, thus increasing the risk of developing caries.

Dental Procedures

While regular check-ups and cleaning are highly recommended during pregnancy, major dental procedures (e.g., wisdom tooth removal, bleaching) that are *not* urgent should be postponed till after delivery. As the first trimester is the most critical period of the baby's development, dental treatment, if necessary, is best performed in the second trimester to minimise any potential risks. Treatment in the third trimester is *not* recommended because of the *unfavourable supine position* of the mother, which may impede cardiac venous return.

Amalgam Fillings (Silver Fillings)

There has been a concern about mercury toxicity during the placement or removal of amalgam fillings in pregnant women, although there has been *no evidence* to prove this relationship. It is thus recommended that unnecessary procedures involving amalgams should be avoided. Alternative filling materials, such as tooth-coloured restorations, may be used.

Dental Radiographs

Dental X-rays have very low radiation dosages and pose little harm. However, to be cautious, dental radiographs should be taken during pregnancy only if there is an emergency. Dental emergencies include severe infections that can lead to sepsis and dental trauma. A *lead apron* over the abdomen should be worn to protect the fetus from radiation when dental radiographs are taken.

Pyogenic Granuloma (Also Known as Oral Pregnancy Tumour/ Pregnancy Epulis) (Fig. 21.2)

This is a benign growth at the gingival margin that may enlarge substantially and bleed easily upon trauma. It results from an extreme inflammatory response to local irritation, such as plaque, and is most common in the second trimester. Large pyogenic granulomas may be uncomfortable and make speech and eating difficult.

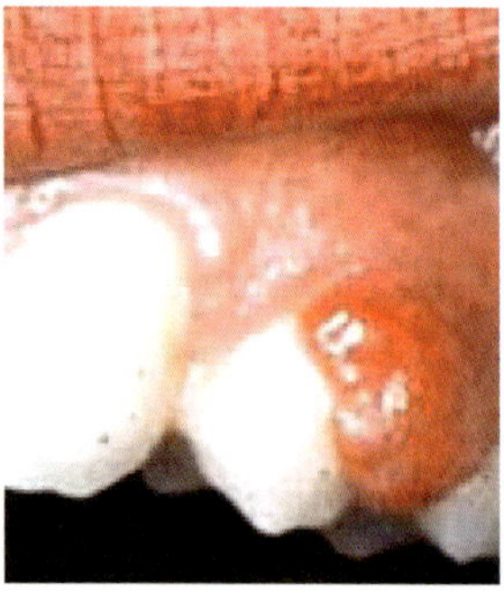

Fig. 21.2 Pyogenic granuloma.

Management

Pyogenic granulomas usually resolve after delivery *without* intervention. However, if they cause discomfort or affect speech or eating, they may be excised surgically by a periodontist under local anaesthesia. Maintaining good oral hygiene and regularly receiving professional cleaning reduce the risk of pyogenic granulomas.

Does Epidural Cause Backache?

Studies have failed to establish a link between long-term backache and epidural analgesia.

Back Pain in Pregnancy

Some studies report back pain in >60% of pregnant women. In most cases, back pain is due to mechanical factors caused by altered posture, muscle weakness, joint laxity, vertebral facet joint irritation or fluid retention. Rarer causes include degenerative spondylolisthesis or disc herniation. Treatment includes analgesics, physiotherapy or referral to the orthopaedic surgeon.

Exercise in Pregnancy

Exercise is safe in an uncomplicated pregnancy. It is not associated with miscarriage, fetal anomalies, preterm delivery, PPROM, stillbirth or neonatal death. All pregnant women are advised to remain fit during pregnancy by exercising if there are no obstetric or medical contraindications.

Contraindications to Exercise in Pregnancy

Pregnant women with medical conditions should consult their healthcare provider regarding advice on exercise.

These are some conditions for which pregnant women should **not** exercise:

	Absolute Contraindications	Relative Contraindications
Medical conditions	• Significant cardiac disease • Restrictive lung disease • Poorly controlled medical conditions, e.g., hypertension, type 1 diabetes, thyroid disease, asthma • Severe anaemia	• Unevaluated cardiac arrhythmias • Mild to moderate cardiac disease • Chronic bronchitis/mild to moderate respiratory disease • Malnutrition/severely underweight • Eating disorders • Anaemia • Heavy smoker • Orthopaedic limitations
Obstetric conditions	• Cervical incompetence • IUGR • PTL • PPROM • Multiple pregnancies • Unexplained vaginal bleeding • Persistent APH • Placenta praevia/placenta accreta spectrum (PAS) • Pre-eclampsia/pregnancy-induced hypertension	• History of spontaneous preterm delivery/miscarriage/IUGR • Recurrent pregnancy loss (RPL)

Benefits of Exercise in Pregnancy

- Exercise helps in the woman's psychological well-being.
- Improves cardiovascular health
- The calories spent help to prevent excessive weight gain during pregnancy.
- Prevents obesity.
- Reduces obesity-associated adverse outcomes, e.g., gestational diabetes mellitus, pre-eclampsia, risk of caesarean section and postpartum weight gain.

Amount of Exercise

Pregnant women should have at least 150 minutes of moderate-intensity physical activity each week. They are recommended to have at least 20–30 minutes of moderate-intensity physical activity per day for at least three days per week, ideally for most of the week.

There should be a gradual progression of activity, by increasing either the frequency of exercise per week, the duration of each session or the intensity of each section. For women who are highly inactive or unfit, the progression of physical activity should be slower.

Types of Exercise

These exercises should be a variety of aerobic and resistance training activities.

- *Aerobic exercises:* Brisk walking, dancing, swimming, stationary cycling. Low-impact aerobics, jogging or modified yoga/pilates sessions designed specifically for pregnant women can also be explored.
- *Resistance training activities:* Squats, lunges, push-ups, exercises with light dumb-bells/weights, resistance band exercises.

Avoid activities with a high risk for injuries, e.g., contact sports, sports with a high risk of falls, skydiving, horseback riding, downhill skating, ice hockey, kick-boxing, soccer, hot yoga/pilates or scuba diving.

Reference for Exercise During Pregnancy

Maternal Age (years)	Fitness Level/Body Mass Index (BMI)	Heart Rate Range (beats/minute)
<20	Regardless of fitness level or BMI	140–155
20–29	Low fitness level Active fitness level BMI >25 kg/m^2	129–144 135–150 102–124
30–39	Low fitness level Active fitness level BMI >25 kg/m^2	128–144 130–145 101–120

Source: Perinatal Society of Singapore, Guidelines on Physical Activity & Exercise in Pregnancy, 10 January 2022. Adapted from PARmed-X for Pregnancy 2015.

Precautions During Exercise in Pregnancy

- Stay well-hydrated before and after exercise.
- Be in a cool environment. Avoid exercise in excessively warm weather.
- Wear loose clothing.
- Perform "warm-up" and "cool-down" exercises.
- Maintain continuous breathing during the exercise.

- Avoid lying supine (after 20 weeks of gestation).
- Avoid excessive abdominal exercises.
- Avoid the Valsalva manoeuvre.

Stop exercises if the woman has the following:

- o Chest pain/shortness of breath (SOB) before exertion/excessive SOB that persists despite rest
- o Contraction pain/vaginal bleeding/leaking liquor
- o Muscle weakness
- o Calf pain/swelling
- o Giddiness/syncope
- o Headache

Postpartum Exercise

Women can resume exercise after delivery once they are deemed safe by their obstetricians. This depends on the mode of delivery and the presence of complications.

- Perform *pelvic floor exercises* (PFEs) to reduce the risk of urinary incontinence.
- Regular aerobic exercises can be carried out as they do not affect breastfeeding or infant growth.

Acne and Facial Treatments in Pregnancy

Acne can either improve or worsen during pregnancy. It tends to worsen during early pregnancy and then improve as the pregnancy progresses. Acne treatment safe in pregnancy includes topical benzoyl peroxide, azelaic acid and low-concentration salicylic acid preparations. If acne is more severe, topical antibiotics, e.g., clindamycin lotion, and oral antibiotics, e.g., erythromycin, clindamycin, penicillin or cephalosporins, can be considered. **Avoid** using topical or oral retinoids, high-concentration salicylic acids, oral tetracyclines, Bactrim and fluoroquinolones. Some women may find that their skin is more sensitive during pregnancy. Inform the therapist to use products that are suitable for sensitive skin.

Food, Smoking and Alcohol in Pregnancy

Foods That Are Safe to Eat or Avoid in Pregnancy

Food Group	Safe to Eat	Avoid Eating
Fruits and vegetables	Washed fruits and vegetables	Unwashed fruits and vegetables
	Cooked sprouts	Raw sprouts, e.g., alfalfa, clover, radish and mung bean
	Pasteurised juice	Unpasteurised juice
Dairy	Eggs that are fully cooked	Eggs that are not fully cooked, are runny or are without a firm yolk and egg white
	Pasteurised eggs	Raw unpasteurised eggs
	Store-bought and pasteurised: • Mayonnaise • Dressings • Sauces • Cookie dough • Other products made with eggs	Products containing raw unpasteurised eggs include: • Raw batter, filling or cookie dough • Eggnog • Homemade Caesar salad dressing • Béarnaise, hollandaise and aioli sauces • Homemade mayonnaise • Homemade ice cream • Tiramisu, mousse, meringue
	Pasteurised milk	Unpasteurised milk
	Pasteurised cheeses	**Unpasteurised cheeses,** including feta, Brie, Camembert, blue-veined cheeses, queso blanco, queso fresco, panela
Meat	Hot dogs and lunch meats heated until steaming hot	Cold hot dogs and lunch meats
	Refrigerated smoked seafood in a cooked dish, such as a casserole	Refrigerated smoked seafood, including salmon, trout, whitefish, cod, tuna, mackerel
	Fully cooked meats and poultry	• Avoid undercooked or raw meat and poultry to reduce the risk of food-borne infections such as listeriosis, toxoplasmosis, campylobacteria or salmonella infection. • Refrigerated pâtés or meat spreads • Liver/liver products
	Pre-stuffed whole poultry that has been purchased frozen and cooked frozen without defrosting first	Pre-stuffed poultry that has been purchased fresh and raw
Seafood	Up to 12 oz a week (two average meals) of fully cooked fish with low levels of mercury*, including: Shrimp, canned light tuna, salmon, pollock, catfish, cod, tilapia, whitefish, fish sticks Up to 6 oz a week of albacore (white) tuna or tuna steaks, which have more mercury than canned light tuna do	Fish with **high concentrations of mercury***: King mackerel, shark, swordfish, tilefish **Raw fish** found in foods such as sushi and sashimi Fish exposed to industrial pollutants
	Fully cooked shellfish	**Raw shellfish,** including oysters, mussels, clams, scallops

Source: https://www.publichealth.va.gov/infectiondontpassiton/womens-health-guide/food-borne-illness/index.asp.

Do's

i) ***Folic acid supplementation***

Folic acid is a type of vitamin B needed to form blood cells and develop the fetal nervous system. It has been shown to reduce the chance of fetal neural tube defects. Take folic acid daily for the first 12 weeks of pregnancy.

ii) Eat a variety of healthy food, including food rich in iron, calcium and folate.

Don'ts

i) ***Smoking***

Smoking is associated with adverse maternal and fetal outcomes, such as miscarriage, IUGR, placental abruption and PTL. In addition, it is associated with attention deficits in children and an increased risk of sudden infant death syndrome (SIDS).

Refer to Chapter 11: *Medical Disorders in Pregnancy.*

ii) ***Alcohol consumption***

Alcohol consumption in pregnancy is linked to infants showing behavioural and learning difficulties. Excessive alcohol consumption is associated with fetal alcohol syndrome (FAS), where the infant may have varying effects, including multiple fetal anomalies and decreased intellectual development.

Refer to Chapter 11: *Medical Disorders in Pregnancy.*

iii) ***Diet***

Do not focus on the weight-loss regime during pregnancy.

Special Considerations for Vegetarians/Vegans in Pregnancy

In addition to routine folic acid and vitamin D supplementation, consider iodine, omega-3 fatty acid and vitamin B12 supplementation.

iv) ***Caffeine***

A high caffeine level has a risk of low birth weight in the fetus. Pregnant women should be informed about other sources of caffeine, such as tea, colas, chocolate and over-the-counter drugs (e.g., headache and pain relief remedies, alertness drugs and some diuretics). It is recommended to have <200 mg of caffeine per day.

- 1 mug of instant coffee = 60–80 mg of caffeine
- 1 mug of filtered coffee = 140 mg of caffeine
- 1 cup of tea = 30–50 mg of caffeine

Ideal Weight Gain in Pregnancy

BMI (kg/m^2) — Institute of Medicine (IOM) Guidelines

BMI <18.5	Underweight	Weight gain 12.5–18.0 kg
BMI 18.5–24.9	Normal weight	Weight gain 11.5–16.0 kg
BMI 25.0–29.9	Overweight	Weight gain 7.0–11.5 kg
BMI ≥30.0	Obese	Weight gain 5.0–9.0 kg

Hair Colouring, Straightening and Perming in Pregnancy

The concern about exposure to hair dye and hair-straightening agents is that chemicals may be absorbed into the bloodstream at the time of use. Most chemicals are cleared from the bloodstream quickly. Unfortunately, there have been very few studies on using such hair products during pregnancy to quantify the risk of hair dye to a developing fetus. The dose used for dyeing hair is very low.

Therefore, hair colouring, straightening, perming and bleaching are generally safe during pregnancy. Painting nails is also safe. Avoid gel manicures.

House Paint in Pregnancy

Pregnant women may have occupational exposure to paint or be exposed to paint at home. The data from various studies are *insufficient* to show a cause-and-effect relationship between paint exposure and fetal harm. However, because oil-based paints and paint thinners contain several aromatic organic solvents, exposure to these products should be limited or avoided, particularly during the first trimester of pregnancy. Brief exposure to water-based paints and similar compounds in a well-ventilated area should *not* pose a significant risk to the fetus.

Insecticides in Pregnancy

Most insecticides are readily absorbed, even with limited exposure. Pregnant women probably should *not* apply pesticides in the home or the garden. They should avoid the use of fumigants.

Massage/Aromatherapy in Pregnancy

Avoid excessive skin contact with essential oils, especially in the first trimester, as they are absorbed through the skin into the bloodstream.

Sauna/Jacuzzi/Hot Tub Use in Pregnancy

Hyperthermia is *contraindicated* as there is an increased chance of miscarriage and birth defects such as spinal cord and brain malformations.

Sexual Intercourse in Pregnancy

Sexual intercourse is safe in uncomplicated pregnancies. Most sexual positions are safe if the woman adopts one in which she is comfortable.

Sex is best avoided in the following scenarios:

- Symptoms or signs of threatened miscarriage, e.g., contraction pain/ vaginal bleeding
- Presence of placenta praevia/placenta accreta spectrum (PAS)
- Threatened PTL
- PPROM
- *Untreated* sexually transmitted infections (STIs)

Tattoos, Eyebrow Threading in Pregnancy

The safety of the ink is unknown when injected into the skin. There exist the risk of local infection or allergy and a small risk of transmission of blood-borne infections such as HIV and hepatitis B or C. Eyebrow threading is safe in pregnancy as *no* chemicals are involved.

Use of Mosquito Repellents Containing DEET in Pregnancy

Skin repellents containing 50% DEET are safe in pregnancy as <10% of DEET is absorbed through the skin. There is *no* evidence of harm in animal studies.

Use of Over-the-Counter (OTC) Slimming Pills in Pregnancy

Avoid them as there are *no* safety data regarding their use in pregnancy. Losing weight in pregnancy can affect fetal growth.

Ionising Radiation Exposure in Pregnancy

Avoid ionising radiation exposure in pregnancy unless the benefits outweigh the risks of radiation to the fetus. Ionising radiation can cause developmental malformation, abnormal brain function, intellectual disability, stunted growth, fetal anomalies and childhood cancers.

Ultrasound and MRI scans without contrast are *not* associated with radiation and are safe to use in pregnancy. Gadolinium use in MRI should be limited to conditions where the benefits outweigh the risks, because of the possible theoretical risk of fetal harm.

Fetal Radiation Doses Associated With Common Imaging Modalities

Examination	Fetal Dose (mGy)
X-ray	
Cervical spine	<0.001
Chest (two views)	0.0005–0.01
Lumbar spine	1.0–10
Any extremity	<0.001
Pelvis	0.7
Abdomen	0.1–3.0
IVU	5–10
Double-contrast barium enema	1.0–20
CT head/neck	0.001–0.01
CT chest/pulmonary angiography	0.01–0.66
CT abdomen	1.3–35
CT pelvis	10–50
PET/CT whole-body scintigraphy	10–50
MMG (two views)	0.001–0.01
Ultrasound (US)	**No radiation exposure**
MRI	**No radiation exposure**

IVU, intravenous urogram; CT, computerised tomography; MMG, mammogram; HSG, hysterosalpingogram; MRI, magnetic resonance imaging.

Threshold of Radiation Exposure

Depending on the type of radiological investigation, women who had radiation exposure may not have significant exposure. Hence, inadvertent exposure, even in the first trimester, may not necessarily be an indication to terminate the pregnancy. The highest risk of CNS effects and intellectual disability with radiation exposure is between 8 and 15 weeks of gestation.

Effects of Radiation Exposure on the Fetus

Dose	Pre-implantation Period (0–2 weeks after conception)	Organogenesis (2–8 weeks after conception)	Early Fetal Period (8–15 weeks after conception)	Late Fetal Period (16–25 weeks after conception)	26 weeks onwards
<100 mGy	Fetal anomalies, fetal growth restriction or miscarriage has **not** been seen with radiation exposure of <50 mGy and up to <100 mGy (0.1 Gy/10 rads).				
>100 to 500 mGy	Exposure to ≥100 mGy can result in the death of the embryo. Embryos that survive are unlikely to have congenital abnormalities or other non-cancer health effects, regardless of the radiation exposure dose ("All or None" effect).	Radiation exposure of >100 mGy can increase the risk of childhood cancer. Possible IUGR. Increased risk of fetal anomalies, e.g., skeletal and eyes.	Radiation exposure of >100 mGy can increase the risk of childhood cancer. Possible IUGR. Risk of microcephaly.	Radiation exposure of >100 mGy can increase the risk of childhood cancer.	Radiation exposure of >100 mGy can increase the risk of childhood cancer.
>500 mGy		Possible increased risk of miscarriage. May have an increased risk of fetal anomalies, e.g., neurological and motor deficits. Likely to have IUGR.	Severe intellectual disability can occur during this period if doses are >500 mGy. Prevalence of IQ of <70 is 40% at the exposure of 1,000 mGy. Possible increased risk of miscarriage. Likely to have IUGR.	Prevalence of IQ of <70 is 15% at the exposure of 1,000 mGy. Possible increased risk of miscarriage. Possible IUGR. May have an increased risk of fetal anomalies.	Miscarriage and neonatal death may occur.

Source: Adapted from Table 1.1 of the National Council on Radiation Protection and Measurements' Report No. 174, "Preconception and Prenatal Radiation Exposure: Health Effects and Protective Guidance" [NCRP2013].

Sleeping Position in Pregnancy

Women are recommended to avoid falling asleep supine from 28 weeks of pregnancy as there may be an association between a supine sleeping position and stillbirth in late pregnancy (≥28 weeks of gestation). Women should *sleep on their side from 28 weeks of gestation* for any sleep episode, including daytime naps, returning to sleep after any awakenings or sleeping at night. They can sleep either on their left or on their right side. It is common to change position while sleeping; some pregnant women may wake up on their backs. This is acceptable as long as they start every sleep lying on their side.

Legs Cramps/Oedema in Pregnancy

Leg cramps can affect up to 50% of pregnant women in their third trimester. The aetiology of leg cramps is unclear; however, it has been attributed to electrolyte imbalances, reduced or excessive activity and metabolic disorders. In addition, there is no clear evidence of the efficacy of supplementation (e.g., calcium, magnesium, vitamin B or C); however, in some small studies, some women have benefitted from these supplements to relieve their leg cramps.

Leg oedema is a common presenting complaint in pregnancy. Causes include physiological oedema (hormone-induced sodium retention, dependent oedema, enlarging uterus causing inferior vena cava compression and reducing femoral vein outflow). It is important to distinguish unilateral from bilateral leg oedema. If the patient presents with unilateral oedema, it will be pertinent to exclude DVT. If the patient presents with bilateral leg oedema, it will be essential to exclude pre-eclampsia. Rarer causes of bilateral leg oedema include cardiac, liver or renal failure or hypoalbuminaemia.

Part 2

Investigations in Obstetrics

CHAPTER 22

Routine Antenatal Investigations

Refer to Chapter 28: *Laboratory Values in Pregnancy and Interpretation of Results.*

Test	Purpose	Management
Full blood count		
Haemoglobin (Hb) RCOG criteria for anaemia • **First trimester** Hb <110 g/L (<11.0 g/dl) • **Second and third trimesters** Hb <105 g/L (<10.5 g/dl) • **Postpartum** Hb <100 g/L (<10.0 g/dl)	Check for anaemia.	Consider serum ferritin, B12, folate and thalassaemia screen. Screen partner's FBC. Refer to Chapter 11 for more details on the management of anaemia in pregnancy.
Mean corpuscular volume (MCV) **If MCV <80** — thalassaemia screen (Hb electrophoresis and alpha gene probe)		Refer to Chapter 23: *Approach to Prenatal Screening for Thalassaemia*. In Singapore, we can refer the patient to National Thalassaemia (NTR) for confirmed thalassaemia cases. NTR provides counselling and screening of other family members.
Total white cell (TW) count	Check for infection.	In pregnancy, TW can be normal up to 17 × 10^9/L.
Platelet count	Check for thrombocytopenia.	Platelet count is low if <140 × 10^9/L. Refer to Chapter 11 for more details on thrombocytopenia in pregnancy.
Others		
Blood group and antibodies **Rhesus status**	Check the partner's Rh status.	If **Rhesus negative**, administer prophylactic anti-D at 28–30 weeks of gestation, if the partner is Rhesus positive. Consider additional anti-D if any sensitising events occur antenatally and within 72 hours after birth if the baby's blood group is Rhesus positive. If any blood group antibodies are detected — refer to Chapter 24: *Approach to Management of Red Cell Antibodies in Pregnancy*.

(Continued)

Test	Purpose	Management
Hepatitis B surface antigen (HBsAg)	If HBsAg is positive, reflex hepatitis B e antigen (HBeAg) will be performed.	Negative — continue routine antenatal care. **Positive** — refer to Chapter 15: *Infections in Pregnancy*.
Human immunodeficiency virus (HIV)		
Syphilis screen		Negative — continue routine antenatal care. **Positive** — refer to Chapter 15: *Infections in Pregnancy* and Chapter 51: *Sexually Transmitted Infections*.
Rubella IgG antibodies for immunity		**IgG positive** — continue routine antenatal care. **IgG negative** — for rubella immunisation [measles, mumps and rubella (MMR) vaccine — live vaccine] ***postnatally*** if the patient is agreeable. Avoid conception for 28 days after MMR vaccination.
Urine FEME and culture	Screen for asymptomatic bacteriuria.	Refer to Chapter 11 on "Urinary Tract Infections (UTIs) in Pregnancy".
Oral glucose tolerance test (OGTT)	For women with previous gestational diabetes mellitus (GDM), screen at booking with a 75 g 2-point OGTT. Repeat a 75 g 3-point OGTT at 24–28 weeks if the initial OGTT is normal. Screen for GDM in other patients with a 3-point 75 g OGTT at 24–28 weeks.	Refer to Chapter 11: *Hyperglycaemia in Pregnancy*". ***KKH:*** We perform universal screening for GDM for all patients at 24–28 weeks. ***NICE Guidelines:*** Screen for GDM at 24–28 weeks for patients with risk factors for GDM. For patients with GDM in previous pregnancies, screen at booking. If the OGTT is normal, repeat OGTT at 24–28 weeks.
Group B streptococcus (GBS) screen — lower vaginal and anorectal swab		Swab at 35–37 weeks (or 3–5 weeks before the anticipated delivery date). For twins, GBS screen at 32–34 weeks of gestation. Intrapartum antibiotics if GBS positive for vaginal deliveries or if SROM before the caesarean section Refer to Chapter 15: *Infections in Pregnancy*.

CHAPTER 23

Approach to Prenatal Screening for Thalassaemia

Haemoglobinopathies are inherited disorders of haemoglobin (Hb) involving haeme or globin. These may be divided into thalassaemia and structural haemoglobinopathies.

- *Thalassaemia* is a spectrum of inheritable haemoglobinopathies that result from a lack of normal adult haemoglobin chains. It may range from mild to life-threatening forms. It is transmitted in an **autosomal recessive** pattern.
- *Structural haemoglobinopathies* include *sickle cell anaemia (HbSS)*, its variant *haemoglobin SC (HbSC) disease* and *HbE disease*. HbE is attributed to both a lack of normal haemoglobin and structurally abnormal haemoglobin chains.

The incidence of thalassaemia in Singapore is 4%. Three common thalassaemia traits of most significant clinical concern locally are alpha-thalassaemia, beta-thalassaemia and HbE traits.

The incidence of alpha-thalassaemia, beta-thalassaemia and HbE traits is 3%, 1% and 0.5%, respectively.

The antenatal screening programme is essential for the early detection of life-threatening haemoglobinopathies in the fetus, to allow for appropriate genetic counselling to prospective parents and to offer informed management choices.

Alpha-Thalassaemia

- Caused by mutations in the alpha-globin gene along the short arm of chromosome 16. **96% are caused by gene deletions, while 2.8% are**

caused by point mutations (which include the Hb Constant Spring mutation and the Hb Quong Sze mutation).

- The clinical severity of alpha-thalassaemia depends on the number of functional alpha-globin genes unaffected by gene deletion or mutation.

Nomenclature	Genotype	Phenotype
Alpha-2 thalassaemia (α+) Silent alpha-thalassaemia carrier	One gene deleted (αα/α–)	– Normal phenotype – MCV low or normal
Alpha-1 thalassaemia (α°) Alpha-thalassaemia trait	Two genes deleted (αα/––) commoner in the Asian population or (α–/α–) commoner in the Black population	– Asymptomatic – Clinically similar to the beta-thalassaemia trait – Mild microcytic anaemia – Few HbH inclusion bodies – Normal Hb electrophoresis
HbH disease	Three genes deleted (α–/––)	– Moderately severe anaemia: Hb 7–10 g/dl – Chronic haemolysis with moderate pallor, jaundice, splenomegaly
HbH CS disease** ***HbH Constant Spring disease Refer to the section *Constant Spring*	Two genes deleted + Constant Spring point mutation (αCSα/––)	– Much more severe than the HbH disease – Severe anaemia, severe splenomegaly, jaundice – Higher rates of transfusion and splenectomy
Hb Bart's hydrops	Four genes deleted (––/––)	– Almost solely amongst Chinese. – Can be lethal to the fetus because of the hydropic state, resulting in fetal anaemia, cardiac failure, intrauterine death or stillbirth. It can also cause maternal mirror syndrome and severe maternal morbidity, including pre-eclampsia, antepartum haemorrhage and postpartum haemorrhage. – However, treatment is now possible with stem cell transplant in the child. **Options if the fetus is diagnosed with Bart's hydrops:** 1. Expectant management with comfort care. – High risk of intrauterine (IUD) or Neonatal (NN) death. 2. Termination of pregnancy.

(*Continued*)

Nomenclature	Genotype	Phenotype
		3. Fetal blood sampling followed by *intrauterine* transfusion — may resolve the cardiac failure. Results in a live birth in 90% of cases. – *Risks of intrauterine transfusion (10%)*: Preterm premature rupture of membranes (PPROM), placenta abruption, non-reassuring fetal status (NRFS), 3–5% fetal loss, cord haematoma/bleeding. – *Post-delivery*, the child needs lifelong regular blood transfusions approximately every 4–5 weeks and iron chelation therapy. There are risks associated with frequent blood transfusions and the risk of developmental delay, growth restriction or stunted growth. – *Stem cell transplant in the child* is usually done in the second year of life and requires a donor (can be related or unrelated). There are transplant-associated risks, e.g., graft-versus-host disease, chemotherapy, severe infection, marrow suppression, toxicity or death.

<u>Constant Spring</u>.

- A clinically significant type of **point mutation** in **alpha-thalassaemia** that converts the stop codon into glutamine, resulting in a longer alpha-globin chain.
- Results in unstable mRNA, which is degraded before protein synthesis, as well as in the production of unstable alpha-globin chains, resulting in a lack of functional alpha-globin chains.

Nomenclature	Genotype	Phenotype
Silent Constant Spring carrier	One gene mutated ($\alpha\alpha/\alpha CS\alpha$)	– Normal phenotype
Homozygous Constant Spring	Two genes mutated ($\alpha CS\alpha/\alpha CS\alpha$)	– Similar to the alpha-thalassaemia trait
HbH Constant Spring	Two genes deleted + Constant Spring point mutation ($\alpha CS\alpha/--$)	– Much more severe than the HbH disease – Severe anaemia, severe splenomegaly, jaundice – Higher rates of blood transfusion and splenectomy

Beta-Thalassaemia

Caused by mutations in the beta-globin gene along chromosome 11.

- 96% caused by point mutations, 2% attributed to deletion mutations.
- Results in a reduced (β_+) or complete absence (β^o) of beta-globin chain synthesis.
- Most beta-thalassaemic syndromes locally are caused by a complete absence of beta-globin chain synthesis — (β^o).
- Inadequate beta-globin chain production results in decreased amounts of normal adult haemoglobin (HbA) with subsequent increased production of HbA2 and HbF.
- This leads to an imbalance in the globin chain, forming unstable alpha-globin tetramers, which interact with erythrocyte membranes and shorten their lifespan.
- A low MCV of <80 fl has a high sensitivity but low specificity (a cut-off of MCV <80 fl captures 99.7% of all beta-thalassaemias, but only 11.4% of microcytic anaemia with MCV <80 fl have beta-thalassaemia).
- Hb electrophoresis of beta-thalassaemia will show elevated HbA2 levels (3.4–10%) and HbF levels.
- A low MCV (microcytosis) could also reflect iron-deficiency anaemia, but it is postulated that thalassaemia has a higher degree of microcytosis in comparison to iron-deficiency anaemia.
- Patients with low MCV levels *without* beta-thalassaemia should still be assessed for alpha-thalassaemia and HbE traits.

Nomenclature	Genotype	Phenotype
Beta-thalassaemia trait	(β^o/β) or (β^+/β)	- Asymptomatic - Mild anaemia - Microcytosis, target cells
Beta-thalassaemia intermedia	(β^+/β^o) or (β^+/β_+)	- Moderately severe anaemia (Hb 7–9 g/dl) - Normal growth rates - Bone marrow hyperplasia - Splenomegaly with blood sequestration requiring splenectomy - Transfusion-independent except during infection or pregnancy
Beta-thalassaemia major	(β^o/β^o)	- Present clinically at 3–6 months of age as HbA requires adequate beta-globin genes - Severe anaemia (Hb 3–4 g/dl) requiring monthly blood transfusions and iron chelation therapy - Iron overload may lead to cardiomyopathies and endocrinopathies.

HbE Trait

- Commonest in the Malay population, which accounts for 96% of the HbE trait.
- Caused by lysine replacing glutamate on codon 26.
- Attributed to both a lack of normal haemoglobin chain production and structural defects in normal adult haemoglobin chains.
- 20% of patients with the HbE trait may not exhibit microcytosis below the discrimination level.

  ***HbE/beta-thalassaemia disease** — 25% chance of inheriting HbE/beta-thalassaemia disease in a couple with one having the HbE trait and the other a beta-thalassaemia carrier.
- A wide spectrum of clinical syndromes, which may range from mild anaemia to severe transfusion-dependent states.
- Up to 50% may require regular, frequent blood transfusions.
- Up to 40% may require splenectomy.

  ***HbE disease**
- The heterozygous HbE trait will resemble a person with the beta-thalassaemia trait.
- The homozygous HbE trait will have a clinical syndrome of mild anaemia.

Alpha-Thalassaemia/Beta-Thalassaemia Co-Inheritance

- A diagnosis of the beta-thalassaemia trait does *not* preclude co-existing alpha-thalassaemia.
- A parent with a silent alpha-thalassaemia carrier ($\alpha\alpha/\alpha-$) or ($\alpha\alpha/--$) and a parent with the beta-thalassaemia trait (β^{+}/β) or (β°/β) have a 25% chance of heterozygous alpha-thalassaemia/beta-thalassaemia co-inheritance.
- However, because of mechanisms resulting in a more balanced alpha-globin and beta-globin chain synthesis, patients with this inheritance are compatible with a healthy lifestyle.

Sickle Cell Disease

- ***Autosomal recessive*** inheritance pattern.
- Commonest in Africa, the Caribbean, the Middle East, India and America.
- Mutation in codon 6 of the beta-globin gene (glutamic acid > valine).
- A mutated form of haemoglobin polymerises in deoxygenated conditions and results in the sickling of erythrocytes. These sickled erythrocytes undergo haemolysis because of membrane rigidity and fragility, resulting in widespread vaso-occlusion.
- **Comprises a spectrum that includes**
  (i) Sickle cell anaemia (HbSS, homozygous HbS)
  - 90% HbS, 2–10% HbF, minimal HbA2, no HbA
  - Usually detected at birth
  - Manifests clinically at age 6 months because of initial high concentrations of HbF (fetal Hb)
  - Four major clinical conditions
    (i) Haemolytic anaemia
    (ii) Vaso-occlusion
    (iii) Infection
    (iv) End organ damage
      - Kidney, spleen, heart, lung, central nervous system, bone, eye, peripheral vascular system

  (ii) Sickle cell trait (HbAS)
  - 40% HbS, 60% HbA
  - Usually asymptomatic

  (iii) Variants (of which HbSC is most significant)
  - *HbSC*
    - Greatest clinical significance with moderate–severe clinical features
    - Better outcomes than sickle cell disease (HbSS) because of longer survival of HbSC compared to HbSS
  - *HbS-B*
    - Clinically similar to HbSS and HbSC diseases

- *HbS-B_+*
  - Mild–moderate severity
- *HbS-HbE*
  - Rare

Prenatal Invasive Testing for Thalassemia
- Chorionic villus sampling (CVS) or amniocentesis.
- If both parents have the alpha-thalassaemia trait, CVS is the preferred mode of prenatal invasive testing.

Table of Thalassaemic Inheritance

Parent 1	Parent 2	Risk of Transmission	Action
Normal ($\alpha\alpha/\alpha\alpha$)	Alpha-2 thalassaemia ($\alpha\alpha/\alpha-$)	• 50% normal • 50% alpha-2 thalassaemia	Reassure
Alpha-2 thalassaemia ($\alpha\alpha/\alpha-$)	Alpha-2 thalassaemia ($\alpha\alpha/\alpha-$)	• 25% normal • 25% alpha-1 thalassaemia • 50% alpha-2 thalassaemia	Reassure
Normal	Alpha-1 thalassaemia o Homozygous ($\alpha-/\alpha-$) or o Heterozygous ($\alpha\alpha/--$)	• If homozygous ($\alpha-/\alpha-$), all will be alpha-2 thalassaemia • If heterozygous ($\alpha\alpha/--$) 50% normal 50% alpha-1 thalassaemia	Reassure
Alpha-1 thalassaemia Heterozygous ($\alpha\alpha/--$)	Alpha-1 thalassaemia Heterozygous ($\alpha\alpha/--$)	• **25% Bart's hydrops** • 50% alpha-1 thalassaemia • 25% normal	*Refer* for genetic counselling. *Offer* prenatal invasive testing.
Alpha-1 thalassaemia Homozygous ($\alpha-/\alpha-$)	Alpha-1 thalassaemia Homozygous ($\alpha-/\alpha-$)	• All alpha-1 thalassaemia	Reassure

(Continued)

(*Continued*)

Parent 1	Parent 2	Risk of Transmission	Action
Alpha-1 thalassaemia Homozygous (α–/α–)	Alpha-1 thalassaemia Heterozygous ($\alpha\alpha$/– –)	• **50% HbH disease** • 50% alpha-2 thalassaemia	*Refer* for genetic counselling. *Offer* prenatal invasive testing.
Normal ($\alpha\alpha/\alpha\alpha$)	Silent Constant Spring carrier ($\alpha\alpha/\alpha$CSα)	• 50% normal • 50% silent Constant Spring carrier	Reassure
Silent Constant Spring carrier ($\alpha\alpha/\alpha$CSα)	Silent Constant Spring carrier ($\alpha\alpha/\alpha$CSα)	• **25% homozygous Constant Spring disease** • 50% silent Constant Spring carrier • 25% normal	*Refer* for genetic counselling. *Offer* prenatal invasive testing.
Alpha-1 thalassaemia Heterozygous ($\alpha\alpha$/– –)	Silent Constant Spring carrier ($\alpha\alpha/\alpha$CSα)	• **25% HbH Constant Spring disease** • 25% alpha-1 thalassaemia • 25% Constant Spring carrier • 25% normal	*Refer* for genetic counselling. *Offer* prenatal invasive testing.
Normal	Beta-thalassaemia trait (β^o/β) or (β^+/β)	• 50% beta-thalassaemia trait • 50% normal	Reassure
Beta-thalassaemia trait (β^o/β) or (β_+/β)	Beta-thalassaemia trait (β^o/β) or (β^+/β)	• **25% beta-thalassaemia major** • 50% beta-thalassaemia carrier • 25% normal	*Refer* for genetic counselling. *Offer* prenatal invasive testing.
Beta-thalassaemia trait (β^o/β) or (β_+/β)	HbE carrier	• **25% HbE beta-thalassaemia disease** • 25% beta-thalassaemia carrier • 25% HbE trait • 25% normal	*Refer* for genetic counselling. *Offer* prenatal invasive testing.
Normal	HbE trait	• 50% HbE trait • 50% normal	Reassure
HbE trait	HbE trait	• 25% homozygous HbE • 50% HbE trait • 25% normal	Reassure

(Continued)

Parent 1	Parent 2	Risk of Transmission	Action
Alpha-2 thalassaemia ($\alpha\alpha/\alpha-$)	Beta-thalassaemia trait (β°/β) or (β^{+}/β)	• 25% co-inheritance alpha–beta-thalassaemia • 25% beta-thalassaemia trait • 25% alpha-2 thalassaemia • 25% normal	Reassure
Alpha-1 thalassaemia ($\alpha\alpha/--$)	Beta-thalassaemia trait (β°/β) or (β_{+}/β)	• 25% co-inheritance alpha–beta thalassaemia • 25% beta-thalassaemia trait • 25% alpha-1 thalassaemia • 25% normal	Reassure
Alpha-2 thalassaemia ($\alpha\alpha/\alpha-$)	Co-inheritance alpha–beta-thalassaemia	• **25% HbH disease** • 25% co-inheritance alpha–beta-thalassaemia • 25% alpha-1 thalassaemia • 12.5% beta-thalassaemia • 12.5% normal	*Refer* for genetic counselling. *Offer* prenatal invasive testing.
Alpha-1 thalassaemia ($\alpha\alpha/--$)	Co-inheritance alpha–beta thalassaemia	• **25% Bart's hydrops** • 25% co-inheritance alpha–beta-thalassaemia • 25% alpha-1 thalassaemia • 12.5% beta-thalassaemia • 12.5% normal	*Refer* for genetic counselling. *Offer* prenatal invasive testing.
Beta-thalassaemia trait (β°/β) or (β^{+}/β)	Co-inheritance alpha–beta-thalassaemia	• **25% beta-thalassaemia major or intermedia**	*Refer* for genetic counselling. *Offer* prenatal invasive testing.
Co-inheritance alpha–beta-thalassaemia	Co-inheritance alpha–beta-thalassaemia	• **50% Bart's hydrops** • **Beta-thalassaemia major or intermedia**	*Refer* for genetic counselling. *Offer* prenatal invasive testing.
HbE trait	Co-inheritance alpha–beta-thalassaemia	• **25% HbE beta-thalassaemia disease**	*Refer* for genetic counselling. *Offer* prenatal invasive testing.

Algorithm for Prenatal Thalassaemia Screening

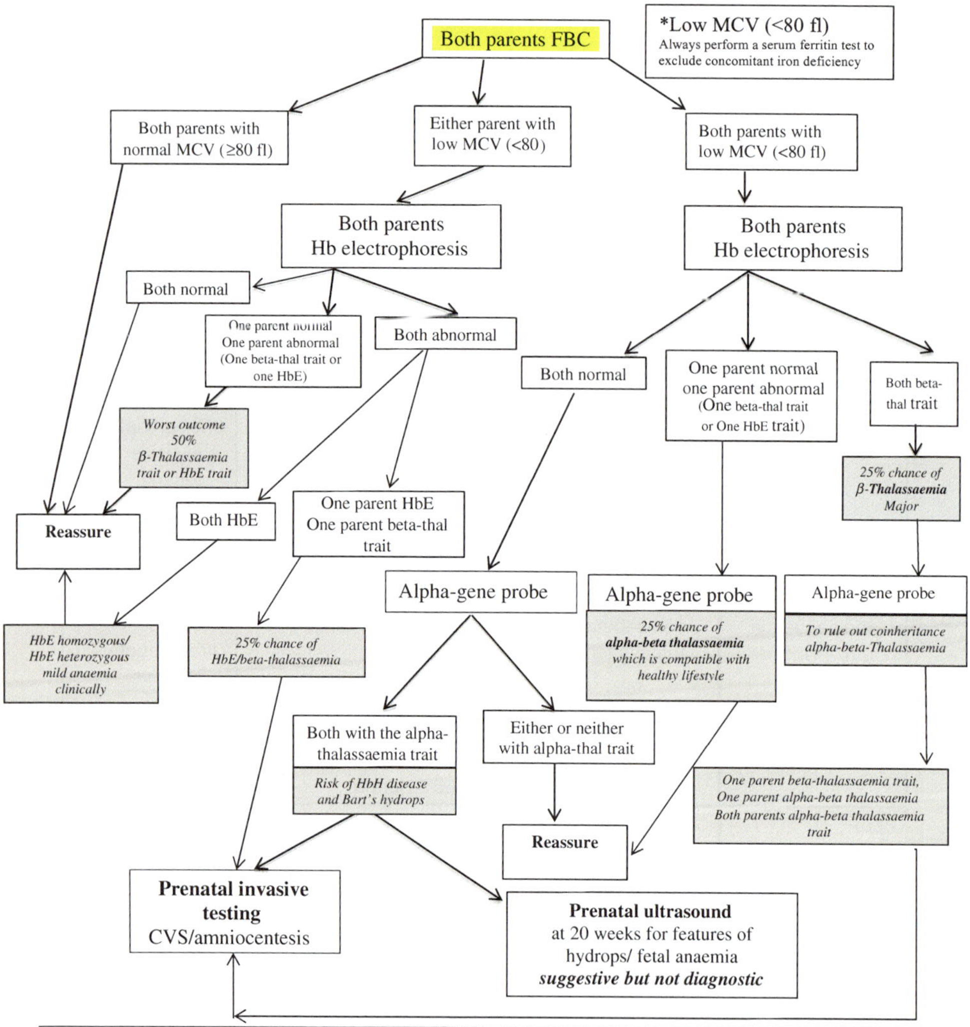

Ultrasound features suggestive of Hb Bart's hydrops foetalis

- Cardio-thoracic ratio >0.5, placental thickening >2 SD, dilated umbilical vein, subcutaneous oedema, ascites, hepatosplenomegaly, oligohydramnios, cord oedema seen in 1/3 of affected pregnancies by weeks 17–18. These are strongly suggestive of Hb Bart's hydrops.
- Fetal anaemia can be predicted based on a Doppler ultrasound scan: fetal MCA/PSV > 1.5 MoM.
- Ultrasound cannot be used to detect beta-thalassaemia major as it only manifests clinically between 3 and 6 months of life.

CHAPTER 24

Approach to Management of Red Cell Antibodies in Pregnancy

Red cell antibodies are present in about 1–2% of pregnant women. All pregnant women should check their blood group and antibody status at booking and again at 28 weeks of gestation. Screening is important to identify women with abnormal red cell antibodies who will have higher-risk pregnancies. This allows clinicians to appropriately manage this group of patients to prevent adverse maternal and perinatal outcomes for their current and future pregnancies.

Importance of performing blood group and antibody tests in pregnancy:

1. To reduce the chance of haemolytic disease of the fetus and newborn (HDFN), e.g., in a rhesus-negative mother carrying a rhesus-positive fetus.
   - We need to administer prophylactic anti-D immunoglobulin at 28–30 weeks of gestation, after any sensitising events and again within 72 hours of the delivery if the baby is rhesus-positive.
   - This is to prevent rhesus isoimmunisation and adverse consequences in current and future pregnancies.
2. To ensure that compatible blood/blood products are transfused to avoid blood transfusion reactions.
3. Autoimmune haemolytic anaemia due to auto-antibodies to the I antigen that develop after infections such as mycoplasma. Paroxysmal cold haemoglobinuria can occur because of auto-antibodies to the P antigen.
4. Confers resistance to certain parasites, e.g., malaria.
   - *Plasmodium falciparum*: Blood group O confers greater resistance to severe malaria, whereas women with blood group A are at a higher risk of developing severe malaria.
   - Duffy antigen negativity confers resistance to *Plasmodium vivax*.

Pathophysiology of Red Cell Antibodies

Maternal alloantibodies can develop as a result of:

1. Pregnancy
2. Previous blood/blood product transfusion
3. History of solid organ/tissue transplant
4. Fetomaternal haemorrhage (FMH)
5. Shared needles from intravenous drug use

Special note: Rh-negative mothers who have been given prophylactic anti-D will have a positive antibody test for anti-D. It is crucial to differentiate iatrogenic from rhesus isoimmunisation causes for positive anti-D results. Iatrogenic anti-D can remain in the maternal circulation for up to 12 weeks.

Transplacental passage of significant maternal red cell antibodies can have adverse maternal, fetal and neonatal effects.

For the ***mother***: Need close antenatal monitoring. If fetal hydrops occurs, it can cause mirror syndrome. The woman will require antigen-negative or cross-matched blood for transfusion. Hence, this can cause a delay in providing blood and blood products.

For the ***fetus***: It can result in HDFN, causing severe fetal anaemia. Without treatment, severe fetal anaemia will cause fetal hydrops, preterm delivery or perinatal death. The fetus may need *intrauterine* transfusion (IUT) or preterm delivery.

For the ***neonate***: Hyperbilirubinaemia, neonatal jaundice and anaemia can occur. The neonate may require phototherapy or exchange transfusions for severe neonatal jaundice to reduce the risks of kernicterus. Blood transfusions may be needed if the neonate is anaemic. If left untreated, the neonate may suffer kernicterus, heart failure and death.

If delivered preterm, the neonate will also have problems associated with prematurity.

Types of Red Blood Cell Antibodies

1. Anti-D
2. Anti-c

3. Anti-K
   The risk of fetal anaemia is highest with anti-D, anti-c and anti-K antibodies.
4. Antibodies that can also cause significant fetal anaemia include:
   - Anti-E
   - Anti-Fy^a
   - Anti-Jk^a
   - Anti-C
   - Anti-Ce
   - Warm-acting Anti-M antibodies (can cause fetal anaemia even at low titres)

There are other blood antibodies that can cause mild or moderate haemolysis. Management should be individualised and in consultation with a maternal–fetal specialist.

Management of Red Cell Antibodies in Pregnancy

Once red blood cell antibodies are identified:

1. *Obtain history from the woman*
   - Obstetric history
   - Fertility history: Potential non-paternity or IVF (donor sperm pregnancy)
   - Risk factors for alloantibody development: History of blood transfusion/transplant/fetomaternal haemorrhage
   - Presence of blood antibodies and titres in previous pregnancies
   - Previous history of HDFN
   - History of *intrauterine* transfusion (IUT): Gestation of IUT and delivery, pregnancy outcomes
   - Previous unexplained severe neonatal jaundice, any phototherapy required
   - History of neonatal anaemia requiring blood transfusion/exchange transfusion
2. Send blood for antibody identification

3. Perform antibody titres
4. Consider paternal red cell antigen phenotype testing or fetal genotyping via cell-free DNA (cfDNA)
   A. *Paternal red cell antigen phenotype testing*
      - This can be done for Kell, C, c, E, e, M and other blood antibodies. However, it is a sent-out test to HSA and the cost varies depending on the type and number of antigens required.
      - If the father is homozygous for the implicated antigen, there is **no role** for cfDNA except for the D antigen. This is because paternal red cell phenotyping *cannot* determine homozygosity for the D antigen.
   B. *Fetal genotyping via cfDNA*
      - Only for D, C, c, E and K
      - **Indicated if**
        - o The paternal antigen status is unknown OR
        - o The father is heterozygous for the implicated antigen OR
        - o The father is homozygous for the D antigen
5. **Monitoring** of red cell antibody titres

   Monitoring of blood antibody titres is required if

   Clinically significant red cell antibodies are present and

   ✓ Paternal antigen is positive OR

   ✓ cfDNA shows fetal K/D/c is positive OR

   ✓ The woman **declined** paternal phenotype/fetal genotype testing

Red cell antibody	Management
D	If the titre is **<1:32**: Repeat titres four weekly till 28 weeks, then two weekly till delivery. Do not give anti-D (Rhogam) for sensitised pregnancies. If unsure of alloimmunisation, give antenatal anti-D.
Kell/c+E and M (warm reacting)	Refer to a maternal–fetal specialist for close monitoring. Repeat the antibody screen at 28 weeks of gestation.
C/c/E/e	If the titre is **<1:32**: Repeat titres four weekly till 28 weeks, then two weekly till delivery.
Other red cell antibodies	Repeat titres at 28 weeks.

6. **Refer to a maternal–fetal specialist for antenatal monitoring if**
   ✓ Previous history of HDFN/IUT (refer by 18 weeks of gestation) OR
   ✓ Previous unexplained severe neonatal jaundice or anaemia requiring blood transfusion/exchange transfusion (refer by 18 weeks of gestation) OR
   ✓ At **ANY** red cell antibody titres of:
      o Kell
      o Anti-M (warm reacting)
      o Anti c+E

   OR

   Definition of a significant titre is a titre of ≥1:32 or >2-fold rise in titres
   ✓ At significant titres of:
      o Anti-D
      o Anti-E/anti-e
      o Anti-C/anti-c
      o Any other red blood cell antibodies
   - Fetal surveillance is via Doppler ultrasound for middle cerebral artery peak systolic velocity (MCA-PSV) and ultrasound features of fetal anaemia or hydrops.
   - <u>MCA-PSV</u> is predictive of moderate or severe fetal anaemia with a 100% sensitivity and a false positive rate of 12%.
   - If <u>MCA-PSV is >1.5 MoM</u> or there are features of fetal anaemia, invasive testing is required via cordocentesis for fetal haemoglobin or haematocrit followed by intrauterine transfusion (IUT).
   - IUT is usually <u>not</u> performed after 34 weeks of gestation.
   - Delivery should be considered instead if ≥34 to 35 weeks of gestation.
   - Anti-D prophylaxis should be given after invasive testing to non-sensitised rhesus-negative women.
7. ***Timing of delivery***
   - A multidisciplinary collaboration involving a maternal–fetal specialist, neonatologist and haematologist.
   - If the antibody titre has been stable *without* fetal anaemia, consider delivery between 37 and 38 weeks of gestation.
   - If the fetus is at moderate or high risk of HDFN, but MCA-PSV is <1.5 MoM, suggest delivery by 37 weeks of gestation.

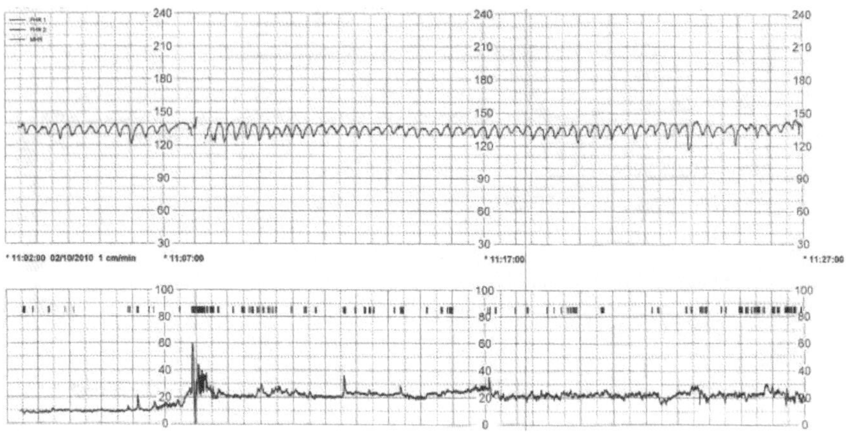

Figure showing sinusoidal trace on CTG.

- If IUT has been performed, delivery is usually arranged 7–10 days after the last IUT.
- For women requiring IUT, delivery should be considered after 34–35 weeks.
- Ensure that cross-matched blood is available for the woman during the delivery.
- Continuous intrapartum CTG monitoring during labour.
- Fetal anaemia can present on CTG in different ways.
    - o *Sinusoidal trace* — occurs rarely but is typical of severe fetal anaemia with haemoglobin <5 g/dl.
    - o *Bradycardia* — suggestive of sudden fetal decompensation, which indicates massive fetomaternal haemorrhage.
    - o *Reduced variability ± decelerations* — indicate a slow but prolonged period of fetomaternal haemorrhage in hydrops fetalis.
    - o *Occasional decelerations but otherwise normal CTG* — indicate small amounts of bleeding that resolve.

CHAPTER 25

Prenatal Screening for Chromosomal Defects and Invasive Diagnostic Tests

When offering genetic testing for chromosomal abnormalities to patients, it is necessary to have pre-test and post-test genetic counselling by appropriately trained medical practitioners/genetic counsellors.

Prenatal Screening Tests for Chromosomal Abnormalities

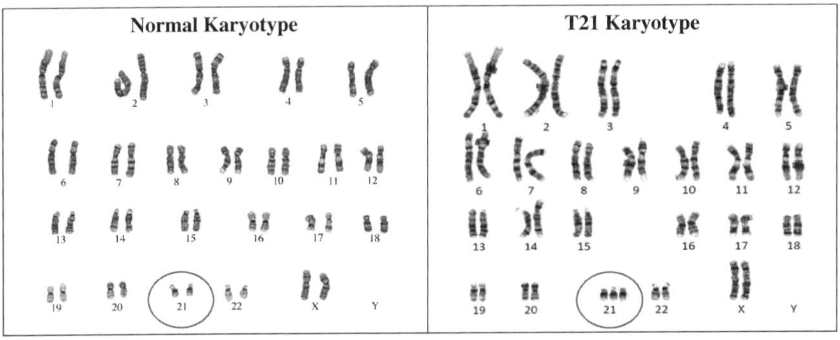

Introduction — Pre-Test Counselling

- Down syndrome, also known as trisomy 21 (T21), is the most common chromosomal disorder.
  - o Individuals with T21 have IQ in the mildly-to-moderately low range, characteristic facial features and other health issues such as cardiac defects (e.g., septal defects, Tetralogy of Fallot, patent

ductus arteriosus) and gastrointestinal problems (e.g., duodenal atresia, annular pancreas and Hirschsprung disease).

- Two other chromosomal disorders that are relatively common in pregnancies are trisomy 18 (T18, also known as Edward syndrome) and trisomy 13 (T13, also known as Patau syndrome).
  - Pregnancies affected by T18 and T13 are at increased risk of miscarriage, severe structural defects and stillbirth, and babies that do survive typically have a severe intellectual disability and long-term medical problems.
- T21, T18 and T13 account for approximately 50% of all chromosomal disorders found in pregnancies.
- All pregnancies are at risk of chromosomal disorders regardless of maternal age or family history. It is for this reason that screening is routinely offered to all pregnant women.

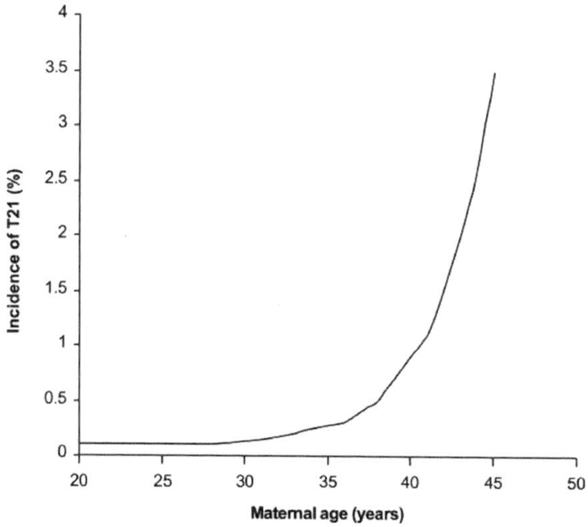

Graph showing correlation between maternal age and incidence of T21

Source: Hultén MA, Patel SD, Tankimanova M, et al. On the origin of trisomy 21 Down syndrome. Mol Cytogenet. 2008;1:21. Published 2008 Sep 18. doi:10.1186/1755-8166-1-21

- **Screening tests are NOT diagnostic.** Most women with screen-positive results have unaffected pregnancies.
- **Screening is optional** as not every pregnant woman finds value in pursuing testing. Proper pre-test counselling involving discussion of the benefits and limitations of various screening options is therefore integral to helping women decide which screening testing is useful to them, if any.

Screening Test Options for Down Syndrome (Trisomy 21)

<table>
<tr><th>Test</th><th>Description</th><th>Abnormal Result</th><th>Timing in Pregnancy</th><th>Detection Rate for T21</th><th>False Positive Rate</th><th>Management of Abnormal Results</th></tr>
<tr><td>Maternal age</td><td>The risk of T21, T18, T13 and other aneuploidies in pregnancy increases with maternal age.</td><td><table><tr><th>Age</th><th>Risk of T21</th></tr><tr><td>20</td><td>1:1,667</td></tr><tr><td>30</td><td>1:952</td></tr><tr><td>35</td><td>1:250</td></tr><tr><td>40</td><td>1:100</td></tr><tr><td>45</td><td>1:30</td></tr></table></td><td>—</td><td>30%</td><td>—</td><td>Offer further screening or diagnostic tests</td></tr>
<tr><td>Age + nuchal translucency (NT)
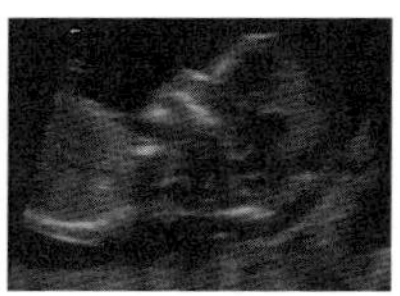
nuchal translucency (NT)</td><td>Ultrasound scan of the width of the translucent gap at the back of the fetal neck</td><td>Thickened NT

Associations with thickened NT:
1. Normal variant
2. Chromosomal disorders
3. Single-gene disorders, e.g., RASopathies when NT is ≥3.5 mm
3. Cardiac defects and other structural abnormalities, e.g., diaphragmatic hernia, renal anomalies, body stalk disruption, abdominal wall defects
4. Increased risk of twin–twin transfusion syndrome in monochorionic twins</td><td>First trimester 11+0 to 13+6 weeks of gestation (CRL 45–84 mm)</td><td>80%</td><td>5%</td><td>As per KKH's protocol

Thickened NT >97th centile: Arrange for a fetal cardiac ultrasound at 15–16 weeks of gestation

NT ≥3.5 mm: Offer diagnostic testing, including for chromosome microarray analysis (CMA — 4% yield when the karyotype is normal) and single-gene disorders such as RASopathies</td></tr>
</table>

Test	Description	Abnormal Result	Timing in Pregnancy	Detection Rate for T21	False Positive Rate	Management of Abnormal Results
Combined first-trimester screen (cFTS) 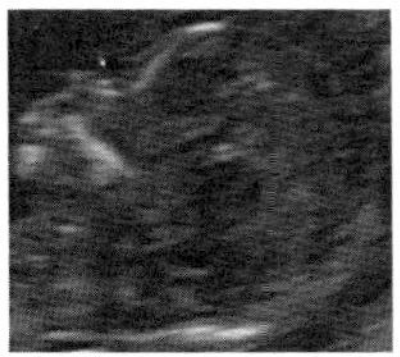 Nasal bone (NB)	Ultrasound scan for NT and NB Blood test: free βHCG, PAPP-A Maternal age	Thickened NT Structural abnormality The cut-off for a high-risk result is 1:300.	First trimester 11+0 to 13+6 weeks of gestation, (CRL 45–84 mm) Blood test from 9 weeks	90%	5%	As per KKH's protocol ***High risk (≥1:300):*** Offer further testing through non-invasive prenatal testing (NIPT), chorionic villus sampling (CVS), amniocentesis ***Intermediate risk*** (1:301 to 1:1,000): Offer NIPT ***Low risk*** (<1:1,000): No further testing is offered *NT >97th centile*: Arrange for a fetal cardiac ultrasound at 15–16 weeks of gestation. NT ≥3.5 mm: Offer diagnostic testing, including for CMA (4% yield when the karyotype is normal) and single-gene disorders such as RASopathies. ***Low PAPP-A <0.415 MoM*** is associated with fetal growth restriction (FGR) and small for gestational age (SGA): serial growth scans to watch for FGR and SGA. *Low PAPP-A* is also associated with T21, pre-eclampsia and stillbirth. **PAPP-A/free βHCG <0.2 MoM:** Increases risk of atypical chromosome problems

(Continued)

(Continued)

Test	Description	Abnormal Result	Timing in Pregnancy	Detection Rate for T21	False Positive Rate	Management of Abnormal Results
Triple screen (maternal serum screening, MSS)	βHCG, AFP, uE3	High risk	Second trimester, up to a head circumference of 220 mm	60%	5%	Offer NIPT or amniocentesis
Quadruple screen	βHCG, AFP, uE3, **inhibin A**	High risk	Second trimester 15–20 weeks of pregnancy	75%	5%	Offer NIPT or amniocentesis
Non-invasive prenatal testing (NIPT)	Cell-free DNA (cfDNA) testing of maternal blood that is placental in origin.	High risk **Causes of false-positive NIPT:** 1. Co-twin demise/vanishing twin (the duration that cfDNA from the placenta of the vanished twin can remain detectable in maternal blood is unpredictable) 2. cfDNA from the placenta – Confined placental mosaicism (aneuploid placenta and euploid fetus) 3. cfDNA from the mother – Maternal aneuploidy, e.g., sex chromosome aneuploidy (SCA), maternal copy number variation or mosaicism	After 10 weeks of pregnancy	>99%	0.1%	**High-risk NIPT:** Offer chorionic villus sampling (CVS)/amniocentesis for diagnostic testing. Chromosome-specific risk of mosaicism through CVS: 2% for T21, 4% for T18, 22% for T13 and 59% for monosomy X. **No-call results for NIPT (occur in 2–3% of samples)** **Causes:** 1. <u>Low fetal fraction</u> ■ Early gestation at the time of the test <9–10 weeks ■ High BMI ■ Twin pregnancy with lower fetal fraction per fetus ■ *Race*: Black, South Asian ■ Autoimmune conditions, e.g., systemic lupus erythematosus ■ Fetal aneuploidy/triploidy/mosaicism ■ IVF pregnancy ■ Maternal medication, e.g., low-molecular-weight heparin (LMWH)

Test	Description	Abnormal Result	Timing in Pregnancy	Detection Rate for T21	False Positive Rate	Management of Abnormal Results
NIPT		– Maternal malignancies, e.g., leukaemia, lymphoma – History of organ transplant/recent blood transfusion in the mother 4. Copy number variation 5. Technical/human error **Causes of false-negative NIPT:** 1. Low fetal fraction 2. Confined placental mosaicism (euploid placenta and aneuploidy/mosaic fetus) 3. Copy number variation 4. Euploid vanishing twin 5. Technical/human error **Sex Chromosome Aneuploidy (SCA)** **Causes of inconclusive results:** 1. Maternal SCA or mosaicism 2. Placental SCA or mosaicism 3. Copy number variation in chromosomes X and Y 4. Vanishing twin 5. Technical reasons				2. Technical and biological factors that affect sample quality (e.g., demised co-twin/vanishing twin, consanguinity, maternal organ transplant, maternal malignancy, copy number variation, mosaicism, biological relationship of the egg donor to the fetus) **Management of no-call NIPT results:** 1. Check if the NIPT laboratory allows repeat testing (the likelihood of success with a second blood draw is 75–80%). 2. Check if cFTS has been done. If not, advise cFTS as an alternative form of screening. 3. Low fetal fraction is associated with an increased risk of chromosomal disorders, so diagnostic testing may be offered.

Maternal Serum Markers in Fetal Aneuploidies and Open Neural Tube Defects

	Condition	Biochemical Marker
First trimester (cFTS)	Trisomy 21	High free βHCG Low PAPP-A
	Trisomy 18 and 13	Low free βHCG Low PAPP-A
Second trimester (triple screen)	Trisomy 21	High hCG Low uE3 Low AFP
	Trisomy 18	Low hCG Low uE3 Low AFP
	Open neural tube defects	High AFP

By taking the pregnant woman's blood, the levels of various biochemical markers can be measured to assess the risks of various conditions in pregnancy.

Maternal Serum Markers and Adverse Obstetric Outcomes

	Result	Spontaneous Miscarriage	Preterm Labour	FGR	Intrauterine Death (IUD)	Gestational Hypertension	Placental Abruption
PAPP-A	↓	+	+	+	+	+ (and pre-eclampsia)	–
	↑	–	–	–	–	–	–
free βHCG	↓	+	–	–	–	–	–
	↑	–	+	–	+	+	–
AFP	↓	–	–	–	–	–	–
	↑	+	+	+	+	–	+
uE3	↓	+	–	+	+	–	–
	↑	–	–	–	–	–	–
Inhibin A	↓	–	–	–	–	–	–
	↑	–	+	+	+	+	–

Comparison of Tests Available at KK Hospital for Singleton Pregnancies

	cFTS	NIPT	Triple Screen/ MSS
Method	Blood test and ultrasound	Blood test	Blood test
When can it be done	11 to 13+6 weeks	After 10 weeks	15–20 weeks
What will be tested	T21 T18 T13	T21 T18 T13	T21 T18
Additional conditions tested for	Structural defects such as acrania, alobar holoprosencephaly, and abdominal wall defects that may be obvious even in the early stages of pregnancy	Other chromosomal conditions such as SCAs, 22q11 deletion syndrome, other microdeletions/duplications, rare autosomal trisomies and even single-gene disorders may also be tested through certain panels → not routinely practised partly because of the rarity of these conditions and limited performance data.	Open neural tube defects
Detection rate for T21	90%	99%	65%
Detection rate for T18	97%	98%	60%
Detection rate for T13	92%	99%	N/A
False positive rate	5%	0.1%	5%

Prenatal Invasive Diagnostic Tests

Some patients may choose to obtain diagnostic results for chromosomal disorders, especially if their screening tests show high risk for T21, T18 or T13, if structural defects are seen in the fetus through prenatal ultrasound or if there is a known risk of inherited genetic disease.

A detailed assessment of the fetal structures is also routinely performed around 20 weeks of pregnancy. Although a majority of chromosome defects are specifically screened for through the cFTS and NIPT, the presence of a structural abnormality in the fetus suggests that CVS/amniocentesis can be considered for diagnostic testing for a wider range of chromosomal/ single-gene disorders.

Diagnostic Testing

There are three primary modalities of obtaining tissue for diagnostic testing:

1) A sample of the chorionic villi from the placenta through chorionic villus sampling (CVS)
2) Amniotic fluid though amniocentesis
3) Fetal blood sampling through cordocentesis

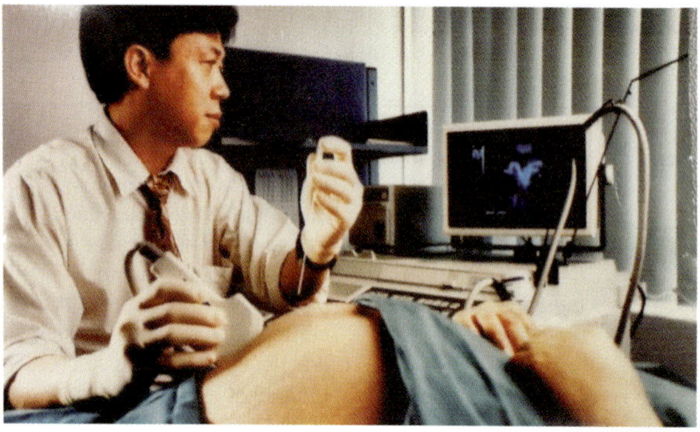

	CVS	Amniocentesis	Cordocentesis
Sample obtained	Chorionic villi from the placenta 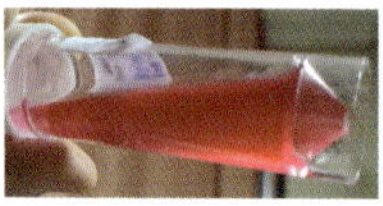	Amniotic fluid ~20 ml (primarily cells from the amnion or cells from the skin, gastrointestinal tract or bladder of the fetus) 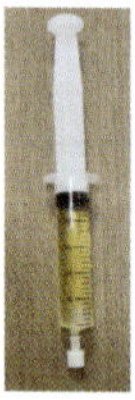	Fetal blood from umbilical vessels (usually from the umbilical cord insertion site at the placenta or intrahepatic vein fetal blood sampling)
Method	Transabdominal **Transcervical**	Transabdominal	Transabdominal
Timeframe	11–14 weeks	16–24 weeks (after 20 weeks if diagnosing fetal infection)	18–24 weeks (after 20 weeks if diagnosing fetal infection)
Benefits	Earlier diagnosis Shorter duration of maternal anxiety Lower risk of termination of pregnancy if done for an abnormal result	Higher accuracy	Higher accuracy

(*Continued*)

	CVS	Amniocentesis	Cordocentesis
Limitations	Lower accuracy due to possible maternal cell contamination or confined placental mosaicism May need amniocentesis at a later date (if the result indicates possible maternal contamination or confined placental mosaicism)	Later diagnosis Increased anxiety and stress waiting for a diagnosis to be made Second-trimester termination is less desirable if the amniocentesis result is abnormal.	Later diagnosis Higher risk of complications
Uses	Chromosomal and genetic disorders – Can be used to detect single-gene conditions such as cystic fibrosis, haemophilia and muscular dystrophies and haemoglobinopathies, e.g., thalassaemia, sickle cell anaemia.	Chromosomal and genetic disorders Diagnose fetal infection, e.g., CMV and toxoplasmosis (refer to Chapter 15: *Infections in Pregnancy*) Amnioreduction in polyhydramnios Assessment of fetal lung maturity (rarely done)	Chromosomal and genetic disorders Blood disorders (i.e., fetal haemolytic disease) Fetal infections, e.g., CMV toxoplasmosis or rubella. Fetal platelet count Fetal anaemia Isoimmunisation *In utero* transfusion
Risks and complications	1 in 300 risk of miscarriage and maternal cell contamination (centre-dependent) 0.5% risk of miscarriage for singletons and 1% risk of miscarriage for twins (RCOG) Uterine infection (rare) (<0.1%) Vaginal bleeding. Risk of fetal limb defects if done before 10 weeks of gestation Transplacental haemorrhage Culture failure 0.5% Mosaicism 1%	1 in 300 risk of miscarriage and maternal cell contamination (centre-dependent) 0.5% risk of miscarriage for singletons and 1% risk of miscarriage for twins (RCOG) Preterm premature rupture of membranes Vaginal bleeding Injury to the fetus (rare as the procedure is ultrasound-guided) Uterine infection (rare) Chorioamnionitis (0.1%) Risk of fetal club foot if done before 15 weeks of gestation.	*Overall 10% risk of complications*: Fetal loss of 3–5% Preterm premature rupture of membranes Vaginal bleeding Injury to the fetus (rare as the procedure is done under ultrasound guidance) Uterine infection (rare) Chorioamnionitis (0.1%) <u>*Specific risks:*</u> Blood loss from the puncture site. Fetal bradycardia secondary to cord haematoma. Preterm premature rupture of membranes. Preterm delivery Placental abruption Fetomaternal haemorrhage

Additional Information

In women with HIV, invasive prenatal tests should ideally be performed when the HIV viral load is <50 HIV RNA copies/ml. If the woman is not on combination antiretroviral therapy (cART) and it is not possible to defer the invasive test, she should be started on cART that includes raltegravir and be given a single dose of nevirapine 2–4 hours before the procedure (BASHH guidelines 2020).

In women with hepatitis B, invasive diagnostic testing can be offered, but they should be informed that the risk of mother-to-child transmission of HBV may be increased with maternal HBV DNA of >6 IU/ml. Antiviral therapy (tenofovir) may be required to reduce the viral load before the invasive procedure. Avoid inserting the needle through the placenta to minimise the risk of intra-amniotic bleeding, which can be a risk factor for vertical transmission.

In women with hepatitis C, there are reassuring but limited data that amniocentesis does not increase the risk of vertical transmission. There are no data available for CVS. Hence, amniocentesis is suggested over CVS. Avoid inserting the needle through the placenta to reduce the risk of intra-amniotic bleeding, which can be a risk factor for vertical transmission.

Non-sensitised rhesus-negative mothers need intramuscular anti-D immunoglobulin (Rhogam) after the procedure to prevent Rh isoimmunisation if the partner is Rh-positive. Avoid sexual intercourse or strenuous exercise for 24–48 hours post-procedure. Inform the patient to return if she is unwell or has fever/chills, fresh vaginal bleeding, watery or foul-smelling vaginal discharge, contraction pain/severe abdominal pain or skin redness/warmth.

Biological samples obtained from these procedures can then be sent for the following tests:

	What it Detects	Turnaround Time
PCR	T21, T18, T13, X and Y	2–3 days
Karyotype	T21, T18, T13, X and Y Deletions/duplications >10 Mb Balanced/unbalanced translocations and inversions	Approximately 2 weeks
CMA (SNP array)	T21, T18, T13, X and Y Deletions/duplications >100 kb Absence of heterozygosity	Approximately 2–3 weeks

1) Karyotyping

a. Karyotype analysis detects T21, T18, T13 and other aneuploidies, rearrangements, deletions and duplications more than 5–10 Mb in size. These chromosome disorders can also be associated with health and intellectual problems.

2) CMA

a. **Benefits**
   i. CMA can detect deletions and duplications 100 times smaller than the karyotype.
   ii. It can be performed on uncultured tissues or cultured cells, reducing the risk of culture failure.

b. CMA provides
   i. Additional 1.7% yield in pregnancies that had CVS/amniocentesis done for the indication of advanced maternal age or positive aneuploidy screen and a normal karyotype.
   ii. Additional 6% yield if the indication of testing was a structural abnormality in the fetus and a normal karyotype. The yield increases to 10% if multiple organ systems are affected in the fetus.

c. Indications for which CMA can be **considered**
   i. Whenever invasive testing is performed

d. Indications for which CMA is **recommended**
   i. Any fetal anomaly (FA)
   ii. NT ≥3.5 mm
   iii. Stillbirth

e. **Limitations**
   i. CMA is **unable** to detect translocations/inversions that are visible through karyotype analysis.
   ii. CMA is **unable** to detect duplications or deletions <100 kb.
   iii. CMA is **unable** to detect single-gene disorders.
   iv. CMA is **unable** to detect mitochondrial disorders, uniparental disomy or low-level mosaicism.
   v. CMA may potentially find copy number variants that are of uncertain significance. This may be because the finding has not been seen before or has variable expressivity or incomplete penetrance. Interpreting such variants of uncertain significance

(**VOUS**) is challenging prenatally because of limited phenotypic information and may cause additional patient anxiety.

3) Single-gene disorders

Targeted variant analysis, customised panels of genes or whole exome sequencing for single-gene disorders.

→ The types of laboratory tests for which the samples can be used depend on the indication for testing and should be carefully considered in consultation with a maternal–fetal medicine specialist.

a. **Targeted variant testing:** If a specific variant is known in family members that indicates that the pregnancy is at increased risk of the genetic condition, targeted testing for the familial variant(s) can be performed.
   i. For example, if both parents are known alpha-thalassaemia carriers and their genetic variant has already been identified, targeted testing for the identified variants can be performed on the placental villi or amniotic fluid.
b. **Customised panel testing:** Multigene panel testing can be considered if the fetus is suspected through ultrasound to be affected by a genetic condition but the variant has not been identified. Panel testing allows the analysis of a carefully curated list of multiple genes known to be associated with the condition of interest. The methods used for these panels may include sequencing analysis and other non-sequencing-based methods, and because the list is limited, it allows for greater depth of coverage and can be more cost-effective.
   i. For example, if the prenatal ultrasound suggests skeletal dysplasia in the fetus, a skeletal dysplasia panel that includes multiple genes associated with various types of skeletal dysplasias may be considered.
c. **Whole exome sequencing (WES):** If the range of differential diagnosis based on the prenatal ultrasound finding(s) is broader, whole exome sequencing may be considered instead. Whole exome sequencing allows the protein-coding exons of thousands of genes to be sequenced, thereby increasing the diagnostic yield.
   i. Patients, however, need to be alerted about the higher possibility of VOUS and the possibility of revealing secondary and incidental findings that may lead to further anxiety.

ii. Patients also need to be aware of the limitations of WES, such as the inability to detect all causes of genetic conditions (e.g., triple repeats), and careful pre-test genetic counselling needs to be provided by individuals with relevant qualifications and training in clinical genetics or genetic counselling.

Depending on the indication for testing, the samples can also be used to test for non-genetic/chromosomal conditions such as fetal infection. All testing should be carefully considered with a maternal–fetal medicine specialist.

Not all patients pursue prenatal screening and diagnostic tests solely for decision-making about continuation versus termination of pregnancy. Information from testing is also beneficial for pregnancy management, delivery management recommendations and the patient's psychological preparation for the reality of raising a child with the condition. Detailed explanations about the benefits and limitations of various test options and exploration of the patient's goals and intentions can be discussed during the genetic counselling session to help patients make informed decisions during their pregnancy.

Prenatal Testing for Multiple Pregnancies

Prenatal screening in multiple pregnancies faces additional challenges compared to singletons. It is important to (1) determine chorionicity and (2) perform correct labelling in twins when screening for aneuploidies and fetal anomalies. It is essential to be aware of the impact of a vanishing twin on prenatal testing (*in utero* death of one twin).

Screening Options

1) cFTS is the screening tool of choice for twin pregnancies up to 13+6 weeks.
   a. For a monochorionic pregnancy, the risk calculated is for the pregnancy as a whole.
      The risk of aneuploidies is the same for each fetus.
   b. For a dichorionic pregnancy, each fetus has an individual risk calculated.

2) A triple screen is also an option for twin pregnancies; the risk calculated is for the pregnancy as a whole.
3) NIPT, but with a higher rate of test failure because of a lower "per fetus" fetal fraction than in singletons.

Comparison of Tests Available at KK Hospital for Twin Pregnancies

	cFTS	NIPT (%)	Triple Screen
Detection rate for T21	83%	99	44%
Detection rate for T18	75%	93	Insufficient data
Detection rate for T13	Insufficient data	95	N/A
False positive rate	5%	0.1	5%

Serum screening and NIPT should *not* be performed on triplets and higher-order multiple pregnancies.

In situations such as co-twin demise/vanishing twin where the performance of serum screening and NIPT is called into question, ultrasound measurement of the NT and nasal bone (NB) can be performed instead.

Diagnostic Options

Both CVS and amniocentesis remain options for twin pregnancies.

	CVS	Amniocentesis
MC twins	A single CVS sample is required	Single sac sampling — *except* in discordant growth and anomalies that will require a two-puncture technique
DC twins	A sample is required from both placentas: a two-needle technique is advised, with sampling near cord insertion of each fetus	Sampling of both amniotic sacs is recommended – Two-puncture technique – Single-puncture technique
Risks and complications	The risk of fetal loss in twin pregnancies is 1% (RCOG 2021).	

CHAPTER 26

Ultrasonography and Fetal Doppler in Obstetrics

Dating Ultrasound Scan

First-trimester ultrasound screening is optimal for

- Establishing pregnancy location and fetal viability and excluding early pregnancy complications.
- Accurate assessment of gestational age by the measurement of the crown-rump length (CRL) (Figure 26.1).
- Confirming multiple pregnancies and determining chorionicity.
- Diagnosis of molar pregnancy.
- Evaluation of adnexae.
- Early detection of fetal anomalies:
  Fetal anomalies fall into three main groups according to whether they are detectable in the first trimester:
  1. ***Always detectable*** — anencephaly, body stalk anomaly, omphalocele, gastroschisis, megacystis, alobar holoprosencephaly.

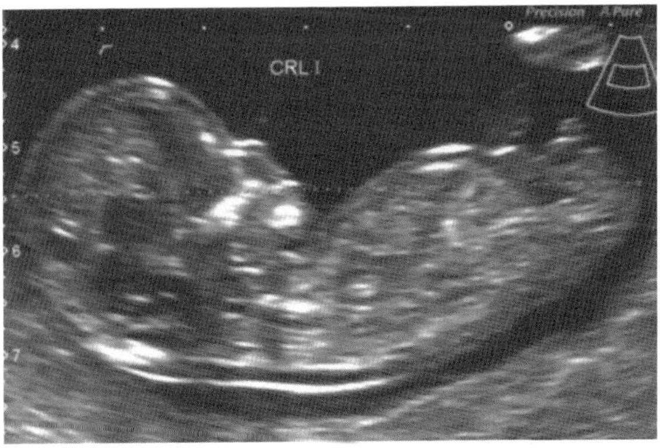

Fig. 26.1 Assessment of gestational age by the measurement of CRL.

2. ***Sometimes/potentially detectable*** — spina bifida, facial cleft, polydactyly, renal agenesis.
3. ***Never detectable*** — microcephaly and agenesis of the corpus callosum (ACC).

Screening Scan

Refer to Chapter 27: *Approach to Management of Abnormal 20-Week Fetal Anomaly Scan.*

Components of the Second-Trimester Ultrasound Examination

- Fetal anatomy — An ultrasound scan between 18 and 22 weeks is optimal for surveying the fetal anatomy and the placental location.
- Placenta — For placental location and relationship to the internal cervical os.
- Fetal biometry.
- Amniotic fluid assessment.

The prevalence of fetal birth defects is around 2–4%, with congenital malformations accounting for 20–30% of neonatal deaths. A routine second-trimester scan is a screening test to detect fetal structural anomalies, which may be followed by genetic evaluation.

The purpose of the screening scan is for:

- Reproductive choice.
- Parents to prepare for any treatment/disability/palliative care or consider termination of pregnancy.
- Management of the pregnancy/delivery in a tertiary centre.
- Intrauterine fetal therapy.
- Management of placenta praevia — placenta praevia complicates 0.3–0.5% of pregnancies. However, the majority (>90%) of low-lying placentas diagnosed at 20 weeks resolve by term. Thus, a follow-up ultrasound in the third trimester, usually between 32 and 35 weeks, is warranted, as this information may influence the mode of delivery.

Growth Scan

The main objective of the third-trimester ultrasound examination is to provide accurate diagnostic information to optimise antenatal care and improve maternal and perinatal outcomes.

Components of the Basic Third-Trimester Ultrasound Examination

- Fetal size [biometry and estimated fetal weight (EFW)]
- Placental location
- Fetal presentation and lie
- Amniotic fluid assessment

Normal growth is defined by measurements of the head [biparietal diameter (BPD), head circumference (HC)], abdominal circumference (AC) and femur length (FL) within the normal ranges for gestation. The *Z*-score of AC is used to determine the EFW.

Abnormal growth is defined as measurements of the head and/or abdomen and/or limbs falling below the normal ranges (<3rd centile). Fetal development is dynamic, and serial measurements at 2–3-week intervals are needed to define normality and abnormality.

Fetal Doppler Studies in Obstetrics

Fetal Doppler offers a unique non-invasive opportunity to extend our ability to investigate fetal haemodynamics. It is used to interrogate fetal, fetoplacental and uteroplacental circulations. Routine Doppler in *low-risk* populations *does not* improve the outcome for the mother or baby.

Common indications for Doppler flow velocimetry studies:

Fetal indications:

- Abnormalities of growth for both intrauterine growth restriction (IUGR) and excessive fetal growth (fetal macrosomia)
- Fetal anomalies (e.g., cystic hygromas, cardiac, thoracic, diaphragmatic, neural tube, renal and abdominal wall)

- Fetal hydrops
- Oligohydramnios and polyhydramnios

<u>Maternal indications:</u>

- Poor obstetric history (e.g., pre-eclampsia, IUGR and previous stillbirth)
- Known maternal risk factors: Hypertension, pre-eclampsia, diabetes, autoimmune disorders (overt and subclinical), thrombophilia (acquired and genetic)
- Multiple pregnancies
- Maternal trauma (fetomaternal haemorrhage)
- Suspected placental abruption
- Known maternal isoimmunisation
- Exposure to parvovirus B19

IUGR complicates 5–10% of all pregnancies and up to 30% of multiple pregnancies. In 60% of these pregnancies, the primary cause is placental insufficiency. Therefore, improvement in identifying the fetus at risk of intrauterine death (IUD) may lead to more successful management strategies.

<u>What to evaluate?</u>

<u>Maternal vessels:</u>

➢ ***Uterine arteries → uterine artery Doppler***

- o Pregnancy is associated with physiologic changes at the level of the uterine vasculature, resulting in a progressive decrease in impedance with advancing gestation. The uterine circulation can be assessed by Doppler velocimetry of the uterine arteries (Fig. 26.2).
- o An increase in the resistance or presence of prediastolic notch predicts association with pre-eclampsia, fetal growth restriction (FGR) and non-reassuring status in labour.
- o Some centres perform uterine artery Doppler in the first trimester to predict the risk of early-onset pre-eclampsia. If the risk of pre-eclampsia is high in the first trimester, low-dose aspirin is started, which has been shown to reduce the risk of pre-eclampsia.
- o In KKH, uterine artery Doppler is performed during the 20-week fetal anomaly screening scan. However, low-dose aspirin started

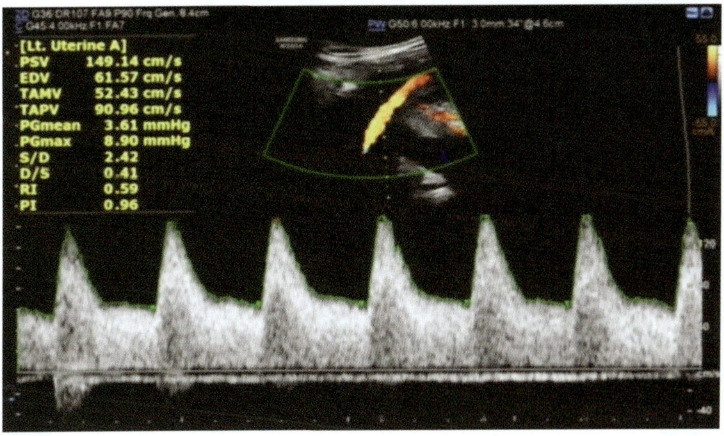

Fig. 26.2 Uterine artery Doppler.

in the second trimester after abnormal uterine artery Dopplers has *not* been shown to reduce the risk of pre-eclampsia.

<u>Fetal vessels:</u>

- ***Umbilical arteries (UA) → UA Doppler***
  - It evaluates blood flow from the fetus to the placenta and, as a result, reflects placental vessel resistance (Fig. 26.3).
  - It is a vital surveillance tool in women diagnosed with FGR. It helps to distinguish FGR caused by placental disease from non-hypoxic or constitutional causes of SGA pregnancies. This is the only measure that provides diagnostic and prognostic information for managing FGR.

A decrease in UA end-diastolic flow (EDF) with elevated resistance indices (high UA pulsatility index) is associated with abnormalities in 30% of fetal vessels (Fig. 26.4).

- Progression of UA Doppler patterns to absent or reverse EDF correlates with the risks of fetal injury or death. Using UA Doppler in high-risk pregnancies (most of them with SGA fetuses) improves perinatal outcomes, with a 29% reduction (2–48%) in perinatal deaths.

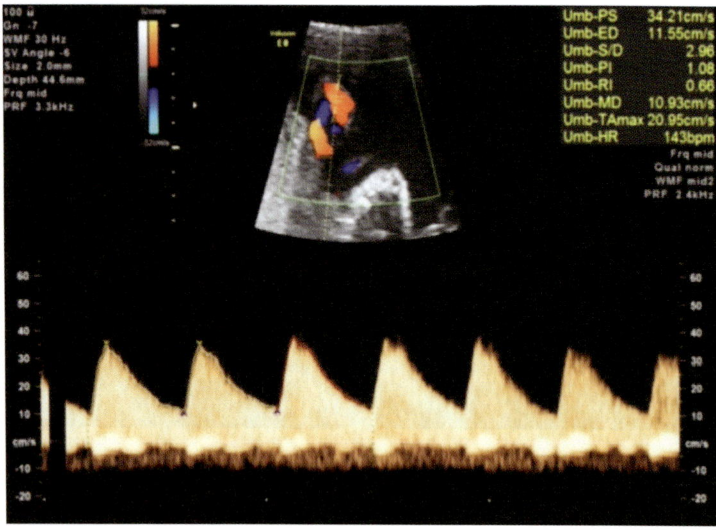

Fig. 26.3 Normal umbilical artery Doppler.

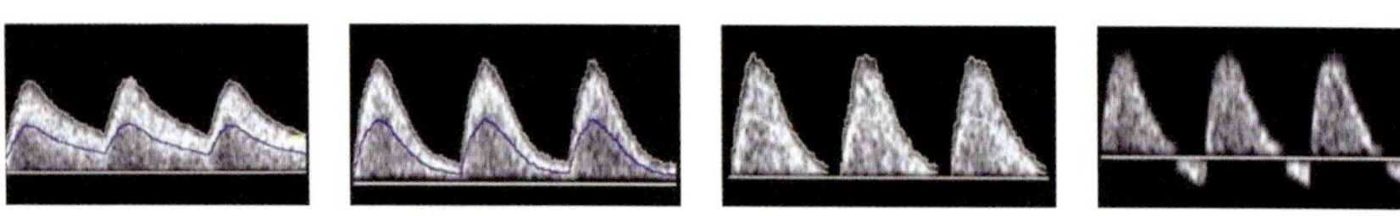

Normal Doppler | Raised UAPI | Absent EDF (AEDF) | Reversed EDF (REDF)

Fig. 26.4 Umbilical artery Doppler showing worsening condition (from right to left).

- ➢ **Middle cerebral arteries (MCA) → MCA Doppler**
  - o MCA peak systolic velocity (PSV) measurements can be done from 16–18 weeks of gestation up to 35 weeks (Fig. 26.5).
  - o Raised MCA PSV is the surrogate marker of fetal anaemia and hypoxia. It is measured for conditions such as red cell antibody alloimmunisation, parvovirus infection, twin-to-twin transfusion, fetomaternal haemorrhage, alpha-thalassaemia and FGR fetus.
  - o FGR due to placental insufficiency is associated with chronic hypoxia, triggering a blood flow centralisation process to maintain blood flow to critical organs such as the brain, chest and adrenal

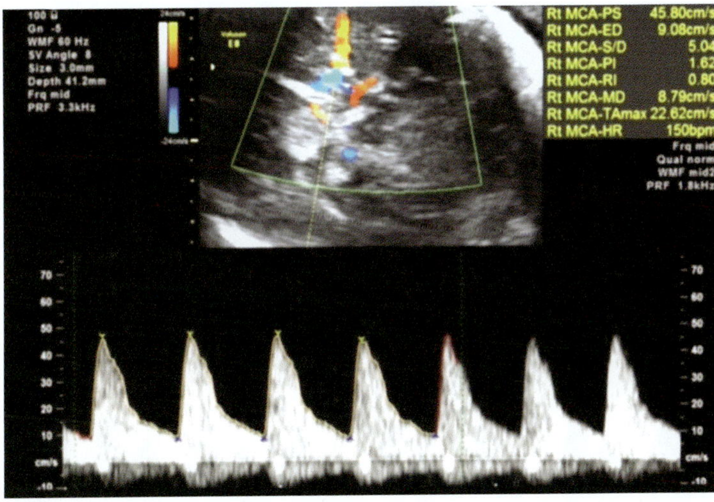

Fig. 26.5 MCA Doppler.

glands. This "brain-sparing" process has been identified as a reduction in the pulsatility index in the middle cerebral artery (MCA PI).

➢ **Ductus venosus (DV) → fetal DV Doppler**
- It is the *strongest single Doppler parameter* to predict the *short-term risk* of fetal death in early-onset FGR.
- DV flow waveforms become abnormal only in advanced stages of fetal compromise, considered sufficient to recommend delivery at any gestational age after completion of antenatal steroids. The sensitivity for fetal loss is 40–70% (Fig. 26.6).
- Changes in DV blood flow reflect fetal heart compliance and its ability to cope with preload.
- A decreased or reversed a-wave in DV results from decreased forward flow in atrial systole.

➢ **Umbilical Vein (UV) → UV Doppler**
- Umbilical venous flow is a non-pulsatile continuous flow pattern in pregnancies after the first trimester.

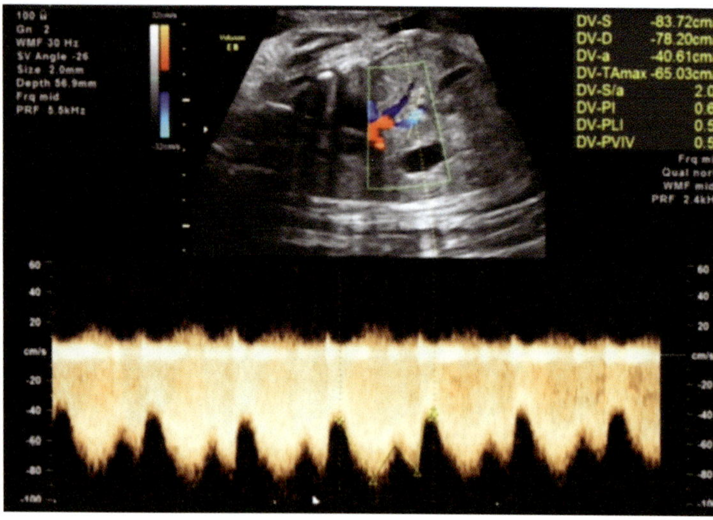

Fig. 26.6 Fetal DV Doppler.

- Pulsations in the umbilical vein reflect increased central venous pressure (CVP) and are pathological. They are often seen at the late stage of a growth-restricted hypoxic fetus and are associated with fetal acidaemia and risk of perinatal mortality.

Table 26.1 Antenatal Doppler Changes and Their Clinical Significance

Vessel	Doppler waveform	Pathophysiology	Clinical significance
Umbilical artery	Reduced/absent/ reversed EDF	Failure of villous trophoblast invasion	Increased resistance in uteroplacental circulation
Middle cerebral artery	Increased peak systolic velocity	Dilatation of cerebral vessels	Brain sparing in anaemia/ hypoxia
Ductus venosus	Absent/reversed “a” wave	Poor fetal heart compliance	Fetal acidaemia
Umbilical vein	Pulsatile flow	Raised CVP	Fetal acidaemia

CHAPTER 27

Approach to Management of Abnormal 20-Week Fetal Anomaly Scan

Introduction

- Major fetal anomalies (FAs) are seen in about 2–4% of live births.
- FAs are important causes of perinatal morbidity and mortality and account for 20–30% of perinatal deaths.
- These could be structural or secondary to aneuploidies/single-gene disorders.
- Congenital anomalies can result in long-term physical, mental, visual and auditory disabilities.
- These can have a significant negative impact on the individual, family, healthcare system and society.
- The most commonly involved structures are the heart (CVS) and central nervous system (CNS).
- These anomalies can be isolated or complex.

FA Scan/Screening Ultrasound (US) Scan

- A screening US scan for detecting FAs should be performed between 18+0 and 20+6 weeks.
- The purpose of the screening scan is to diagnose conditions that may:
  1. Benefit from antenatal/postnatal treatment.
  2. Require postnatal treatment at a specialist centre to improve outcomes.
  3. Indicate a poor prognosis with a high risk of neonatal death.
  4. Lead to a discussion regarding options of terminating or continuing with the pregnancy.

- Overall, the US scan can pick up ~60–70% of FAs, with the rest detected postnatally.
- Detection rates vary depending on the FA.
  It can range from 50% for cardiac defects to almost 98% for anencephaly.
- The US scan cannot assess hearing, vision and intellectual capacity, nor the possibility of future behavioural problems and developmental delay.
- Prenatal detection of FAs allows for optimal antenatal management, providing parents with opportunities for additional imaging, genetic testing and information regarding prognosis and management options.

Causes of FA

- **Genetics** — chromosomal, e.g., aneuploidy, single-gene disorders, genetic syndromes
- **Drugs** (refer to Chapter 18: *Medications in Pregnancy and Lactation*)
  - Retinoids, e.g., isotretinoin
  - Anti-convulsants, e.g., sodium valproate
  - Mood stabilisers, e.g., lithium
  - Angiotensin-converting-enzyme (ACE) inhibitors, e.g., enalapril
  - Anticoagulants, e.g., warfarin, radioactive iodine
  - Immunosuppressive agents, e.g., mycophenolate mofetil
  - Chemotherapy agents, e.g., methotrexate
- **Substance abuse** — illicit drugs, smoking and alcohol
- **Non-consumption of folic acid**
- **Infections during pregnancy** (refer to Chapter 15: *Infections in Pregnancy*) — Toxoplasmosis, CMV, syphilis, rubella, herpes simplex virus (HSV), varicella-zoster virus (VZV)
- **Oligohydramnios**
- **Maternal medical conditions** — type 2 DM, hyperandrogenism
- **Maternal hyperthermia**
- **Environmental exposure** — ionising radiation
- **Mechanical causes** — amniotic bands, uterine fibroids (rare)
- **Idiopathic**

Evaluation of FAs

History

- Age, marital status. Consanguinity.
- Past obstetric history to ascertain gravidity and parity — it is important to identify any previous baby with FAs, neonatal death, stillbirth or recurrent miscarriages.
- Mode of conception — spontaneous or assisted reproductive technology (ART).
- Family history.
  - Congenital abnormalities (cardiac, renal, etc.)
  - Early infant or neonatal death
  - Learning disabilities
  - Familial syndromes
- Detailed *maternal* medical and surgical history.
  - Type 2 DM
  - Epilepsy
  - Autoimmune conditions, e.g., systemic lupus erythematosus (SLE)
  - Tuberous sclerosis
  - Myotonic dystrophy
  - Velocardiofacial syndrome (22q11.2 microdeletion)
  - *Folate deficiency*: inflammatory bowel disease, coeliac disease, malabsorptive disease, previous bariatric surgery
- Detailed *paternal* medical history.
- Dietary habits: look for any risk factors for folate deficiency.
- Exposure to teratogens.
  - Medication
  - Infection — e.g., TORCH infections (toxoplasmosis, rubella, CMV and herpes simplex), VZV
    - Check the patient's rubella immunity status
    - Check for symptoms of CMV or toxoplasmosis infection
  - Ionising radiation
  - Illicit drugs
  - Alcohol — fetal alcohol syndrome (FAS)
  - Toxins, pesticides

- Antenatal history.
  - Singleton or multiple pregnancies
  - Gestation at booking and estimated delivery date (EDD)
  - Fetal aneuploidy screening results

Examination

- Body mass index (BMI) — normal: BMI: 18.5–24.9.
- Evidence of detected phenotypic abnormalities in the parents to rule out an autosomal dominant/chromosomal trait — e.g., single incisor/hypotelorism in a parent may be a mild manifestation of holoprosencephaly; microtia or mild underdevelopment of facial structures may suggest Treacher Collins syndrome.

Investigations

- When FA is detected, *genetic testing* must be offered.
- *Chromosomal microarray analysis* (*CMA*) is a technology used to detect clinically significant microdeletions or duplications and should be the testing modality of choice if the patient decides to pursue further testing.
- As there are constant advancements in genetic testing technology, the recommended testing modality may change in the near future — e.g., *whole exome sequencing* (*WES*) is a method that has been used increasingly frequently in recent years.
- Other specific tests may be required depending on the FA — e.g., testing amniotic fluid for CMV/toxoplasma PCR for ventriculomegaly.

General Management for FA

- Refer to a tertiary centre for multidisciplinary team (MDT) management with a maternal–fetal specialist, neonatologist, genetic counsellor, paediatric cardiologist, paediatric surgeon, neurosurgeon, palliative medicine specialist and medical social worker (MSW).
- Appropriate counselling for the patient on the FA, prognosis, impact on pregnancy, maternal/fetal risks and post-delivery outcomes (both immediate and long-term).
- Discuss the option of termination of pregnancy (TOP) (legally allowed before 24 weeks in Singapore) versus continuing with the pregnancy.

- If the woman continues the pregnancy, antenatal or postnatal testing may be performed.
- If a decision is made for TOP, *postmortem examination and genetic testing* of the fetus should be offered to aid counselling for the subsequent pregnancy.
- Refer to MSW for emotional support as required.

Central Nervous System (CNS)

Fetal Anomaly	Condition/Associations	Management/Delivery/Prognosis/ Recurrence
Acrania–exencephaly–anencephaly sequence (1 in 1,000 at 12 weeks) Can be diagnosed on the first-trimester screening scan at 11–12 weeks (cannot be diagnosed before 11 weeks as skull ossification is *not* complete)	Absent cranial vault and cerebral hemispheres At 12 weeks, acrania is suspected if there is an absence of the normally ossified skull and distortion of the brain (exencephaly). At >16 weeks, the brain is destroyed (anencephaly). CNS or other defects found in 50% of cases, e.g., cleft lip/palate, spina bifida in 25% of cases Associated with other scan findings: – Polyhydramnios in 50% of cases in the second and third trimesters – Fetal hydrops – Placental abruption Associated with cord prolapse or postdate pregnancy. Elevated levels of maternal serum alpha-fetoprotein	• Lethal condition with death within the first week of life • Discuss options of TOP versus continuing pregnancy • Exclude maternal DM • Mode of delivery (MOD) based on obstetric indications if continuing with the pregnancy • Peri-conception folic acid 5 mg/day (3 months before conception and up to 12 weeks of gestation) reduces recurrence risk by ~75%. <u>Recurrence risk</u>: • If one previously affected sibling: 5% • If two previously affected siblings: 10%
Ventriculomegaly (1 in 100 at 20 weeks, 1 in 1,000 births) *Male*: Risk of X-linked hydrocephalus, especially if moderate to severe ventriculomegaly Hydrocephalus	Bilateral or unilateral dilated lateral ventricles ≥10 mm ***Mild:*** 10–12 mm ***Moderate:*** 13–15 mm ***Severe:*** >15 mm Diagnosis of hydrocephalus can be made when there is severe ventriculomegaly and obstruction is seen or can be inferred. – Can be a normal variant if mild ventriculomegaly – Chromosomal defects (T21, T18, T13) in 10% of cases	• Need to exclude other FAs • Offer genetic testing • Maternal CMV/toxoplasma screen or amniocentesis for CMV/toxoplasmosis PCR • Maternal testing for anti-platelet antibodies in cases of evidence of cerebral haemorrhage • MRI scan of the fetal brain at ≥32 weeks for a diagnosis of abnormalities of neuronal migration • Repeat the US scan at 28–34 weeks to assess for progression or regression • Timing and MOD as per obstetric indication

(*Continued*)

(*Continued*)

Fetal Anomaly	Condition/Associations	Management/Delivery/Prognosis/Recurrence
	– Cerebral/non-cerebral defects and genetic syndromes found in 50% of cases – Congenital infections: CMV, toxoplasmosis – Intracranial haemorrhage	• Deliver via caesarean section if fetal head circumference >40 cm • The prognosis depends on the severity, progression and presence of other anomalies. • Isolated *severe* ventriculomegaly: 10-year survival 60%, severe mental handicap 50% • Isolated *moderate* ventriculomegaly: most have a favourable prognosis, but the risk of neurodevelopmental delay is increased. • Isolated *mild* ventriculomegaly: normal outcome <u>Recurrence risk:</u> • 4–50% depending on the cause • If isolated: <1%. Increases to 5% if there is a history of affected fetus/sibling • Part of infection — no increased risk • Part of trisomies — 1% • X-linked hydrocephaly — 50% of males • Associated with alloimmune thrombocytopenia and no treatment — 100%
Encephalocele (1 in 5,000 births)	Cranial bone defect with herniated fluid-filled or brain-filled cyst Usually *occipital* (85%), but can be parietal (15%), rarely frontal Chromosomal defects (T18, T13) in 10% of cases Cerebral/non-cerebral defects and genetic syndromes in >60% of cases *Most common genetic syndromes*: Meckel–Gruber syndrome, Walker–Warburg syndrome, amniotic band syndrome	• Offer genetic testing. • Deliver via caesarean section at 38 weeks to avoid trauma to the exposed brain. • Will require postnatal surgery. • Peri-conceptional folic acid 5 mg/day. • Prognosis depends on the size of the defect, contents of the sac, location, presence of hydrocephalus, infection and underlying chromosomal/genetic issues. • Mortality for posterior encephalocele is >50% and for posterior meningocele and anterior encephalocele is about 20%. • Neurological handicap in >50% of survivors. <u>Recurrence:</u> • If isolated: 3–5% • If part of trisomies: 1% • If part of autosomal recessive conditions: 25%

(*Continued*)

Fetal Anomaly	Condition/Associations	Management/Delivery/Prognosis/ Recurrence
Holoprosencephaly (1 in 10,000 births)	Incomplete cleavage of the forebrain *Four types:* alobar, semilobar, lobar, syntelencephaly (middle interhemispheric fusion) Associated with CNS and craniofacial defects. Facial deformities are usually present, e.g., cleft lip/ palate, deformed nose/ proboscis and hypotelorism/ cyclops deformities. The primary cause of malformation is suspected to be multifactorial, with genetic and environmental components. *Chromosomal defects* (T18, T13) in >50% of cases *Genetic syndromes* in 20% of cases *Congenital infections:* CMV/toxoplasmosis, syphilis, rubella, HSV *Associated environmental factors*: maternal DM, usage of certain drugs such as retinoic acid, alcohol or lithium; drug and alcohol abuse	• Offer genetic testing • MDT management • Discuss the option of TOP versus continuing the pregnancy • Fetal MRI may be useful in the confirmation of cases of lobar holoprosencephaly. • Alobar and semilobar — usually lethal in the first year of life • Lobar — life expectancy may be normal but usually with severe developmental delay and visual impairment *Recurrence risk:* • If isolated: 6% • If part of trisomies: 1% • If part of genetic syndromes: 25–50%
Microcephaly (1 in 1,000 births)	Ratio of fetal head circumference to abdominal circumference <3rd centile Sloping forehead present because of the disproportion of the frontal lobes and face Associated with a history of consanguinity, other FAs, congenital infections: CMV, toxoplasmosis, Zika virus Chromosomal abnormalities (T21, T18, T13) are rare. Genetic syndromes are very common, usually single-gene defects with either an autosomal recessive or X-linked inheritance pattern.	• Offer genetic testing • MDT management • Maternal CMV/toxoplasma screen for fetal infections. Consider testing for Zika infection. • Exclude DM, FAS • MRI fetal brain at ≥32 weeks for a diagnosis of abnormalities of neuronal migration • US scans every 4 weeks for monitoring • The risk of neurodevelopmental delay increases with the decreasing head circumference. • The prognosis depends on aetiology and other associated anomalies. *Recurrence risk:* • If no associated structural defects: 5–10% • If it is a familial form of isolated microcephaly: 25%

Cardiac

- Cardiac defects are the most common FAs, occurring in 0.4–1% of all live births and 2% of patients with DM.
- A cardiac scan may be performed at 15–16 weeks for early detection.
- MDT management with a maternal–fetal specialist, paediatric cardiologist, cardiothoracic surgeon, neonatologist and geneticist.
- A fetal 2D echocardiogram may be performed by a paediatric cardiologist.
- Anomalies that are difficult to diagnose antenatally on the US: transposition of great arteries (TGA), aortic coarctation, tetralogy of Fallot (ToF), atrioventricular (AV) septal defect, aortic stenosis.

Fetal Anomally	Condition/Associations	Management/Delivery/Prognosis/ Recurrence
AV Canal Defects – 5% of congenital heart defects	Group of congenital cardiac defects involving the AV septum and AV valves (mitral and tricuspid valves) Results from the failure of superior and inferior endocardial cushions to fuse correctly during cardiac development *Types of defects:* 1. Complete 2. Partial 3. Transitional 4. Intermediate Strong association with T21	• Offer genetic testing • MDT management — including a paediatric cardiologist and a cardiothoracic surgeon • Surgical repair required postnatally • Significant morbidity and mortality if the defect is uncorrected • The management approach depends on the defect type if other anatomic and haemodynamic abnormalities (such as relative ventricular size, AV valve regurgitation, right or left ventricular outflow obstruction) and other cardiac defects are present. • The overall mortality rate for surgical repair of complete AV canal defects is 3%, 10-year survival >90%. • The prognosis is excellent for cases of repaired partial and transitional AV canal defects (similar to that of the general population). • Long-term follow-up is required with a cardiologist with expertise in congenital heart disease (CHD).
Hypoplastic left heart syndrome • 2–3 cases per 10,000 live births • Accounts for 2–3% of all CHD • Major congenital cardiac cause of neonatal mortality	Left-sided heart structures are underdeveloped with significant left ventricle (LV) hypoplasia, stenosis/atresia of the mitral and/or aortic valves and hypoplasia of the ascending aorta and aortic arch. Survival is dependent on a patent ductus arteriosus (PDA) for systemic perfusion and an unrestrictive atrial septal defect	• Offer genetic testing • MDT management — including a paediatric cardiologist and a cardiothoracic surgeon • Discussion of options: TOP versus continuing pregnancy • Counselling on the choice of postnatal interventions: comfort measures versus staged palliative surgical repair after initial medical management

(*Continued*)

Fetal Anomaly	Condition/Associations	Management/Delivery/Prognosis/Recurrence
	(ASD) for adequate mixing of oxygenated and deoxygenated blood. *Causes are likely multifactorial* – Genetic – Abnormal fetal development of mitral or aortic valves results in altered flow and consequent hypoplasia of LV.	• For delivery at a tertiary centre with a neonatal intensive care unit (NICU) • 6-year survival rates: 60–70% • For children who survive till 1 year of age, long-term survival is approximately 90%. However, there is a high risk of significant morbidity, including neurodevelopmental delay, thrombotic complications and exercise intolerance.
Ventricular septal defect (VSD) – 4 per 1,000 live births	May occur at: 1. Septum of AV canal 2. Muscular septum 3. Parietal band or distal conal septum May be isolated or with other CHD defects	• MDT management — including a paediatric cardiologist and a cardiothoracic surgeon. • Postnatally, a close follow-up for cardiac failure is required in the first few weeks of life for neonates with moderate to large defects. • Management depends on the size of the defect, the degree of shunting and the likelihood of spontaneous closure. • *Asymptomatic and small defect*: no intervention. • *Symptomatic* — usually moderate to large defects: medical therapy for heart failure. • Surgical closure is recommended when medical therapy is inadequate or there is evidence of elevated pulmonary artery pressure or valvar involvement.
Tricuspid regurgitation – Present in 7% of normal fetuses	Abnormal backflow of blood into the right atrium during right ventricular contraction due to valvular leakage <u>Classified into</u> Trivial, mild, moderate or severe — depending on the phase of systole in which it occurs and peak velocity May be an isolated finding in an otherwise normal fetus May also be associated with aneuploidy and with both cardiac and extra-cardiac defects If severe, need to watch for atrialisation of the right ventricle (RV) — Ebstein anomaly	• Offer genetic testing if severe or persistent • MDT management — including a paediatric cardiologist and a cardiothoracic surgeon • Follow-up with US scans to monitor for progression • Management depends on the degree of severity

(*Continued*)

(*Continued*)

Fetal Anomaly	Condition/Associations	Management/Delivery/Prognosis/ Recurrence
Ebstein anomaly – 1 in 20,000 live births	Congenital malformation characterised by variably malformed and displaced tricuspid valve leaflets that are partly attached to the tricuspid valve annulus and partly attached to the right ventricular endocardium — resulting in tricuspid valve regurgitation and right heart enlargement. – Associated with maternal lithium usage.	• MDT management — including a paediatric cardiologist and a cardiothoracic surgeon. • Symptomatic children should be evaluated early for surgical repair. • Prognosis depends on the severity of the lesion. • Severe malformations with cyanosis in neonates and the presence of heart failure have a guarded prognosis.
Coarctation of the aorta – 4 in 10,000 live births – 4–6% of all CHD	Underlying pathogenesis is unknown Prenatal diagnosis is challenging — difficult to detect aortic narrowing as only 10% of fetal cardiac output flows through the thoracic aorta. Possible genetic predisposition — association with Turner syndrome.	• Offer genetic testing: especially for Turner syndrome • MDT management • Postnatal interventions include surgery and catheter-based interventions. • Choice of which depends on the age of the patient and the morphology of the underlying lesion • 10-year survival following repair is >90%. • However, long-term survival is reduced compared to that of the general population.
Tetralogy of Fallot (ToF) – 4 in 10,000 live births – 7–10% of all CHD	<u>*Four anatomic features:*</u> 1. Right ventricular (RV) hypertrophy 2. VSD 3. Overriding aorta 4. RV outflow tract (RVOT) obstruction Usually isolated finding, but may be associated with Down syndrome (DS), Alagille syndrome or DiGeorge syndrome May also be associated with other cardiac anomalies in 40% of patients	• Offer genetic testing • MDT management • Need for medical intervention is dependent on the degree of RVOT obstruction. • Primary complete repair recommended for most infants with ToF • Surgical correction has resulted in excellent long-term survival, particularly for patients who had operations at a young age — survival >90% 25 years after repair.
Transposition of Great Arteries (TGA) – 2.3–4.7 per 10,000 live births	Ventriculoarterial discordant lesion – Aorta arises from the RV – Pulmonary artery from the LV <u>*Two types:*</u> dextro and levo One of the more difficult CHD defects to diagnose antenatally on the fetal US	• Arterial switch operation (ASO) is the standard for surgical repair of D-TGA. • 90% mortality rate in the first year of life if untreated • Peri-operative mortality <1% for simple D-TGA, 4% for complex D-TGA • Long-term survival post-repair is >95% at 15–25 years following surgery

(Continued)

Fetal Anomaly	Condition/Associations	Management/Delivery/Prognosis/ Recurrence
	Underlying pathophysiology likely due to abnormal growth and development of the bilateral subarterial conus Not associated with any genetic abnormality, rarely occurs in other family members Less frequently associated with non-cardiac anomalies compared with other CHD defects	• Risk of mild long-term neurodevelopmental delay because of peri-operative factors and slightly reduced exercise capacity • Patients require long-term follow-up.
Congenital heart block (CHB)	Anti-Ro and anti-La antibodies cause heart block via fetal myocarditis and destruction of the conducting fibres in the fetal heart. – Therefore, association with maternal autoimmune conditions, e.g., SLE, Sjogren syndrome. – If ventricular rate <60/min: there is a high risk of fetal hydrops and congestive cardiac failure. It can affect brain development and function.	• MDT management — including a paediatric cardiologist and a paediatric electrophysiologist. • Counsel on the risk of intrauterine death (IUD), fetal hydrops, possible need for a postnatal pacemaker and risk of neonatal death. • Test for anti-Ro/SSA and anti-La/SSB antibodies in fetuses with a heart block and structurally normal heart. • Maternal use of oral (PO) hydroxychloroquine 400 mg once daily to reduce the risk of the fetus developing a heart block. • Monitor 1–2 weekly from 18 to 26 weeks. • Trial of vaginal delivery is possible as long as fetal well-being can be monitored in some way. • However, CTG monitoring in fetuses with a complete heart block is challenging to interpret. • For delivery at a tertiary centre with a NICU. • Infants with a complete heart block may require the insertion of a pacemaker, especially if the heart rate at delivery is <55 beats/min. • The *recurrence* rate is 17%.
Supraventricular tachycardia (SVT)	Characterised by a regular rate between 220 and 260 bpm, rarely as high as 300 bpm May be sustained for hours/ days but is more commonly intermittent This is the *most common* fetal tachycardia Accounts for up to 90% of cases	• MDT management — including a paediatric cardiologist and a paediatric electrophysiologist • Monitor for mirror syndrome in the mother if hydrops present • The mainstay of management is to slow the rate adequately to allow for good cardiac output. • *First-line therapy*: digoxin

(Continued)

(*Continued*)

Fetal Anomaly	Condition/Associations	Management/Delivery/Prognosis/ Recurrence
	Early signs: haemodynamic compromise, including biatrial enlargement and AV valve regurgitation Late signs: cardiomegaly and decreased systolic function, resulting in hydrops fetalis The most common mechanism is re-entrant tachycardia.	• Second-line therapy: flecainide, sotalol, amiodarone • Even if abnormal rhythm persists, a slower rate should prevent hydrops from developing or, if already present, help in the resolution of hydrops. • *<30 weeks*: transplacental drug therapy • *At 30–36 weeks*: transplacental drug therapy is reasonable, but the presence of mirror syndrome and pre-eclampsia (PE) are indications for delivery. • *At term*, the primary decision resolves around where and how to deliver the baby, rarely role for transplacental drug therapy unless hydrops is present • Trial of vaginal delivery is possible as long as fetal well-being can be monitored in some way. • For delivery at a tertiary centre with a NICU • The mortality rate of fetuses with SVT and hydrops is >50%.

Spine/Neck

Fetal Anomaly	Condition/Associations	Management/Delivery/Prognosis/ Recurrence
Spina bifida ***Types:*** **1. Open spina bifida (also known as spina bifida cystica)** – Occurs in 6 per 10,000 births **2. Spina bifida occulta**	Incomplete closure of the spinal cord or its coverings *Three types of open spina bifida*: a. Myelomeningocele – Cystic pouch containing nerve fibres and cerebrospinal fluid (CSF) – 75% of all cases – Can occur anywhere along the spinal cord – Most commonly in the lumbar and sacral areas – Higher the level: more loss of function b. Myeloschisis – No pouch, spinal cord and nerves exposed to amniotic fluid	• Offer genetic testing. • MDT management. • Discuss options of TOP versus continuing pregnancy. • Follow-up scans every four weeks to monitor for any evolution of ventriculomegaly, possible kyphoscoliosis and development of talipes. • Fetal surgery for closure of spina bifida may be performed *in utero* (open surgery requiring hysterotomy or via fetoscopy) — reduces the need for postnatal shunt placement and may improve motor and urologic function. • Deliver at a tertiary centre with neonatal intensive care

(Continued)

Fetal Anomally	Condition/Associations	Management/Delivery/Prognosis/Recurrence
	c. *Meningocele* – Cystic pouch containing CSF only, no nerves *Sites of spina bifida:* lumbosacral (65%), sacral (24%), thoracolumbar (10%), cervical (1%) Elevated maternal alpha-fetoprotein levels Associated with Arnold-Chiari II malformation — caudal displacement of the brain stem and obliteration of the cisterna magna Chromosomal abnormalities (mainly T18), single mutant genes, maternal DM or ingestion of anti-epileptic drugs are found in ~10% of cases. The risk of non-chromosomal syndromes is low.	and paediatric surgery service available. • Deliver via caesarean section if HC >40 cm or biparietal diameter ≥12 cm. • Peri-conception folic acid 5 mg/day (3 months before conception and up to 12 weeks of gestation) reduces recurrence risk by ~75%. • The 5-year mortality rate is 35%, with 20% dying during the first 12 months of life. 25% of fetuses are stillborn. • Survivors usually have paralysis in the lower limbs and dual incontinence. Intelligence is often normal. *Recurrence risk:* • An affected parent or one affected sibling: 5% • Two affected siblings: 10% • Three affected siblings: 20%
Sacrococcygeal teratoma (SCT) (1 in 20,000 births — most frequent fetal teratoma) SCT type 2 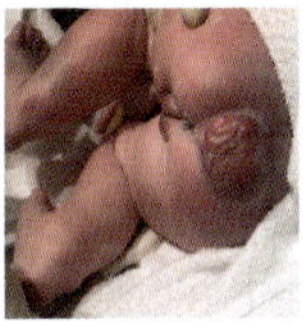	Mixed solid and cystic tumours, which are extremely vascular May be entirely external, partially internal and external or mainly internal Hydronephrosis may occur because of ureteric compression for internal tumours. Large tumours may result in fetal anaemia and thrombocytopenia, fetal heart failure, hydrops, placentomegaly, polyhydramnios and maternal mirror syndrome.	• Assess fetal cardiac function and monitor for fetal anaemia with the measurement of fetal middle cerebral artery peak systolic velocity (MCA PSV). • Fetal anaemia is present if MCA PSV ≥1.5 MoM. • Monitor for hydrops and polyhydramnios. If hydrops is present, monitor for maternal mirror syndrome. • Fetal surgery, i.e., US-guided laser coagulation of vessels within the tumour, fetal blood transfusions and amnioreduction may be performed where indicated. • Deliver at 38 weeks (earlier if poor growth, fetal hypoxia or hydrops) at a tertiary centre with neonatal intensive care and paediatric surgery service available. • Recommended MOD would be a caesarean section if the tumour is large and there are signs of cardiac failure.

(Continued)

(*Continued*)

Fetal Anomaly	Condition/Associations	Management/Delivery/Prognosis/ Recurrence
		• 50% risk of perinatal mortality — mainly due to the risk of preterm birth of a hydropic infant requiring major neonatal surgery. • Complex surgeries may result in nerve injury and incontinence. • Tumour is usually benign in the neonatal period, but delayed surgery or incomplete excision can result in malignant transformation. • The risk of malignancy is ~10% before 2 months of age to ~80% by 4 months. • <u>Recurrence risk</u> — no increased risk.
Cystic hygroma (1 in 800 pregnancies, 1 in 8,000 live births)	Bilateral symmetrical cystic structures located in the occipital-cervical region of the fetal neck with midline septum (nuchal ligament) present. It is a congenital malformation resulting from lymph accumulation in jugular lymphatic sacs due to the obstruction of the lymphatic system, most commonly in the fetal neck. May be septated or simple. Associated with *chromosomal abnormalities* in ~50% of cases — mainly Turner syndrome. *Genetic syndromes* are found in ~40% of cases. – Most commonly, Noonan syndrome, multiple pterygium syndrome, Fryns syndrome, Neu–Laxova syndrome. *Hydrops* occurs in 60–80% of cases.	• Offer genetic testing. • MDT management. • Deliver at 38 weeks (earlier if hydrops develops) at a tertiary centre with neonatal intensive care and paediatric surgery service available. • Recommended MOD will be a caesarean section if there is hydrops or large cystic hygromas preventing flexion of the head. • The risk of fetal death is 90%. • Increased risk of miscarriage, hydrops, IUD and neonatal death. • In 10% of cases where the fetal karyotype is normal and no other obvious defects are present, the prognosis can be good if the hygromas resolve during pregnancy. <u>Recurrence risk:</u> • No increased risk if isolated or part of Turner syndrome. • If part of the autosomal recessive syndrome: 25%.

Facial

Fetal Anomally	Condition/Associations	Management/Delivery/Prognosis/ Recurrence
Facial cleft — cleft lip/ palate (1 in 700 births)	<u>For *cleft lip*</u> — linear defect extending from one side of the lip into the nostril <u>For *cleft palate*</u> — the defect extends through the alveolar ridge and hard palate, reaching the floor of the nasal cavity or even the floor of the orbit. 25% of cases — cleft lip only 25% of cases — cleft palate only 50% of cases — *both* lip and palate affected *Unilateral* in 75% of cases (more on the left side) and *bilateral* in 25% of cases More common in males than in females and in caucasians *Chromosomal abnormalities* are found in 1–2% of cases — mainly T13 and T18 Unilateral cleft lip is *not* associated with chromosomal abnormalities Associated with any one of >400 syndromes in 30% of cases — most commonly Goldenhar syndrome, Treacher-Collins syndrome, Pierre Robin sequence *Environmental risk factors*: exposure to radiation, viral infections, metabolic abnormalities, teratogenic compounds	• Offer genetic testing if bilateral cleft lip, midline cleft or cleft palate present • <u>*MDT management*:</u> paediatric surgeon, plastic surgeon, Cleft Lip and Palate Association of Singapore (CLAPAS) • Surgical repair is at 3–6 months of age. • Prognosis depends on the presence and type of associated anomalies. • Good prognosis and normal survival if isolated • <u>*Long-term issues:*</u> dental and speech abnormalities, hearing and olfactory problems, midface hypoplasia and psychological problems <u>*Recurrence risk*:</u> • Advise preconception folic acid • Stop smoking/drinking • In isolated cases – If one sibling or parent is affected: 5% – If two siblings are affected: 10% • If it occurs as part of a syndrome, the risk would depend on the mode of inheritance of the syndrome.

Thorax

Fetal Anomally	Condition/Associations	Management/Delivery/ Prognosis/Recurrence
Congenital diaphragmatic hernia (CDH) (1 in 3,500–4,000 births)	Herniation of abdominal viscera into the thorax through a defect in the diaphragm with an associated deviation of the heart from its normal position • 80% occur on the left • 15% on the right • 5% are posterolateral/ anterior retrosternal Polyhydramnios occurs at ≥26 weeks in most cases. Associated with chromosomal defects, mainly T18 or T13 Genetic syndromes are found in 10% of cases — most commonly Fryns syndrome. Defects in other systems — mainly craniofacial and cardiac — found in 20% of cases Assessment of severity is by measurement of the contralateral lung area in a transverse section of the lung-to-head circumference ratio (LHR). This is compared to the LHR in normal babies. Classified as *severe* if the ratio is ≤25%, *moderate* if 26–45% and mild if >45% Possible complications include pulmonary hypoplasia and pulmonary arterial hypertension, which may result in life-threatening respiratory compromise.	• Offer genetic testing • MDT management • Fetal therapy in the form of fetoscopic endoluminal tracheal occlusion (FETO) is available — endoscopic insertion of an inflatable balloon into the trachea with consequent retention of fluid produced by the lungs may stimulate lung growth. A balloon is inserted at 26 weeks and removed endoscopically at 34 weeks. • Monitor for the development of hydrops and associated maternal mirror syndrome. • Deliver at 38 weeks (earlier if poor growth or fetal hypoxia) at a tertiary centre with neonatal intensive care and paediatric surgery service available • May have a vaginal delivery • Risk of fetal death ~5% • If it occurs as part of T18, this is lethal. • If isolated, survival is <15% for *severe* disease, 50% for *moderate* disease and >90% for *mild* disease • Morbidity in survivors includes developmental delay, gastro-oesophageal reflux in 50% of cases and scoliosis in 10% of cases. <u>*Recurrence risk:*</u> • If isolated, there is no increased risk • If part of trisomies: 1% • If part of the syndrome: 25%

(*Continued*)

Fetal Anomaly	Condition/Associations	Management/Delivery/ Prognosis/Recurrence
Congenital pulmonary airway malformation (CPAM) — previously known as congenital cystic adenomatoid malformation (CCAM) (1 in 4,000 births) Differentiate from bronchopulmonary sequestration (BPS), which does not contain cysts, is formed from normal lung tissue and has a feeding vessel from the aorta	Hyperechogenic tumour in the fetal chest, usually presenting at ≥16 weeks May be solid, microcystic (cysts <5 mm in diameter and appear echogenic and solid) or macrocystic (≥1 cyst >5 mm in diameter) >95% are unilateral and usually involve one lobe or segment of the lung Associated with hydrops in <10% of cases Polyhydramnios, due to compressed and obstructed oesophagus, may present at ≥26 weeks. Not associated with chromosomal abnormalities and genetic syndromes Defects in other systems — cardiac, renal, tracheo-oesophageal fistulas — found in 10% of cases	• MDT management • Thoraco-amniotic shunting may be useful in cases of a large cyst causing major mediastinal shift and/or ascites. • In certain cases of hydrops, open fetal surgery with excision of the lesion may be considered with relatively good results. • Some evidence presents that maternal administration of steroids may cause shrinkage of the lesion and resolution of hydrops. • Monitor with serial US scans — look for polyhydramnios and hydrops. • During the early third trimester, >80% of microcystic lesions resolve, but in >80% of these cases, there is no true resolution but purely an inability to detect the lesion by US because the normal lungs also become echogenic. • The lesion can be detected postnatally by chest X-ray or CT scan. • Deliver at 38 weeks (earlier if poor growth, fetal hypoxia or hydrops) at a tertiary centre with neonatal intensive care and paediatric surgery service available. • May have a vaginal delivery. • Survival is >95% if no hydrops is present as surgical excision in the neonatal period is curative and the prognosis is excellent. • Usually lethal if hydrops is found. • <u>*Recurrence risk*</u>: no increased risk.

Abdominal Wall

Fetal Anomaly	Condition/Associations	Management/Delivery/Prognosis/ Recurrence
Body stalk anomaly — also known as limb-body wall complex (1 in 10,000 pregnancies)	A major abdominal wall defect is present with severe kyphoscoliosis *and a short or absent umbilical cord*. The liver is usually directly attached to the placenta without an umbilical cord in between, with major distortion of the spine. More often in the younger age group and cocaine abuser Elevated maternal serum alpha-fetoprotein levels in the second trimester Not associated with chromosomal abnormalities and genetic syndromes. Exencephaly or encephalocele, facial cleft and limb amputations are common.	• Lethal condition either *in utero* or in the early neonatal period • Discuss options of TOP versus continuing pregnancy • Recurrence risk: no increased risk
Exomphalos (also known as omphalocele) • *Only bowel in sac*: – 1 in 100 at 11 weeks – 1 in 800 at 12 weeks – 1 in 2,000 at 13 weeks • *Liver in sac*: – 1 in 3,500 fetuses at 11–13 weeks **To differentiate from gastroschisis*	Midline sac containing bowel or liver with umbilical cord at the apex. High exomphalos may contain the heart (Pentalogy of Cantrell). Low exomphalos may be associated with cloacal abnormality and spina bifida [omphalocele–exstrophy–imperforate anus–spinal defects complex (OEIS complex)]. Associated with chromosomal defects — mainly T18/T13 — in 30–50% of cases. Genetic syndromes such as Beckwith–Wiedemann syndrome are found in 10% of cases. Exomphalos containing bowel only at 11–13 weeks resolves by 20 weeks in 90% of cases.	• Offer genetic testing • Monitor growth through estimation of the fetal weight using the Sieme formula, which uses biparietal diameter, occipitofrontal diameter and femur length, rather than formulas that use the abdominal circumference. • Antenatal surveillance for intrauterine growth restriction (IUGR) and oligohydramnios • Deliver at 38 weeks (earlier if poor growth or fetal hypoxia) at a tertiary centre with neonatal intensive care and paediatric surgery service available • Vaginal delivery is possible unless a giant exomphalos (sac containing >75% of the liver) is present — recommended delivery would be via a caesarean section to avoid rupture and haemorrhage. • Isolated small or moderate exomphalos: survival is >90% • Isolated giant exomphalos: survival is 80% • When associated with other defects, the prognosis would depend on the defect present, e.g., T18 is lethal. • Most cases are sporadic, and recurrence depends on the cause. Recurrence risk: • Isolated finding: no increased risk • Part of trisomies: 1% • Part of Beckwith–Wiedemann syndrome: up to 50%

(Continued)

Fetal Anomaly	Condition/Associations	Management/Delivery/Prognosis/ Recurrence
Gastroschisis (1 in 3,000 births) 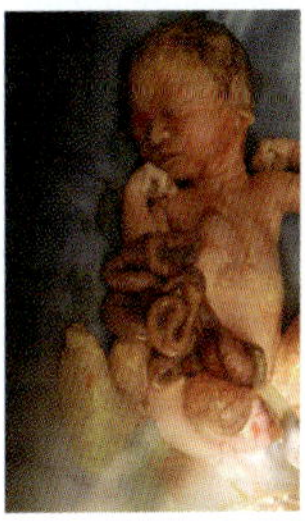	Paraumbilical abdominal wall defect, usually on the right, with associated evisceration of the bowels. The bowels float freely in the amniotic fluid with a normally inserted umbilical cord. 85% are isolated abnormality Increased risk in young women and in cocaine abusers Not associated with chromosomal abnormalities/genetic syndromes The risk of bowel atresias or obstruction secondary to volvulus and/or ischaemia at the hernia orifice occurs in ~10–30% of cases. <u>*Pregnancy complications:*</u> IUGR (30–60%), fetal death (2–4%), spontaneous preterm birth (30%), bowel thickening and dilatation	• MDT management • Monitor growth through estimation of the fetal weight using the Sieme formula, which uses biparietal diameter, occipitofrontal diameter and femur length, rather than formulas that use the abdominal circumference. • Antenatal surveillance for IUGR and oligohydramnios • Deliver at 38 weeks (earlier if poor growth, fetal hypoxia or dilatation of intra-abdominal bowel >20 mm) at a tertiary centre with neonatal intensive care and paediatric surgery service available • Vaginal delivery is possible. • No evidence that a caesarean section is beneficial • Survival is >90%, with the main cause of death being short bowel syndrome. • *Recurrence risk*: 3%

Comparison between Gastroschisis and Omphalocele

Characteristics	Gastroschisis	Omphalocele
Defect size (diameter)	2–3 cm	2–15 cm
Sac	Not present	Always present, may be ruptured
Gestational age at delivery	Preterm	Term
Location of defect	Defect lateral to the umbilicus (usually right side/paraumbilical)	Central defect
Umbilical cord	Adjacent to the defect (left side of the defect)	Attached to sac
Herniated viscera	Small bowel, stomach, colon	Small bowel, stomach, colon, liver
Malrotation	Yes	Yes
Bowel character	Inflammatory, oedematous	Normal
Enteral nutrition	Delayed	Normal
Associated chromosomal/FA	Uncommon	Common
Need for surgery	Urgent	Non-urgent

Gastrointestinal Tract

Fetal Anomaly	Condition/Associations	Management/Delivery/Prognosis/ Recurrence
Duodenal atresia (1 in 5,000 births) – Most common form of intestinal atresia	The "double bubble" sign is a result of an enlarged stomach and duodenal cap — usually diagnosed at >24 weeks. Polyhydramnios found at >24 weeks in 50% of cases *Features include*: – Polyhydramnios – Dilated bowel – Increased bowel echogenicity Associated with chromosomal defects — mainly T21 — in 30% of cases Other defects, such as cardiac, renal and vertebral, in 10–20% of cases	• Offer genetic testing • Amnioreduction may be necessary if there is polyhydramnios associated with cervical shortening or symptomatic, e.g., shortness of breath (SOB), unable to lie supine • Deliver at 38 weeks at a tertiary centre with neonatal intensive care and paediatric surgery service available • Survival rate >95% <u>*Recurrence risk:*</u> • No increased risk if isolated • If part of T21: 1%
Oesophageal atresia (1 in 3,000 births)	Small or "absent" stomach with polyhydramnios at >25 weeks. ***Absent*** *stomach bubble* on the scan Difficult diagnosis and only suspected prenatally in ~40% of cases as there is usually a tracheo-oesophageal fistula in >80% of cases; therefore, the stomach may look normal Associated with chromosomal defects with T18 in 20% and T21 in 1% May be associated with other defects — usually cardiac — in 50% of cases May be seen as part of VACTERL (vertebral defects, anal atresia, cardiac defects, tracheo-oesophageal fistula, renal anomalies and limb abnormalities) association	• Offer genetic testing • Discuss options of TOP versus continuing with the pregnancy • Amnioreduction may be necessary if there is polyhydramnios associated with cervical shortening or the patient is symptomatic (SOB, unable to lie supine). • Deliver at 38 weeks at a tertiary centre with neonatal intensive care and paediatric surgery service available • Survival is dependent on gestation at delivery and the presence of other anomalies. • If isolated and born >32 weeks without aspiration pneumonitis, post-op survival is >95% <u>*Recurrence risk:*</u> • No increased risk if isolated • If part of trisomies: 1%
Meconium peritonitis (1 in 3,000 births)	Intra-abdominal hyperechogenic areas (peritoneal calcifications) result from *in utero* perforation of the bowels, leading to local sterile chemical peritonitis. Dilated bowel loops, ascites and meconium pseudocyst may also be found. No association with chromosomal abnormalities/ genetic syndromes The risk of cystic fibrosis is 75%.	• DNA studies for cystic fibrosis if both parents are carriers • CMV/toxoplasma screen for fetal infections • Deliver at 38 weeks at a tertiary centre with neonatal intensive care and paediatric surgery service available • In *simple* peritonitis, the outcome is good and surgical intervention is not required. • In *complex* peritonitis (associated with bowel dilatation and ascites), the prognosis is poor and neonatal mortality is >50%. • <u>*Recurrence risk:*</u> no increased risk if isolated

Urinary Tract

Fetal Anomally	Condition/Associations	Management/Delivery/ Prognosis/Recurrence
Horseshoe kidney — renal fusion anomaly (1 in 400 births)	Fusion of lower poles of both kidneys in front of the descending aorta — normal bladder and amniotic fluid volume More common in males Found in 30% of cases of Turner syndrome and 20% of cases of T18 Also associated with caudal regression syndrome Other defects include hydronephrosis and genital anomalies Extra-renal defects such as CNS, cardiac or skeletal are found in 30% of cases.	• Offer genetic testing • Requires postnatal follow-up because of significant risk of infections, hydronephrosis and nephrolithiasis (70%) • Good prognosis if isolated <u>Recurrence risk:</u> • No increased risk if isolated or part of Turner syndrome • If part of T18: 1% recurrence risk
Hydronephrosis (1 in 500 births)	Dilatation of the collecting system of the kidney with normal ureters and bladder. Classified into <u>mild, moderate and severe</u> based on the dimensions and involvement of renal pelvis/calyces/ cortex – *Mild*: ≥4–7 mm – *Moderate*: 8–10 mm – *Severe*: >10 mm If isolated, there is a low risk of association with chromosomal defects Abnormalities of the contralateral kidney, such as multicystic kidney, ectopia and renal agenesis, may be present. Associated syndromes in 5% of cases	• MDT management. • The condition usually remains stable or resolves in the neonatal period. • In 20% of cases, there may be underlying ureteropelvic junction obstruction or vesicoureteric reflux, which requires postnatal follow-up and possibly surgery. • Moderate hydronephrosis is usually progressive, and surgery is necessary in >50% of cases during the first 2 year of life. • <u>Recurrence:</u> no increased risk if isolated.
Multicystic kidneys (1 in 1,000 births)	Kidneys are replaced by multiple irregular cysts of variable size with intervening hyperechogenic stroma — unable to visualise the renal pelvis. Can be unilateral (80%), bilateral or segmental. If bilateral, there is anhydramnios and the bladder is "absent". Abnormalities of the contralateral kidney present in 25% of cases. Bilateral polycystic kidneys are usually inherited. – <u>*Adult:*</u> autosomal dominant – <u>*Paediatric:*</u> autosomal recessive Associated with chromosomal defects — mainly T18 — in 3% of unilateral lesions and 15% of bilateral ones. Associated with syndromes in 10% of cases such as brachio-oto-renal syndrome, VACTERL association, short-rib polydactyly syndrome and Meckel–Gruber syndrome.	• Offer genetic testing • Serial US scans to monitor for oligohydramnios • Postnatally for unilateral cases, usually expectant management as the kidney gradually shrinks and may disappear • Parents and family should be scanned to exclude autosomal dominant branchio-oto-renal syndrome. • If bilateral, lethal *in utero* or in the neonatal period because of pulmonary hypoplasia from anhydramnios • Normal prognosis if unilateral • <u>Recurrence risk:</u> 1–2% if isolated

(*Continued*)

(*Continued*)

Fetal Anomally	Condition/Associations	Management/Delivery/ Prognosis/Recurrence
Pelvic kidney (1 in 1,000 births)	Visualisation of the kidney in the pelvis above the bladder with empty renal fossa on the affected side and adrenal gland filling the space. Amniotic fluid volume and bladder normal. No associated increase in chromosomal defects/genetic syndromes.	• May be asymptomatic postnatally • Increased risk of traumatic injury, UTI, renal calculi formation • Good prognosis • *Recurrence risk:* no increased risk
Renal agenesis (1 in 2,000 births for unilateral, 1 in 5,000 births for bilateral)	Non-visualisation of one or both kidneys. – If *unilateral*, bladder and amniotic fluid will be normal. The contralateral kidney may have compensatory hypertrophy. – If *bilateral*, anhydramnios present. Usually diagnosed after 16 weeks. The majority of cases are sporadic and are isolated anomalies. Chromosomal defects such as T18 are found in 1–2% of cases. Associated syndromes are found in 10% of cases — such as Fraser syndrome, VACTERL association, MURCS association.	• Lethal if bilateral — usually in the neonatal period because of pulmonary hypoplasia from anhydramnios • If bilateral, discuss options of TOP versus continuing pregnancy • Females should have an US of the pelvis performed postnatally to assess for abnormalities in Müllerian structures • Normal prognosis if unilateral. May be associated with vesicoureteric reflux, an increased risk of renal dysfunction, proteinuria, hypertension and a high risk of dialysis *Recurrence risk:* • If non-syndromic: 3% • In 15% of cases, one parent has unilateral renal agenesis. In these families, the risk of recurrence increases.

Extremities/Skeletal

Fetal Anomaly	Condition/Associations	Management/Delivery/Prognosis/ Recurrence
Clubfoot — talipes equinovarus (1 in 1,000 births)	The sole is not perpendicular to the lower leg bones. Bilateral in 30–50% of cases Isolated finding in >50% of cases and mostly idiopathic It is a common finding in T18 and T13 and also commonly associated with prolonged oligohydramnios, brain abnormalities, spina bifida, skeletal and neuromuscular disorders. More than 250 genetic syndromes include clubfoot as one component.	• Offer genetic testing. • *MDT management* — including a paediatric orthopaedic surgeon. • No antenatal management options. • Antenatal care as per routine obstetric care. • Postnatally, may be observed or managed with physiotherapy, serial casting or surgery in severe cases. • Good prognosis if isolated. • In 90% of cases, a good long-term function is achieved by manipulation and serial application of casts. • Operative intervention is usually limited. • Surgery is necessary in about 10% of cases. Of these, >1/3 require more than one operation. *Recurrence risk:* • If one sibling with clubfoot: 3% • If one sibling and parent with clubfoot: 25%
Polydactyly 1 in 100 births in Blacks 1 in 700 births in Whites	>5 digits with or without bony phalanx in hand or foot *Most common*: post-axial where supernumerary digits of the hand are found on the lateral (ulnar) surface of the fifth digit More common in males than in females — 2:1 ratio. Found in 75% of fetuses with T13 Usually isolated finding with autosomal dominant inheritance. May be associated with genetic syndromes such as Meckel–Gruber syndrome, Bardet–Biedl syndrome, short-rib polydactyly syndrome, Ellis–van Creveld syndrome	• Offer genetic testing • Consult a clinical geneticist • Good prognosis in isolated cases *Recurrence risk:* • If isolated familial: 50% • If part of T13: 1% • If part of autosomal recessive syndromes: 25%
Skeletal dysplasia (1 in 4,000 births)	There is a wide range of skeletal dysplasias *3 most common types are:* 1. Thanatophoric dysplasia 2. Osteogenesis imperfecta type II 3. Achondroplasia	• Offer genetic testing • MDT management with a maternal–fetal specialist • Refer to a tertiary centre • If lethal type, counsel on options of TOP versus continuing pregnancy

(*Continued*)

(Continued)

Fetal Anomally	Condition/Associations	Management/Delivery/Prognosis/ Recurrence
	The assessment of long bones may show shortening, abnormal shape, reduced echogenicity or the absence of extremities. A systematic examination of the limbs, head, thorax and spine needs to be performed.	• Monitor for IUGR with serial US scans • 25% are stillborn and 30% die in the neonatal period • Recurrence risk depends on the mode of inheritance.
Achondroplasia (1 in 25,000 births)	Short limbs, short hands and fingers, large head with frontal bossing and depressed nasal bridge, and lumbar scoliosis Limb shortening and typical facial features are apparent at >22 weeks. Due to mutation in the *FGFR3* gene with autosomal dominant inheritance	• Offer genetic testing • Recommended delivery via caesarean if head circumference >40 cm • For homozygotic type: lethal due to severe pulmonary hypoplasia • For heterozygotic type: intelligence and life expectancy are normal. Respiratory limitations due to a small thorax and the development of a stenotic vertebral canal (with peripheral neurological deficits) may decrease the quality of life. Recurrence risk: • With one affected parent: 50% • With both parents affected, 50% risk of heterozygous achondroplasia, a 25% risk of homozygous achondroplasia and a 25% chance of an unaffected child • Low recurrence risk if *de novo* mutation

Lethal FAs

Definition

1. A condition that invariably leads to fetal death *in utero*
2. A condition that invariably leads to death *in utero* or in the newborn period, regardless of attempted supportive treatment
3. A condition that usually leads to death *in utero* or in the newborn period
4. A condition that has been associated with death *in utero* or in the newborn period

Types of Lethal FAs

- **Chromosomal**: T18, T13, triploidy
- **CNS:** Anencephaly/acrania, holoprosencephaly, hydranencephaly, severe congenital hydrocephalus with absent/minimal brain growth, complex or severe cases of myelomeningocele, large encephaloceles, exencephaly, iniencephaly
- **CVS:** Acardia, hypoplastic left heart
- **Renal:** Autosomal recessive polycystic kidney disease, bilateral renal agenesis/Potter syndrome, multicystic/dysplastic kidneys
- **Skeletal dysplasia:** Thanatophoric dysplasia, osteogenesis imperfecta type 2, achondrogenesis, sirenomelia
- **Abdominal wall:** Pentalogy of Cantrell, body stalk anomaly
- **Respiratory**: Severe congenital diaphragmatic hernia with hypoplastic lungs
- **Others**: Non-immune hydrops with major cardiac defects, Harlequin fetus, inoperable conjoined twins

Soft Markers on US Scan

- Soft markers are non-specific US findings that typically reflect normal variation in fetal anatomy and are not abnormalities per se.
- They may point to a small-to-moderate increased risk of underlying chromosomal abnormalities.
- They may be transient and resolve with advancing gestational age or postnatally, often with no clinical sequelae.
- **Descriptions of soft markers on US scan:**
  - *Short/absent nasal bone*: Nasal bone length ≤2.5 mm or a gestational age threshold of <5th centile or <0.75 MoM for gestational age.
  - *Aberrant right subclavian artery* (*ARSA*): Right subclavian artery arises directly from the aortic arch instead of from the brachiocephalic artery.
  - *Increased cervical skin*: Thickened skin in the back of the fetal neck ≥6 mm.
  - *Echogenic bowel score 2*: Increased echogenicity of the fetal bowel.
  - *Mild to moderate ventriculomegaly*: Dilated ventricles with a diameter of 10–15 mm.

- *Mild hydronephrosis:* Renal pelvic dilatation with a diameter of 4–6 mm at 16–27 weeks.
- *Shortened long bones* (*femur/humerus*): Observed-to-expected length ratio <0.9 for femur/humerus.
- *Single umbilical artery* (*SUA*): US scan showing two instead of three vessels in the umbilical cord.
- *Choroid plexus cysts* (*CPC*): Small (<10 mm) sonolucent structures with well-delineated borders within the choroid plexus of the cerebral lateral ventricles, which may be unilateral single simple cysts or septated, bilateral or multiple cysts.
- *Echogenic intracardiac focus* (*EIF*): Punctate echogenic area (as bright as bone and seen in two imaging planes) that is typically seen in the left cardiac ventricle but may be seen in either or both ventricles.

- When CPC or EIF is present in isolation, this represents a *normal variant* and further testing is *not* recommended.
- For the other soft markers, further testing with either amniocentesis or NIPT should be offered.
- If NIPT was previously done and was low risk, but an isolated soft marker is subsequently found, there is no need to offer invasive testing solely to test for DS as NIPT trumps soft markers.
- When ≥2 soft markers are present, offer genetic testing.

Soft markers where testing beyond DS needs to be offered and other associations:

- *ARSA:* Karyotype and DiGeorge syndrome
- *Increased cervical skin:* Karyotype, CMA, Noonan syndrome
- *Echogenic bowel score 2:* Given an association with congenital infection, send maternal blood for CMV/toxoplasma IgM and IgG. If amniocentesis is performed, send for karyotype and CMV/toxoplasma PCR. It is also associated with cystic fibrosis, intra-amniotic bleeding (fetus swallowing blood), IUGR and other gastrointestinal pathology. Perform a third-trimester growth scan.
- *Ventriculomegaly:* Karyotype, CMA, CMV/toxoplasma PCR
- *Short femur/humerus:* Karyotype, CMA
- *SUA:* Third-trimester scan for fetal growth because of the possible association with IUGR

US Features of Aneuploidies

- **Down Syndrome (T21):** Nasal hypoplasia, increased prenasal and nuchal fold thickness, cardiac defects, duodenal atresia, short femur, sandal gap, clinodactyly or mid-phalanx hypoplasia of the fifth finger
- **Edward syndrome (T18):** Strawberry-shaped head, absent corpus callosum, enlarged cisterna magna, facial cleft, micrognathia, nuchal oedema, cardiac defects, diaphragmatic hernia, oesophageal atresia, omphalocele, renal abnormalities, myelomeningocele, IUGR, shortening of the limbs, radial aplasia, overlapping fingers and talipes or rocker bottom feet
- **Patau syndrome (T13):** Holoprosencephaly, microcephaly, facial/cardiac abnormalities, enlarged and echogenic kidneys, omphalocele, post-axial polydactyly
- **Turner syndrome:** Large cystic hygromas, generalised oedema, mild pleural effusions and ascites, cardiac abnormalities, horseshoe kidney

US Features of Intra-Uterine Infection (IUI)

- IUGR
- Ascites
- Hydrops
- *CNS:* Ventriculomegaly, intracranial calcifications, hydrocephaly, microcephaly
- Cardiac anomalies
- *Gastrointestinal tract:* Hepatosplenomegaly, echogenic bowel
- Placentomegaly
- Abnormal amniotic fluid volume

Assessment of Liquor Volume

- Deepest vertical pocket (DVP) — vertical measurement of the deepest pocket of amniotic fluid, which is free of fetal parts
- Amniotic fluid index (AFI) — the sum of DVP in four quadrants

Polyhydramnios — *Mild:* DVP 8–11 cm, *moderate:* DVP 12–15 cm, *severe:* DVP ≥16 cm

Two major causes of polyhydramnios:

1. *Reduced fetal swallowing*, e.g., anencephaly, gastrointestinal obstruction (duodenal atresia), compressive pulmonary disorders (congenital diaphragmatic hernia)
2. *Increased fetal urination*, e.g., maternal DM, hyperdynamic fetal circulation due to fetal anaemia (alloimmunisation, parvovirus B19 infection, SCT)

- US scans every 1–3 weeks to monitor the fetal condition and cervical length and for the serial assessment of the amniotic fluid volume

Oligohydramnios — DVP <2 cm or AFI <5 cm
When diagnosed at <24 weeks, three major causes need to be considered:

1. *Urinary tract abnormalities*, e.g., bilateral renal agenesis, multicystic/polycystic kidneys
2. *Preterm pre-labour rupture of membranes* (PPROM)
3. *Uteroplacental insufficiency*

- US scans every 1–3 weeks to monitor growth and for the serial assessment of the amniotic fluid volume

Other Findings on Screening Scan

- Placental localisation is also performed at the 20-week screening scan.
- 90% of low-lying placentas found at the 20-week screening scan resolve during the third trimester following the development of the lower uterine segment.
- Beware of placenta accreta in patients with a low-lying placenta and a history of previous caesarean section/s or uterine instrumentation, e.g., evacuation of the uterus — further US scans or MRI may be required in the third trimester to assess for the presence of placenta accreta.
- Doppler assessment of uterine artery blood flow may be performed.
- *Bilateral uterine artery notching* is associated with an increased incidence of pregnancy-induced hypertension, pre-eclampsia (PE) and IUGR. The patient should be advised on home blood pressure (BP) monitoring and symptoms and signs of PE. The fetus should be monitored with serial growth scans every 3–4 weeks from 24 weeks

onwards. Starting low-dose aspirin (LDA) to reduce the risks of PE and IUGR may be considered. However, efficacy is reduced when low-dose aspirin is started after 16 weeks of gestation.

Role of First Trimester Screening Scan

- Mainly assesses nuchal translucency (NT).
- NT is the clear space at the posterior fetal neck, between the spine and the skin edge — recommended to be assessed when the crown-rump length (CRL) of the fetus is 45–84 mm (corresponding to 11–13+6 weeks of gestation).
- Thickened NT is defined as ≥97th centile for gestational age by CRL in KKH.
- Other structures that can be assessed: nasal bone (present or absent), bladder, CNS, abdominal wall, cardiac, face and limbs.
- Conditions that may be detected on the first-trimester screening scan: cystic hygroma, megacystis (enlarged bladder), acrania/anencephaly, holoprosencephaly, abdominal wall defects, major abnormalities of fetal contour such as body stalk anomaly, major cardiac malformations, facial clefts, limb anomalies.
- With these findings, early confirmatory genetic testing via chorionic villus sampling (CVS) may be offered if found before 14 weeks or amniocentesis from 16 weeks onwards.

FA Found on the Third Trimester Scan

- New FAs detected on third-trimester scans were most frequently of the urinary tract, e.g., renal pelvis dilatation.
- Other FAs include CNS, e.g., ventriculomegaly, fetal ovarian cysts and skeletal dysplasia.
- The period for follow-up with repeat scans is usually short as the patient is already in the third trimester.
- The primary focus for management would be counselling regarding postnatal follow-up and investigations.

CHAPTER 28

Laboratory Values in Pregnancy and Interpretation of Results

Normal physiological adaptations during pregnancy can alter biochemical results. This should be taken into consideration before interpreting the results.

The results of biochemical tests during pregnancy may differ from the normal non-pregnant reference ranges. Hence, physiological adaptations of pregnancy can be interpreted as pathological or pathological findings may not be recognised. This can lead to the mismanagement of patients.

In general, most of the serum analytes have lower concentrations than in the non-pregnant state because of increased intravascular volume, while the free fractions, such as ionised calcium, remain unchanged. Serum total calcium, phosphate and magnesium are low in pregnancy because of the expanded intravascular space. It is uncommon for an analyte to be elevated; thus, this is a useful point to note to avoid errors in interpreting laboratory results during pregnancy.

Some serum analytes such as leucocyte and alkaline phosphatase (ALP) continue to rise in pregnancy. Haemoglobin and haematocrit reduce because of physiological dilution in pregnancy. The increase in renal blood flow causes a reduction in serum urea, creatinine and uric acid.

All markers of liver function are reduced because of the expansion of extracellular fluid except ALP. Serum albumin, alanine transaminase (ALT), aspartate transaminase (AST) and total albumin levels are lower in pregnancy. ALP is elevated because of ALP from the placenta or bone or liver isoenzymes.

TSH levels tend to decrease in the first trimester, return to pre-pregnant values in the second trimester and rise slightly in the third trimester. Free T4 and T3 usually decrease slightly in pregnancy.

The summary below will serve as a quick reference; however, it is not exhaustive.

Haematology

	Non-pregnant Adult	First Trimester	Second Trimester	Third Trimester	Comments on the Effect of Pregnancy
Haemoglobin (g/dl)	12.0–15.8	11.0–13.9	10.5 –14.8	10.0–15.0	↓ nadir at 30–34 weeks of gestation. Anaemia in pregnancy is defined: *First trimester*: Hb <110 g/L (<11.0 g/dl). *Second and third trimesters*: Hb <105 g/L (<10.5 g/dl). *Postpartum* Hb: <100 g/L (<10.0 g/dl).
Haematocrit (%)	35.4–44.4	31.0–41.0	30.0–39.0	28.0–40.0	↓ nadir at 30–34 weeks of gestation.
MCV (fl)	80–100	80–100			↔ no change.
White blood cell ($\times 10^9$/L)	3.5–9.1	5.7–13.6	5.6–14.8	5.9–16.9	WBC ↑ because of a rise in neutrophils.
Neutrophils ($\times 10^9$/L)	1.4–4.6	3.6–10.1	3.8–12.3	3.9–13.1	Neutrophils ↑ by 35% 24 hours after steroid administration. It is associated with a 25% ↓ in lymphocyte count. The effect is transient and returns to baseline within 3 days.
Lymphocytes ($\times 10^9$/L)	1.0–4.5	1.1–3.6	0.9–3.9	1–3.6	Lymphocytes ↓ in the first and second trimesters and ↑ in the third trimester.
Platelets ($\times 10^9$/L)	165–415	174–391	155–409	146–429	↓ or ↔ The incidence of gestational thrombocytopenia is up to 15%.
APTT (s)	26.3–39.4	24.3–38.9	24.2–38.1	24.7–35.0	↓
PT (s)	12.7–15.4	9.7–13.5	9.5–13.4	9.6–12.9	↓
INR	0.9–1.04	0.89–1.05	0.85–0.97	0.80–0.94	↓
Fibrinogen (g/L)	2.3–5	2.4–5.1	2.9–5.4	3.7–6.2	↑ significantly by 1.5–3-fold.
Antithrombin III (%)	70–130	89–114	88–112	82–116	↓
Protein S, total (%)	70–140	39–105	27–101	33–101	↓ Testing should not be done during pregnancy. The ideal time to perform the test is ≥3 months after delivery and stopping breastfeeding.

(*Continued*)

(*Continued*)

	Non-pregnant Adult	First Trimester	Second Trimester	Third Trimester	Comments on the Effect of Pregnancy
Ferritin (ng/ml)	10–150	6–130	2–230	0–166	Generally ↓. Iron deficiency is defined as serum ferritin <30 ng/ml.
Transferrin (μmol/L)	2.5–5	3.1–4.2	2.7–5.4	3.5–6.5	↔
Transferrin saturation (%)	22–46	Not reported	10–44	5–37	↓
Folate (nmol/L)	12–41	6–34	1.8–54	3–47	↓ or ↔
Vitamin B12 (pmol/L)	206–713	87–323	96–484	73–388	↓

Biochemistry

	Non-pregnant Adult	First Trimester	Second Trimester	Third Trimester	Comments on the Effect of Pregnancy
Urea (mmol/L)	2.5–7.5	2.8–4.2	2.5–4.1	2.4–3.8	↓ by the first trimester.
Creatinine (μmol/L)	65–101	52–68	44–64	55–73	↓ Creatinine >77 μmol/L (0.87 mg/dl) is considered outside the normal range for pregnancy. eGFR is *not* valid for use in pregnancy.
Potassium (mmol/L)	3.5–5.0	3.6–5.0	3.3–5.0	3.3–5.1	↔, ↓ by mid-pregnancy, can range from 3.3 to 4.1.
Sodium (mmol/L)	136–145	133–148	129–148	130–148	↔, ↓ by mid-pregnancy, can range from 130 to 140.
Chloride (mmol/L)	102–109	101–105	97–109		↔
Bicarbonate (mmol/L)	22–30	20–24			↓
Uric acid (mmol/ml)	180–350	140–230	140–290	210–380	↓ in the first and second trimesters. Hyperuricemia is **not** diagnostic of pre-eclampsia, although elevated levels may be seen in pre-eclampsia.
Urine spot protein-to-creatinine ratio (urine PCR) mg/mmol creatinine	<0.15	<0.3			↑ in pre-eclampsia and renal disorders: ≥0.3. Perform urine PCR to quantify proteinuria if the urine dipstick shows albumin ≥1+.

(Continued)

	Non-pregnant Adult	First Trimester	Second Trimester	Third Trimester	Comments on the Effect of Pregnancy
24-hour urine total protein (g/24 hour) *NICE guidelines do **not** recommend routine use of the 24-hour urinary collection. Consider use for women with renal complications.*	<0.15		<0.3		↑ in pre-eclampsia and renal disorders: ≥0.3. The gold standard for quantification of proteinuria. However, it is more cumbersome and time-consuming.
24-hour creatinine clearance (mL/min)	70–140	140–162	130–169	119–139	↑
Bilirubin (μmol/L)	0–17	4–16	3–13	3–14	↔
Bile acids (μmol/L)	0.3–4.8	0–4.9	0–9.1	0–11.3	Significant rise after a meal, so measuring fasting bile acid levels is best. Serum bile acid >100 μmol/L is an indication for delivery in obstetric cholestasis.
AST (IU/L)	7–40	10–28	11–29	11–30	↓ in the upper limit of normal.
ALT (IU/L)	0–40	3–30	2–33	2–25	↓ in the upper limit of normal.
Gamma-glutamyl transpeptidase (GGT) (IU/L)	11–50	5–37	5–43	3–41	↔/↓ in the second and third trimesters.
ALP (IU/L)	30–130	32–100	43–135	133–418	↑ 2- to 3-fold by 20 weeks (mainly due to placental source but may be due to bone or liver isoenzymes).
Albumin (g/L)	41–53	31–51	26–45	23–42	↓
Total protein (g/L)	67–86	62–76	57–69	56–67	↓
Amylase (IU/L)	20–96	24–83	16–73	15–81	↔
Lipase (U/L)	0–160	0–104	0–140	5–148	↔

Inflammatory Markers

	Non-pregnant Adult	First Trimester	Second Trimester	Third Trimester	Comments on the Effect of Pregnancy
C-reactive protein (CRP) (mg/L)	0.2–3.0	Not reported	0.4–20.3	0.4–8.1	May ↑ in the second trimester.
Erythrocyte sedimentation rate (ESR) (mm/hour)	0–20	4–57	7–47	13–70	↑. Do not measure in pregnancy as it is a non-specific test.
Lactate (mmol/L)	0.5–2.2	*No established reference values in pregnancy* >2: Possible manifestation of hypoperfusion in the presence or absence of hypotension. ≥4: Consistent with but **not** diagnostic of septic shock.			↔. May ↑ during labour.
Procalcitonin (μg/L)	<0.09	***No established reference values in pregnancy*** o **<0.5**: Suggests low risk of severe sepsis or septic shock but cannot exclude any infection. o **<2**: May require repeat testing in 6–24 hours if sepsis is clinically suspected. o **>2**: Represents a high risk of severe sepsis or septic shock.			↔. Elevated procalcitonin levels can be seen in systemic bacterial infections and sepsis but cannot definitively confirm or exclude any infection or sepsis. Levels should decrease by approximately 50% over 24 hours, following physiological control of systemic infections. It also helps determine the initiation and discontinuation of antibiotic therapy.

Endocrine

Glucose	Non-pregnant Adult	First Trimester	Second Trimester	Third Trimester	Comments on the Effect of Pregnancy
Fasting glucose (mmol/L)+ Glycaemic targets for patients with DM in pregnancy: **Fasting:** 4.4–5.5 mmol/L **2 hours postprandial:** 5.5–6.6 mmol/L	4.2–5.5	≤5.0	≤5.0	≤5.0	10% ↓. Corticosteroids induce an ↑ in fasting blood glucose to >5 mmol/L for 5 days after the first course. A standard two-dose course of steroids may result in an abnormal glucose challenge test within 7 days of administration. Administration of an intravenous beta-agonist for

(*Continued*)

Glucose	Non-pregnant Adult	First Trimester	Second Trimester	Third Trimester	Comments on the Effect of Pregnancy
					tocolysis may also cause a ↑ in serum glucose. If antenatal steroids/beta-agonist were given, monitor the blood sugar profile closely. Start on an insulin sliding scale or IV insulin infusion with a dextrose drip.
HbA1C (%)	4–6	4–6	4–6	Third	↓ in the second trimester and ↑ in the third trimester. HbA1c is not a reliable indicator of glycaemic control in the second and third trimesters because of physiological changes in pregnancy. It can lead to reduced HbA1c in women without diabetes. Aim for HbA1c <6.5% before conceiving or during pregnancy.
Free T4 (pmol/L)	7–16	11.4–19.5	10.1–15.4	8.9–14.9	↓ slightly in the second and third trimesters. There is a rise in total T4 but a decrease in free T4 because of increased thyroid-binding globulin (TBG) and prolonged half-life of TBG.
Free T3 (pmol/L)	2.6–5.7	3–7	3–5.5	2.5–5.5	↓ There is a rise in total T3 but a decrease in free T3 because of increased TBG and prolonged half-life of TBG.
TSH (mIU/L)	0.3–4.3	0.1–2.5	0.2–3.0	0.3–3.0	↔ Transient decrease in TSH from 8 to 14 weeks as HCG shares a common α unit with TSH and HCG cross-reacts with and stimulates TSH receptors. Subsequently, as HCG levels fall, serum TSH rises slightly to or within the normal range.
Prolactin (μg/L)	0–20	36–213	110–330	137–372	↑ throughout pregnancy, reaching a peak at delivery. The magnitude of the rise in prolactin is variable.

Lipid Profile

It is <u>not</u> usually performed during pregnancy as cholesterol levels are increased by 50% and remain high for at least 1 month postpartum. Triglycerides increase by 300% during pregnancy and may remain high for at least 1 month postpartum but may normalise earlier in breastfeeding women.

A lipid profile should be done ≥6 to 8 weeks after delivery and after stopping breastfeeding. If the woman had complications post-delivery or surgeries, e.g., caesarean section, wait for ≥3 months before doing the test as cholesterol is used for wound healing. Hence, results might not be reliable if obtained earlier.

	Non-pregnant Adult	First Trimester	Second Trimester	Third Trimester	Comments on the Effect of Pregnancy
Cholesterol, total (mmol/L)	<5.2	3.7–5.4	4.6–7.7	5.7–9.0	↑ with gestational age (50% rise). Especially in the second and third trimesters, mainly because of a rise in LDL-cholesterol due to elevated maternal oestrogen levels.
HDL-cholesterol	1.04–1.55	1.04–2.02	1.35–2.25	1.24–2.25	↑
LDL-cholesterol	<2.6	1.6–4.0	2.0–4.8	2.6–5.8	↑
VLDL-cholesterol	0.16–1.0	0.26–0.46	0.34–0.60	0.54–0.93	↔
Triglycerides	<1.7	0.45–1.8	0.85–4.3	1.5–5.1	↑ with gestational age, especially in the second and third trimesters, because of elevated maternal oestrogen levels.

Tumour Markers

	Non-pregnant Adult	First Trimester	Second Trimester	Third Trimester	Comments on the Effect of Pregnancy
CA 125 (U/ml)	<35	0–51.5	0–30.8	0–56.3	May ↑ till 16 weeks. Refer to Chapter 60: *Tumour Markers in Gynaecology and Pregnancy*.
Alpha-fetoprotein (AFP) (μg/L)	<15	19–119	96–302	160–550	↑ from about 14 to 32 weeks in pregnancy. Used as part of the aneuploidy screening test for Down syndrome. Refer to Chapter 60: *Tumour Markers in Gynaecology and Pregnancy*.

CHAPTER 29

An Overview of Serum Human Chorionic Gonadotrophin (HCG)

Human chorionic gonadotrophin (HCG) is a hormone produced by syncytiotrophoblast cells of the placenta during pregnancy. Smaller amounts of HCG are produced in the pituitary gland, liver and colon.

Measurement of serum βHCG levels is useful in the following clinical situations:

1. Diagnosis and management of pregnancy and pregnancy-related problems, e.g., pregnancy of unknown location (PUL), ectopic pregnancy, miscarriage and gestational trophoblastic disease (GTD).
2. Biochemical markers in first- or second-trimester aneuploidy screening.
3. Tumour markers in some gynaecological malignancies, e.g., germ cell tumours (GCTs). They are used to monitor treatment response after chemotherapy and detect tumour recurrence.

Sources of HCG

Benign causes:

a) *Pregnancy*

Syncytiotrophoblasts produce regular HCG, which promotes progesterone production by the corpus luteum until placental progesterone production is established after 12 weeks of gestation.

Extra villous cytotrophoblasts produce HCG-h, which promotes the invasion of extravillous cytotrophoblast into the uterine wall to form anchoring villi and into the spiral arteries to create high-flow, low-resistance vessels.

b) *Pituitary gland*

The normal pituitary gland produces a small amount of HCG-h (1–32 IU/L). It may occur before ovulation in peri-menopausal or menopausal women and cause false positive results.

c) *In response to or recovery from chemotherapy-induced gonadal suppression*

As chemotherapy results in gonadal suppression, pituitary hCG can be seen immediately after treatment when the LH level is high, resulting in a false positive result.

d) *Exogenous HCG injections*

These can be given as part of assisted reproductive technique (ART) protocols.

Malignant causes:

e) ***GCT of the ovary***, e.g., embryonal carcinoma.

f) *GTD*

Serum βHCG levels of >200,000 IU/L strongly suggest GTD.

HCG-h promotes trophoblast growth and invasion. Invasion may be **controlled** in implantation of a normal pregnancy and molar pregnancies or **uncontrolled** as in malignant choriocarcinoma.

g) *Non-trophoblastic malignancy*

Breast, germ-cell, bladder, renal, prostate, lung, gastrointestinal, head, neck, haematological and neuroendocrine origins.

Types of βHCG Tests

The earliest time for a positive HCG test is about 8 days after conception. However, this is only possible in about 5% of women. Most women have a positive HCG test 11–12 days after conception, i.e., days 25–26 of their last menstrual period (LMP).

Serum βHCG	Urine βHCG
Quantitative test	Qualitative test (positive or negative)
Higher sensitivity and specificity Longer turnaround time	More convenient, affordable Faster turnaround time
Lowest detectable level is 1.2 IU/L	Lowest detectable level is 25 IU/L
Possible false negative result from the "hook effect" – Extreme high HCG levels may cause the antibodies to be saturated and result in an artefactually low HCG value → the laboratory should perform dilution before testing.	Possible false negative result due to diluted urine
Possible false positive results due to: – Recent exposure to mononucleosis – IgA deficiency syndrome – History of GTD/gestational trophoblastic neoplasia (GTN)	Possible false positive result due to the presence of blood or protein in the urine

βHCG Levels in Pregnancy

βHCG usually increases by at least 63% in 48 hours in a normal pregnancy, although the possibility of an ectopic pregnancy cannot be excluded.

If βHCG decreases by >50%, the diagnosis is likely a non-viable pregnancy (could be intrauterine or extrauterine). Advise to repeat urine pregnancy test 14 days after second serum βHCG or to repeat another serum βHCG if the second value is high (NICE guidelines).

If βHCG decreases by <50% or increases by <63%, ectopic pregnancy cannot be excluded. There is a high index of suspicion for ectopic pregnancy until HCG levels return to non-pregnant levels or ultrasound confirms a non-viable intrauterine pregnancy.

Gestation via the Last Menstrual Period	Levels of HCG (IU/L)
3	5–50
4	5–426
5	18–7,340
6	1,080–56,500
7–8	**7,650–229,000**
9–12	**25,700–288,000**
13–16	13,000–254,000
17–24	4,060–165,400
25–40	3,640–117,000

The decline of βHCG to undetectable levels after pregnancy or termination can take 7–60 days. The decline is rapid for the first few days (half-life 9–31 hours), then more slowly (half-life 55–64 hours).

Trending βHCG levels are used for managing molar pregnancies and following the termination of normal or ectopic pregnancies to ensure that treatment has been successful.

βHCG Levels in Spontaneous Miscarriage

βHCG rises sub-optimally or falls in miscarriages (does not increase by >63% over 48 hours). The βHCG level returns to negative 2–4 weeks after surgical evacuation of the uterus.

The persistent elevation of βHCG should always raise the suspicion of GTN if retained products of conception have been excluded.

Serum βHCG is not routinely done after a spontaneous miscarriage unless there is persistent vaginal bleeding or if the diagnosis is uncertain.

Serum βHCG is no longer required after future pregnancies following a history of GTD unless in women who have received chemotherapy (RCOG 2020).

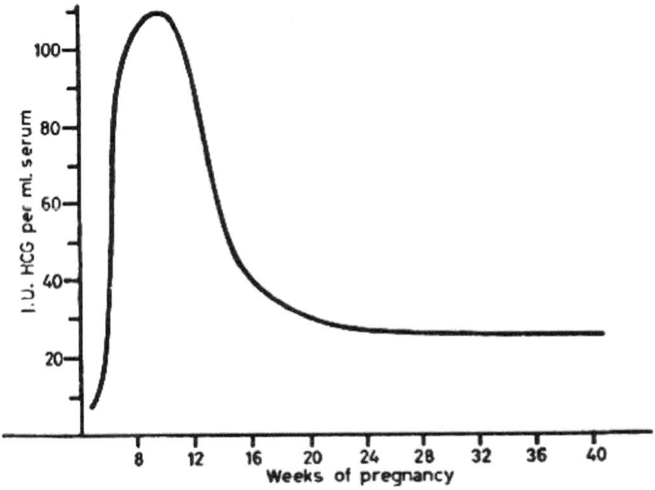

βHCG levels in pregnancy.

βHCG levels rise exponentially in the first trimester of pregnancy, doubling every 24 h during the first 8 weeks. After that, they peak around 10 weeks; then, the levels decrease until the 16th week of gestation, remaining fairly constant until term.

βHCG Levels in GTD

Levels of >200,000 IU/L usually suggest GTD.

Follow-up after GTD

1. **Complete mole**
   - If βHCG normalises *within* 56 days of the pregnancy event — follow up for 6 months from the date of molar evacuation.
   - If βHCG normalises *after* 56 days of the pregnancy event — follow up for 6 months after the normalisation of βHCG levels.
2. **Partial mole**
   - Follow-up until two consecutive serum βHCG levels taken at least 4 weeks apart are normal (KKH protocol).

***Persistent GTD*:** 15% after complete mole; 0.5% after partial mole.

Suspect persistent GTD if:

i. Serum βHCG reaches a plateau (a decline of <10% for four values over 3 weeks).

ii. Serum βHCG rises (an increase of >10% of three values over 2 weeks).
iii. Persistence of detectable serum βHCG for >6 months after molar evacuation. In total, 90% of persistent GTD are invasive moles and <10% are choriocarcinomas.

For further management of GTD, refer to Chapter 9: *Approach to Gestational Trophoblastic Disease* (GTD).

βHCG Levels in Ectopic Pregnancy (EP)

- **Discriminatory zone** — an intrauterine gestational sac (IUGS) should be visible via a transvaginal ultrasound scan (TVUS) at a βHCG level of **1,500 IU/L.**
- Conversely, no IUGS at βHCG >1,500 is termed PUL, and a diagnosis of ectopic pregnancy must be excluded.
- Most ectopic pregnancies have suboptimal βHCG rise, BUT a normal rise in βHCG does not exclude an ectopic pregnancy as ~20% of ectopic pregnancies can have a normal βHCG rise.

βHCG Trending After Medical Treatment for Ectopic — Methotrexate (MTX)

- Do βHCG on days 4 and 7 after MTX and then weekly till negative to rule out persistent trophoblastic disease.

Trending of βHCG Levels After Surgery for Ectopic Pregnancy

- Do *serum* βHCG 1 week after *salpingostomy*, then weekly βHCG till the level is undetectable to exclude persistent trophoblastic disease.
- Do a *urine* pregnancy test 3 weeks after *salpingectomy* to exclude persistent trophoblastic disease.

Persistently Elevated βHCG After Treatment of Ectopic Pregnancy

- Failure of MTX treatment (15–25%).
- Rare incidence of heterotopic pregnancy (concomitant intrauterine and ectopic pregnancy): ranging from fewer than 1 in 30,000 in spontaneous pregnancies to 1 in 100–500 for ART pregnancies.

Part 3

Gynaecology

CHAPTER 30

Gynaecological Emergencies and Surgical Complications

Gynaecological emergencies refer to conditions of the female reproductive system that threaten the woman's life, sexual function or fertility.

The **general approach** includes an assessment of the haemodynamic status and resuscitation if necessary. Because of the urgent nature, history taking, physical examination and investigations should occur concurrently. Always do a urine pregnancy test (UPT) in women of reproductive age as this will help narrow the differential diagnoses.

Resuscitation — General Guidelines

- Exclude pregnancy in reproductive-aged females
  - Check the last menstrual period (LMP) and perform a UPT
- Check for drug allergies
- **A**irway: give high-flow oxygen
- **B**reathing
- **C**irculation
  - Two large-bore intravenous (IV) cannulas
  - IV fluids — up to 2 litre (L) crystalloids (Hartmann's) and 1.5 L colloids can be infused rapidly until blood is available (ensure no contraindications to aggressive fluid replacement)
  - Insert indwelling urinary catheter (IDC) for strict input and output (I/O) monitoring
  - Estimation of blood loss (if applicable)
- Regular monitoring of vital signs
- Early escalation to senior staff, code blue activation if necessary

- Involvement of the anaesthetic team for haemodynamic support
- Admit to an intensive care unit or a high dependency unit
- If the woman is in pain, remember to give appropriate analgesia after excluding an acute abdomen.

Gynaecological emergencies

1 Ectopic Pregnancy (EP)

a. EP occurs when a developing blastocyst becomes implanted at a site other than the endometrium of the uterine cavity. Most occur in the fallopian tube (96%).
b. Other sites include cervical, interstitial (proximal segment of the fallopian tube embedded within the muscular wall of the uterus), caesarean scar, ovary and abdomen.
c. Rarely, a heterotopic pregnancy can occur where both an intrauterine pregnancy and an EP are present.
d. A ruptured EP can lead to massive haemoperitoneum and life-threatening haemodynamic compromise.
e. **Symptoms:** Per vaginal bleeding (PVB) preceded by amenorrhoea and/or abdominal pain. Shoulder pain due to diaphragmatic irritation by blood in the peritoneal cavity may be present.
f. **Physical findings:** Abdominal tenderness ± guarding, adnexal tenderness, PVB on speculum examination.
g. **Red flags:** Haemodynamic instability, pallor, poor peripheral perfusion, distended abdomen, signs of peritonitis (rebound tenderness/guarding), massive PVB.
h. **Investigations:**
   i. *Blood tests*: full blood count (FBC), type and screen (check rhesus status), βHCG ± urea, electrolytes and creatinine (UECr) and liver function test (LFT) if planned for methotrexate (MTX) therapy.
   ii. *Transabdominal/transvaginal (TA/TV) US of the pelvis*:
      - Determine the location of the pregnancy and whether the EP has ruptured.
      - If βHCG is >1,500 IU/L, an intrauterine gestational sac should be visualised on a TVUS.

- *Signs of EP*: presence of an adnexal mass or gestational sac/yolk sac/embryo at an ectopic site.
- The presence of echogenic fluid (indicative of blood) in the pouch of Douglas or abdomen is consistent with a ruptured EP.

i. **Approach to immediate management of EP:**

(For further management, refer to Chapter 8: *Approach to Ectopic Pregnancy.*)

Options for *unruptured EP* include *expectant, medical and surgical. Ruptured EP* usually requires surgical management with salpingectomy.

i. **Surgery criteria:** Haemodynamically unstable, suspected tubal rupture or if MTX treatment is contraindicated or unsuccessful.
   - Surgical options include salpingectomy versus salpingostomy.
   - Both salpingectomy and salpingostomy have similar fertility outcomes in subsequent pregnancies if the contralateral tube is normal.

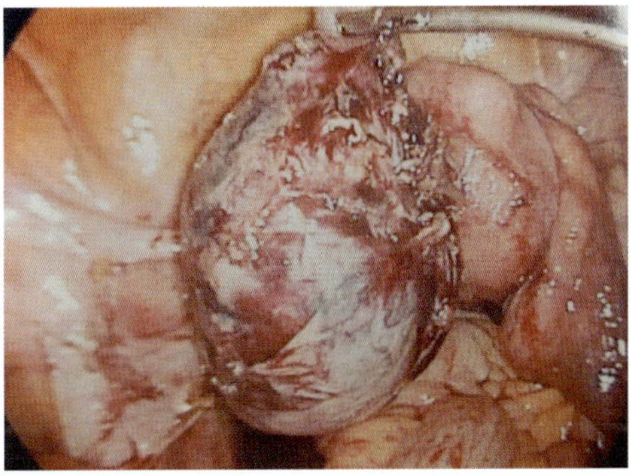

Left salpingectomy for left tubal pregnancy

1. *Salpingectomy* = removal of the fallopian tube
   a. *Indications for salpingectomy*: Uncontrolled bleeding, ruptured tube, damaged tube, large tubal pregnancy or if the patient desires permanent sterilisation
2. *Salpingostomy* = incising the tube to remove the tubal gestation but leaving the remaining tube
   a. *Salpingostomy* is preferred for women who desire future fertility and in whom the contralateral tube is absent or

damaged. However, this method has the risk of persistent trophoblastic tissue.

b. The patient will need regular follow-up to ensure that bHCG returns to negative and should be counselled on the possibility of needing MTX or a second surgery if there is persistent trophoblastic tissue.

ii. Laparoscopic surgery is the standard surgical approach (diagnostic laparoscopy keep in view (KIV) salpingostomy/salpingectomy KIV laparotomy). However, an open approach may be required if the patient is haemodynamically unstable.

iii. **Long-term management of EP**
   - Counsel on contraception if the pregnancy was unplanned and unintended.
   - If the patient is keen to conceive, advise her to wait until she has recovered from surgery and her menses has resumed before trying to conceive (TTC).
   - Avoid pregnancy for the next 3 months for patients who have received MTX.

2 Inevitable Miscarriage

a. This refers to a dilated cervical os in the presence of vaginal bleeding and abdominal cramps before 24 weeks of gestation.
b. Massive PVB can be life-threatening, leading to severe anaemia requiring transfusion of blood or blood products.
c. **Symptoms:** Abdominal pain, PVB, passage of products of conception.
d. **Physical findings:** Lower abdominal tenderness, speculum and vaginal examination (VE) to assess the cervical os, amniotic membranes may be seen and bulging through the os, presence of products of conception or active bleeding.
e. **Red flags:** Pallor, poor peripheral perfusion, massive PVB.
f. **Investigations:**
   i. *Blood tests*: FBC and T&S ± PT/PTT, vaginal swabs for infection, urine FEME and culture.
   ii. *TA/TVUS*: The intrauterine gestational sac is located in the lower endometrial cavity/cervical canal; the cervical os (internal/external) may be dilated.

g. **Approach to immediate management of impending miscarriage:** Expectant or surgical management (evacuation of the uterus). Surgical management is indicated if the patient is haemodynamically unstable or actively bleeding.
h. **Long-term management of miscarriage:**
   i. Counsel on contraception if the pregnancy was unplanned and unintended.
   ii. Offer referral to a medical social worker (MSW) or a counsellor for grief or emotional counselling (if indicated).
   iii. The patient can start trying to conceive once her menses resume (typically in 4–6 weeks) and she is emotionally ready.
   iv. Consider work-up if recurrent miscarriage or second-trimester miscarriage
   (refer to Chapter 6: *Approach to Recurrent Pregnancy Loss*).

3 Ovarian Cyst Accidents

a. **Ovarian cyst accidents** include cyst rupture, haemorrhage and torsion.

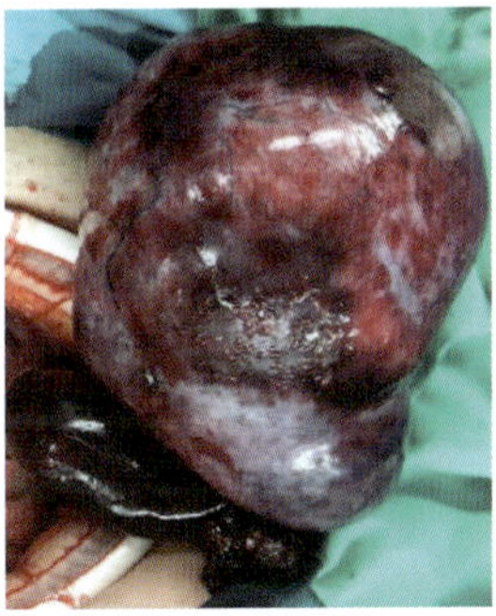

Ovarian torsion with necrosis

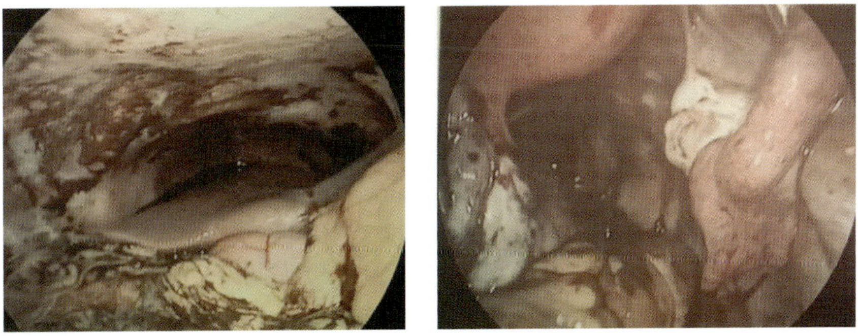

Ruptured endometriotic cyst with contents extending into the upper abdomen

b. **Ovarian cyst rupture and haemorrhage** may cause significant haemoperitoneum and haemodynamic instability. Ruptured corpus luteal/haemorrhagic cysts are a common cause of ovarian cyst rupture.
c. **Ovarian torsion** is defined as a partial or complete rotation of the ovarian vascular pedicle, causing obstruction to venous outflow and later arterial inflow. **An elusive clinical diagnosis,** ovarian torsion may lead to ischaemia and necrosis of the ovary/tube [which would warrant a salpingo-oophorectomy (SO) if noted intra-operatively], resulting in a loss of ovarian function and reserve. Therefore, prompt diagnosis is vital to preserve ovarian and/or tubal function and to prevent other associated morbidities, e.g., sepsis.
d. **Symptoms:** Acute lower abdominal pain, usually severe and of sudden onset. This may be associated with a loss of appetite, nausea or vomiting. With any adnexal pathology, there may be referred pain down the cutaneous distribution of the obturator nerve (the medial aspect of the thigh down to the knee).
   i. *Ovarian cyst rupture/haemorrhage:* Pain may be worsened by movement because of peritoneal irritation from the free peritoneal fluid.
   ii. *Ovarian torsion:* Pain may be waxing and waning. Pain may be worsened by movement because of peritoneal irritation by inflammed ovarian mass.
      a. **Physical findings:** Elevated pulse rate, abdominal tenderness with rebound tenderness/guarding, adnexal tenderness and a possibly palpable mass.
      b. **Red flags:** acute abdomen, pallor, poor peripheral perfusion.
      c. **Investigations**
         a. *Blood tests*: FBC T&S, KIV ovarian tumour markers (if suspicious of malignancy)
         b. *Imaging*:
            i. *TA/TV ultrasound scan*:
               1. *US features of ovarian cyst rupture/haemorrhage:* Ovarian cyst with typical mixed, often heterogeneous, internal echoes suggestive of blood clots. Normal ovaries but site-specific tenderness and free fluid in the pouch of Douglas may be suggestive of ovarian cyst rupture.

2. *US features of ovarian torsion:* Unilateral enlarged oedematous ovary, uniform peripheral cystic structures (representing follicles displaced by ovarian oedema), a co-existent mass within the affected ovary, free pelvic fluid, lack of venous or arterial flow and a twisted vascular pedicle. The mass may be displaced superiorly and towards the midline, usually anterior to the uterus. Colour Doppler examination may demonstrate a lack of arterial or venous flow or a twisted vascular pedicle ("whirlpool sign").

ii. *Computer tomography scan of the abdomen and pelvis (CTAP):* Typically done to investigate abdominal pain.
   1. CT features of ovarian torsion include an enlarged ovary, deviation of the uterus to the twisted side, engorged blood vessels on the twisted side, a small amount of ascites and obliteration of fat in the torted adnexa.
   2. If the adnexae appear normal on TA/TVUS, consider CTAP in cases of an acute abdomen to exclude non-gynaecological causes of abdominal pain.
   3. *Note of caution:* Finding an ovarian cyst does not always mean that this will be the cause of the presenting symptoms.

d. **Approach to immediate management of ovarian cyst accidents**
   a. Laparoscopy may be necessary in cases where the diagnosis is in doubt or for haemodynamic compromise.
   b. *Ovarian cyst rupture/haemorrhage*
      i. *Expectant management*: Analgesia and observation with haemoglobin (Hb) trending, follow-up with interval US pelvis in 8 weeks (within day 2–10 of menses) to assess for resolution
      ii. *Consider laparoscopy if*:
         1. Haemodynamic compromise
         2. Diagnostic uncertainty or likelihood of torsion
         3. No relief of symptoms after 24–48 hours of presentation
         4. Increasing haemoperitoneum on ultrasound or a falling haemoglobin (Hb)
   c. *Ovarian torsion*
      i. There should be a high index of suspicion and a low threshold for surgical management, especially in young women.

Expectant management with observation may be misleading if the pain improves because of nerve tissue damage by necrosis rather than the resolution of the pathological process.

ii. The goal of surgical evaluation is to confirm torsion and assess ovarian viability: Diagnostic laparoscopy KIV ovarian detorsion/cystectomy KIV Salpingo-oophorectomy (SO) KIV laparotomy.

iii. Salpingo-oophorectomy (SO) is indicated if:
(1) The ovary is non-viable after detorsion
(2) Suspicious of malignancy
(3) The patient is menopausal

e. **Long-term management of ovarian cysts**

i. Post-surgery, the specimen should be sent for histology.

ii. Surgery should *not* be delayed to await a frozen section during office hours as a torted ovary may become non-viable, resulting in a SO and loss of the ovary. Moreover, a necrotic ovary/tube can result in negative histology because of extensive necrosis, which makes interpretation impossible.

iii. In premenopausal women with recurrent cyst haemorrhage or rupture, suppression of ovulation with COCP may be considered.

iv. In women with endometriotic cysts, medical treatment, e.g., Visanne®, may be offered to prevent cyst recurrence.

4 Heavy Menstrual Bleeding (HMB) Causing Anaemia

a. **HMB** is defined as excessive bleeding that occurs regularly, every 24–35 days, and affects a woman's physical, social and emotional well-being or quality of life; it is also defined as a prolonged flow for >7 days. For academic purposes, it is defined as bleeding >80 ml per menstrual cycle.

b. Excessive menstrual bleeding can be life-threatening because of severe anaemia.

c. **Symptoms:** Heavy or prolonged PVB. Anaemic symptoms (fatigue, non-vertiginous giddiness, breathlessness on exertion, syncope, palpitations, chest pain) require urgent attention.

d. **Physical findings:** Pallor, goitre, palpate the abdomen for masses, speculum examination to assess the cervix (malignancy/prolapsing polyp/mass) and bleeding, VE to assess uterus size and presence of adnexal masses.

e. **Red flags:** Haemodynamic instability, pallor, massive PVB
f. **Investigations:**
   i. *Blood tests*: FBC, group & crossmatch (GXM), thyroid function test (TFT), anaemia work-up [serum ferritin, folate, vitamin B12, Hb electrophoresis], ± UECr, especially if haemodynamic instability/ severe anaemia/patient has co-morbid conditions.
   ii. ECG
   iii. US pelvis to assess for other acute gynae pathology, especially if the patient has abdominal pain (which may be due to dysmenorrhoea).
g. **Approach to immediate management of HMB:**
   i. Medical management in the acute setting:
      1. Intramuscular (IM) progesterone 100 mg stat
      2. IV/oral (PO) tranexamic acid (TXA) 1 g three times a day (TDS)
   ii. Replacement of blood products (1 unit of PCT increases Hb by 1 g/dl), generally advised to keep Hb >8 g/dl if there is no cardiovascular history and no anaemic symptoms. If the patient is iron deficient, consider IV iron to boost iron stores, followed by oral iron 5–7 days later to maintain iron levels.
   iii. Rarely, emergency uterine artery embolisation (UAE) or hysterectomy may be required for acute life-threatening bleeding.
h. **Long-term management of HMB**
   i. Once the patient has been stabilised, consider endometrial biopsy to exclude endometrial hyperplasia/cancer if there are risk factors.
   ii. Discuss long-term options to treat HMB
      1. *Non-hormonal medical options:* TXA (anti-fibrinolytic), NSAIDs
      2. *Hormonal medical options:* Cyclical oral progestogens, combined oral contraceptive pill (COCP), Depo-Provera, gonadotrophin-releasing hormone (GnRH) agonist, Mirena® intra-uterine contraceptive device (IUCD)
      3. *Surgical options:* Endometrial ablation, UAE, myomectomy or hysterectomy
   iii. Maintain Hb levels (encourage an iron-rich diet and supplement with oral iron as necessary)

5 Pelvic Inflammatory Disease (PID)

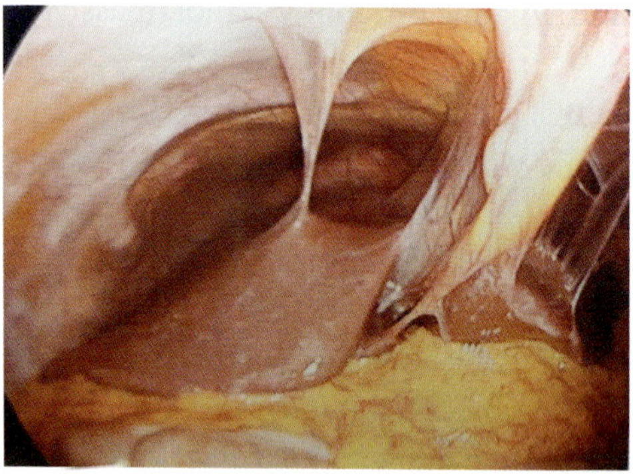

Fitz-Hugh–Curtis syndrome

a. **PID** refers to an acute infection of the upper genital tract (cervix, uterus, fallopian tubes, ovaries). It represents a spectrum of infections and can present acutely (ranging from mild symptoms to life-threatening sepsis) or with long-term sequelae such as chronic pelvic pain, subfertility or EP (this chapter will focus on *severe acute PID*).
(Refer to Chapter 50: *Pelvic Inflammatory Disease* for further management.)
b. **Symptoms:** Lower abdominal pain, fever, chills, foul-smelling vaginal discharge, abnormal uterine bleeding. RHC pain may be due to Fitz-Hugh–Curtis syndrome and is a sign of chronic infection.
c. **Physical examination:** Fever, tachycardia, lower abdominal tenderness, purulent endocervical discharge, cervical excitation and/or adnexal tenderness on bimanual examination.
d. **Red flags:** Signs of septic shock
e. **Investigations:**
   i. *Blood tests*: FBC, C-reactive protein (CRP), UECr, PT/PTT — if concerned about disseminated intravascular coagulation (DIC) or planning for interventional radiology (IR)-guided aspiration of a tubo-ovarian abscess (TOA), septic work-up including blood cultures, consider a full STI screen (HIV, syphilis, hepatitis B and C).

ii. Swabs in high-risk groups:
   1. *VP3 swab*: *Gardnerella*, *Candida* and *Trichomonas*
   2. *Gonorrhoea and Chlamydia PCR*

iii. <u>*Others:*</u> Urine FEME and culture, if indicated

iv. US pelvis to assess for TOA

v. CTAP if acute abdomen to rule out complications, e.g., ruptured TOA or non-gynaecological causes of pain

f. **Approach to immediate management of acute PID:**

i. *Medical*: IV ceftriaxone 1 g every morning (OM) + IV metronidazole 500 mg every 8 h + PO doxycycline 100 mg twice a day (BD) for 14 days

ii. Consider image-guided abscess drainage if:
   1. Haemodynamically unstable
   2. Large size of the abscess (>5 cm) and amenable to drainage (as per the interventional radiologist)
   3. No improvement with antibiotics after 48–72 hours (send fluid aspirate for aerobic and anaerobic cultures)

iii. *Surgery is the last resort* reserved for clinically deteriorating patients despite antibiotics. Surgery is often complex, given the extensive involvement of various intra-abdominal organs and the inflammed nature of the affected tissues. Given the anatomic distortion, this can be done via an open or laparoscopic approach and depends on the operator's skill and experience. The abscess cavity and associated infectious/inflammatory fluid and debris are drained/resected, and the peritoneal cavity is copiously irrigated, lessening the patient's overall infectious/inflammatory burden. In **severe cases**, a Salpingo-oophorectomy (SO) or even a total hysterectomy and bilateral SO may need to be performed.

g. **Long-term management of PID:**

i. For patients with PID who test positive for STI, sexual partners should be notified of the need for evaluation and treatment.

ii. Counsel on possible long-term sequelae, including chronic pelvic pain, subfertility and EP. This occurs because of scarring and adhesion formation that accompany the healing of infected and damaged tissues.

6 Ovarian Hyperstimulation Syndrome (OHSS)

a. **OHSS** is the most serious complication of ovarian hyperstimulation for assisted reproduction technologies (ARTs). It occurs when the ovaries are hyperstimulated and exposed to human chorionic gonadotrophin (hCG), resulting in the release of pro-inflammatory mediators, mainly vascular endothelial growth factor (VEGF). Hence, there is increased vascular permeability and third spacing, mainly into the abdominal cavity.
b. 6–8% of patients undergoing IVF treatment will experience mild forms of OHSS. The severe form affects <1% of patients.
c. *Severe OHSS* is a life-threatening condition because it can cause venous or arterial thromboembolic events because of haemoconcentration, including stroke.
d. In *critical OHSS*, the functions of vital organs and systems are adversely compromised. *Complications*, e.g., anuria with acute renal failure, cardiac arrhythmias, respiratory insufficiency, reduced liver perfusion and function, DIC or venous thromboembolism (VTE), may result in death.
e. **Symptoms:** Abdominal pain/bloating, nausea/vomiting, breathlessness, diarrhoea, anuria/oliguria.
f. **Physical findings:** Dry mucosa, reduced breath sounds, abdominal distension and tenderness, clinical ascites.
g. **Red flags:** Haemodynamic instability, desaturation (indicating compromised pulmonary function), neurological deficits.
h. **Investigations:**
   i. *Blood*: FBC, renal panel, LFT, PT/APTT, serum βHCG (to determine if the patient has conceived, usually at least 14 days after embryo transfer), CRP (for the severity of OHSS)
   ii. *US pelvis*: Enlarged ovaries, ascites
   iii. *Chest X-ray* (*CXR*) if respiratory symptoms, desaturation or suspected pleural effusion
   iv. *2D-echocardiography* (*2D-ECHO*) if cardiac problems/pericardial effusion are suspected
   v. *CT pulmonary angiogram* (*CTPA*) *or US Doppler of the lower limbs* if pulmonary embolism or deep vein thrombosis (DVT), respectively, is suspected

i. **Approach to immediate management of OHSS:**
   i. The pathophysiological process of OHSS is self-limited, and increased vascular permeability regresses spontaneously.
   ii. Multidisciplinary care, e.g., the anaesthetist, intensive care team
   iii. <u>*Goals of treatment*:</u>
      1. Supportive care
      2. Analgesia
      3. Correcting the fluid and electrolyte imbalance
      4. Monitoring for and managing secondary complications, e.g., acute renal failure, ascites and pleural effusion
      5. VTE thromboprophylaxis
   iv. <u>*Monitoring*:</u> Daily weight and abdominal girth measurements, strict input and output monitoring. Consider invasive monitoring with central venous pressure monitoring.
   v. <u>*Management*:</u>
      1. Oral hydration guided by thirst is the most physiological way of hydration if the patient can tolerate it orally. If not, start intravenous crystalloids. Aim 2 L/day.
      2. Consider colloids IV albumin 20% 100 ml every 6–12 hours.
      3. Correct electrolyte imbalance.
      4. Abdominal drainage for ascites causing significant pain or respiratory compromise.
      5. Thoracocentesis or chest drains for symptomatic pleural effusions.
      6. Prophylactic VTE thromboprophylaxis (mechanical or pharmaceutical methods, e.g., TED stockings, LMWH) for all hospitalised and outpatients with VTE risk factors.
      7. Symptom relief and analgesia (avoid NSAIDs as they may compromise renal function), anti-emetics as necessary.

j. **Long-term management of OHSS:** If the patient is pregnant, there is an increased risk of pre-eclampsia and preterm delivery during the pregnancy.

7 Sepsis in an Immunocompromised Individual

a. Chemotherapy is a standard treatment for various gynaecological malignancies and has led to increased survival and reduced recurrence rate in gynaecological cancer patients. However, chemotherapy often causes myelosuppression, increasing the risk of neutropenia. This makes the patient susceptible to conventional and opportunistic pathogens. Life-threatening multi-organ dysfunction can quickly evolve in these patients.

b. **History taking:**
   i. *Presenting complaint:* Symptoms may be non-specific, and signs may be muted because of the immunocompromised state.
   ii. *Cancer history:* Type of cancer, FIGO stage, recurrence status, previous or current treatment (surgery/chemotherapy/radiotherapy)
   iii. Previous infections (blood, urine cultures), recent antimicrobial use

c. **Red flags:** *Signs of sepsis:* Hypothermia, tachycardia, tachypnoea, hypoxia, hypotension, oliguria, impaired consciousness
   i. **Febrile neutropenia** is defined as a single temperature of ≥38.3°C or temperature of ≥38.0°C sustained over an hour and an absolute neutrophil count (ANC) of $<0.5 \times 10^9$/L or expected to fall below 0.5×10^9/L over the next 48 hours.

d. **Investigations**
   i. *Blood tests*: FBC–ANC count (in KKH, neutropenia is defined as $<1.0 \times 10^9$/L), CRP, procalcitonin, renal panel, LFT, PT/APTT, lactate, blood cultures and cultures obtained from other suspected sites of infection (e.g., urine, catheters).
   ii. *Imaging*: CXR, CTAP (if abdominal symptoms are present).

e. **Approach to immediate management of neutropenic sepsis:**
   i. Ascertain the localising source of infection, if possible, e.g., genitourinary, gastrointestinal (GI), lung, skin or central nervous system source, to direct investigations and target treatment.
   ii. Initiate the SEPSIS 1-hour bundle
      1. Measuring the lactate level
      2. Obtaining a blood culture before the administration of antibiotics
      3. Administering broad-spectrum IV antibiotics

4. Beginning rapid administration of 30 ml/kg crystalloid fluid for hypotension or lactate ≥4 mmol/L
5. Administering vasopressors if the patient is hypotensive during or after fluid resuscitation to maintain mean arterial pressure (MAP) at ≥65 mmHg within 1 hour of sepsis recognition

iii. *Antibiotics:* IV piperacillin/tazocin 4.5 g every 6 hours ± IV amikacin 15–20 mg/kg every 24 hours (if not better after 48 hours) ± IV vancomycin 25–30 mg/kg/dose (max 2 g) × 1 then 15 mg/kg/dose (max 1 g) every 12 hours (if catheter-related bloodstream infection or MRSA positive is suspected).

iv. Consider granulocyte colony-stimulating factor (G-CSF) for patients with ANC $<1 \times 10^9$/L

v. *A fungal screen and antifungal cover* should be considered ≥96 hours after the anti-bacterial treatment is started if the patient is still febrile and neutropenic.

vi. Update the medical oncologist and refer to an infectious disease (ID) physician if there is a persistent fever.

vii. Look out for complications: renal and liver impairment, septic shock.

viii. Continue IV antibiotics for at least 2–3 days. **Stop vancomycin** if there is *no evidence* of MRSA or coagulase-negative *staphylococci*, and **stop amikacin** if there is *no evidence* of Gram-negative organisms.

ix. The duration of antibiotics depends on the presence and type of pathogen and clinical condition.

1. If ANC $\geq 0.5 \times 10^9$/L, afebrile ≥48 hours and cultures negative: consider switching to oral antibiotics.
2. If ANC $\leq 0.5 \times 10^9$/L but stable patient: continue antibiotics until the patient has been afebrile for 5–7 days.
3. For specific infections, e.g., pneumonia or urinary tract infections: treat according to the pathogen and based on the institution's antimicrobial guidelines.

f. **Long-term management of patients with neutropenic sepsis:**

– Confirm follow-up plans with the medical oncologist and gynaecological oncologist for the treatment of the patient's cancer.

8 Sexual Assault

a. **Sexual assault** is defined as any sexual act performed by one person on another without consent.
b. Evaluation is urgent and time-sensitive (especially if the offence has taken place within 72 hours), as any delay in an examination may result in a loss of vital forensic evidence. A police report should be made as formal forensic specimens **cannot** be collected without a report.
c. The approach includes assessment and treatment of physical injury with a particular focus on the genitalia, forensic evaluation, evaluation of STI, psychological assessment and support.
d. The **history** must be obtained in a sensitive and supportive manner. This should include the circumstances of the assault, use of force, details of the assault, the type of penetration, use of contraception and ejaculation.
e. **Physical examination** should be detailed and objective. A head-to-toe approach should be taken to look for any trauma, including in the anogenital region. Use a body diagram for documentation. Consider photo documentation. Remember to document negative findings as well.

Recommended time frames for evidence collection for DNA profiling

Site of specimen	Time for swab (upper limit) (hours)
Oral cavity	24
Anus	72
Bite marks	96
Vagina	120

f. **Approach to immediate management of sexual assault:**
   i. Forensic evaluation should be offered to victims of sexual assault. The sexual assault kit issued by law enforcement includes **forensic samples for DNA profiling and STI screening**. Consider empiric treatment for STI if appropriate.
   ii. The police are updated to follow up on the investigation of the case.
   iii. **Screening for pregnancy:** The pregnancy risk following an episode of sexual assault with unprotected sexual intercourse (UPSI) is 5%. Women who *do not* wish to conceive should be offered emergency contraception **(EC)** after UPSI that has taken place on any day of a natural menstrual cycle. Pregnancy testing is advised if the

next menstrual period is delayed by >7 days, lighter than usual or associated with atypical abdominal pain.

iv. Provide **adequate analgesia for** associated traumatic injuries.

v. Offer **prophylactic treatment for the prevention of STI:** PO azithromycin 1 g single dose, IM/IV ceftriaxone 500 mg single dose, PO metronidazole 2 g single dose.

vi. Consider **prophylactic treatment for those at risk of HIV transmission.** Start antiretroviral therapy [PO dolutegravir 50 mg every 24 hours + PO tenofovir 300 mg/PO emtricitabine 200 mg (Truvada) one tablet every 24 hours] as early as possible if the patient is seen within 48–72 hours of exposure. The patient needs a follow-up with an ID specialist.

vii. All patients are given follow-up appointments with the **MSW** for psycho-emotional counselling and support. Referrals to psychology or psychiatry should be made where necessary.

g. **Long-term management of sexual assault:**

i. Arrange subsequent follow-up in 6 weeks. During the visit, check the LMP and any symptoms of STI or pregnancy, ensure adequate psycho-social support and monitor side effects and adherence to post-exposure prophylactic medication if prescribed.

O&G Surgical Complications

a. The mortality rate for gynaecological surgeries is 0.2% within 30 days of admission and 0.5% within 90 days. Death rates are higher for women with malignancy.

b. *General surgical risks*:

i. Adverse reactions to drugs

ii. Infectious complications (surgical site, respiratory, urinary)

iii. Risks of transfusion of blood and blood products if required

iv. Anaesthetic risks: acute coronary syndrome, stroke, death

v. VTE

c. Complications of gynaecological surgery include haemorrhage, infection and injury to surrounding organs such as the bowel, bladder, ureters, vessels and nerves.

d. **History:** Type of surgery, indication, date of surgery, intra-operative findings, presence of any complications (intra-operative or post-operative) and post-operative recovery.
e. **Management**
   i. Inform the primary surgeon, the surgical team and the head of department (HOD).
   ii. Multidisciplinary team management, including general surgery, urology, IR or ID specialists, as indicated
   iii. Risk identification — root cause analysis
   iv. Duty of candour
   v. Debriefing the patient and family
   vi. Documentation — incident report
   vii. Audit and re-audit
   viii. Learn from the incident and adopt a no-blame culture.
   ix. Collate and disseminate learning points to all relevant stakeholders.

Possible Complications of O&G Surgery

1 Hysteroscopy Dilatation and Curettage (D&C) or Transcervical Resection of Polyp or Myoma (TCRP/TCRM)

a. Bleeding
   i. From cervix (due to trauma from tenaculum/vulsellum)
   ii. From uterus
b. Uterine perforation and resulting complications, e.g., injury to bladder/ureters/bowels
c. Infection (endometritis, pelvic abscess, intra-abdominal sepsis)
d. Asherman syndrome
e. Fluid overload with complications such as subsequent hyponatraemia, hypo-osmolality, hypothermia, pulmonary oedema, cerebral oedema or heart failure (higher risk in older patients and patients with renal or cardiac co-morbidities)

2 Evacuation of Uterus/Surgical Termination of Pregnancy

a. Retained products of conception (may cause bleeding and infection)
b. Bleeding from cervix due to trauma from tenaculum/vulsellum forceps
c. Uterine perforation

d. Infection
e. Asherman syndrome
f. Uterine arteriovenous malformation (AVM)

3 Laparoscopic Surgeries

a. Laparoscopic injuries frequently occur during the blind insertion of needles, trocars and cannula through the abdominal wall; hence, the greatest risk is from the start of the procedure until visualisation within the peritoneal cavity has been established. In addition, the risk is increased in obese or significantly underweight women and in those with previous midline abdominal incisions.
b. *Bleeding*
   i. From the secondary port site (due to injury of the inferior epigastric vessels)
   ii. Vault dehiscence (post-hysterectomy) can cause vaginal bleeding
   iii. Damage to large vessels, e.g., iliac vessels or inferior vena cava
c. *Infection*
d. *Uterine perforation* (if a uterine manipulator was used)
e. *Injury to surrounding structures* (e.g., bowels, ureters and bladder), GI or urinary fistula formation
f. *Adhesions*
g. *Port site hernia*
h. *Nerve injuries* (e.g., femoral, ilioinguinal, pudendal, obturator, lateral cutaneous, iliohypogastric and genitofemoral nerves). Risk factors include patient malpositioning, incorrect placement of self-retaining retractors, haematoma formation and direct nerve entrapment or transection.
i. *Lower limb compartment syndrome*: Lithotomy position requires hip flexion of at least 90°. Venous obstruction in the inguinal region may result, thereby lowering venous return, which allows interstitial fluid to accumulate, causing oedema and increased compartment pressure.

4 Open Abdominal Surgeries

a. Bleeding
b. Infection
c. Wound complications (infection, haematoma, dehiscence)

d. Incisional hernia
e. Adhesions
f. Intestinal obstruction
g. Injury to surrounding structures (e.g., bowel and bladder), GI or urinary fistula formation

5 Urogynaecological (UG) Procedures

a. *Vaginal hysterectomy risks*: bleeding, infections, injury to bladder and bowel, urinary retention, constipation, vaginal vault dehiscence, vault haematoma, VTE
b. *Specific UG surgical risks*:
   i. *Pelvic floor repair* (PFR): recurrence of cystocele or rectocele
   ii. *Sacrospinous fixation* (SSF): recurrent vault prolapse, prolene thread extrusion in the vagina, buttock claudication pain
   iii. *Mid-urethral sling*: infection and rejection of tape, mesh erosion or extrusion, voiding difficulty, *de novo* detrusor overactivity, failure of the procedure, dyspareunia
   iv. *Mesh implants*: erosion into urethra/bladder, extrusion out of vagina, rejection, infection and pain, temporary voiding difficulty, *de novo* detrusor overactivity or stress incontinence, recurrence of prolapse, dyspareunia

6 Oncological Procedures

a. *Cervical excisional procedures*, e.g., loop electrosurgical excisional procedure (LEEP) and cone biopsy of the cervix
   i. Bleeding
   ii. Infection
   iii. Uterine perforation — higher risk if the uterus is acutely anteverted or the patient is menopausal
   iv. Cervical stenosis
   v. Cervical incompetence — risk of second-trimester miscarriage and preterm birth in future pregnancies
   vi. Injury to surrounding structures, e.g., bowels, bladder, ureters
   vii. Recurrence of disease

b. *Lymph node dissection*
   i. Risk of lymphoedema due to lymphatic obstruction — 10 to 20% after pelvic lymph node dissection

7 Caesarean Section

- Maternal Complications

a. *Early complications* (include peri- and post-procedural conditions within 30 days after a caesarean delivery)
   i. *Fever/infection* — endometritis, respiratory tract infection or extensive atelectasis, urinary tract infection
   ii. *Wound complications* — infection, haematoma, dehiscence, scarring
   iii. *PPH* — causes include uterine atony, retained products of conception, lacerations of intra-abdominal vessels (uterine and ovarian vessels) or extra-abdominal arterial or venous vessels, coagulopathy
   iv. *Injury to surrounding structures* such as the bladder, ureters or bowels
   v. *GI complications* — ileus, intestinal obstruction, bowel perforation
   vi. *VTE*

b. *Late complications*
   i. *Adhesions* — may lead to pain or GI complications such as intestinal obstruction
   ii. *Incisional hernia*
   iii. *Caesarean scar niche* — may cause abnormal uterine bleeding, dysmenorrhoea, chronic pelvic pain, dyspareunia, subfertility
   iv. *In the subsequent pregnancy*:
      1. Higher chance of requiring a caesarean section
      2. Caesarean scar pregnancy
      3. Placenta accreta spectrum (PAS)
      4. Uterine dehiscence or rupture
      5. Unexplained stillbirth

- Fetal complications
  - Risk of injury to fetus (<1%) e.g. lacerations, fractures
  - Risk of respiratory distress, transient tachypnoea of the newborn (TTNB)

CHAPTER 31

Primary and Secondary Amenorrhoea

WHO Classification of Anovulatory Disorders

Type 1 — *hypogonadotrophic hypogonadism*
- Females with low levels of endogenous gonadotrophins and oestrogen.
- This includes hypogonadotrophic hypogonadism, hypopituitarism and hypothalamic amenorrhoea.

Type 2 — *normogonadotrophic normogonadism*
- Females with normal levels of gonadotrophins and oestrogen.
- They present with anovulation associated with a variety of menstrual disorders.

Type 3 — *hypergonadotrophic hypogonadism*
- Females with high levels of gonadotrophins and low levels of oestrogen.
- Primary ovarian insufficiency (POI).

Primary Amenorrhoea

Definition:
- Absence of menses by ≥16 years of age in the *presence* of normal secondary sexual characteristics OR
- Absence of menses by ≥13 years of age in the *absence* of secondary sexual characteristics

Evaluate for primary amenorrhoea if:
- Absence of menses 3 years after thelarche OR
- Absence of menses 5 years after thelarche if thelarche occurred before 10 years of age

Evaluation of Primary Amenorrhoea

History:

- Stage and sequence of secondary sexual characteristics, if any (thelarche, pubarche, growth spurt)
- *Family history*: Menarche, delayed puberty, early menopause, infertility, chromosomal/genetic conditions
- *Past medical/surgical history*: Cancer, chemotherapy, radiotherapy, head trauma/surgery
- Sexual activity
- Medication history
- Eating habits and exercise level
- Social history
- Psychosocial stress
- Symptoms of hyperprolactinaemia or thyroid disorders
- Any vasomotor symptoms
- History of headache, nausea, anosmia
- Abdominal symptoms, e.g., pain, bloatedness, diarrhoea, constipation
- Symptoms of hyperandrogenism — virilisation/hirsutism

Physical examination:

- Vitals, BMI
- Growth chart
- Use Tanner staging to stage pubertal development
- *Hyperandrogenism signs*: Assess hirsutism with the modified Ferriman–Gallwey score
- Thyroid examination
- Galactorrhoea
- *Abdominal examination*: Masses, haematometra
- External examination for imperforate hymen ± pelvic examination for Müllerian abnormalities
- Hypercortisolism signs, e.g., buffalo hump, striae
- *Skin examination*: Acne, acanthosis nigricans
- Visual field examination
- Palpate for gonads (if relevant)

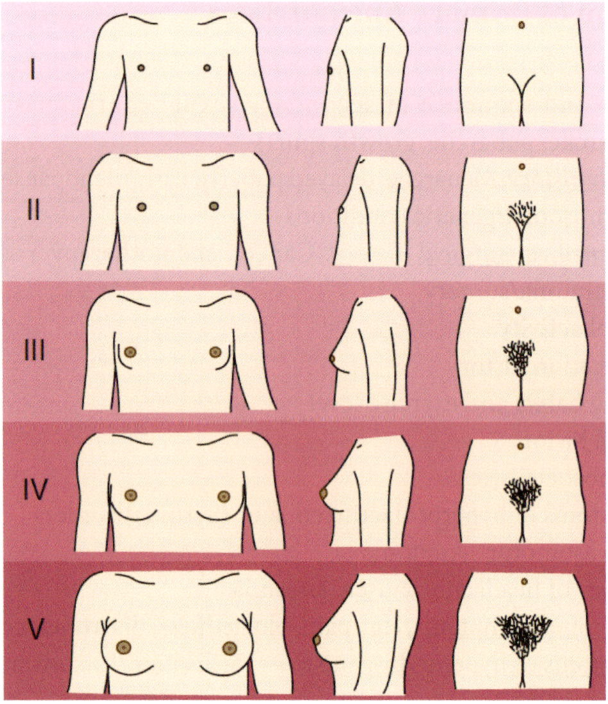

Source: Early Puberty: Adulthood Metabolic Consequences & Childhood Nutritional Determinants — scientific figure on ResearchGate. Available from: https://www.researchgate.net/figure/2-Female-Tanner-stages_fig2_258327803 [accessed 24 April, 2022].

Table 31.1 Tanner Staging

Tanner stage	Breast development	Pubic hair
I	Prepubertal — elevation of papilla only.	Prepubertal — none.
II	Breast bud forms.	Sparse hair along the labia.
III	Breast and areola enlarge. The breast tissues create a small cone.	Dark, coarser pubic hair but mainly over the central area. Sparse over the mons pubis.
IV	Breasts in a "mound" form. Projection of areola and papilla.	Pubic hair is in the triangular adult shape but smaller.
IV	Fully formed breasts.	Pubic hair is adult in shape, quantity and type. Spread to inner thighs.

Investigations:

- Urine pregnancy test (UPT) to exclude pregnancy
- Transabdominal (TA) ± transvaginal (TV) ultrasound (US) scan of the pelvis to assess the pelvic anatomy
- *Hormonal profile*
  - o FSH, LH, E2 (oestradiol)
  - o Thyroid function test (TFT)
  - o Prolactin
  - o Total testosterone
- *Others if indicated*:
  - o DHEA-S
  - o 17-Hydroxyprogesterone
  - o Karyotype
  - o Fragile X genetics
  - o Bone mineral density (BMD)
  - o Magnetic resonance imaging (MRI) scan of the pituitary gland
  - o Computer tomography (CT)/MRI scan of the brain

Causes and Management of Primary Amenorrhoea

***Goals of treatment*:**

1. Treat the underlying cause
2. Prevent complications
3. Puberty induction (if required)
4. Fertility management
5. Psychosocial aspect

Algorithm for the Evaluation of Primary Amenorrhoea

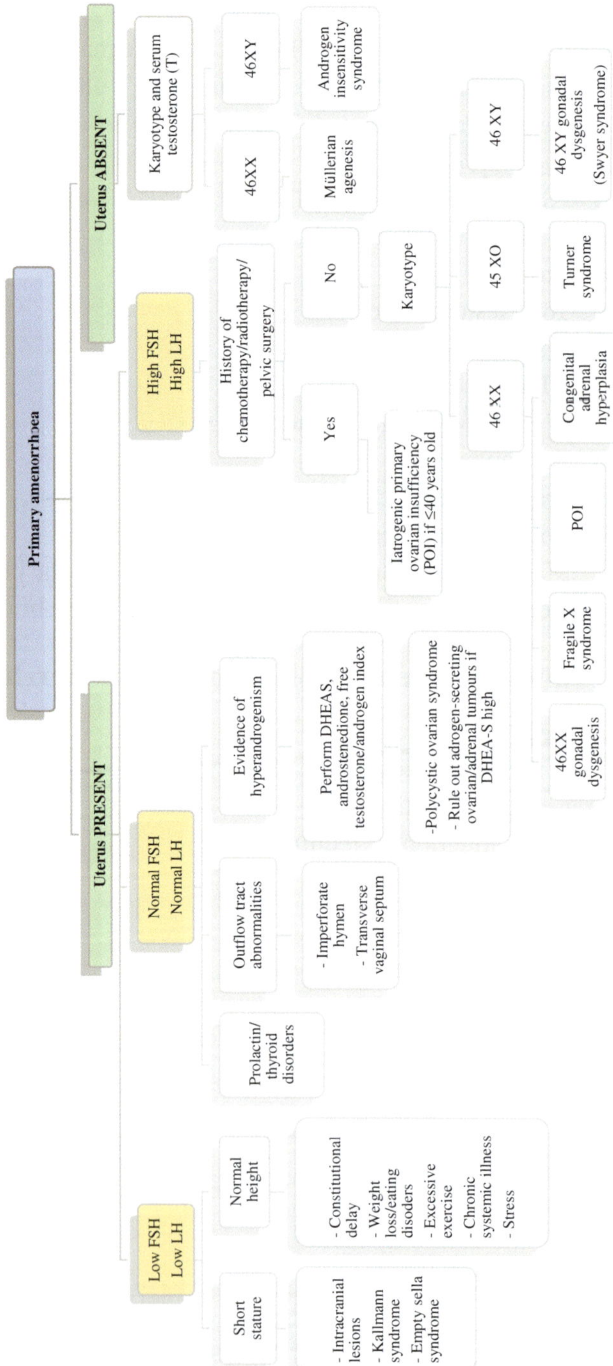

Condition	Cause	Features and Investigations	Management
Constitutional delay	Most common cause of delayed puberty.	• Height is appropriate for bone age. • All stages of development are delayed. • Family history of constitutional delay. • ***Karyotype:*** 46XX. • Female internal and external genitalia.	• Reassure. • Continue follow-up.
Hypothalamic causes			
Functional hypothalamic amenorrhoea	There is suppression of GnRH pulsatility. ***Causes:*** 1. Excessive exercise 2. Weight loss/dieting 3. Stress 4. Critical illness 5. Chronic diseases, e.g., coeliac disease, inflammatory bowel disease	• Low BMI. • May have breast development. • Low FSH, LH and E2. • ***Karyotype:*** 46XX. • Female internal and external genitalia.	• Treat the underlying cause. • Do a pituitary MRI to rule out other causes before diagnosing hypothalamic amenorrhoea. • Gain weight if low BMI. To aim for 30 kcal/kg lean body mass. • May need induction of puberty.
Hypogonadotrophic hypogonadism	There is a deficiency in the action, production or secretion of GnRH. ***Causes:*** ***Congenital*** 1. Kallmann syndrome (failure of embryonic migration of GnRH neurons from the olfactory bulb to the hypothalamus, occurs in 1 in 120,000 females) 2. Genetic syndromes, e.g., Prader–Willi. ***Acquired*** 1. Tumours 2. Radiation/surgery 3. Medical conditions, e.g., haemochromatosis 4. *Drugs*: Steroids, narcotics 5. *Infection*: Meningitis, encephalitis, tuberculosis 6. Trauma	• No breast development. • Normal pubic hair. • Low FSH, LH and E2. • ***Karyotype:*** 46XX. • Female internal and external genitalia. *Kallmann syndrome*: • Anosmia/hyposmia.	• Treat the underlying cause. • Removal of CNS tumours. • May need induction of puberty. • *Kallmann syndrome*: Needs long-term hormone replacement therapy (HRT).

(*Continued*)

(*Continued*)

Condition	Cause	Features and Investigations	Management
Pituitary causes			
Prolactinoma	Microadenoma or macroadenoma	• Galactorrhoea. • Incomplete breast development. • Normal pubic hair. • Low FSH, LH and E2. • ***Karyotype:*** 46XX. • Female internal and external genitalia.	Refer to Chapter 57: *Approach to Galactorrhoea and Hyperprolactinaemia*.
Drug-induced hyperprolactinaemia	E.g., anti-psychotics, anti-depressants	• Galactorrhoea. • Incomplete breast development. • Normal pubic hair. • Low FSH, LH and E2. • ***Karyotype:*** 46XX. • Female internal and external genitalia.	
Ovarian/genetic causes			
Primary ovarian insufficiency (POI)		• High FSH and LH and low E2. • ***Karyotype:*** 46XX. • Female internal and external genitalia.	Refer to Chapter 53: *Menopause and POI*.
Turner syndrome/ monosomy X	Occurs in 1 in 2,500 females. Lethal in >95%. Up to 25% will enter puberty spontaneously, but only 10% will progress through puberty, and only 1% will develop ovulatory cycles.	• Short, webbed neck, widely spaced nipples, cardiac defects (e.g., coarctation of the aorta), hypothyroidism, cubitus valgus. • Breast and pubic hair development usually does *not* occur. • High FSH and LH and low E2. • ***Karyotype:*** 45X0, can have mosaicism. • Mosaicism can include 45X/46XX, 45X/46XY and 45X/47XXX. • Female internal and external genitalia.	• Multidisciplinary team (MDT) care. • Healthy lifestyle and diet. • *Growth hormone therapy:* Aim to gain height. Initiate as early as possible. • <u>*Screen for complications:*</u> – Cardiac abnormalities. – Osteoporosis. – Risk of hypertension, diabetes mellitus. • Puberty induction. • Long-term HRT. • *Gonadectomy* is required if there is a Y chromosome because of the risk of malignancy. • Fertility: – Donor oocytes (need cardiac clearance for pregnancy).

(Continued)

Condition	Cause	Features and Investigations	Management
Androgen insensitivity syndrome (AIS)	A mutation of the androgen receptor on the long arm of chromosome X results in complete or partial insensitivity to androgen. It is an X-linked recessive condition. Incomplete AIS can result in ambiguous genitalia.	• Tall. • Normal breast development. • No/sparse pubic hair. • Normal/high FSH, high LH and normal E2. • Testosterone in the normal male range. • ***Karyotype:*** 46XY. • Short blind-ending vagina.	• MDT care. • Psychological counselling. • Discuss gender identity. • *Gonadectomy* because of the risk of malignancy — 5%. • Long-term HRT. • Develop a functional vagina. • Fertility. – Surrogacy with donor oocytes. – Adoption.
46 XY gonadal dysgenesis/Swyer syndrome	10–20% are due to SRY gene mutations.	• No breast development. • No pubic hair. • High FSH and LH and low E2. • ***Karyotype:*** 46XY. • Streak gonads — non-functional. • Female internal and external genitalia.	• MDT care. • Psychological counselling. • Discuss gender identity. • *Gonadectomy* because of the risk of malignancy. • Puberty induction. • Needs long-term HRT. • Fertility with donor oocytes and HRT.
46XX gonadal dysgenesis	Streak ovaries. Many mutations have been identified, such as in FSH receptors.	• No breast development. • Normal pubic hair. • High FSH and LH and low E2. • ***Karyotype:*** 46XX. • Streak gonads — non-functional. • Female internal and external genitalia.	• MDT care. • *Gonadectomy* because of the risk of malignancy. • Puberty induction. • Needs long-term HRT.
Polycystic ovarian syndrome (PCOS)		• Normal FSH, LH and E2. • ***Karyotype:*** 46XX. • Female internal and external genitalia.	Refer to Chapter 36: *Polycystic Ovarian Syndrome (PCOS)*.

(Continued)

(Continued)

Condition	Cause	Features and Investigations	Management
Outflow tract causes			
Müllerian agenesis/ Mayer–Rokitansky–Kuster–Hauser (MRKH) syndrome	There is marked underdevelopment of the Müllerian duct. Occurs in 1 in 5,000 females.	• Normal breast development. • Normal pubic hair. • Normal FSH, LH and E2. • ***Karyotype:*** 46XX. • Ovaries present. • The uterus is absent or rudimentary. • Short and blind-ending vagina. • US kidneys, ureter and bladder (KUB) and spine X-ray.	• MDT care. • Psychological support. • Creating a functional vagina. – Vaginal dilators: 95% success rate. – *Surgery:* Vecchietti procedure, McIndoe procedure, sigmoid vaginoplasty, Davydov procedure. • Need to exclude other congenital anomalies, e.g., urinary tract (absent kidney) or skeletal anomalies. • *Discuss fertility options:* – Surrogacy. – Adoption. – Uterine transplant.
Transverse vaginal septum	This could be due to failure of canalisation or fusion between the urogenital sinus and the Müllerian duct. Occurs in 1 in 30,000–80,000 women.	• Cyclical abdominal pain due to haematocolpos. • Normal breast development. • Normal pubic hair. • Normal FSH, LH and E2. • ***Karyotype:*** 46XX. • Female internal and external genitalia.	• MDT care. • Perform an MRI pelvis to assess the anomaly. • Surgical resection of the septum.
Imperforate hymen	Aetiology is unknown. Occurs in 1 in 2,000 females.	• A blue bulge at the introitus. • Haematocolpos. • Normal breast development. • Normal pubic hair. • Normal FSH, LH and E2. • ***Karyotype:*** 46XX. • Female internal and external genitalia.	• Perform a cruciate incision in the hymen. It should be done after the onset of puberty. • Drain any haematocolpos.

Secondary Amenorrhoea

Definition:

- Cessation of regular menses for ≥3 months OR
- Cessation of irregular menses for ≥6 months

Fewer than 9 menstrual cycles per year in women with oligomenorrhoea (cycle length >35 days) also warrant investigations.

Evaluation for Secondary Amenorrhoea

History:

- Menstrual history, including the last menstrual period (LMP)
- *Family history*: Early menopause, infertility, chromosomal/genetic conditions
- *Past medical history*: Pelvic inflammatory disease, cancer, chemotherapy, radiotherapy, head trauma
- *Past surgical history*: Uterine surgeries, e.g., dilatation and curettage, evacuation of the uterus
- Sexual activity
- *Past obstetric history*: Obstetric catastrophes, postpartum haemorrhage
- *Medication history*: especially hormonal treatment
- Eating habits and exercise level
- Social history
- Psychosocial stress
- Symptoms of hyperprolactinaemia or thyroid disorders
- Any vasomotor symptoms
- History of headache, nausea, anosmia
- Abdominal symptoms, e.g., pain, bloatedness, diarrhoea, constipation
- Symptoms of hyperandrogenism — virilisation/hirsutism

Physical examination:

- Vitals, BMI
- *Hyperandrogenism signs*: Assess hirsutism with the Ferriman–Gallwey score
- Thyroid examination
- Galactorrhoea
- Abdominal examination
- Speculum/vaginal examination (if the patient is sexually active)

- Hypercortisolism signs, e.g., buffalo hump, striae
- *Skin examination*: Acne, acanthosis nigricans
- Visual field examination

Investigations:

- UPT to exclude pregnancy.
- Ultrasound scan of the pelvis to assess the pelvic anatomy.
- *Hormonal profile*
  - FSH, LH and E2.
  - Thyroid function test (TFT).
  - Prolactin.
- *Others if indicated*
  - Total testosterone, DHEAS, free androgen index.
  - 17-Hydroxyprogesterone.
  - Sex-hormone binding globulin (SHBG).
  - Karyotype.
  - Fragile X genetics.
  - Bone mineral density (BMD).
  - *To investigate Asherman syndrome*: Saline infusion sonohysterography (SIS), hysterosalpingogram (HSG) or diagnostic hysteroscopy, keep-in-view adhesiolysis.
  - MRI of the pituitary gland.
- *Progestogen challenge test*
  - Give oral norethisterone/dydrogesterone 10 mg bd for 7–10 days.
  - If there is withdrawal bleeding with progestogens, this indicates the presence of endogenous oestrogen.
  - If there is *no* withdrawal bleeding with progestogen, it could be due to hypoestrogenism or outflow tract disorders, e.g., Asherman syndrome.
  - Consider performing an oestrogen/progestin withdrawal test.
    - Give oestradiol 1 mg/day for 30 days, then add progesterone from days 20–30 OR
    - Give 1 month of the combined hormonal contraceptive pill.
    - If there is still no withdrawal bleeding, it is highly suggestive of intrauterine adhesions.

Algorithm for the Evaluation of Secondary Amenorrhoea

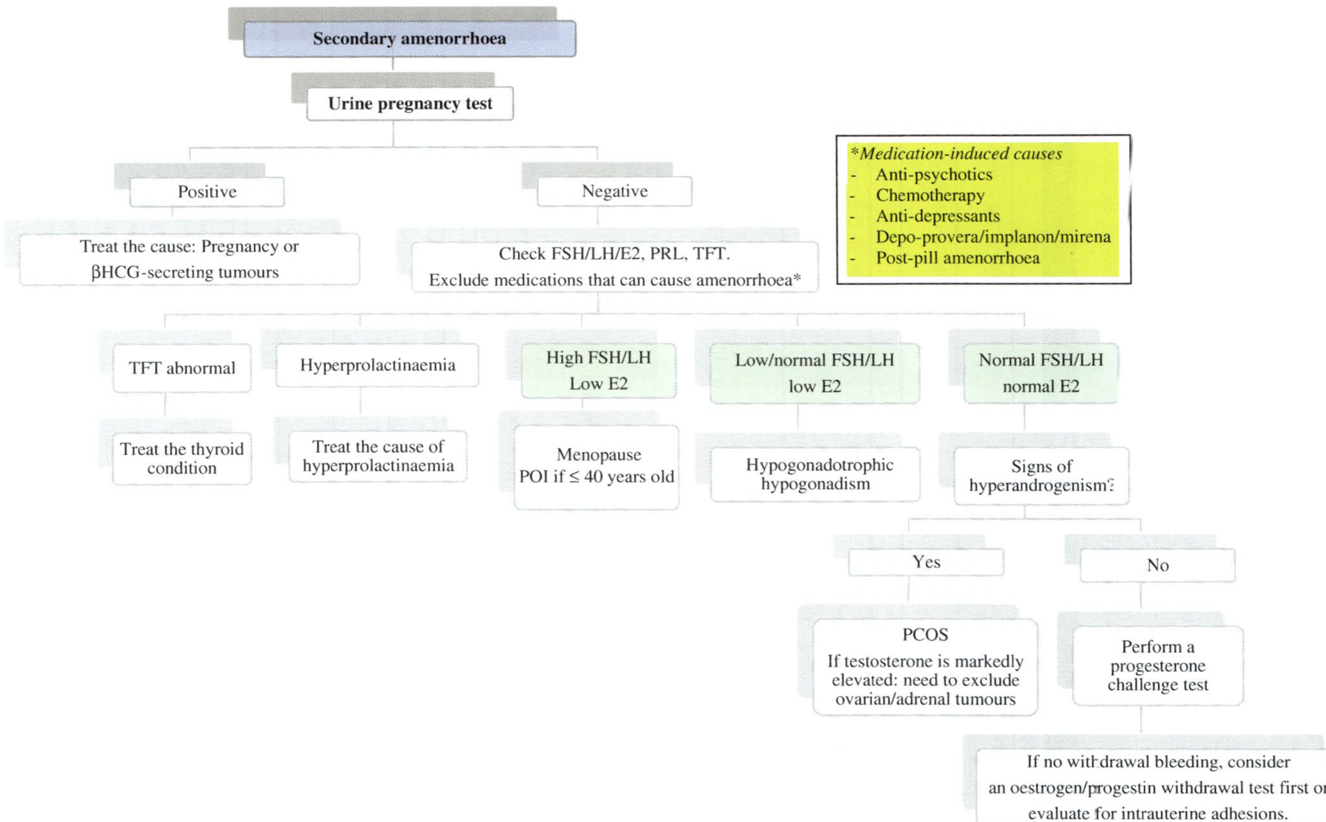

Causes and Management of Secondary Amenorrhoea

The causes of secondary amenorrhoea are like those of primary amenorrhoea.

<u>*Goals of treatment:*</u>

1. Treat the underlying cause
2. Prevent complications
3. Fertility management

Condition	Cause	Management
Hypothalamic causes		
Functional hypothalamic amenorrhoea		Refer to the above.
Hypogonadotrophic hypogonadism		Refer to the above.
Pituitary causes		
Prolactinomas		Refer to Chapter 57: *Approach to Galactorrhoea and Hyperprolactinaemia.*
Drug-induced hyperprolactinaemia		
Hypopituitarism	***Causes*** ***Congenital:*** 1. Structural abnormality of the pituitary ***Acquired:*** 1. Trauma 2. Tuberculosis 3. Thalassaemia, chronic transfusions 4. Sarcoidosis 5. Pituitary tumours/treatment 6. Sheehan syndrome	– Treat the underlying cause. – Replace the necessary hormones, e.g., HRT, hydrocortisone.
Ovarian/genetic causes		
Primary ovarian insufficiency (POI)		Refer to Chapter 53: *Menopause and Primary Ovarian Insufficiency.*
Turner syndrome/ monosomy X		Refer to the above.
Polycystic ovarian syndrome (PCOS)		Refer to Chapter 36: *Polycystic Ovarian Syndrome.*
Outflow tract disorders		
Asherman syndrome or intrauterine adhesions	*Risk factors*: – Pregnancy – Retained products of conception – Dilatation and curettage – Evacuation of uterus – Postpartum curettage – Hysteroscopic myomectomy – Uterine infection – Uterine compression sutures for postpartum haemorrhage (PPH) due to uterine atony	**Primary prevention:** – *Surgical technique*: Targeted resection rather than blind curettage. – Using gel adhesion barriers can reduce the risk of adhesions in the short term, but data on fertility is lacking. **Treatment options:** – Hysteroscopic adhesiolysis. <u>*To prevent the recurrence of adhesions:*</u> – Oestrogen therapy. – Intrauterine contraceptive device (IUCD). – Intrauterine catheter.

CHAPTER 32

Abnormal Uterine Bleeding and Adolescent Abnormal Uterine Bleeding (AUB)

The normal menstrual cycle lasts between 21 and 35 days, with menstrual flow lasting 2–8 days. Cycle variation (the difference between the shortest and longest cycle) is generally up to 7 days in women 26–41 years old and up to 9 days in women 18–25 years old and 42–45 years old.

Definition of Irregular Menstrual Cycles

1st year post menarche: irregular menses is considered normal

- >1 to <3 years post menarche: <21 or >45 days
- >3 years post menarche to perimenopause: <21 or >35 days or <8 cycles per year
- >1 year post menarche: >90 days for any 1 cycle

Definition of Abnormal Uterine Bleeding (AUB)

There was near unanimity for the International Federation of Gynaecology and Obstetrics (FIGO) to recommend discarding the term "dysfunctional uterine bleeding" and using AUB instead.

AUB is defined as any menstrual bleeding from the uterus that is abnormal either in volume (excessive duration or heavy flow), in regularity or in timing (delayed or frequent), or bleeding that is out of schedule, i.e., intermenstrual bleeding (IMB), post-coital bleeding (PCB) or post-menopausal bleeding (PMB).

Acute AUB = excessive AUB bleeding that requires immediate intervention to prevent further blood loss.

Chronic AUB = AUB that has been present for the majority of the past 6 months.

FIGO AUB classification also recommends other terminologies that replace the earlier ones.

Heavy menstrual bleeding (HMB), previously known as menorrhagia, is an excessive menstrual blood loss (MBL) leading to interference with a woman's physical, emotional, social and material quality of life, which can occur alone or in combination with other symptoms. Adverse outcomes are more significant in women with total MBL exceeding 80 ml or menses duration exceeding 7 days.

IMB = uterine bleeding that occurs between clearly defined cyclic and predictable menses

PCB = non-menstrual genital tract bleeding immediately (or shortly) after intercourse

PMB = non-menstrual genital tract bleeding after the menopause

FIGO PALM-COEIN Classification of AUB

- **PALM:** Polyp, adenomyosis, leiomyoma (further divided into submucosal fibroids, L_{SM}, and other fibroids, L_O), malignancy and hyperplasia
- **COEIN:** Coagulopathy, ovulatory dysfunction, endometrial, iatrogenic.
  Not yet classified.

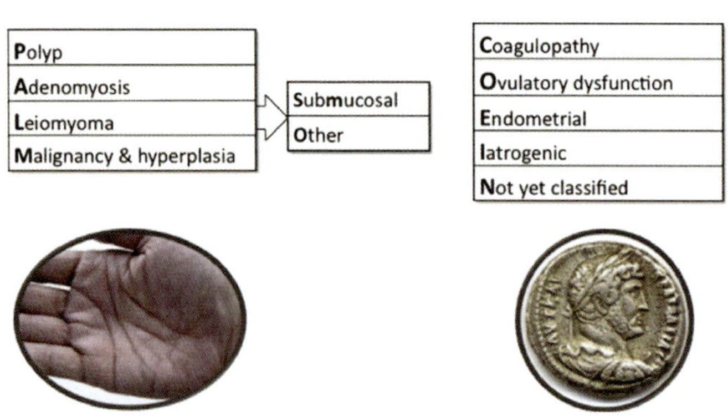

Source: Munro MG, Critchley HO, Broder MS, Fraser IS; FIGO Working Group on Menstrual Disorders. FIGO classification system (PALM-COEIN) for causes of abnormal uterine bleeding in nongravid women of reproductive age. *Int J Gynaecol Obstet.* 2011;113(1):3-13. doi:10.1016/j.ijgo.2010.11.011.

Approach to AUB

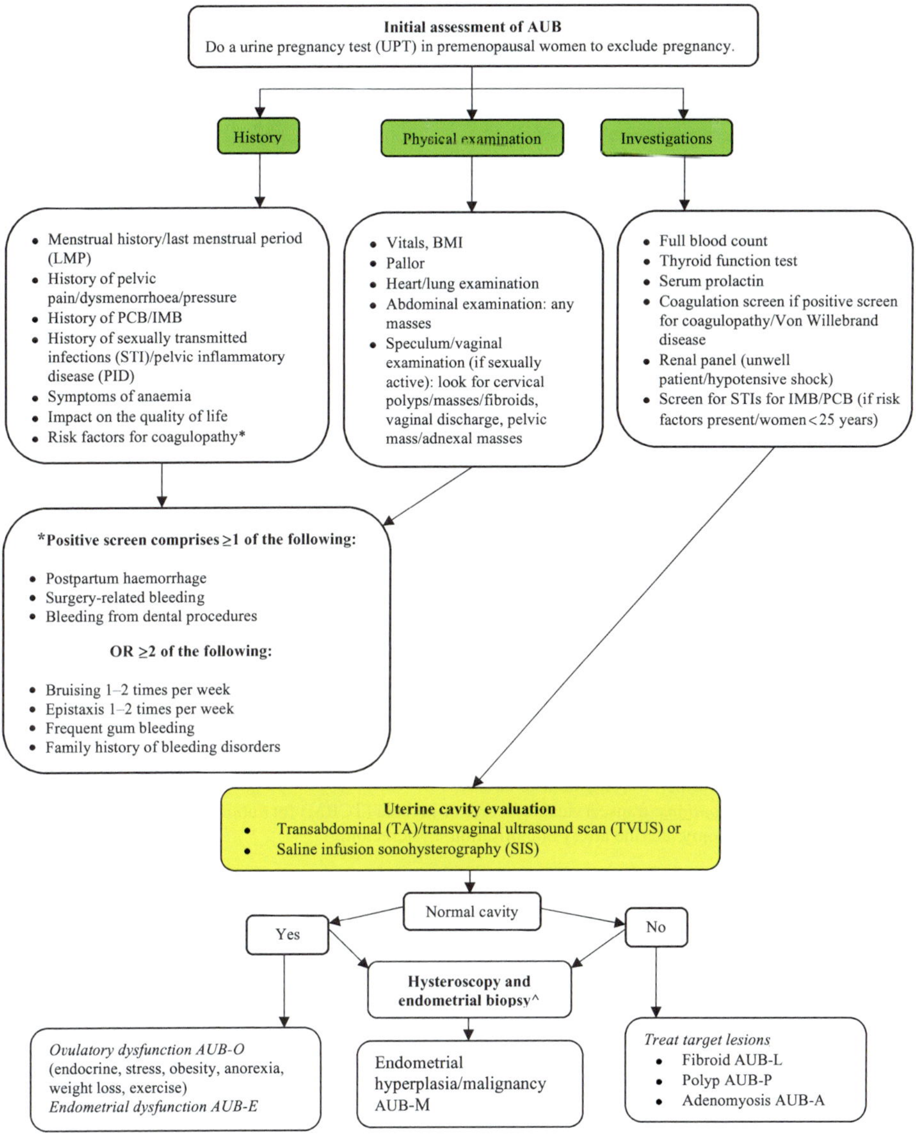

^Perform endometrial biopsy if risk factors present for endometrial hyperplasia/cancer
Age >40 years, history of anovulatory cycles/(PCOS) tamoxifen use,
AUB that has failed medical treatment, obesity/hypertension/diabetes/metabolic syndrome
Family history of breast, endometrial, ovarian, colorectal cancer

Treatment for AUB

A. If the woman has **no identified pathology, fibroids <3 cm in diameter, or suspected or diagnosed adenomyosis**

→ **Consider a levonorgestrel-releasing intrauterine system (LNG-IUS), e.g., Mirena®, as the first line treatment**

↓

If a woman with HMB declines an LNG-IUS or it is not suitable, consider

- *Non-hormonal*: Tranexamic acid/NSAIDs
- *Hormonal*: Combined hormonal contraception/cyclical oral progestogens

If treatment is unsuccessful, the woman declines pharmacological treatment OR symptoms are severe

- Perform investigations to diagnose the cause of HMB, if not yet done
- Alternative treatment choices, including:
  - Pharmacological options *not* already tried
  - *Surgical options*: Transcervical resection of myoma (TCRM) for submucosal fibroids, myomectomy, endometrial ablation, hysterectomy

Refer to Chapter 46: *Endometriosis and Adenomyosis* for more information on management of adenomyosis.

B. If the woman has **fibroids of ≥3 cm in diameter**

↓

Pharmacological:

- *Non-hormonal*: tranexamic acid/NSAIDs
- *Hormonal*: combined hormonal contraception/cyclical oral progestogens
- Ulipristal acetate – *no longer used* because of the risk of liver failure

If the above treatment is unsuccessful:

- Consider further investigations to re-assess
- *Surgical options*: transcervical resection of myoma (TCRM) for submucosal fibroids, myomectomy, uterine artery embolisation, hysterectomy

Refer to Chapter 45: *Fibroids, Fibroids in Pregnancy, Fibroid Variants and Leiomyosarcoma* for further information.

Types of Medications and Effects on Fibroid Size/ HMB/Fertility

Treatment	Effect on fibroid size	Decrease in HMB	Effect on fertility
1. First-line treatments (pharmacological)			
Tranexamic acid (TXA)	Nil	30–50%	No effect
NSAIDs (e.g., mefenamic acid)	Nil	20–40%	No effect
Combined oral contraceptive (synthetic oestrogen)	—	40%	Contraceptive
Combined oral contraceptive Qlaira® (natural oestrogen)	—	88% after six cycles	Contraceptive
Oral progestogen (high-dose)	Nil	60%	No effect
Intrauterine progestogen (LNG-IUS)	Decrease 30%	70–100%	Contraceptive
GnRH analogues (3–6 months with/without add-back hormone replacement therapy)	Decrease 30%	60–100% (causes amenorrhoea in 80–90% of women)	Contraceptive
Progestogen-only implant (Implanon®) or progestogen-only injectable (Depo-Provera)®	—	30–100% (causes amenorrhoea in 15–20%)	Contraceptive
2. Second-line treatments (minimally invasive uterus-conserving surgery)			
Hysteroscopic fibroid resection	Excision and removal of intracavitary fibroids	50–80%	Improved if submucous fibroid excised
Endometrial ablation	No effect	80%	Not suitable if fertility is desired
Transcervical resection of endometrium	Will be able to excise and remove intracavitary fibroids	80–100%	No effect
Laparoscopic myomectomy	Excise subserosal and non-deeply embedded intramural fibroids	No effect or may decrease up to 30%	May improve fertility
Uterine artery embolisation (UAE)	Decrease 30%	60–80%	Not suitable if fertility is desired
3. Third-line treatments (major surgical procedures)			
Myomectomy (Laparoscopic/ Abdominal)	Excise subserosal, intramural and intracavitary lesions	60–80%	May improve
Hysterectomy	Complete cure	Complete cure	Permanent, irreversible contraception

Goals of Treatment for HMB

- Alleviate acute bleeding. Give intramuscular progesterone 100 mg stat.
- Avoid concurrent use of tranexamic acid and oral progestogens because of the risk of venous thromboembolism (VTE)/stroke.
- Prevent future episodes of non-cyclic bleeding. Aim to give a bleed that is predictable in timing and amount.
- Decrease the risk of long-term complications, e.g., development of endometrial cancer.

A Medications Used for Management of AUB

1. **NSAIDs**, e.g., mefenamic acid 500 mg three times a day (TDS). Add antacids for gastric protection.
2. **Antifibrinolytic agents**, e.g., *tranexamic acid* (500 mg–1 g TDS) Side effect — can cause VTE.
3. **Combined oestrogen and progestogen preparation**

   Combined oral contraceptive pill (COCP) — refer to Chapter 52: *Contraception.*

   Qlaira® (oestradiol valerate/dienogest)

   Progyluton®

   Qlaira®

   - First oral therapy approved for HMB with contraceptive effects.
   - A dosing regimen of 26 + 2 (i.e., 26 days of active pills and 2 days of placebo pills), which provides good cycle control.
   - Reduces MBL by 88% after six cycles of treatment.
   - Rapid and significant reduction of MBL by 70% after two cycles.
   - Low discontinuation rate of 3% with a favourable safety profile.

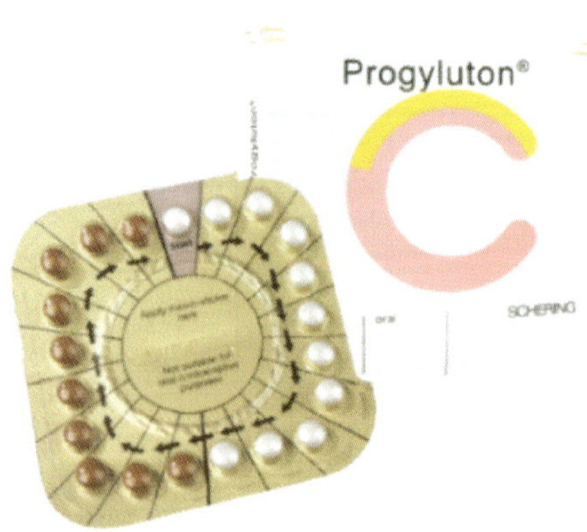

Progyluton®

- Cyclical sequential combined hormonal replacement therapy with 2 mg oestradiol valerate for the first 11 days and 2 mg oestradiol valerate with 0.5 mg norgestrel for the next 10 days
- Regulates the menstrual cycle and does *not* affect endogenous hormone production
- Does *not* interfere with ovulation
- Can be used by pre- and perimenopausal patients

4. **Cyclical progestogen (at least 10–14 days per cycle)**
   - Norethisterone 10 mg BD
   - Provera 10 mg BD
   - *Side effects:* VTE/stroke with high-dose progestogens
5. **LNG-IUS/Mirena®**
   - Releases 20 μg of LNG daily, which affects the endometrium locally
   - Lasts 5 years
   - Low local hormonal effect in the endometrium, which provides shorter and lighter menses and reduces dysmenorrhoea
   - 20% amenorrhoea after 1 year, 75–95% decrease in objectively measured MBL
   - 20% intermittent per-vaginal spotting in the first 6 months
   - Lower risk of pelvic inflammatory disease and ectopic pregnancy compared with copper IUCD

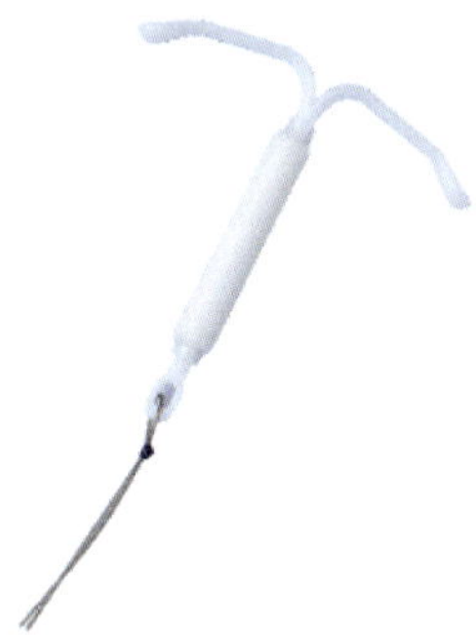

Mirena® intrauterine contraceptive device

Compliance rate	Mirena/LNG-IUS	No treatment
At 1 year	68% continued with Mirena	32% had a hysterectomy
At 5 years	58% continued with Mirena	42% had a hysterectomy
Cost–benefit analysis	Mirena was 40% cheaper than a hysterectomy	

6. **Gonadotrophin-releasing hormone analogue (GnRHa)**
   - Continuous treatment with GnRHa causes down regulation of the pituitary gland and a subsequent decrease in gonadotrophins and ovarian steroids.

- o Causes amenorrhoea (90%).
- o *Side effects* are related to hypoestrogenism and post-menopausal in type (hot flushes, insomnia, mood swings).
- o *Not recommended* for more than 6 months of continuous usage because of the risk of osteoporosis unless with hormonal add-back therapy.
- o Subcutaneous injection Zoladex (goserelin) 3.6 mg monthly, subcutaneous injection Lucrin (leuprorelin) 3.75 mg monthly/ 11.25 mg 3-monthly, intra-muscular injection decapeptyl (triptorelin) 3.75 mg 4–6 weekly.

7. **Depo-Provera®**
   - o Intramuscular Depo-Provera 150 mg every 3 months
   - o Induce endometrial atrophy and amenorrhoea
   - o Irregular bleeding in the first 3 months
   - o *Side-effects:* abdominal bloating, breast tenderness, weight gain, depression, water retention

B Surgical Management of AUB

- **As a last resort for patients with failed medical treatment**

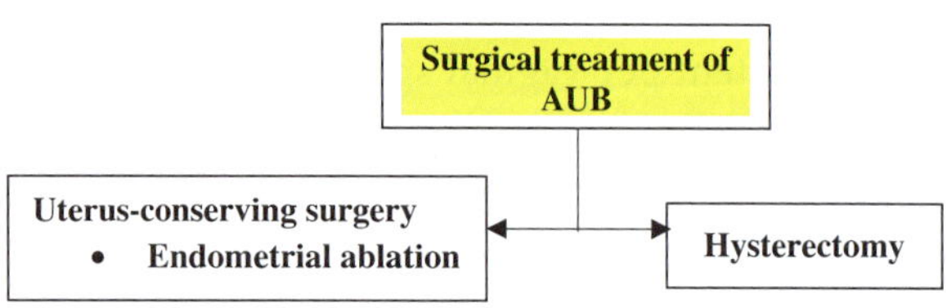

Endometrial Ablation

Prerequisite:

- o HMB is severe enough to affect the quality of life.
- o The woman has completed her family.
- o Uterine cavity length <10 cm
- o With benign endometrial biopsy histology
- o *Indications*:
  - ▪ Failed medical treatment (including Mirena LNG-IUS) for HMB
  - ▪ Wish to conserve the uterus
- o **Techniques of Endometrial Ablation**
  1) **First-generation techniques**

- Done under direct hysteroscopic vision using electrocautery (either monopolar or bipolar).
  - ➢ Transcervical resection of the endometrium [TCRE]
  - ➢ Ablation (rollerball) of the endometrium

<u>*Disadvantages:*</u>

- Experienced operator required.
- The risk of complications depends on the operator's experience (e.g., uterine perforation) and the method (e.g., dilutional hyponatraemia or fluid overload if using glycine uterine distension).

2) **Second-generation techniques**
   - ➢ Thermal balloon endometrial ablation (Thermachoice®)
   - ➢ Impedance bipolar radiofrequency ablation (NovaSure®)
   - ➢ Hydrothermablation (HydroThermAblator®)
   - ➢ Endometrial cryotherapy (Her Option®)

   <u>*Advantages:*</u>
   - Performed as a day surgery procedure
   - Some can be under local anaesthetic (with or without sedation)

Hysterectomy

<u>*Indications:*</u>

- o Other treatment options have failed or are inappropriate
- o Non-compliance with medical treatment
- o Women have completed their families
- o Desire for amenorrhoea
- o Concurrent gynaecological pathology

<u>Adolescent AUB</u>

Incidence and facts

1. The mean age of menarche is about 11–12 years old in Singapore.
2. 50% of girls have irregular periods in the first year after menarche. This is normal and is part of the transition to puberty. This is due to the *immature* hypothalamic–pituitary–ovarian (HPO) axis.
3. 50% of cycles are anovulatory.
4. 20% of girls have irregular periods up to 5 years of menarche.

Presenting complaints

1. Unexpected and often heavy vaginal bleeding
2. Irregular periods >45-day cycle or frequent menses occurring <21-day cycle
3. Prolonged vaginal bleeding

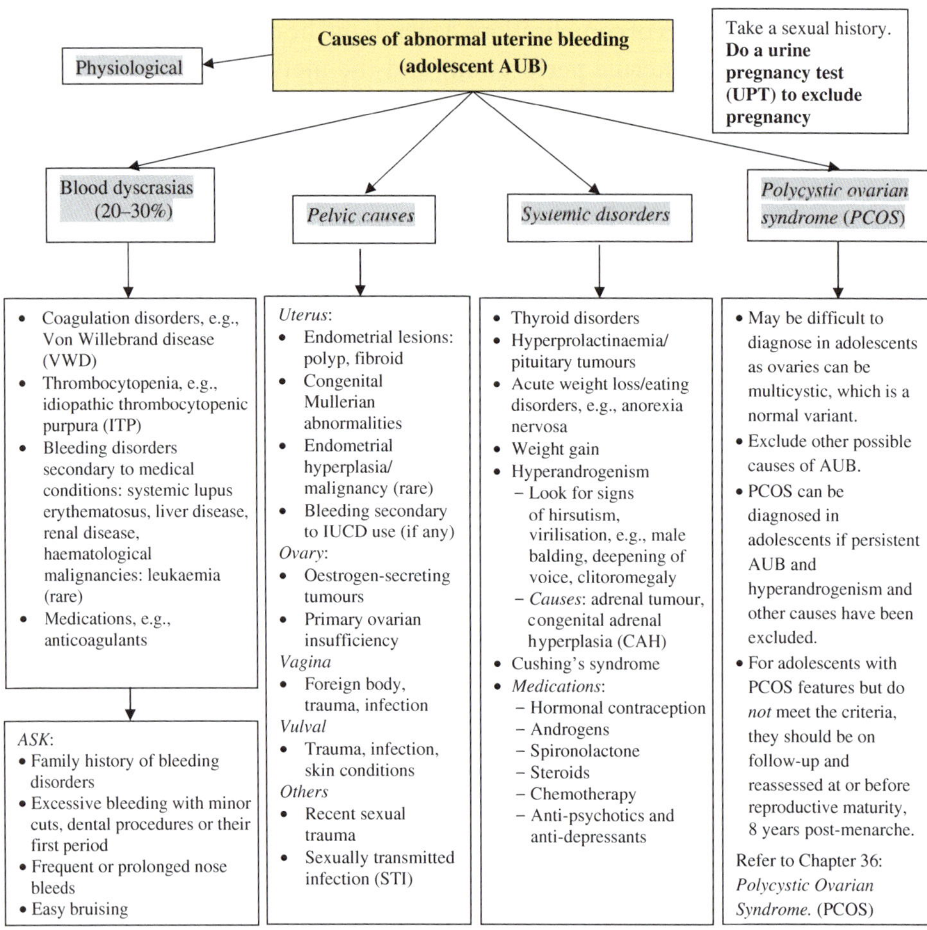

Investigations of Adolescent AUB

1. *Full blood count (FBC)* — useful to reveal anaemia and thrombocytopenia.
2. *Prothrombin time (PT), activated partial thromboplastin time (aPTT) and bleeding time* — if blood dyscrasias and clotting disorders are suspected.
3. *Urine pregnancy test (UPT)* — must be performed even in patients who deny sexual activity, especially if there is a high index of suspicion.
4. *Cervical swabs* — to exclude chlamydia and gonorrhoea infection, especially if sexual activity is confirmed.
5. *Thyroid function test (TFT)* — to screen for thyroid disease.
6. *Serum prolactin* — to screen for hyperprolactinaemia.
7. *Dehydroepiandrosterone sulfate (DHEAS), free testosterone* — to evaluate for PCOS.
8. *VWF Ag (Von Willebrand factor antigen), VWF RCo (Von Willebrand factor ristocetin cofactor) and factor VIII* — if Von Willebrand disease is suspected.
9. *Pelvic ultrasound scan:* to exclude pelvic pathology such as fibroids and polycystic ovaries.
10. *Hysteroscopy and uterine curettage* — **rarely indicated** in adolescents. This procedure is usually reserved for women with significant and prolonged haemorrhage unresponsive to medical therapy.

Management of Adolescent AUB

1. *Oral haematinics* if haemoglobin is <11 g/dl.
2. *Oral tranexamic acid* (TxA) (250 mg TDS) to treat heavy bleeding days.
3. If bleeding persists, *add oral NSAIDs* (e.g., mefenamic acid 250 mg TDS).

4. Consider *hormonal treatment,* e.g.,
   A. *Combined oral contraceptive pill* (COCP).
   B. *Cyclical progesterone*: e.g., dydrogesterone or medroxyprogesterone acetate 10 mg BD for 21 days. Alternatively, progestogens can be given for 12–14 days each month.

CHAPTER 33

Premenstrual Syndrome (PMS) and Premenstrual Dysphoric Disorder (PMDD)

Type	Definition
Physiological premenstrual disorder	Cyclical symptoms during the luteal phase, which are relieved by menstruation. There is no impact on the quality of life.
Premenstrual syndrome (PMS)	Cyclical symptoms that cause significant impairment to the woman during the luteal phase of the menstrual cycle, and symptoms are completely relieved by the end of menstruation.
Premenstrual dysphoric disorder (PMDD)	A severe form of PMS. _Diagnosis is by the DSM-V criteria_ • A: Affects most menstrual cycles; at least five symptoms must be present in the final week before the onset of menses, which start to improve within a few days after the onset of menstruation and become minimal or absent in the week post menstruation. • B: ≥1 of the following symptoms must be present: 1) Marked affective lability (e.g., mood swings, feeling suddenly sad or tearful or increased sensitivity to rejection). 2) Marked irritability or anger or increased interpersonal conflicts. 3) Markedly depressed mood, feelings of hopelessness or self-deprecating thoughts. 4) Marked anxiety, tension or feelings of being keyed up or on edge. • C: ≥1 of the following symptoms must additionally be present to reach a total of five symptoms when combined with symptoms from criterion B above. 1) Decreased interest in usual activities. 2) Subjective difficulty in concentration. 3) Lethargy, easy fatigability or marked lack of energy. 4) Marked change in appetite; overeating or specific food cravings. 5) Hypersomnia or insomnia. 6) A sense of being overwhelmed or out of control. 7) Physical symptoms such as breast tenderness or swelling; joint or muscle pain, a sensation of "bloating" or weight gain. • D: The symptoms are associated with clinically significant distress or interference with work, school, usual social activities or relationships with others. • E: Rule out other psychiatric disorders. • F: Criterion A should be confirmed by prospective daily ratings during at least two symptomatic cycles. • G: The symptoms are *not* attributable to the physiological effects of a substance/drug or another medical condition.

Epidemiology

Clinically significant PMS affects 3–8% of women with regular menstrual cycles. True PMDD only affects 2% of this group.

Risk Factors

Genetics: Preliminary evidence that PMDD is associated with genetic variation in the oestrogen receptor alpha gene, *ESR1*.

Environmental: Smoking, history of traumatic events or anxiety disorders.

Clinical Features of PMS

Symptoms occur in the luteal phase, worsen as menstruation approaches and resolve within the first few days of menstruation *without* recurrence until at least day 12 of the cycle.

***Physical*:** Breast swelling and discomfort, abdominal bloating, oedema, weight gain, headaches, extreme fatigue, deterioration in asthma, migraine or epilepsy.

***Psychological*:** Aggression, anger, irritability, tearfulness, low mood, anxiety, altered eating habits, disturbed sleep, relationship difficulties, occupational problems.

*Important to exclude organic causes before diagnosing PMS/PMDD.

***Differentials include*:** Premenstrual exacerbation of an underlying medical/psychiatric disorder (e.g., hyper/hypothyroidism, depression, migraine), progestogen-induced premenstrual disorder and perimenopause period.

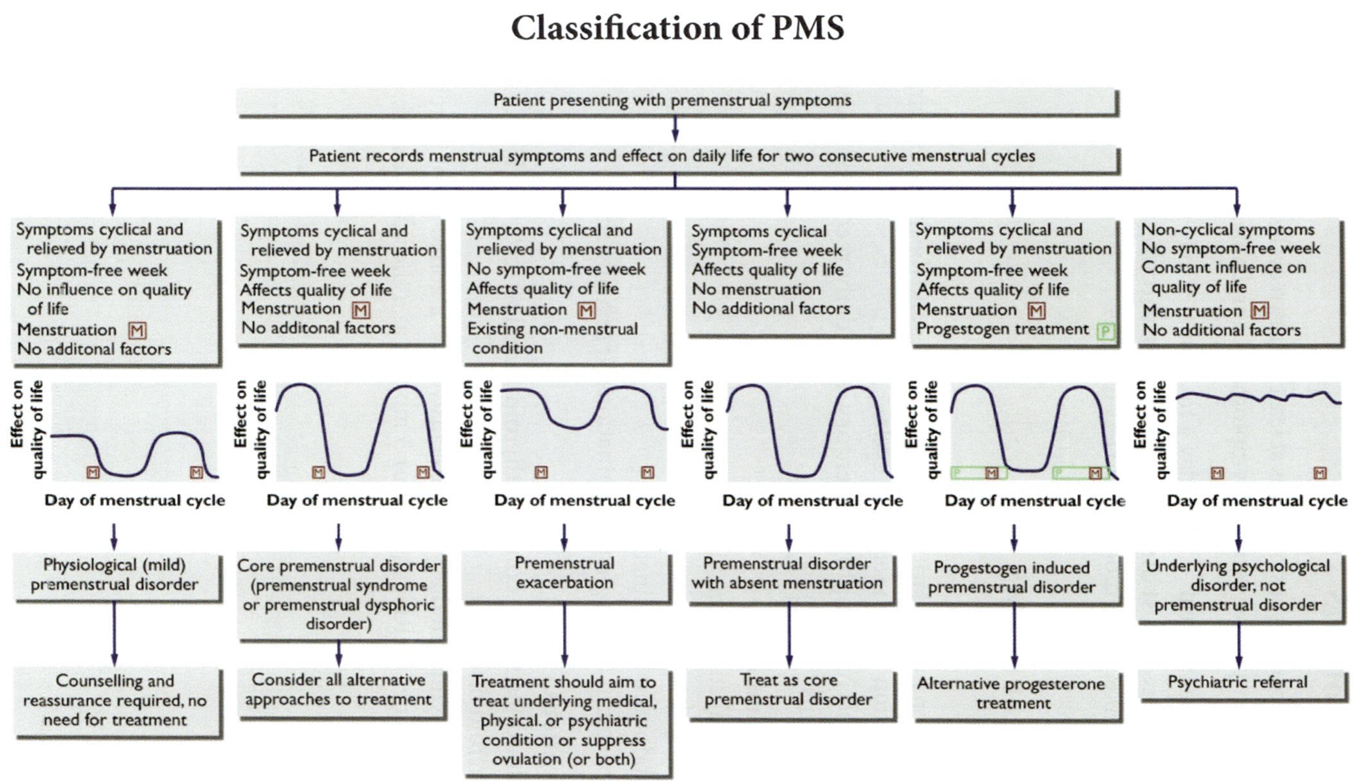

Source: Management of Premenstrual Syndrome: Green-top Guideline No. 48. *BJOG*. 2017;124(3):e73–e105. doi:10.1111/1471-0528.14260.

Diagnosis of PMS

Prospective recording of symptoms at least over two cycles, using a symptom diary as a retrospective recall of symptoms, is unreliable.

Symptom-free interval — from day 4 to 12 of a 28-day menstrual cycle.

If symptoms **persist throughout** the menstrual cycle, then an alternative diagnosis is likely, e.g., mood or anxiety disorder.

Assessment of PMS

History:

- Focus on the regularity of menstrual cycles and the timing of symptoms in relation to the menstrual cycle.
- Prospective symptom inventory, e.g., daily record of severity of problems (DRSP).

Physical examination:

- General condition, vital signs.
- Any goitre.
- Abdominal examination.
- Speculum and vaginal examinations (if sexually active).

Investigations:

- Blood tests, e.g., consider thyroid function tests (TFT) to exclude thyroid disorders.
- If the symptom diary is inconclusive, use a gonadotrophin-releasing hormone (GnRH) agonist for 3 months as a therapeutic trial.

DAILY RECORD OF SEVERITY OF PROBLEMS

Please print and use as many sheets as you need for at least two FULL months of ratings.

Name or Initials ____________________

Month/Year ____________________

Each evening note the degree to which you experienced each of the problems listed below. Put an "x" in the box which corresponds to the severity: 1 - not at all, 2 - minimal, 3 - mild, 4 - moderate, 5 - severe, 6 - extreme.

Enter day (Monday-"M", Thursday-"R", etc) >																																
Note spotting by entering "S" >																																
Note menses by entering "M" >																																
Begin rating on correct calendar day >		1	2	3	4	5	6	7	8	9	10	11	12	13	14	15	16	17	18	19	20	21	22	23	24	25	26	27	28	29	30	31
1 Felt depressed, sad, "down" or "blue", or felt hopeless; or felt worthless or guilty	6																															
	5																															
	4																															
	3																															
	2																															
	1																															
2 Felt anxious, tense, "keyed up" or "on edge"	6																															
	5																															
	4																															
	3																															
	2																															
	1																															
3 Had mood swings (i.e. suddenly feeling sad or tearful) or was sensitive to rejection or feelings were easily hurt	6																															
	5																															
	4																															
	3																															
	2																															
	1																															
4 Felt angry or irritable	6																															
	5																															
	4																															
	3																															
	2																															
	1																															
5 Had less interest in usual activities (work, school, friends, hobbies)	6																															
	5																															
	4																															
	3																															
	2																															
	1																															
6 Had difficulty concentrating	6																															
	5																															
	4																															
	3																															
	2																															
	1																															
7 Felt lethargic, tired or fatigued; or had lack of energy	6																															
	5																															
	4																															
	3																															
	2																															
	1																															
8 Had increased appetite or overate; or had cravings for specific foods	6																															
	5																															
	4																															
	3																															
	2																															
	1																															
9 Slept more, took naps, found it hard to get up when intended; or had trouble getting to sleep or staying asleep	6																															
	5																															
	4																															
	3																															
	2																															
	1																															
10 Felt overwhelmed or unable to cope; or felt out of control	6																															
	5																															
	4																															
	3																															
	2																															
	1																															
11 Had breast tenderness, breast swelling, bloated sensation, weight gain, headache, joint or muscle pain, or other physical symptoms	6																															
	5																															
	4																															
	3																															
	2																															
	1																															
At work, school, home or in daily routine, at least one of the problems noted above caused reduction of productivity or inefficiency	6																															
	5																															
	4																															
	3																															
	2																															
	1																															
At least one of the problems noted above caused avoidance of or less participation in hobbies or social activities	6																															
	5																															
	4																															
	3																															
	2																															
	1																															
At least one of the problems noted above interfered with relationships with others	6																															
	5																															
	4																															
	3																															
	2																															
	1																															

Source: Management of Premenstrual Syndrome: Green-top Guideline No. 48, *BJOG*, 2017;124(3):e73–e105. doi:10.1111/1471-0528.14260.

Management of PMS

RCOG Algorithm for Treatment of PMS

First line	Exercise, cognitive behavioural therapy, vitamin B6. Combined new-generation contraceptive pill (cyclical or continuous regimen). Continuous or luteal phase (days 15–28) *low-dose* selective serotonin reuptake inhibitors (SSRIs), e.g., citalopram/escitalopram 10 mg.
Second line	Oestradiol patches (100 mg) + micronised progesterone (oral/vaginal 100 or 200 mg on days 17–28) OR levonorgestrel-releasing intrauterine system (LNG-IUS 52 mg). Continuous or luteal phase *higher dose* SSRIs, e.g., citalopram/escitalopram 20–40 mg.
Third line	GnRH analogues + add-back hormone replacement therapy (continuous combined oestrogen + progesterone, e.g., 50–100 mg oestradiol patches or 2–4 doses of oestradiol gel combined with micronised progesterone 100 mg/day or tibolone 2.5 mg daily.
Fourth line	Surgical treatment ± HRT (Hormone Replacement Therapy).

For complicated cases, multidisciplinary team care (MDT) is recommended — general practitioner (GP), gynaecologist, psychiatrist, psychologist and dietician.

If a primary psychiatric disorder is diagnosed, refer to a psychiatrist.

- **Lifestyle measures:** Exercise and weight loss.
- **Cognitive behavioural therapy (CBT).**
- ***Hormonal treatment:***
  1. **Combined oral contraceptive pill (COCP)** — first line treatment.
     - Use drospirenone-containing COCP (e.g., Yaz/Yasmin).
     - A continuous regimen is preferred.
     - Also preferred for women requiring contraception.

2. **Percutaneous oestradiol with cyclical progestogens** on days 10–12 of the menstrual cycle.
   - Progestogens can be oral/vaginal/LNG-IUS.
   - Using oral or vaginal micronised progesterone 100/200 mg daily is less likely to have PMS-like symptoms.
3. **GnRH agonist** — highly effective for severe PMS.
   - *Side effects* related to hypoestrogenism such as hot flushes and osteoporosis.
   - The efficacy of GnRHa is maintained when used with add-back therapy (low-dose oestrogen and progesterone or tibolone). However, it is essential that oestrogen and progesterone are given continuously and *not* cyclically, as the latter may reproduce PMS symptoms.
   - Annual bone mineral density (BMD) scan while on long-term treatment. Stop treatment if BMD decreases significantly.
4. **Danazol** 200 mg twice a day — used to treat breast symptoms during the luteal phase of the cycle.
   - However, there are *virilising side effects* for the woman, e.g., hirsutism and deepening of the voice, which may *not* be reversible.
   - Contraception should be used while on danazol because of potential virilising effects on female fetuses, e.g., clitoromegaly, labial fusion and urogenital sinus abnormalities.

- ***Non-hormonal treatment***
  1. ***SSRIs — Selective serotonin reuptake inhibitors***
     - SSRIs can be given to women who do *not* need contraception.
     - If SSRI is taken during the luteal phase, it can be stopped at any time. However, if taken continuously, gradual withdrawal of SSRIs is needed to prevent withdrawal symptoms.
     - Luteal phase therapy has the benefits of being more cost-effective and having fewer side effects. However, a higher dose of SSRI may be needed in some women to treat physical symptoms adequately.
     - *Side effects of SSRIs:* Nausea, fatigue, insomnia, somnolence and sexual dysfunction.

  - *Examples of SSRIs:* Fluoxetine 20–60 mg/day, sertraline 50–150 mg/day, paroxetine 20–30 mg/day, citalopram 20–30 mg/day.
  - PMS symptoms will abate during pregnancy: SSRIs should be discontinued before and during pregnancy. Most studies indicate that SSRIs are *not* major teratogens. However, some small studies show an increased risk of cardiac defects and postpartum haemorrhage (PPH) with paroxetine.

2. ***Diuretics***, e.g., spironolactone.
   - Physical symptoms, e.g., weight gain, mood changes.

- ***Complementary therapies***
  - Some benefits shown with chasteberry, evening primrose oil, vitamin B6, calcium and vitamin D.
  - The only herbal supplement that has been reported to be effective in small placebo-controlled trials is *Vitex agnus-castus.*
- ***Surgery***
  - Surgery, i.e., total hysterectomy ± bilateral salpingo-oophorectomy (TH±BSO), may be considered for women who have failed medical treatment or need long-term GnRHa or if any underlying gynaecological pathology is present.
  - Use GnRHa before surgery as a therapeutic trial and ensure that hormone replacement therapy (HRT) is tolerated.

CHAPTER 34

Dysmenorrhoea

Causes (see Table 34.1)

1. ***Primary*** — absence of pelvic pathology, usually peri-menarche.
2. ***Secondary*** — pelvic pathology is present.
   a. Endometriosis — most common cause
   b. Adenomyosis
   c. Fibroids, endometrial polyps
   d. Ovarian cysts
   e. Pelvic inflammatory disease (PID)/Sexually Transmitted Infections (STIs)
   f. Intrauterine or pelvic adhesions
   g. Congenital obstructive Müllerian anomalies — non-communicating accessory uterine cavity with functioning endometrium
   h. Cervical stenosis
   i. Pelvic congestion syndrome
   j. Haematometra/pyometra
   k. Use of copper intrauterine contraceptive device (IUCD)

***Factors to consider in the management of dysmenorrhoea*:**

1) Impact of condition(s) on the patient's quality of life
2) Need for contraception
3) Desire for fertility
4) Contraindications to hormonal therapy or NSAIDs
5) Patient's preference and co-morbidities

Table 34.1 Features of Primary and Secondary Dysmenorrhoea

	Primary dysmenorrhoea	Secondary dysmenorrhoea
Pathophysiology	No pelvic pathology.	Presence of pelvic pathology.
Incidence	Up to 50%.	20–90% (variable).
History		
Age	16–25 years old (improves with older age).	30–45 years old (worsens with older age).
Onset	Within 6–12 months of menarche.	After menarche.
Duration	8–72 hours during menses.	Dependent on the underlying pathology.
Risk factors	Early menarche (<12 years old). Low BMI. Family history.	Dependent on the underlying pathology.
Symptoms	Crampy/dull pain in the lower quadrants of the abdomen. Occurs at the onset or a few days before the onset of menses and lasts for 1–3 days. *Associated with* nausea/vomiting, fatigue, backache, dizziness and diarrhoea. No other gynaecological, renal or gastrointestinal (GIT) symptoms.	Onset after ovulatory cycles become established. Crampy, intermittently intense menstrual pain or continuous dull aching pain in the lower abdomen. *Associated with* nausea, fatigue, diarrhoea and headache. *Co-existing gynaecological symptoms*: Heavy menstrual bleeding (HMB), dyspareunia, vaginal discharge, intermenstrual bleeding (IMB), post-coital bleeding (PCB), chronic pelvic pain (CPP). Possible bowel/urinary symptoms.
Response to NSAIDs or combined oral contraceptive pills (COCPs)	YES — if *not* improving after 3–6 months of treatment, investigate for secondary causes and treatment non-compliance.	YES, but it may require further treatment. If *not* responding to treatment, exclude other GI, urologic, musculoskeletal and psychosocial causes of pain → consider referral to other specialities.
Clinical exam	Normal pelvis.	Fixed retroverted uterus, thickened uterosacral ligaments, endometriotic nodules on a vaginal examination, enlarged tender uterus and adnexal masses. Cervical excitation or abnormal vaginal discharge may be seen.
Investigations	Normal ultrasound scan of the pelvis.	Ultrasound of the pelvis shows gynaecological pathology, e.g., adenomyosis, fibroids, ovarian cysts, hydrosalpinx. Genital swab cultures for PID/STI.
Prognosis	Good.	Dependent on aetiology.

Management of Dysmenorrhoea

Assess
- Severity of pain
- Menstrual flow
- Relief with painkillers

Investigate if clinically indicated

Ultrasound pelvis ± serum CA125

Primary dysmenorrhoea
Normal ultrasound scan
Normal CA125 ≤35 U/ml

Normal uterus

Secondary dysmenorrhoea
Pelvic pathology on ultrasound scan ±
Raised CA125 >35 U/ml

Adenomyosis (enlarged uterus)

Endometriosis

Cyclical NSAIDs (e.g., mefenamic acid 500 mg TDS during dysmenorrhoea)
- COCP

No response after 3–6 months

Refer to OB-GYN for further evaluation, keep-in-view diagnostic laparoscopy (for secondary dysmenorrhoea).

Refer to Chapter 46: *Endometriosis and Adenomyosis* for further management.

Refer to OB-GYN for further evaluation.

1. Cyclical NSAIDs
2. Visanne® (1 tablet daily)
   - 2 mg dienogest (progestin)
   - Effectively reduces painful symptoms of endometriosis
   - Efficacy in pain reduction comparable to gonadotrophin-releasing hormone agonists (GnRHa)
   - Inhibits gonadotrophin secretion, which, when given continuously, leads to a hypo-oestrogenic state and initial decidualisation of endometrial tissue, followed by atrophy of endometriotic lesions
   - Inhibits proliferation of endometrium-like tissue directly
   - Can start on any day of menstrual cycle and must be *continuous* regardless of vaginal bleeding/spotting
3. COCP
4. Progestogens – oral/Mirena®/Depo-Provera
5. GnRHa
6. Surgery (diagnostic/therapeutic laparoscopy)

Refer to Chapter 46: *Endometriosis and Adenomyosis* for further management.

CHAPTER 35

Chronic Pelvic Pain (CPP)

Definition of Chronic Pelvic Pain (CPP)

- Intermittent or constant pain in the woman's lower abdomen or pelvis for at least 6 months, not occurring exclusively with menstruation, intercourse or pregnancy (RCOG).
- It occurs in 1 in 6 women.

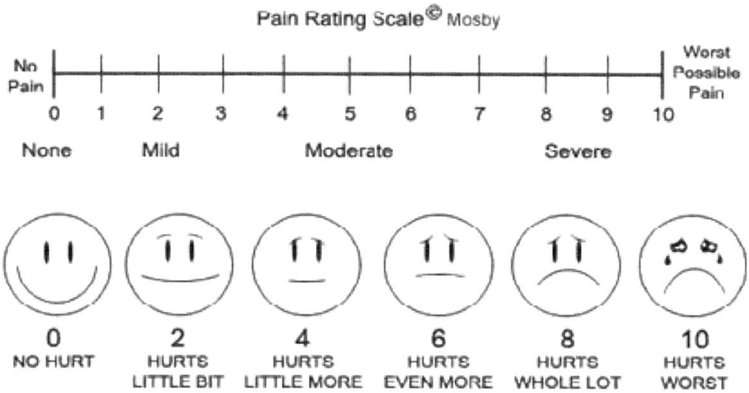

Pain score chart

History

- *Abdominal pain*: site of pain, onset, character, radiates to which area, associated symptoms, duration of pain, exacerbating or relieving factors, the severity of pain
- *Menstrual history*: last menstrual period (LMP), menstrual flow, intermenstrual bleeding (IMB), postcoital bleeding (PCB)
- Dysmenorrhoea, dyspareunia, dyschezia, per-vaginal (PV) discharge

- History of pelvic inflammatory disease (PID)/sexually transmitted infections (STIs)
- Dysuria, nocturia, incomplete voiding
- Change in bowel habits
- Headache
- Past medical/surgical history, especially abdominal surgeries
- Family history of malignancy
- Previous medications or investigations
- *Social history*: occupation, the impact on her quality of life, mood, sexual intercourse and relationships
- History of sexual abuse

Risk Factors

- PID/STI
- Sexual abuse
- Anxiety or depression
- Drug or alcohol abuse

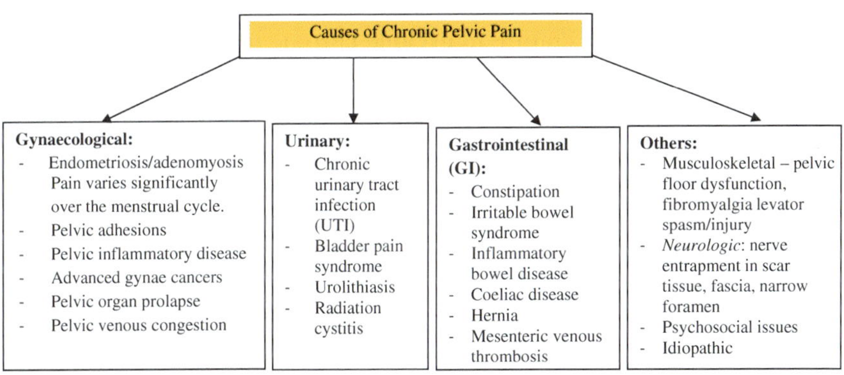

Physical Examination

- Vitals, BMI
- *Abdominal examination*: any distension, tenderness, signs of acute abdomen, masses, surgical scars
- *Speculum examination*: gynaecological pathology, e.g., endometriotic nodules, presence of pelvic organ prolapse, vaginal discharge

- <u>*Vaginal examination*</u>: bulky uterus/mobility of uterus/retroverted uterus, presence of adnexal masses/tenderness, cervical excitation, tender/thickened uterosacral ligaments, pouch of Douglas tenderness
- ±Digital rectal examination
- Tender trigger points in the abdomen/pelvic floor
- Tender symphysis pubis/sacroiliac joints → suggests a musculoskeletal origin

Investigations for CPP

- Tailor according to clinical signs and symptoms
- *Daily pain diary for two to three menstrual cycles*: identify provoking factors or temporal association
- Transabdominal (TA)/transvaginal (TV) ultrasound (US) scan of the pelvis to exclude pelvic pathology, e.g., endometriotic cyst, adenomyosis
- Screen for pelvic infection (refer to Chapter 50: *Pelvic Inflammatory Disease*) — offer to sexually active women, especially the high-risk group (age < 25 years old)
- Urine FEME and culture to exclude chronic urinary tract infection (UTI)
- Consider a computer tomography (CT) scan of the abdomen/pelvis or magnetic resonance imaging (MRI) scan of the pelvis, if indicated
- Laparoscopy (diagnostic/therapeutic) to exclude pelvic endometriosis, and adhesions — if other treatment options have failed

Management of CPP

- Treat the underlying cause

Refer to OB-GYN if

- Evidence of pelvic pathology, e.g., endometriosis or adenomyosis
- Failed first-line medical treatment
- Chronic pelvic pain related to the menstrual cycle

Multidisciplinary team care: Refer to other specialties if suspicious of non-gynaecological pathology, e.g., surgeons, urologist, gastroenterologist, neurologist, psychiatrist, pain specialist

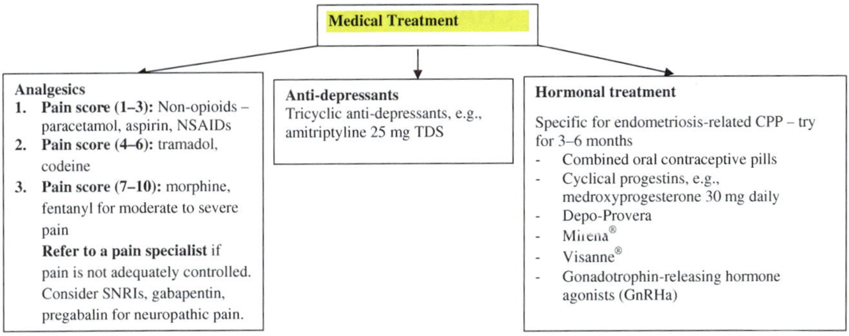

NSAIDs, *non-steroidal anti-inflammatory drugs;* **SNRIs**, *serotonin and norepinephrine reuptake inhibitors*

- Offer therapeutic trial with hormonal treatment for 3–6 months before performing a diagnostic laparoscopy
- Laparoscopic versus laparotomy approach — depends on the aetiology, presence of pelvic masses and their sizes, surgeon's expertise

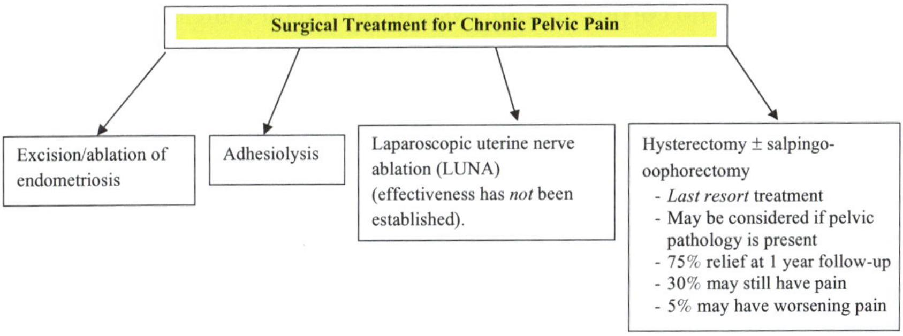

Other Treatments Options for CPP

- Pelvic floor therapy, cognitive behavioural therapy (CBT), sex therapy — if dyspareunia is present
- Acupuncture
- Transcutaneous electrical nerve stimulation (TENS)
  - It helps to reduce pain and dyspareunia if administered intravaginally.

CHAPTER 36

Polycystic Ovarian Syndrome (PCOS)

Definition Based on the Rotterdam Criteria

1. **Polycystic ovarian morphology (PCOM) (ideally by TV ultrasound scan)**
   - Previously, the definition in the Rotterdam Criteria was ≥12 follicles 2–9 mm throughout the entire ovary and/or ovarian volume ≥10 ml in at least one ovary

   Now defined as
   - ≥20 follicles in at least one ovary or increased ovarian volume ≥10 ml or follicle number per section ≥10 in at least one ovary — to ensure no corpus luteum, cysts or dominant follicles are included in the ovarian volume calculations (ESHRE PCOS guideline 2023)
2. **Oligo- or anovulation**
3. **Clinical and/or biochemical signs of hyperandrogenism**
   Clinical: hirsutism, acne or male balding pattern
   Biochemical: high serum androgen concentration

Fulfilment of **two of the three** criteria above is diagnostic of polycystic ovarian syndrome (PCOS). Other causes have to be excluded, e.g. adrenal tumours, Cushing's syndrome, 17-OH progesterone deficiency.

In women <8 years post-menarche, do not use the ultrasound criteria to diagnose PCOS as there is a high incidence of multi-follicular ovaries at this age.

Some studies propose screening for PCOS using serum anti-Mullerian hormone (AMH):

AMH level of 24.5 pmol/L or 3.44 ng/L is diagnostic of PCOS.

Advantage of AMH: It is not dependent on the menstrual cycle.

Disadvantage of AMH: There are no standardised assays or established cut-off levels based on age and ethnicity. AMH should not be used as a single test to diagnose PCOS. AMH peaks between 20–25 years old, is lower in those with higher BMI, may vary across menstrual cycle and may be suppressed by current/recent COCP use.

Epidemiology — Occurs in 5–10% of women

High-risk patients include:

- Women with anovulatory infertility
- Obesity or insulin resistance
- Type I or II diabetes mellitus (DM)
- First-degree relatives with PCOS

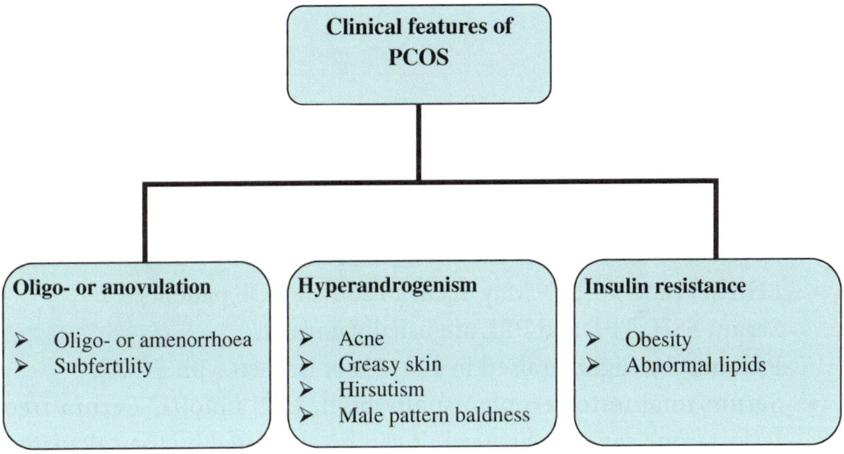

Assessment of PCOS

History

Menstrual history: Usually **oligomenorrhoea or secondary amenorrhoea**

Obstetric history: Possible subfertility, recurrent miscarriages, gestational diabetes

Past medical history: Possible DM, hyperlipidaemia or cardiovascular disease

Others: Complains of daytime fatigue, hypersomnolence, weight gain, hirsutism, acne or male pattern balding

Family history: PCOS/DM/metabolic syndrome

Physical Examination

Blood pressure (BP)/body mass index (BMI) — obesity is common
Acanthosis nigricans
Acne
Hirsutism — assess using the modified Ferriman–Gallwey score (a score of 4-6 should be used to detect hirsutism, may vary based on ethnicity)

Investigations

- ***Hormonal blood tests*** *— follicle-stimulating hormone (FSH), luteinising hormone (LH), prolactin (PRL), oestradiol (E2), testosterone, thyroid function test (TFT) done on days 2–3 of the menstrual cycle or at presentation in women with amenorrhoea.*
- Reversal of the FSH/LH ratio is no longer needed to diagnose PCOS.
- LH:FSH ratio >3:1 → May occur in some PCOS patients.
  Serum FSH, TFT and PRL are usually normal.
  PRL may be slightly raised in 10–15% of women with PCOS.
- Serum total testosterone: usually high, ≥2.5 nmol/L. Serum free testosterone can also be used. It can be estimated by the calculated free androgen index.
- If serum testosterone is ≥5 nmol/L or there is clinical evidence of hyperandrogenism: To do *serum 17-hydroxyprogesterone* to rule out non-classical congenital adrenal hyperplasia (CAH).
- Androgen-secreting tumours of the ovaries should also be excluded with an ultrasound scan of the pelvis.
- Raised serum-free testosterone and low sex-hormone-binding globulin (SHBG) levels — if there is clinical suspicion of Cushing's syndrome, this should be further investigated.

- **OGTT** if obese (BMI ≥30), age ≥40 years or has a strong family history of DM.
- ***Ultrasound scan of pelvis* (*required for PCOS diagnosis*)**
  Typical ultrasound scan features of polycystic ovaries
- Lipid profile at diagnosis.

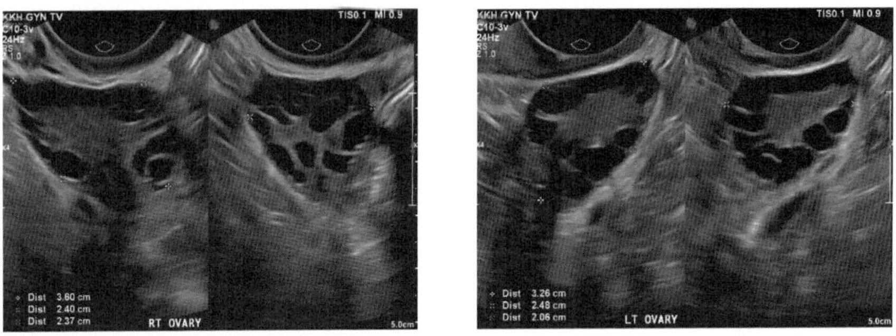

The appearance of polycystic ovaries containing ≥20 follicles arranged at the periphery of a dense stroma core.

Implications of PCOS

1. Anovulation: results in anovulatory cycles, which is a risk factor for endometrial hyperplasia/malignancy.
2. Subfertility due to anovulation.
3. Hyperandrogenism: can affect cosmesis.
4. Cardiovascular health: increased risk of DM, hypertension, hyperlipidaemia, metabolic syndrome, obesity, obstructive sleep apnoea (OSA).
5. Depression and mood: They can affect a woman's quality of life and relationships. They may increase the risk of eating disorders.

Management of PCOS

Goals of management:

1. Treat menstrual irregularity → Prevent endometrial hyperplasia/ malignancy

2. Suppress hyperandrogenism
3. Facilitate ovulation in women keen on fertility
4. Reduce hyperinsulinaemia and optimise general health
5. Screen for mood disorders

Management options

Treatment should be individualised based on the severity of symptoms and the woman's desire for fertility.

Conservative

Lifestyle modifications and screening of cardiovascular risk factors

- Regular BP check, lipid panel, OGTT
- Stop smoking
- Weight loss through diet and exercise

Weight loss of 5–10% has been reported to result in the spontaneous resumption of ovulation, improvement in fertility and impact on metabolic status.

Refer to dietician/weight management clinics/bariatric surgeon as indicated.

Consider metformin in PCOS women with BMI ≥ 25 kg/m^2 to improve anthropometric and metabolic outcomes.

Medical

a. *Menstrual regulation*
   i. Using combined oral contraceptive pills (COCPs): Diane-35 if concurrent treatment for hirsutism and acne is required, but there is a higher risk of venous thromboembolism (VTE).
   BMI ≥35 is a contraindication for COCP use.
   ii. Cyclical or 3-monthly progestogens to induce withdrawal bleeding to reduce the risk of endometrial hyperplasia and cancer.
   iii. Mirena® intrauterine contraceptive device (IUCD) in women with heavy menstrual bleeding/endometrial hyperplasia/fertility-sparing management of endometrial cancer.

b. *Subfertility*

First-line ovulation induction (OI) agent: letrozole or clomiphene citrate

- Letrozole is preferred to clomiphene.

Comparison of Letrozole and Clomiphene Citrate for Ovulation Induction

	Letrozole (first line for PCOS)	Clomiphene citrate
Mode of action	Aromatase inhibitor	Selective oestrogen receptor modulator (SERM)
Starting dose	2.5 mg every morning (OM) on days 2–6 × 5/7 Stepwise increment by 2.5 mg to a maximum of 7.5 mg OM × 5/7	50 mg OM on days 2–6 × 5/7 Stepwise increment by 50 mg to a maximum of 150 mg OM × 5/7
	To do a urine pregnancy test on day 1 of menses	
Ovulation rate	60%	50%
Live birth rate	25%	20%
Side effects	Fatigue, dizziness	Hot flushes, mood symptoms, blurring of vision
Pros	Monofollicular development Less vasomotor and mood symptoms	Reduced hirsutism and hyperandrogenism
Cons	Greater drop in antral follicular count (AFC) and AMH Lower E2 in the mid-luteal phase → thinner ET	Higher risk of multiple pregnancies (rate 3–8%) and ovarian hyperstimulation syndrome (OHSS) (rate 1%) More side effects

Metformin:

Usually for type 2 DM/impaired glucose tolerance/obesity. May be used alone if the woman has no other infertility factors beside anovulatory disorders but is less effective than the other ovulation agents. Efficacy is similar to that of laparoscopic ovarian drilling for inducing ovulation.

Dose: metformin 500 mg twice a day (BD)/three times a day (TDS)

Mechanism of action:
Reduces insulin resistance → aids in weight loss
Reduces ovarian androgen production and serum-free testosterone levels
Restores ovulation
Side effects: mainly gastrointestinal — diarrhoea, nausea, vomiting, indigestion, flatulence, abdominal discomfort

Second-line OI agent: gonadotrophins
Indicated in women who have failed oral OI agents. It can be used alone or as part of the superovulation and intrauterine insemination (SO-IUI) protocol.

c. *Insulin resistance*
   Metformin: no evidence that it confers a long-term benefit. Can use in women with impaired glucose tolerance.
d. *Hirsutism/androgen-related alopecia*
   Cosmesis: laser/intense pulsed light (IPL) treatment, mechanical hair removal
   Anti-androgens, e.g., spironolactone or finasteride: consider if failed 6 months of COCP/cosmetic treatment.
   Topical eflornithine cream
   COCP
e. *Weight loss* — metformin and other weight loss agents, e.g., orlistat or liraglutide injections
f. *Medical co-morbidities* — refer to respective specialists

Surgical

- *Bariatric surgery*
  Indications: BMI ≥40 or in women with BMI 35.0–39.9 with at least one co-morbid condition, e.g., DM, hypertension, hyperlipidaemia, OSA, gastroesophageal reflux disease, non-alcoholic fatty liver disease
- *Endometrial evaluation*
  Have a high index of suspicion for endometrial hyperplasia/cancer
  Indication: abnormal uterine bleeding (AUB), thickened endometrium or risk factors for endometrial cancer

- **<u>Other fertility treatments</u>**

  Laparoscopic ovarian drilling (2nd line treatment)

  The exact mechanism of action is unknown.

  Indication: Clomid-resistant patients, women with high LH or normal BMI, concomitant gynaecological pathology requiring laparoscopic surgery.

  Using monopolar diathermy, cauterise the ovary at four points per ovary for 4 seconds at 40 watts.

Advantages and Disadvantages of Laparoscopic Ovarian Drilling

Advantages	Disadvantages
– Once-off, minimally invasive surgery – Normalises endocrinological and ultrasound abnormalities – Ovulation is restored for many years – Pregnancy, live-birth rates similar to those of gonadotrophin OI – No increase in multiple pregnancies or OHSS rates – May improve acne and hirsutism	– Involves surgical/anaesthetic risks – Post-operative adhesions – Reduces ovarian reserve – Normalises elevated AMH and AFC

Superovulation and Intrauterine Insemination (SO-IUI) — refer to a reproductive medicine specialist
Risk of OHSS, 30% risk of multiple pregnancies

***In vitro* fertilisation (IVF)** — refer to a reproductive medicine specialist
5–10% risk of OHSS

<u>*Strategies to reduce the risk of OHSS:*</u>

- o Gonadotrophin-releasing hormone (GnRH) antagonist cycle
- o Lower gonadotrophin dose
- o Careful monitoring during ovarian stimulation to adjust the dose
- o Agonist trigger
- o May need to defer embryo transfer (ET) and freeze embryos if the woman has severe or critical OHSS

Commonly Used Medications for the Treatment of PCOS

Drug	Example	Active ingredient	Mechanism	Efficacy for			Indications	Contraindications
				Hirsutism	Menstrual irregularity	Insulin lowering		
COCP	Diane 35 Yasmin	Ethinyl oestradiol 35 μg + cyproterone acetate 2 mg Ethinyl oestradiol 30 μg + drospirenone 3 mg	Suppress ovarian function	+	+	Nil	Menstrual irregularity, hirsutism	Contraindicated in patients with venous thrombosis, uncontrolled hypertension BMI ≥35 Refer to Chapter 52: *Contraception* for the full list of contraindications.
Progestin	Provera Duphaston	Medroxy-progesterone acetate Dydrogesterone	Suppress gonadotrophin		+	Nil	Menstrual irregularity	Less efficacious than COCP
GnRH agonists (GnRHa)	Lucrin Depot	Leuprolide acetate depot	Suppress gonadotrophin	+	+	Nil	Alternative to COCP	Contraindicated in patients with osteoporosis
Anti-androgens	Spironolactone Cyproterone acetate Finasteride	Spironolactone Cyproterone acetate Finasteride	Competitive inhibitor of androgen receptor binding Competitive 5α-reductase inhibitor	+	+/−	Nil	Severe hirsutism	Use only with effective contraception because of adverse effects on the fetus. Spironolactone-contraindicated in kidney or liver failure.
Biguanide	Metformin	Metformin	Reduces hepatic glucose production	Nil	+/−	+	Obesity and insulin resistance; type II DM	Efficacy poor without weight control

CHAPTER 37

Approach to Gynaecological Cancers

In Singapore, cancer ranks as the top cause of death. Gynaecological cancers such as cancers of the uterus, ovary and cervix were ranked 4th, 6th and 10th, respectively, among the 10 most frequent cancers in Singaporean females from 2017–2021 (source: Singapore Cancer Registry Annual Report 2021).

Special Considerations

Fertility-Sparing Treatment in Gynaecological Oncology

As women delay childbearing, there is an increase in cancer diagnoses in women still desiring fertility. Fertility-sparing treatment is becoming more important, but it should not compromise survival. Currently, fertility-sparing treatments are possible for specific early-stage endometrial cancer, cervical cancer, ovarian cancer and, rarely, vulval cancer. Set criteria have to be fulfilled before we can offer the fertility-sparing option to patients. Management of these patients requires a multidisciplinary approach involving a gynaecological oncologist, fertility specialist, medical social worker and maternal–fetal medicine specialist during pregnancy. There will be a case discussion at the tumour board meeting to review the investigations and results and discuss suitability for fertility-sparing management.

KKH has a multidisciplinary weekly onco-fertility clinic run by a gynaecological oncologist and a fertility specialist.

The team will have a detailed discussion with the patient regarding the following aspects:

- Gold standard treatment for the type of cancer.
- The fertility-sparing treatment.
- Need for compliance with follow-up.

- Oncological risks, e.g., risk of progression to a higher stage/more aggressive disease, affecting her prognosis and lifespan.
- Impact of treatment on fertility.
  - *Chemotherapy*, especially involving alkylating agents, such as cyclophosphamide, is cytotoxic. Hence, it can decrease ovarian reserve, causing primary ovarian insufficiency and early menopause. The extent of damage depends on the type of chemotherapy, the dose, the duration and the patient's age.
  - *Pelvic and abdominal radiotherapy* can cause direct damage to the ovaries, resulting in decreased follicles and primary ovarian insufficiency. It can also affect uterine function, causing myometrial damage, fibrosis and atrophy of the uterus. As a result, there is an increase in pregnancy-related complications, e.g., miscarriages, preterm labour, intrauterine growth restriction, low birth weight and placental abnormalities.
- Baseline evaluation of fertility prospects.
- The fertility-preservation options available for the patient.
- High likelihood of requiring assisted reproductive techniques (ARTs).
- Consider inheritance of genetic predisposition to malignancy.
- Completion surgery once the woman has completed the family.

Fertility-Preservation Options for Women With Gynaecological Malignancy

Various fertility-preservation methods have *not* been shown to increase the risk of the offspring having cancer unless there is a genetic predisposition to cancer.

1. ***Embryo cryopreservation***
   - This is the most established method of fertility preservation.
   - It requires 10–14 days of oocyte preservation before oocyte pick-up.
   - In Singapore, the patient has to be married before this can be offered.
   - The success rate depends on the patient's age. The older the woman, the higher the number of frozen embryos to increase the chance of a live birth, but the oocyte yield is lower per cycle.

2. ***Oocyte cryopreservation***
   - It has a fairly good success rate, with approximately four to five oocytes needed to get one live birth. In subfertile patients, approximately 10 to 15 oocytes are generally needed to get one live birth. This depends on the patient's age, ovarian reserve and presence of subfertility factors. The success rate is higher in younger women.
   - All future pregnancies with preserved oocytes require *in vitro* fertilisation (IVF). There is no increase in aneuploidies or fetal abnormalities as compared to "fresh" oocytes.
   - This option is *contraindicated* in *prepubescent girls* as stimulation is difficult on immature ovaries and transvaginal scans cannot be performed for follicular tracking or oocyte retrieval procedures.

3. ***Ovarian tissue cryopreservation***
   - Limited data are available compared to oocyte cryopreservation.
   - It has the following benefits:
     - o Eliminates the need for oocyte stimulation and avoids the risks involved.
     - o May resume ovarian function.
     - o Potential chance of spontaneous pregnancies if the ovary is reimplanted into the pelvic cavity.
   - However, two surgeries are required: One for removal of the ovary or ovarian cortex stripping, and another for reimplantation after cancer remission. Ovarian function can take time to return, up to 18 weeks post-surgery. There is also the theoretical risk of replanting the original malignancy, e.g., ovarian cancer or occult metastatic tumour cells of the primary malignancy. Therefore, it is recommended to have a histological examination of the frozen-thawed ovarian tissues for malignancy before reimplantation.

4. ***Gonadotrophin-releasing hormone (GnRH) agonist***
   - There are *conflicting results* regarding the use of GnRH agonists for fertility preservation.
   - The aim is to reduce chemotherapy-induced ovarian damage.

- The issue is that dormant primordial follicles do *not* express GnRH receptors, gonadotrophins, follicle-stimulating hormone (FSH) or luteinising hormone (LH) receptors. Hence, using GnRH agonists does *not* protect against the loss of ovarian reserve.

5. ***Ovarian transposition***
   - The evidence of efficacy is *poor*. The risk of ovarian failure is approximately 25% to 50%.
   - Transposition following the division of the ovarian ligament is the preferred method, with the ovaries repositioned to at least 3 cm above the upper border of the radiation field.
   - Complications include radiation scatter risk, remigration of the ovaries, ovarian torsion, ovarian cysts, adhesions and metastatic ovarian deposits in advanced tumours.

Cancer in Pregnancy

Some women develop cancer while pregnant, and the incidence is 1 in 1,000 pregnancies. The most common cancers during pregnancy are cervical, breast and melanoma. The patient should be cared for and counselled by a multidisciplinary team, including a gynaecological oncologist, maternal–fetal medicine specialist, neonatologist, anaesthetist, medical social worker or psychiatrist. Management decisions are based on a few factors, including the gestational age at diagnosis, the stage of disease, the mother's autonomy regarding treatment options and future childbearing desire. The benefits of treatment to the mother should be weighed against the risks of treatment in pregnancy.

Genetic Predisposition Syndromes in Gynaecological Oncology

Generally, about 20% of ovarian and 5% of endometrial cancers are hereditary. The most common genetic predisposition syndromes are hereditary breast and ovarian cancer (HBOC) and Lynch syndrome (also known as hereditary nonpolyposis colorectal cancer, HNPCC). In addition, other syndromes, e.g., Peutz–Jeghers syndrome (PJS) and Cowden syndrome, may be associated with gynaecological cancers (Table 37.1).

Table 37.1 Genetic Syndromes Associated With Gynaecological Cancers

Syndrome	Genetics/inheritance	Associated cancer and lifetime risks	Screening strategies	Risk-reducing strategies
Hereditary Breast and Ovarian Cancer (HBOC) – Carrier frequency 1:500, 1:40 in Ashkenazi Jews	Autosomal dominant (AD) inheritance *Involves tumour suppressor genes*: BRCA 1 gene on chromosome 17 BRCA 2 gene on chromosome 13	• ***Breast Cancer:*** – BRCA 1: 60–80% (usually triple negative). – BRCA 2: 60–80% (usually ER/PR positive, HER2 negative). • ***Ovarian cancer:*** Usually high-grade serous/endometrioid, primary fallopian tube/peritoneal cancer. Increased sensitivity to platinum-based chemotherapy. Can use poly (ADP-ribose) polymerase (PARP) inhibitors. – BRCA 1: 40%. – BRCA 2: 20%. • ***Other cancers:*** – BRCA 2: Pancreatic cancer (3%), prostate, melanoma.	• ***Breast:*** – Clinical breast examination every 6–12 months from age 25 or 10 years before the youngest age of diagnosis in the family (whichever is earlier). – Annual magnetic resonance imaging (MRI) scan of the breast from age 25. – Annual mammogram (MMG) from age 30 or ultrasound (US) scan of the breasts if MMG is unavailable. • ***Ovary:*** – No data show that screening reduces mortality. – Consider 6 monthly US pelvis + CA125 from age 30 or 5–10 years before the youngest age of diagnosis in the family (whichever is earlier).	• *Breast*: – Bilateral risk-reducing mastectomy at 35–40 years old for BRCA 1 carriers, 40–45 for BRCA 2 carriers: Reduces risk by 90%. – Tamoxifen as primary prevention (weak evidence). – If the patient has unilateral breast cancer, contralateral mastectomy reduces the risk. • *Ovary*: – Risk-reducing bilateral salpingo-oophorectomy (RRBSO) at age 35–40 for BRCA 1 carriers, age 40–45 for BRCA 2 carriers: Reduces risk by 80–90% for ovarian/fallopian tube/peritoneal cancer, reduces mortality, but there is still a residual 1–6% risk of primary peritoneal cancer. ➢ Perform intraperitoneal survey, send off peritoneal washings. – Combined oral contraceptive pill (COCP) use: 20% reduction in risk for every 5 years of use.

(*Continued*)

Table 37.1 (*Continued*)

Syndrome	Genetics/inheritance	Associated cancer and lifetime risks	Screening strategies	Risk-reducing strategies
Lynch syndrome or Hereditary Non-polyposis Colorectal Cancer (HNPCC) *Amsterdam II criteria* – Three or more relatives with any Lynch-syndrome-associated cancer (colorectal cancer, cancer of the endometrium, small bowel, ureter or renal pelvis). – One should be a first-degree relative of the other two. – Two or more successive generations should be affected. – One or more should be diagnosed before 50 years old. – Familial adenomatous polyposis should be excluded in the colorectal cancer case(s), if any. – Tumours verified by pathological examination.	AD inheritance *Involves DNA mismatch repair genes* (MLH1, MSH2, MSH6, PMS2) or deletions in the epithelial cell adhesion molecule gene (EPCAM)	*Risk of any cancer: 81%.* • ***Colorectal cancer (20–60%):*** *Usually right-sided colon cancer, can have synchronous and metachronous cancer.* • ***Endometrial cancer (20–57%):*** *Endometrioid/clear cell adenocarcinoma.* • ***Ovarian cancer (10–17%):*** *Often early stage, moderately differentiated, higher risk of synchronous endometrial cancer.* • ***Others:*** *breast cancer (13%, can be 55% for the PMS2 variant, but poor-quality data), stomach, duodenum, pancreas, bladder, ureter/kidney, brain.* • *The prevalence of Lynch syndrome in endometrial cancer is 3% and in ovarian cancer is 1–2%.*	• *Endometrium*: – 1–2 yearly endometrial sampling at age 30–35 or 5–10 years before the earliest age of diagnosis in the family → benefit for survival is uncertain. • *Ovary*: – Annual pelvic examination, US scan of the pelvis ± CA125 6–12 monthly at age 30–35 or 5–10 years before the earliest age of diagnosis in the family → unclear effectiveness. • *Colon*: – Colonoscopy 1–2 yearly at age 20–25 or 2–5 years before the earliest age of diagnosis in the family.	Starting aspirin from age 18 reduces the risk of all cancers. The optimal dose is unknown. • *Endometrium*: – Risk-reducing total hysterectomy and bilateral salpingo-oophorectomy (THBSO) once the patient has completed the family or by a certain age. ➢ ACOG: 40 to 45 years old. ➢ NCCN: Individualise based on gene mutation, family history and desire for fertility. ➢ Ryan NA *et al. Obstet Gynaecol*. 2021;23(1):9–20: For MLH1 and MSH2: do at age 35; for MSH6: do at 40; for PMS2: do at 50 years old. ➢ Unsure whether a two-staged procedure with hysterectomy after childbearing and delayed BSO after menopause will improve the outcome.
Peutz-Jeghers Syndrome (PJS) – Clinical diagnosis with any one of the following: – ≥2 Peutz–Jeghers-type hamartomatous polyps of the gastrointestinal tract	AD Mutation in the serine/threonine kinase 11 (STK11) gene	• ***Gastrointestinal cancer (38–66%):*** Colorectal (40%), stomach (30%), small bowel, pancreas, biliary tree, gallbladder, oesophagus. • ***Breast cancer*** *(30–60%).*	• *Cervix*: – *Annual cervical cancer screening (Pap smear — not human papillomavirus (HPV) as adenoma malignum is not HPV-dependent) from 18 to 20 years old.*	

Syndrome	Genetics/inheritance	Associated cancer and lifetime risks	Screening strategies	Risk-reducing strategies
Peutz-Jeghers Syndrome (PJS) – Characteristic mucocutaneous hyperpigmentation of the mouth, lips, nose, eyes, genitalia or fingers in a person with a family history of PJS – Any number of Peutz–Jeghers polyps in an individual with a family history of PJS in a first-degree relative – Any number of Peutz–Jeghers polyps in a person with the characteristic mucocutaneous pigmentation of PJS		• ***Ovarian cancer (20%):*** Ovarian sex-cord tumours with annular tubules (SCTAT tumours) can be present. • ***Cervical cancer (10%):*** e.g., cervical adenoma malignum. • ***Endometrial cancer*** *(10%).* ***Others:*** lung cancer.	• ***Endometrium/ovary:*** – *Guidelines vary.* – *Annual pelvic examination from 25 years old.* – *± US scan of the pelvis.* – *CA 125 not indicated.* • ***Breast:*** – *Clinical breast examinations every 6 months and annual breast MRI and mammography starting at age 30.*	
Cowden syndrome 1 in 200 000	AD inheritance Mutation in the PTEN gene	• *Breast cancer (70–95%).* • *Endometrial cancer (17–40%).* • *Colorectal cancer (5–17%).* • *Thyroid cancer (20–50%).* • *Renal cell cancer (17–50%).*	• *Cervix:* – *Annual cervical cancer screening (Pap smear — not HPV as adenoma malignum is not HPV-dependent) from 18 to 20 years old.* • *Endometrium/ovary:* – *Consider endometrial biopsy every 1–2 years.* – *Consider US of the pelvis.*	Discuss the option of risk-reducing mastectomy and hysterectomy once childbearing has been completed.

(Continued)

Table 37.1 (*Continued*)

Syndrome	Genetics/inheritance	Associated cancer and lifetime risks	Screening strategies	Risk-reducing strategies
Cowden syndrome			• *Breast*: – *Clinical breast exam every 6–12 months starting at age 25 years or individualised based on the earliest age of breast cancer diagnosis in the family.* – *Annual mammography and breast MRI screening starting at age 30–35 or 5–10 years before the earliest age of diagnosis.*	
Li–Fraumeni syndrome	AD inheritance Mutation in the p53 gene	• >90% risk of cancer by 60 years old. • *Breast cancer* (54%). • *Sarcomas* (15%). • *Brain cancer* (6%). • *Adrenocortical carcinomas.* • Gynaecological cancers are *unusual*: The most common is *epithelial ovarian cancer*.	• *Breast*: – *Annual breast MRI scan from age 20.* • *Soft tissue/bone sarcoma/ brain tumours*: – *Abdominal ultrasound every 6 months from birth to 18 years old.* – *Annual whole-body and brain MRI (age of initiation is individualised).* – *± Colonoscopy.*	–

Carcinoma of the Cervix

Type of cancer	Risk factors	Protective factors	Histological subtypes	Screening	Prognosis
Cervix • 10th most frequent cancer in Singaporean females • Lifetime risk 0.6% • High-risk age group: 40–59 and 80–84 years old	• Age • HPV infection • Multiple sexual partners • Early age of sexual debut • Smoking • Immune suppression • COCP use >5 years • DES exposure • Family history	• Cervical cancer screening • HPV vaccines: Cervarix®, Gardasil® 4 and 9	• Squamous cell carcinoma (80–90%) • Endocervical adenocarcinomas: – HPV-associated (e.g. villoglandular/micropapillary subtypes, mucinous types e.g. intestinal, signet-ring cell and invasive stratified mucin-producing carcinoma (invasive SMILE) – HPV-independent (e.g. gastric, clear cell, mesonephric and endometrioid) • Adenosquamous • Neuroendocrine carcinoma of the cervix (<5%)	• Cervical cancer screening (Pap smear, primary HPV testing or co-testing). Refer to Chapter 38: *PAP Smear Screening, Primary Human Papillomavirus Testing, Co-Testing and Management of Abnormal Cervical Cancer Screening Results*.	***5-year survival rates*** Stage 1: 95% Stage 2: 80% Stage 3: 50% Stage 4: 20%
	Symptoms and physical examination	**Investigations**	**Treatment**	**Fertility-sparing management**	
	Symptoms: • Irregular vaginal bleeding/AUB • PCB • PMB • IMB • Dyspareunia • Vaginal discharge • If advanced: pain, loss of weight/appetite • Abnormal Pap smear ***Physical examination*:** • May be normal in microinvasive disease	• Colposcopy if no gross lesions • Cervical biopsy • Cancer staging: Examination under anaesthesia (EUA), cystoscopy, proctoscopy ± hysteroscopy, endocervical curettage, biopsy – Indicated if patient unable to cooperate with bedside examination or suspicion of bladder involvement	*Early-stage disease.* • *1A–2A*: Surgery ± postoperative adjuvant radiotherapy (RT) if indicated. • *1A1*: Simple hysterectomy [+ pelvic lymph node dissection (PLND) if the lymphovascular space is involved]. • *1A2*: Modified radical hysterectomy + PLND. • *1B/2A*: Radical hysterectomy + PLND OR radical pelvic RT (Figure 37.1).	• *Criteria.* – Tumour <2 cm. – Desire for fertility. – Age <40 years old. – *Histological subtypes*: Squamous cell, adenocarcinoma or adenosquamous. – The upper endocervical canal is not involved. – No evidence of lymph node or distant metastasis. • *Stage 1A1*: Cone biopsy if margins clear and no lymphovascular space invasion. • *Stage 1A2–1B1*: Radical trachelectomy and PLND (Figure 37.2).	

(*Continued*)

(Continued)

Cervical cancer	Symptoms and physical examination	Investigations	Treatment	Fertility-sparing management
	• Cervical abnormalities include gross erosion, ulcers or a friable, irregular mass with contact bleeding • Involvement of the vagina, parametrium, pelvic side wall, rectal mucosa in the advanced stage	*Imaging*: • CXR • CT thorax and abdomen • MRI pelvis • PET-CT scan where indicated, e.g., indeterminate or suspicious lymph nodes on CT/MRI scan ***FIGO 2018 staging allows the use of imaging or pathological results to allocate the stage.**	*Locally advanced disease* (2B to 4A): • Chemoradiation, radical RT. *Metastatic/recurrent disease*: • Chemoradiation, chemotherapy, palliative RT, pelvic exenteration (if appropriate) or palliative care.	

AFP, alpha-fetoprotein; AGUS, atypical glandular cells of undetermined significance; AUB, abnormal uterine bleeding; βHCG, beta human chorionic gonadotrophin; BRCA 1, 2, tumour suppression gene: a mutation in this gene is associated with a high risk of breast and other cancers; CA 125, carbohydrate antigen 125; CEA, carcinoembryonic antigen; COCPs, combined oral contraceptive pills; CT, computed tomography; CXR, chest X-ray; DES, diethylstilbestrol; EUA, examination under anaesthesia; GnRHa, gonadotrophin-releasing hormone analogues; HSIL, high-grade squamous intraepithelial lesion; HPV, human papillomavirus; LDH, lactate dehydrogenase; LSIL, low-grade squamous intraepithelial lesion; IMB, intermenstrual bleeding; MRI, magnetic resonance imaging; PAND, para-aortic lymph node dissection; PCB, postcoital bleeding; PET, positron emission tomography; PLND, pelvic lymph node dissection; PMB, post-menopausal bleeding; RT, radiotherapy; SLNB, sentinel lymph node biopsy; THBSO, total hysterectomy bilateral salpingo-oophorectomy; U/S, ultrasound; VIN, vulvar intraepithelial neoplasia.

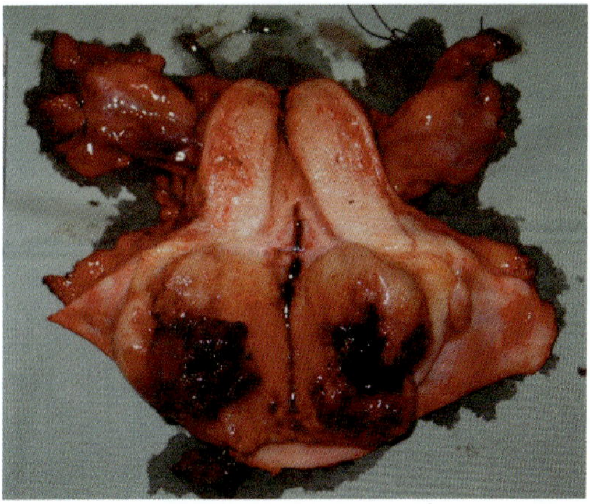

Fig 37.1 Radical hysterectomy BSO specimen for cervical cancer.

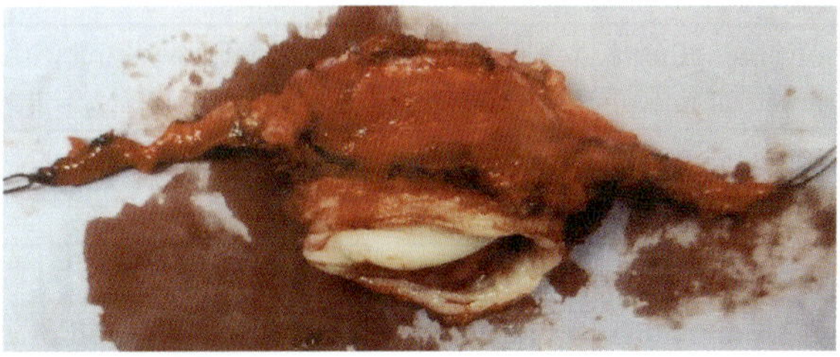

Fig 37.2 Radical trachelectomy specimen for fertility-sparing management of cervical cancer.

FIGO 2018 Staging for *Cervical Cancer*

Stage I: The carcinoma is strictly confined to the cervix (extension to the corpus should be disregarded).	
IA	Invasive carcinoma that can be diagnosed only by microscopy with a maximum depth of invasion ≤5 mm
IA1	Measured stromal invasion ≤3 mm in depth
IA2	Measured stromal invasion >3 and ≤5 mm in depth
IB	Invasive carcinoma with measured deepest invasion >5 mm (greater than Stage IA); lesions limited to the cervix uteri with size measured by the maximum tumour diameter
IB1	Invasive carcinoma >5 mm depth of stromal invasion and ≤2 cm in greatest dimension
IB2	Invasive carcinoma >2 cm and ≤4 cm in greatest dimension
IB3	Invasive carcinoma >4 cm in greatest dimension
Stage II: The cervical carcinoma invades beyond the uterus but has not extended onto the lower third of the vagina or to the pelvic wall.	
IIA	Involvement limited to the upper two-thirds of the vagina without parametrial invasion
IIA1	Invasive carcinoma ≤4 cm in greatest dimension
IIA2	Invasive carcinoma >4 cm in greatest dimension
IIB	With parametrial invasion but not up to the pelvic wall
Stage III: The carcinoma involves the lower third of the vagina and/or extends to the pelvic wall, causes hydronephrosis or non-functioning kidney, or involves pelvic or paraaortic lymph nodes.	
IIIA	Carcinoma involves the lower third of the vagina, with no extension to the pelvic wall.
IIIB	Extension to the pelvic wall and/or hydronephrosis or non-functioning kidney (unless known to be due to another cause)
IIIC	Involvement of pelvic and/or paraaortic lymph nodes (including micrometastases) c, irrespective of the tumour size and extent [with r (imaging) and p (pathology) notations]
IIIC1	Pelvic lymph node metastasis only
IIIC2	Paraaortic lymph node metastasis
Stage IV: The carcinoma has extended beyond the true pelvis or has involved (biopsy proven) the mucosa of the bladder or rectum. A bullous oedema, as such, does not permit a case to be allotted to Stage IV.	
IVA	Spread of the growth to adjacent organs
IVB	Spread to distant organs

Carcinoma of the Uterus (Endometrium)

Type of cancer	Risk factors	Protective factors	Histological subtypes	Screening	Prognosis
Endometrium • Fourth most frequent cancer in Singaporean females • Lifetime risk 2.5% • High-risk age group: 50–69 years old	• Age. • Obesity. • Nulliparity. • PCOS/anovulatory cycle. • Unopposed oestrogen stimulation. • Early menarche, late menopause. • Tamoxifen use. • Family history of uterine, breast or colon cancer — 5% hereditary. • Genetic syndromes, e.g., Lynch syndrome (40–60 times lifetime risk), Cowden syndrome. These are AD inheritance. • Oestrogen-secreting tumours.	• Parity • Breastfeeding • The use of COCP reduces risk by 30–40%. • Use of progestin-only contraceptives	***Type I tumour (80%)*** • Endometrioid subtype, low-grade, usually arise in the background of endometrial hyperplasia. ***Type II tumour (10–20%)*** • High-grade histology, serous, clear cell, squamous and undifferentiated, malignant mixed Müllerian tumour (MMMT). ***Others:*** • Uterine sarcoma: Leiomyosarcoma, endometrial stromal sarcoma (ESS), adenosarcoma. **With the new FIGO 2023 staging, classification is divided into** 1. <u>Non-aggressive subtype:</u> endometrioid grade 1 and 2 2. <u>Aggressive subtypes:</u> endometrioid grade 3, serous, clear cell, mixed carcinoma, undifferentiated, carcinosarcoma, other unusual types, e.g. mesonephric-like and gastrointestinal mucinous type carcinomas. Molecular classification testing is encouraged in all patients.	• No proven screening tool at present. • For women with Lynch syndrome, consider an endometrial biopsy every 1–2 years, beginning at 30–35 years old or 5–10 years before the earliest age of diagnosis in the family.	***5-year survival rates*** Stage 1: 90% Stage 2: 70% Stage 3: 50% Stage 4: 15%

(Continued)

(Continued)

Endometrial cancer (Figure 37.3)	**Symptoms and physical examination**	**Investigations**	**Treatment**	**Fertility-sparing management**
	Symptoms (>80% present in the early stage): • AUB • PMB • IMB/PCB • Persistent post-menopausal vaginal discharge • Pyometra • Haematometra • Abnormal cells on Pap smear (e.g., AGUS smear) ***Physical examination:*** • May be normal • Abdominal or pelvic mass • If advanced: ascites, hepatomegaly	***Laboratory:*** • CA 125 (e.g., in high-grade disease) ***Imaging:*** • CXR • U/S pelvis • CT thorax and abdomen • MRI pelvis or CT pelvis ***Histology:*** • Endometrial biopsy (*gold standard* is hysteroscopy, dilatation and curettage). <u>*Alternative:*</u> Office endometrial sampling with Pipelle® or Explora®.	***Surgery:*** • Staging surgery, THBS±O, bilateral SLNB or PLND (depending on tumour subtype, grade, size and degree of myoinvasion). Extended staging, including PAND and omentectomy in selected cases. • For Stage 2 endometrial cancer, a modified radical hysterectomy is required. • The laparoscopic or laparotomy approach should be individualised. ***Adjuvant radiotherapy:*** • Brachytherapy ± external beam RT based on risk stratification. ***Chemotherapy:*** • Platinum-based drugs, anthracyclines and taxanes for advanced disease or palliation. ***Hormonal treatment:*** • If hormone-receptor-positive.	***Criteria:*** • Age <40 years old. • Grade 1 endometrioid adenocarcinoma. • Clinical and radiological Stage 1A. ***Treatment:*** • Treat underlying risk factors, e.g., weight loss. • <u>*First-line options:*</u> High-dose progestogens, e.g., Megace 160–320 mg daily, Mirena®. • <u>*Other alternatives:*</u> GnRHa, aromatase inhibitors. • Hysteroscopic resection of the tumour (limited to case reports and case series). • Repeat endometrial biopsy at 3 monthly intervals. If failure of regression after 6 months of treatment, advise gold standard treatment. • Refer to a fertility specialist once there is regression. Advise for ART. Consider completion surgery once the patient has completed family. • If failed medical treatment, advise THBS±O and staging surgery.

FIGO 2023 Staging for *Uterine Cancer*

Stage I: Confined to the uterine corpus and ovary	
IA	Disease limited to the endometrium OR non-aggressive histological type, i.e. low-grade endometroid, with invasion of less than half of myometrium with no or focal lymphovascular space involvement (LVSI) OR good prognosis disease IA1: Non-aggressive histological type limited to an endometrial polyp OR confined to the endometrium IA2: Non-aggressive histological types involving less than half of the myometrium with no or focal LVSI IA3: Low-grade endometrioid carcinomas limited to the uterus and ovary
IB	Non-aggressive histological types with invasion of half or more of the myometrium, and with no or focal LVSI
IC	Aggressive histological types limited to a polyp or confined to the endometrium
Stage II: Invasion of cervical stroma with extrauterine extension OR with substantial LVSI OR aggressive histological types with myometrial invasion	
IIA	Invasion of the cervical stroma of non-aggressive histological types
IIB	Substantial LVSI of non-aggressive histological types
IIC	Aggressive histological types with any myometrial involvement
Stage III: Local and/or regional spread of the tumour of any histological subtype	
IIIA	Invasion of uterine serosa, adnexa, or both by direct extension or metastasis IIIA1: Spread to ovary or fallopian tube (except when meeting stage IA3 criteria) IIIA2: Involvement of uterine subserosa or spread through the uterine serosa
IIIB	Metastasis or direct spread to the vagina and/or to the parametria or pelvic peritoneum IIIB1: Metastasis or direct spread to the vagina and/or the parametria IIIB2: Metastasis to the pelvic peritoneum

(*Continued*)

(*Continued*)

IIIC	Metastasis to the pelvic or para-aortic lymph nodes or both IIIC1: Metastasis to the pelvic lymph nodes IIIC1i: Micrometastasis IIIC1ii: Macrometastasis IIIC2: Metastasis to para-aortic lymph nodes up to the renal vessels, with or without metastasis to the pelvic lymph nodes IIIC2i: Micrometastasis IIIC2ii: Macrometastasis
Stage IV: Spread to the bladder mucosa and/or intestinal mucosa and/or distance metastasis	
IVA	Invasion of the bladder mucosa and/or the intestinal/bowel mucosa
IVB	Abdominal peritoneal metastasis beyond the pelvis
IVC	Distant metastasis, including metastasis to any extra- or intra-abdominal lymph nodes above the renal vessels, lungs, liver, brain, or bone

- If available and feasible, molecular classification testing (POLEmut, MMRd, NSMP, p53abn) is encouraged in all patients with endometrial cancer for prognostic risk-group stratification and as factors that might influence adjuvant and systemic treatment decisions.
- FIGO Stages I and II are based on surgical/anatomical and histological findings. In case the molecular classification reveals POLEmut or p53abn status, the FIGO stage is modified in the early stage of the disease.
- FIGO Stages III and IV are based on surgical/anatomical findings. The stage category is not modified by molecular classification; however, the molecular classification should be recorded if known.
- Micrometastases are considered to be metastatic involvement (pN1 (mi)). The prognostic significance of isolated tumor cells (ITCs) is unclear. The presence of ITCs should be documented and is regarded as pN0(i+). According to TNM8, macrometastases are >2 mm in size, micrometastases are >0.2–2 mm and/or >200 cells, and isolated tumor cells are ≤0.2 mm and ≤200 cells.

FIGO 2009 Staging for *Uterine Sarcomas*

Leiomyosarcomas and endometrial stromal sarcomas	
Stage I: Tumour limited to the uterus	
IA	<5 cm
IB	>5 cm
Stage II: Tumour extends beyond the uterus, within the pelvis	
IIA	Adnexal involvement
IIB	Involvement of other pelvic tissues
Stage III: Tumour invades abdominal tissues (not just protruding into the abdomen)	
IIIA	One site
IIIB	More than one site
IIIC	Metastasis to pelvic and/or para-aortic lymph nodes
Stage IV	
IVA	Tumour invades the bladder and/or rectum
IVB	Distant metastasis
Adenosarcomas	
Stage I: Tumour limited to the uterus	
IA	Tumour limited to the endometrium/endocervix with no myometrial invasion
IB	Less than or equal to half myometrial invasion
IC	More than half myometrial invasion
Stage II: Tumour extends to the pelvis	
IIA	Adnexal involvement
IIB	Tumour extends to the extrauterine pelvic tissue
Stage III: Tumour invades abdominal tissues (not just protruding into the abdomen)	
IIIA	One site
IIIB	More than one site
IIIC	Metastasis to pelvic and/or para-aortic lymph nodes
Stage IV	
IVA	Tumour invades the bladder and/or rectum
IVB	Distant metastasis

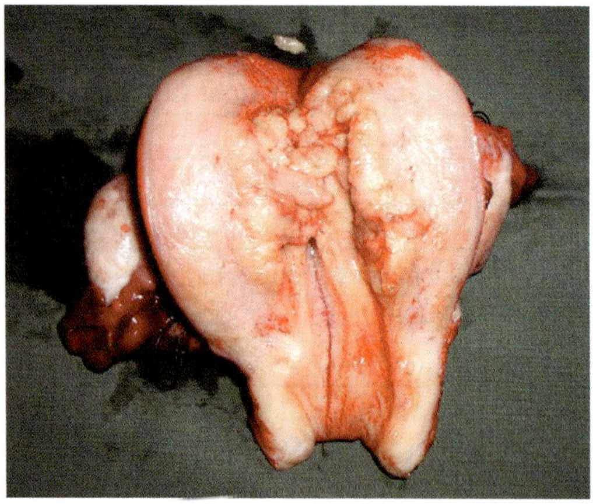

Fig. 37.3 Carcinoma of the endometrium.

Carcinoma of the Ovary

Type of cancer	Risk factors	Protective factors	Histological subtypes	Screening	Prognosis
Ovary • Fifth most frequent cancer in Singaporean females • Lifetime risk 1–2% • High-risk age group: 60–70 years old	• Age. • Nulliparity. • Infertility. • Endometriosis (associated with endometrioid adenocarcinoma and clear cell carcinoma). • Previous history of breast, uterine or colorectal cancer. • Family history of breast, gynaecological or colorectal cancer (5–10% have inherited predisposition of breast and ovarian cancer). • Genetic syndromes, e.g., BRCA 1 and 2, Lynch syndrome, PJS. These are AD inheritance.	• Parity • Pregnancy • Breastfeeding • Use of COCP (20% reduction for every 5 years of use) • Salpingectomy (30% risk reduction) • Tubal ligation (60% risk reduction) • Late menarche/ early menopause	**1. *Primary*** Epithelial ovarian cancers (90%) • Most common subtype is serous (70–80%), followed by endometrioid, clear cell, mucinous, transitional, mixed and undifferentiated. Sex cord-stromal tumours (5–6%) • 70% are granulosa cell tumours. They secrete oestrogen, potentially leading to endometrial hyperplasia and carcinoma. • Other subtypes include: Sertoli–Leydig cell tumours, steroid cell tumours and gynandroblastomas. Malignant germ cell tumours (2–3%) • Occur mostly in young females. • Dysgerminoma is most common. Others: Yolk sac tumour, embryonal carcinoma, polyembryoma, non-gestational choriocarcinoma and immature teratoma. Others • Squamous cell carcinoma (<1%). **2. *Secondary*** Metastasis from other cancers.	• No proven screening tool at present. Most commonly used are CA 125 and U/S pelvis. However, trials have not shown that screening for ovarian cancer is effective. • Women should be counselled on BRCA testing. • For BRCA carriers, RRBSO should be undertaken to reduce risks of ovarian and fallopian tube cancers, but there is a residual 1–6% risk of primary peritoneal carcinoma.	**5-year survival rates** Stage 1: 90% Stage 2: 65–70% Stage 3: 25% Stage 4: 15%

(*Continued*)

(Continued)

	Symptoms and physical examination	Investigations	Treatment	Fertility-sparing management
Carcinoma of ovary (Fig. 37.5)	***Symptoms*** • Asymptomatic • Pelvic or abdominal pain • Abdominal distension • Early satiety • Changes in bowel habit • Urinary frequency • Loss of weight/appetite • Shortness of breath • Abnormal uterine bleeding • Post-menopausal bleeding ***Physical examination:*** • Normal in the early stage <u>In advanced disease:</u> • Cachexia • Abdominal or pelvic mass • Ascites • Pleural effusion	***Laboratory:*** • Ovarian cancer profile (CA125, βHCG, CEA, AFP, LDH. Levels are difficult to interpret in pregnancy). Refer to Chapter 60: *Tumour Markers in Gynaecology and Pregnancy*. ***Imaging:*** • U/S pelvis. • CXR. • CT thorax, abdomen and pelvis. • Histopathology: Cytology of ascitic or pleural fluid. • Biopsy of peritoneal nodules/mass.	***Surgery:*** • Primary upfront staging surgery: Peritoneal washings, THBSO, omentectomy and pelvic or para-aortic lymphadenectomy, debulking surgery (± appendicectomy if mucinous tumour). • Usually the laparotomy approach. Laparoscopy can be done as a diagnostic procedure to obtain specimens for histology and assess resectability or as a re-staging for previously incompletely staged early ovarian cancer. • **Chemotherapy** (<u>*first-line*</u>: platinum-based drug with taxane, <u>*second-line*</u>: doxorubicin, topotecan, etc.) • **Consider neoadjuvant chemotherapy and then interval debulking surgery for Stage 3 or 4** if there is extensive disease or if unable to achieve optimal debulking at the outset or if the patient is a poor surgical candidate. • **Other chemotherapeutic agents** may be considered if failed conventional treatment or recurrent disease (targeted treatment such as bevacizumab).	• 8% of Stage 1 epithelial ovarian cancers <35 years. ***Criteria for fertility-sparing management*** *1. <u>For epithelial ovarian cancer</u>* • <40 years old. • Stage 1 unilateral tumour and Grade 1 or 2. • Histology subtypes: Endometrioid, mucinous or serous. *2. <u>For ovarian germ cell tumours</u>* • Fertility sparing is possible even in advanced cancer if the contralateral ovary is normal. *3. <u>For sex-cord stromal tumours</u>* • Limited data on fertility-sparing management. *<u>Treatment</u>* • Counsel the patient on the risk of contralateral disease, recurrence and mortality. • Discuss regarding fertility preservation • Unilateral salpingo-oophorectomy and surgical staging, e.g., ipsilateral PLND/PAND, omentectomy. • Fertility outcomes have been shown to be successful, and survival is comparable to that of standard treatment. • For Grade 3 tumours and Stage 1C, there is a higher risk of disease relapse with fertility-sparing treatment. • May require adjuvant chemotherapy. • Consider completion surgery once the patient has completed the family.

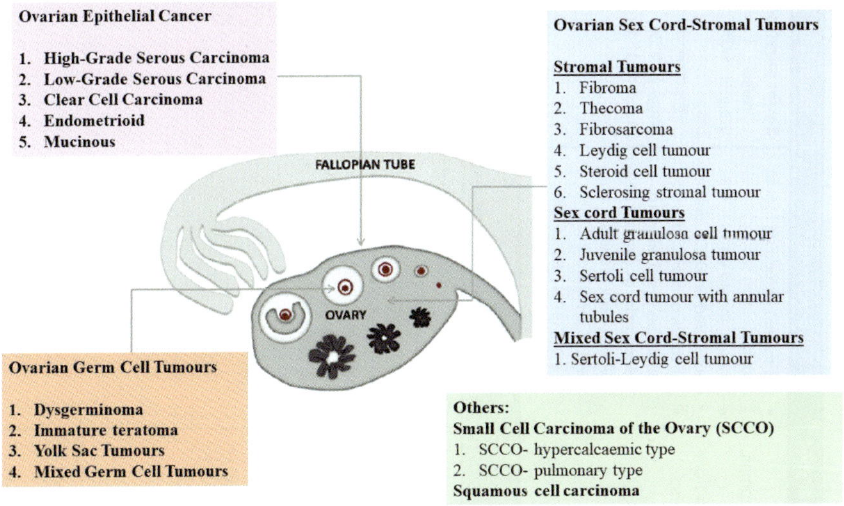

Fig. 37.4 Origin of ovarian cancer subtypes.

Source: Ravindran F, Choudhary B. Ovarian Cancer: Molecular Classification and Targeted Therapy. In: Ho G, Webber K, eds. Ovarian Cancer — Updates in Tumour Biology and Therapeutics. IntechOpen; 2021. Accessed 21 August 2022. https://doi.org/10.5772/intechopen.95967.

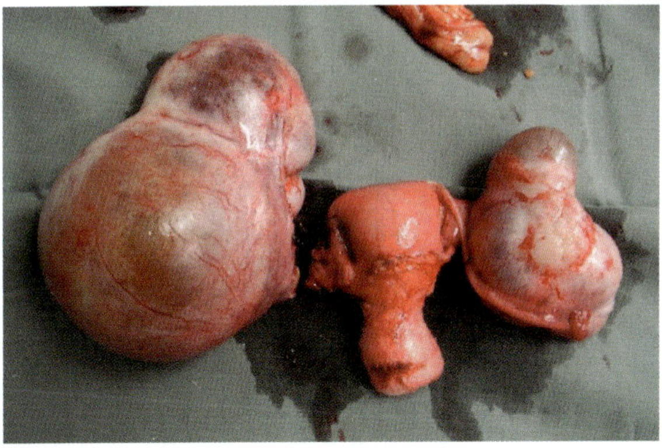

Fig. 37.5 Carcinoma of the ovary.

Carcinoma of the Fallopian Tube

Type of cancer	Risk factors	Protective factors	Histological subtypes	Screening	Prognosis
Fallopian tube • High-risk age group: fifth to sixth decade. • Up to 80% of high-grade serous carcinoma of the ovary or peritoneum may have originated from the fimbrial end of tubes. Hence, high-grade ovarian cancers, fallopian tube cancers and peritoneal cancers are considered collectively and have the same staging system.	• Age • Nulliparity • History of infertility • Family history • Genetic syndromes, e.g., BRCA variants	• Parity • Pregnancy • Breastfeeding • Use of COCP • Salpingectomy/ tubal ligation	• Epithelial, adenocarcinomas, sarcomas • Secondaries from other cancers, especially gynaecological cancers	• No proven screening tool at present. • Women should be counselled on BRCA testing. • For BRCA carriers, RRBSO should be undertaken to reduce risks of ovarian and fallopian tube cancers, but there is a residual 1–6% risk of primary peritoneal carcinoma.	***5-year survival rates*** Stage 1: 90% Stage 2: 65–70% Stage 3: 25% Stage 4: 15%
	Symptoms and physical examination	**Investigations**	**Treatment**	**Fertility-sparing management**	
	Symptoms: • Asymptomatic • *Latzko's triad:* Colicky abdominal pain, serosanguinous vaginal discharge ("hydrops tubae profluens"), abdominal/pelvic mass • Incidental finding in a hysterectomy specimen • AUB • PMB • IMB • Urinary or bowel symptoms • Unexplained abnormal cervical cytology (e.g., AGUS smear) ***Physical examination:*** • Pelvic mass • Profuse watery vaginal discharge • Ascites	***Laboratory*:** • CA 125 ***Imaging*:** • CXR • U/S pelvis • CT thorax, abdomen and pelvis (CTTAP)	Management principles are similar to those of ovarian cancer. Primary debulking surgery, adjuvant chemotherapy or neoadjuvant chemotherapy followed by interval debulking surgery.	Management principles similar to those of ovarian cancer. *Disease confined to one fallopian tube*: Unilateral salpingo-oophorectomy, omental biopsy, ipsilateral pelvic/para-aortic lymph node dissection. Consider completion surgery once the patient has completed the family.	

FIGO 2014 Staging for *Cancer of the Ovary, Fallopian Tube, Peritoneum*

Stage I: Tumour confined to ovaries or fallopian tube(s)	
IA	Tumour limited to one ovary (capsule intact) or fallopian tube; no tumour on the ovarian or fallopian tube surface; no malignant cells in the ascites or peritoneal washings
IB	Tumour limited to both ovaries (capsules intact) or fallopian tubes; no tumour on the ovarian or fallopian tube surface; no malignant cells in the ascites or peritoneal washings
IC	Tumour limited to one or both ovaries or fallopian tubes, with any of the following:
1C1	Surgical spill
1C2	Capsule ruptured before surgery or tumour on the ovarian or fallopian tube surface
1C3	Malignant cells in the ascites or peritoneal washings
Stage II: Tumour involves one or both ovaries or fallopian tubes with pelvic extension (below the pelvic brim) or peritoneal cancer	
IIA	Extension and/or implants on the uterus and/or fallopian tubes and/or ovaries
IIB	Extension to other pelvic intraperitoneal tissues
Stage III: Tumour involves one or both ovaries or fallopian tubes, or peritoneal cancer, with cytologically or histologically confirmed spread to the peritoneum outside the pelvis and/or metastasis to the retroperitoneal lymph nodes	
IIIA1	Positive retroperitoneal lymph nodes only (cytologically or histologically proven):
IIIA1(i)	Metastasis ≤10 mm in greatest dimension
IIIA1(ii)	Metastasis >10 mm in greatest dimension
IIIA2	Microscopic extrapelvic (above the pelvic brim) peritoneal involvement with or without positive retroperitoneal lymph nodes
IIIB	Macroscopic peritoneal metastasis beyond the pelvis up to 2 cm in greatest dimension, with or without metastasis to the retroperitoneal lymph nodes
IIIC	Macroscopic peritoneal metastasis beyond the pelvis more than 2 cm in greatest dimension, with or without metastasis to the retroperitoneal lymph nodes (includes the extension of the tumour to the capsule of the liver and spleen without the parenchymal involvement of either organ)
Stage IV: Distant metastasis excluding peritoneal metastases	
IVA	Pleural effusion with positive cytology
IVB	Parenchymal metastases and metastases to extra-abdominal organs (including inguinal lymph nodes and lymph nodes outside of the abdominal cavity)

Carcinoma of the Vulva

Type of cancer	Risk factors	Protective factors	Histological subtypes	Screening	Prognosis
Vulva • High-risk age group: Post-menopausal women (80% >60 years old)	• Age • HPV infection • Multiple sexual partners • Early age of sexual debut • Smoking • Immunodeficiency • Chronic inflammatory vulvar conditions, e.g., lichen sclerosus, lichen planus • VIN (vulvar intraepithelial neoplasia) – *Subtypes:* Vulvar HSIL (VIN usual type) 5–10% risk, differentiated VIN (dVIN) >50% risk • Paget's disease of the vulva • History of cervical/vaginal cancer • Previous radiation	• HPV vaccines: Cervarix®, Gardasil® 4 and 9	• Squamous cell (75%) • *Others*: Melanoma, adenocarcinoma, basal cell carcinoma, Bartholin's gland tumour, sarcoma, invasive Paget's disease of the vulva	• No proven screening tool at present. • Vulvar cytology cannot replace diagnostic biopsy of suspicious lesions.	**5-year survival rates** Stage 1: >85% Stage 2: 50% Stage 3: 25–40% Stage 4: 15%

(Continued)

Type of cancer	Risk factors	Protective factors	Histological subtypes	Screening	Prognosis
	Symptoms and physical examination	**Investigations**	**Treatment**	**Fertility-sparing management**	
Carcinoma of vulva (Fig. 37.6)	***Symptoms:*** • Asymptomatic • Vulvar lump or ulcer • Vulvar pruritus • Vulvar pain • Bleeding or discharge from the lesion • Dysuria • Lump in groin ***Physical examination:*** • Ulcer, especially long-standing non-healing ulcer • Fleshy/irregular mass or leukoplakia on labia • Pigmented lesions • Enlarged groin nodes	• Colposcopy • Keye's punch biopsy 3–5 mm deep for histology • Pap smear of the cervix ***Imaging:*** • CXR • CT thorax, abdomen • CT or MRI pelvis	*Surgery for early-stage vulvar cancer or resectable locally advanced tumours*: • Radical local excision or vulvectomy ± groin node dissection depending on the stage • May require postoperative radiotherapy *Unresectable tumours that would require a stoma or surgically unfit patients*: • Chemoradiation or primary radiotherapy followed by surgical resection of the residual tumour <u>Prognostic factors:</u> • Age. • Immunocompromised state. • Tumour size. • Presence and number of lymph node metastases. – 5-year survival with no lymph node involvement is >80%. This drops to <50% if lymph nodes are involved and further to 10–15% if pelvic lymph nodes are involved. • Extracapsular involvement of lymph nodes. • Lymphovascular space invasion. • Perineural involvement.	• Early vulvar cancer treated by surgery should *not* affect the ability to conceive. Chemotherapy or radiotherapy can affect the ovarian reserve. Ovarian transposition if radiotherapy is required • Vulvar scarring resulting from surgery or radiotherapy can affect the mode of delivery. A caesarean section may be indicated to avoid perineal trauma.	

FIGO 2021 Staging for *Cancer of the Vulva*

Stage I: Tumour confined to the vulva	
IA	Tumour size ≤2 cm and stromal invasion ≤1 mm*
IB	Tumour size >2 cm and stromal invasion >1 mm*
Stage II: Tumour of any size with extension to the lower one-third of the urethra, lower one-third of the vagina, lower one-third of the anus with negative nodes	
Stage III: Tumour of any size with extension to the upper part of adjacent perineal structures, or with any number of nonfixed, nonulcerated lymph nodes	
IIIA	Tumour of any size with disease extension to the upper two-thirds of the urethra, upper two-thirds of the vagina, bladder mucosa, rectal mucosa or regional lymph node metastases ≤5 mm
IIIB	Regional (inguinal/femoral) lymph node metastases >5 mm
IIIC	Regional (inguinal/femoral) lymph node metastases with extracapsular spread
Stage IV: Tumour of any size fixed to bone, or fixed, ulcerated lymph node metastases or distant metastases	
IVA	Disease fixed to the pelvic bone, or fixed or ulcerated regional (inguinal/femoral) lymph node metastases
IVB	Distant metastases

*The depth of invasion is measured from the basement membrane of the deepest, adjacent, dysplastic, tumour-free rete ridge (or nearest dysplastic rete peg) to the deepest point of invasion.

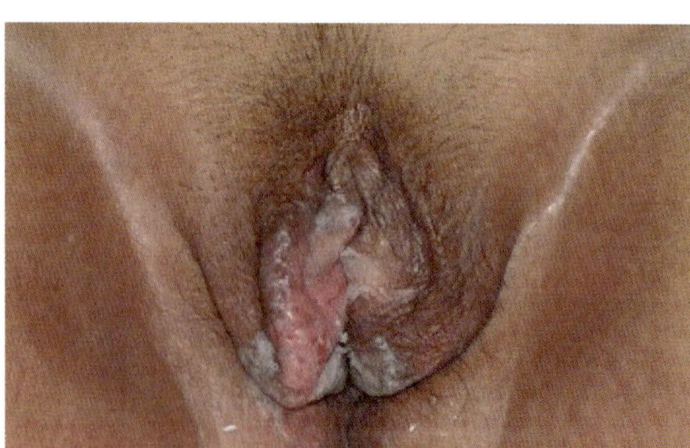

Fig. 37.6 Carcinoma of the vulva.

Carcinoma of the Vagina

Type of cancer	Risk factors	Protective factors	Histological subtypes	Screening	Prognosis
Vagina • Primary vaginal cancer is rare, 1–2% of gynaecological cancers • High-risk age group: Post-menopausal women	• Age • HPV infection • Multiple sexual partners • Early age of sexual debut • Smoking • Immunodeficiency • *Vaginal HSIL*: 2–12% risk of cancer • History of cervical/vulvar cancer • Previous radiation • DES exposure (offspring: increases the risk of clear cell carcinoma)	• HPV vaccines: Cervarix®, Gardasil® 4 and 9	***Primary (20%)*** • Squamous cell (90%) adenocarcinoma (8–10%); others (melanoma, sarcoma, small cell, lymphoma, undifferentiated) ***Metastasis to the vagina from primary cancer (80%)*** • Cervix/endometrium/ovary/vulva • Gestational trophoblastic neoplasia (GTN) • Breast, lymphoma	• No role for routine screening after a hysterectomy for benign gynaecological conditions. • If a hysterectomy was performed for CIN/cervical cancer, vault smears are required for long-term follow-up. • For women with intrauterine exposure to DES: Annual vaginal cytology and mammogram because of slightly increased breast cancer risk.	***5-year survival rates*** Stage 1: 75% Stage 2: 50% Stage 3: 40% Stage 4: 15–20%
	Symptoms and physical examination	**Investigations**	**Treatment**	**Fertility preservation**	
	Symptoms: • Asymptomatic • Vaginal lump • Vaginal itch • Vaginal bleeding or discharge • Urinary symptoms • Tenesmus ***Physical examination:*** • Exophytic lesions	• Colposcopy • Punch biopsy of the lesion ***Imaging:*** • CXR • CT thorax, abdomen • CT or MRI pelvis • PET-CT	• Management is individualised. • *Radiotherapy* is the mainstay of treatment for most cases, especially in the advanced stage. • Concurrent chemotherapy with radiation may be used. Data regarding its use are limited but may potentially improve overall and disease-free survival. • The role of surgery is limited; for early-stage cancer and able to achieve negative margins. *Unresectable tumours that would require a stoma or surgically unfit patients:* • Chemoradiation or primary radiotherapy followed by surgical resection of the residual tumour.	• Ovarian transposition if radiotherapy is required.	

FIGO 2009 Staging for *Cancer of the Vagina*

Stage I: Tumour confined to the vagina.	
IA	The tumour is ≤2.0 cm.
IB	The tumour is >2.0 cm.
Stage II: Tumour has involved the subvaginal tissues but has not extended to the pelvic side wall.	
IIA	Tumour has grown through the vaginal wall but not as far as the pelvic wall and is ≤2.0 cm.
IIB	Tumour has grown through the vaginal wall but not as far as the pelvic wall and is >2.0 cm.
Stage III: Tumour has extended to the pelvic side wall.	
Stage IV: Tumour has extended beyond the true pelvis or has involved the rectal or bladder mucosa. Bullous oedema does not constitute Stage IV.	
IVA	Spread of the growth to adjacent organs and/or direct extension beyond the true pelvis.
IVB	Spread to distant organs.

Metastasis to the Ovary/Krukenberg Tumours

Introduction	• They form approximately ~1–2% of ovarian malignancies. The incidence is higher in Asian countries due to the higher rate of gastric cancer, ~10–20% of ovarian malignancies. • They tend to present at an earlier age than primary ovarian malignancies. • **Krukenberg tumours** were originally defined as ovarian metastases from gastrointestinal cancers that have a signet-ring cell morphology. However, it is now more loosely used to describe any metastasis to the ovary. • There are various routes of spread to the ovary: – Direct spread. – Haematogenous spread. – Lymphatic spread. – Transcoelomic spread.
Histological subtypes	Tumours can metastasise to the ovary from other organs: • <u>*Gynaecological*:</u> Endometrium, cervix, fallopian tube, vulva, vagina • Peritoneum • <u>*Gastrointestinal*:</u> Stomach, small and large intestines, appendix, pancreas, biliary tract • Breast • <u>*Urinary*:</u> renal, bladder • <u>*Rare*:</u> Thyroid carcinoma, melanoma, leukaemia, neuroblastoma The most common primary cancers are stomach, colorectal and breast cancers.
Symptoms and signs	• Similar to those of primary ovarian malignancies. • Abdominal distension or bloatedness, pain.
Diagnosis	• Ovarian metastases can show similar features to primary ovarian malignancies. • It is essential to know if there is a previous history of malignancy. • They are usually bilateral tumours.
Investigations	• Radiologically, they can be multiloculated tumours with necrotic and haemorrhagic areas. • Tumour deposits can also be seen on the surface of the ovary with stromal invasion. • CA125 is *not* useful for distinguishing between primary and metastatic ovarian lesions. • A serum CA125-to-CEA ratio of >25 may help differentiate between primary ovarian and colorectal cancer metastases. • Consider preoperative oesophago-gastro-duodenoscopy (OGD) and colonoscopy if CEA is raised. • Immunohistochemical stains can provide additional information regarding the origin of the ovarian mass. – Primary ovarian carcinomas are associated with positive cytokeratin (CK) 7, CA125, WT1, PAX8 and vimentin. They are negative for cytokeratine 20 (CK20), CEA and gross cystic disease fluid protein-15 (GCDFP-15). Primary mucinous ovarian carcinomas can be positive for CK20 and CEA. – Metastatic colorectal carcinomas are positive for CK20, CEA and CDX2 and negative for CK 7 and CA125. – Metastatic breast carcinomas are positive for GCDFP-15 and negative for vimentin.

(Continued)

Management	• Multidisciplinary approach. • Treat primary cancer. Depending on the stage and prognosis of the primary tumour, cytoreductive surgery of ovarian metastases may be indicated. • Adjuvant chemotherapy may be required post-cytoreductive surgery.
Prognosis	• Prognosis is poorer for patients with non-gynaecological cancers that metastasise to the ovaries than for patients with gynaecological cancers with ovarian metastases.

CHAPTER 38

PAP Smear Screening, Primary Human Papillomavirus Testing, Co-Testing and Management of Abnormal Cervical Cancer Screening Results

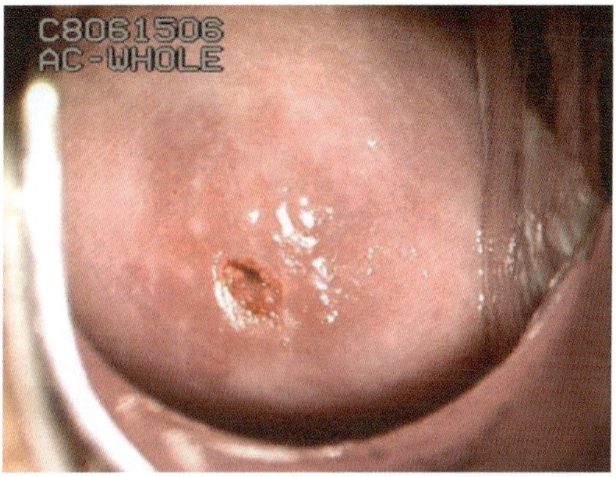

Fig. 38.1 Nulliparous cervix.

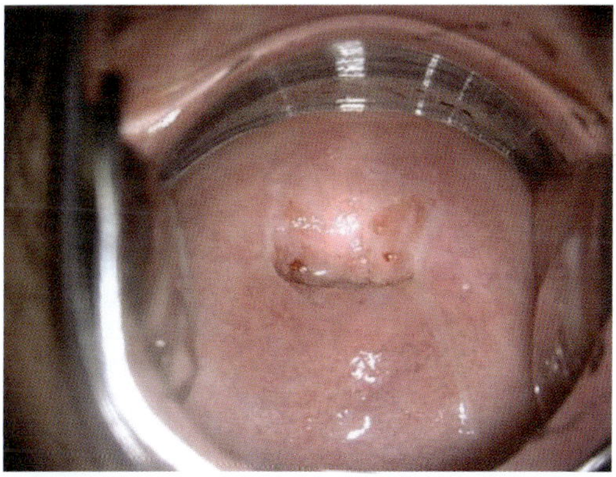

Fig. 38.2 Parous cervix with a slit-shaped os.

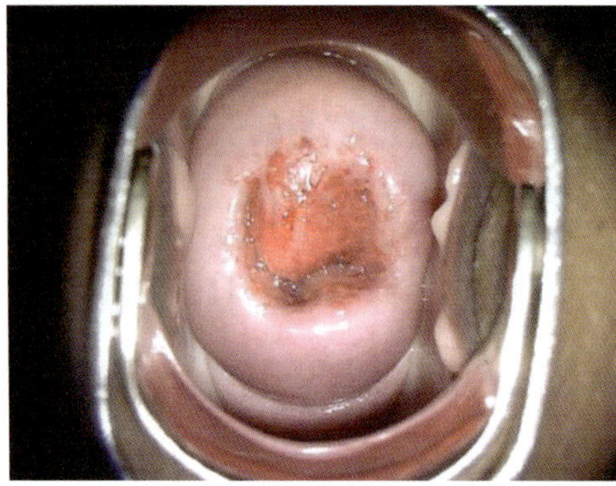

Fig. 38.3 Cervical ectropion.

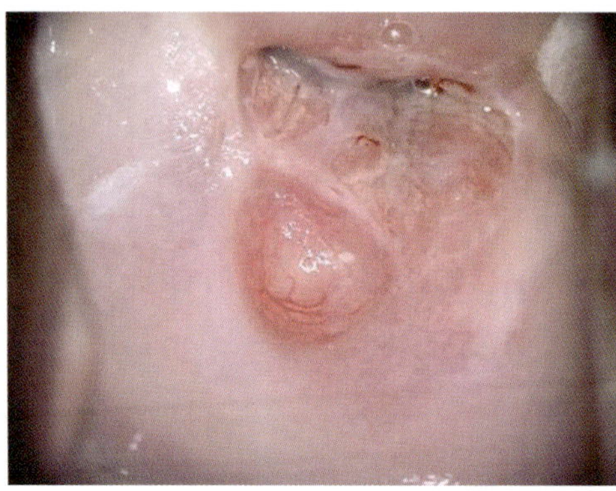

Fig. 38.4 Nabothian cyst/follicle. Note the prominent blood vessels on the surface showing a normal regular branching pattern.

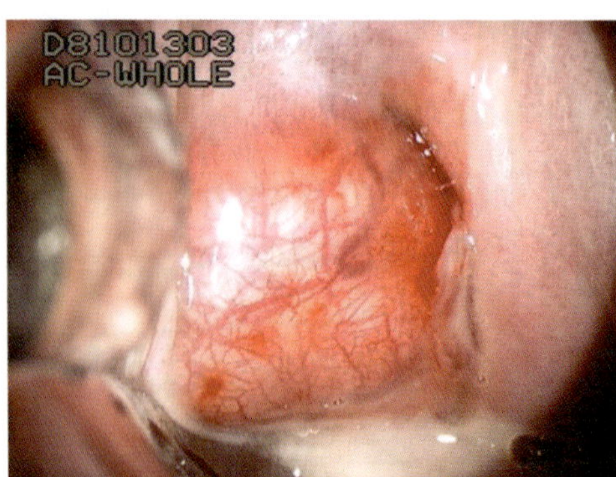

Fig. 38.5 A cluster of nabothian cysts distorting the cervix.

Facts About Cervical Cancer

- Cervical cancer is the fourth most common cancer worldwide, especially in developing countries.
- In Singapore, it is the 10th most frequent cancer, and the age-standardised incidence rate was 6.8 per 100,000 population from 2017 to 2021.
- It is a highly preventable cancer.

Human Papillomavirus (HPV) and Associated Cancers — Cervical and Other Cancers

- HPV causes the majority of cervical cancers. It is a common virus that is transmitted via skin-to-skin contact. The HPV virus affects about 80% of men and women worldwide at some point in their life.
- HPV DNA is found in almost 100% of cervical cancers.
- More than 100 types of HPVs can infect humans.
- 15 HPV types are considered high-oncogenic-risk HPV (hr-HPV). hr-HPVs have also been implicated in causing cancers of the vulva, vagina, anus, penis, head and neck.
- The hr-HPV types 16 and 18 account for 70% of cervical cancers.
- hr-HPV 31, 33, 45, 52 and 58 are responsible for approximately 20% of cervical cancers.

Human Papilloma Virus and Genital Warts

- HPV types 6 and 11 account for 90% of genital warts.
- Genital warts are benign and do not lead to cancer.
- However, genital warts are highly infective and can be persistent and debilitating — refer to Chapter 51: *Sexually Transmitted Infections*.

Clinical Manifestations

- It is not possible to know when a woman is infected with HPV. This is because it can stay dormant for years before becoming active and causing changes in the cervical cells.
  When it stays dormant, it will not be detectable on HPV tests.

- Cervical intraepithelial neoplasia (CIN) usually occurs between the ages of 25 and 40 years.
- Cervical cancer usually presents after 40 years old.

Natural History of hr-HPV Infection and Pathogenesis of Cervical Cancer

- HPV infection of the cervix occurs commonly but is usually transient in young women.
- In 80% of women infected with HPV, the infection regresses spontaneously.
- Persistent hr-HPV infection of the cervix predisposes to the development of pre-cancer and cancer.

The Cervical Epithelium and Cervical Cancers

- The epithelium of the ectocervix (*visible*) is made of squamous epithelium.
- The epithelium of the endocervix (*not visible*) is made of glandular epithelium.
- The epithelium between the endocervix and ectocervix that is transformed from glandular cells to squamous cells is called the transformation zone (TZ).
- The *TZ* of the cervix is prone to carcinogenesis.

CIN and Squamous Cell Carcinoma (SCC)

- CIN are pre-cancers of the squamous epithelium.
- *Three grades of CIN*: CIN I, CIN II and CIN III.
- 60–70% of CIN I will regress spontaneously after 2 years.
- High-grade CIN (CIN II and III) has a significant risk of developing squamous cell carcinoma (SCC).
  The risk of progression to cancer is at least 30–50% over 10 years.

Grade of CIN	Risk of progression to higher grade CIN/cervical cancer
CIN 1	70% regress in 1 year 90% regress in 2 years ~10% progress to carcinoma *in situ* (1% progress to invasive cancer)
CIN 2	60% regress in 3 years 15% progress to CIN 3 in 3 years ~20% progress to carcinoma *in situ* (5% progress to invasive cancer)
CIN 3	30% regress in 2 years (12% progress to invasive cancer)

Source: Rowland, A. and Brady, J., 2020. Colposcopy and cervical intraepithelial neoplasia. Obstetrics, Gynaecology and Reproductive Medicine, 30(5), pp. 133–138.

Adenocarcinoma *in situ* (AIS) and adenocarcinoma — Why does it need special attention?

- Adenocarcinoma develops from the glandular epithelium of the endocervix.
- AIS is a pre-cancer of the endocervical glandular epithelium.
- HPV 18 is responsible for approximately 50% of adenocarcinomas.
- HPV 16 and 18 are responsible for adenocarcinomas in a higher proportion than SCCs, which are associated with more diverse HPV strains.
- **Screening for adenocarcinoma of the cervix is more difficult because:**
  - The endocervix is **not** visible for clinical examination.
  - Unlike the squamous epithelium, the endocervical glandular epithelium does not exfoliate, making Pap smear screening less reliable.
- Hence, adenocarcinoma of the cervix tends to present later when the tumour is bulky.

Cervical Cancer Screening Singapore Programme

Pap Smear Screening

- For over 50 years, Pap smear screening has been the sole screening method for cervical pre-cancers and cancers.

- Pap smear is a screening test to detect cancer or pre-cancerous lesions of the cervix.
- It is a cytological investigation that involves collecting cellular materials from the cervix or vagina.
- It is **not** a diagnostic test. Both false-positive and false-negative results can occur.
- Therefore, Pap smears should **not** be used solely to diagnose or exclude pre-malignant or malignant cervical or vaginal conditions.
- With a normal Pap smear, the risk of high-grade abnormalities is very low within 3 years, approximately 10–66 per 10,000.

Primary hr-HPV Testing

- Cervical hr-HPV tests are now widely available and increasingly used in clinical practice.
- The Cervical Screen Singapore Advisory Committee has adopted HPV testing as a primary modality for cervical cancer screening for women aged 30 years and above.
- It has greater sensitivity and better predictive value of cervical disease but lower specificity than Pap smears.
- A woman who tested negative for hr-HPVs has a very low cervical pre-cancer or cancer risk. The 5-year risk of at least CIN 3 is 0.14%.
- However, as not all hr-HPV-positive women have a cervical disease, using hr-HPV tests for routine screening tends to overcall and increase referrals for further cervical evaluation.

hr-HPV and Pap Smear Co-Testing

- HPV co-testing increases the detection rate of high-grade CIN more than performing cytology alone. However, studies have **not** shown much improvement in sensitivity or protection against future CIN compared to primary HPV testing. Moreover, there are additional costs to HPV co-testing.
- A woman with a negative hr-HPV and a normal Pap smear has a negligible cervical pre-cancer or cancer risk. The 5-year risk of at least CIN 3 is 0.12%.

Who Are to be Screened for Cervical Cancer?

- Under the National Cervical Cancer Screening Programme, all women who have had sex are advised to have their first Pap smear by 25 years old.
- *Frequency of screening*
    - Those aged 25–29 should have a Pap smear every 3 years.
    - Those 30–69 years old should have a HPV test every 5 years.
- HPV testing is *not* recommended for those under 30 years old as the prevalence of HPV is high in this age group, and most people will clear the HPV infection within 2 years.
- *Other screening options for those aged 30 years old and above*:
    - Pap smear every 3 years.
    - Co-testing with HPV and Pap smear every 5 years.
- *Discharge from screening at 69 years of age if*:
    - Three consecutive negative Pap smears OR
    - Two consecutive negative hr-HPV tests, with the latest test within the last 5 years OR
    - Two consecutive negative co-tests, with the latest test within the last 5 years
- Women who have a history of CIN 2/CIN 3/AIS and have been appropriately treated (or the disease has spontaneously regressed) should be routinely screened for at least 20 years following diagnosis, even if this extends screening past age 69 years.

Women Who Have Undergone Hysterectomy

- If a **subtotal** hysterectomy was performed, the woman still has a risk of cervical cancer, so she should continue the routine screening protocol.
- If a **total** hysterectomy was done for CIN 1/2/3, review the excision margins on histology.
    - If margins are negative, do yearly vault smears for 5 years and two yearly subsequently.
    - If margins are involved or inadequately assessed, do vault smears at least yearly.
- If a total hysterectomy was done for a benign uterine condition and the woman had a normal cervical screening history with a benign cervix on histology specimen — <u>stop</u> cytology or HPV screening.

- If the histology is not known — do one baseline vault smear. If this is negative, there is no need for further cytology or HPV screening.

For Immunocompromised Women

Definition:

- o All HIV-positive women
- o All women who had solid organ transplants
- o All women on two or more immunosuppressants

Start screening from 25 years old as per the national guidelines

- o For 25–29 years old: annual Pap smear
- o For 30 years old and above: HPV test every 3 years.

Any positive hr-HPV strain(s) should be referred for colposcopy directly rather than for a cytology triage.

For Women Who Have Not Had Sexual Intercourse

- They *do not* require routine cervical cancer screening but should be referred to an OBGYN for further evaluation if they develop gynaecological symptoms.

High-risk factors for cervical cancer

- Early onset of sexual intercourse
- Multiple sexual partners
- Human papilloma virus (HPV) infection
- Human immunodeficiency virus (HIV) infection
- History of sexually transmitted infections (STIs)
- Immunosuppression, such as on long-term steroids

Bethesda 2014 Cervical Cytology Classification

- **Negative for intraepithelial lesion or malignancy**
- **<u>Other:</u> endometrial cells (in a woman ≥45 years old)**

Epithelial Cell Abnormalities: Squamous Cell

- o Atypical squamous cells of undetermined significance (ASCUS)
- o Atypical squamous cells, cannot exclude HSIL (ASC-H)

- o Low-grade squamous intraepithelial lesion (LSIL) encompassing: HPV effect/mild dysplasia/CIN 1
- o High-grade squamous intraepithelial lesion (HSIL) encompassing: moderate dyskaryosis (CIN 2), severe dyskaryosis (CIN 3) — with features suspicious for invasion (if an invasion is suspected)
- o SCC

Epithelial Cell Abnormalities: Glandular Cell

- o Atypical glandular cells (AGC)
  - endocervical cells (NOS or specify in comments)
  - endometrial cells (NOS or specify in comments)
  - glandular cells (NOS or specify in comments)
- o AGC
  - endocervical cells, favour neoplastic
  - glandular cells, favour neoplastic
- o Endocervical AIS
- o Adenocarcinoma
  - endocervical
  - extrauterine
  - endometrial
  - not otherwise specified (NOS)

Comparison of the WHO and Bethesda System Terminology

WHO histopathologic terms	Bethesda cytology terms
CIN 1/mild dysplasia	LSIL
CIN 2/moderate dysplasia	HSIL
CIN 3/severe dysplasia	HSIL
CIN 3/carcinoma *in situ*	HSIL

Types of Pap smear tests

(a) *Conventional Pap smear* — promptly smear the sample onto a slide and fix the slide with an alcohol fixative.

(b) *Liquid-based thin-layer cytology (used in KKH)* — the cellular material collected is placed into a liquid medium, and the material is transferred to a glass slide in the laboratory.

Sampling devices for Pap smear

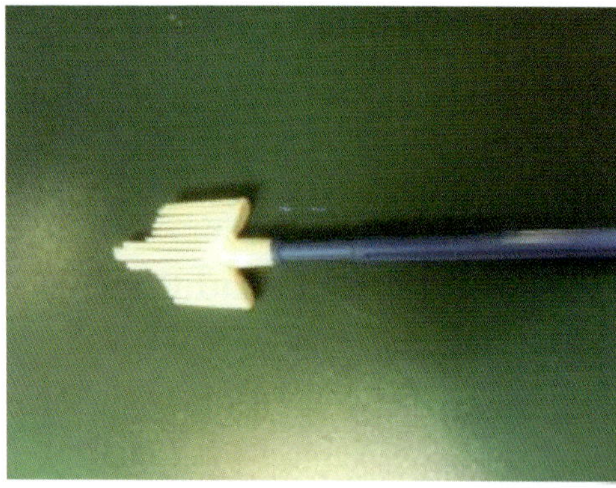

Fig. 38.6 Cytobrush for a Pap smear.

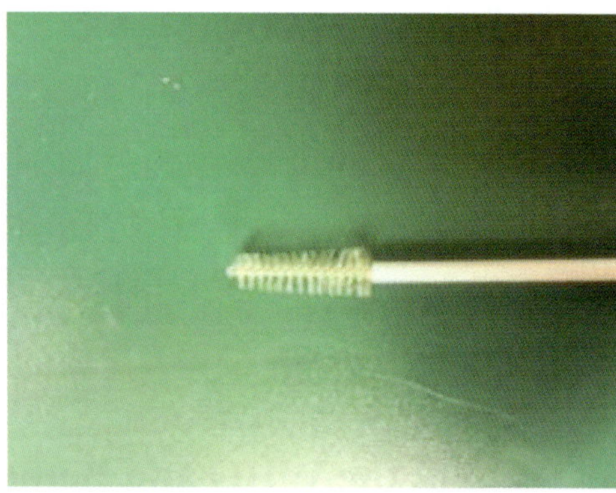

Fig. 38.7 Endocervical brush for a Pap smear.

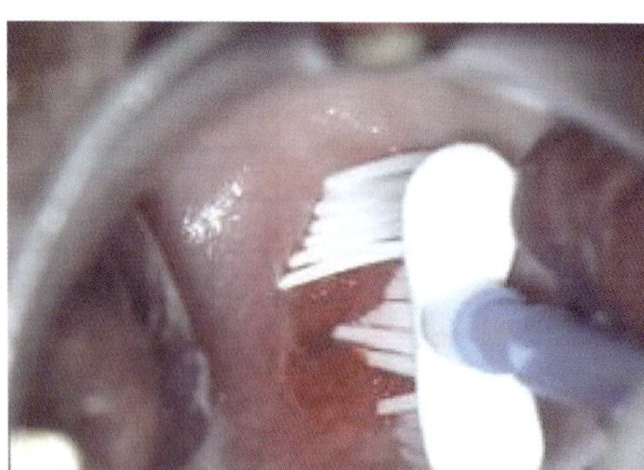

Fig. 38.8 Pap smear with the cytobrush. Care should be taken to sample both the ectocervix and the endocervix.

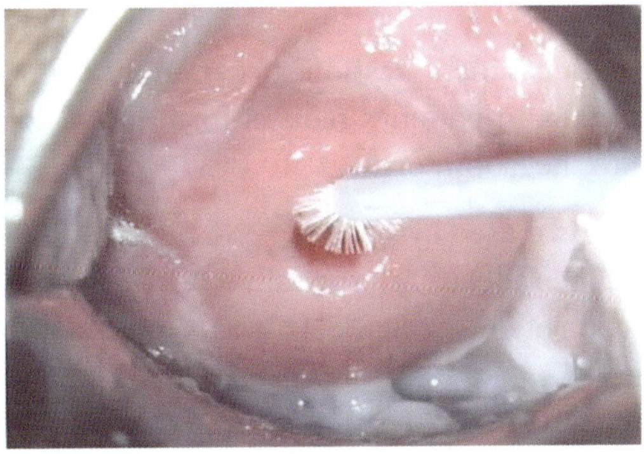

Fig. 38.9 Pap smear with the endocervical brush. The endocervix may need additional sampling with the endocervical brush if the cytobrush cannot reach the endocervix.

How to Obtain Samples for Cervical Smear?

Patient's preparation before the Pap smear

- The ideal sampling date is about 2 weeks after the first day of the last menstrual period.
- Sampling is discouraged during menses and active uterine bleeding.
- Avoid using vaginal medications, vaginal contraceptives or douches for 48 hours before a Pap smear.

Collection technique for liquid-based cytology

i. Insert the central bristles of the brush (either Cervex or Combi brush) into the endocervical canal. Use gentle pressure on the cervix until the lateral bristles bend against the ectocervix.
ii. Maintain gentle pressure and rotate by rolling the stem between the thumb and forefinger.
iii. For the Cervex brush, rotate five times in a clockwise direction.

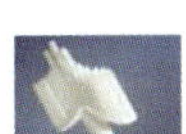

iv. For the Combi brush, rotate two times in a clockwise direction.

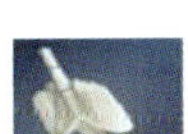

v. Drop the detachable head device into the SurePath™ vial.

vi. Tighten the cap.
vii. Paste the patient's identification sticker on the vial.
viii. Place the vial and patient's request form into a specimen bag for transport to the laboratory.

Advantages of liquid-based cytology

1. Greater specimen adequacy (especially with bleeding or inflammation).
2. Better detection of AGC, ASCUS, LSIL as compared with a conventional Pap smear.
3. Can do concurrent HPV testing.
4. Well-preserved cellular materials. Less fixation and drying artefacts.

Factors Thought to Affect or Interfere with Pap Smear Sampling

1. Menses *do not* affect sample cellularity, but sampling should ideally not be done during heavy menses. Liquid-based methods are less likely to be affected by menses.
   HPV test results are *unaffected* by menses.
2. Gels/lubricants/semen/spermicidal agents/intravaginal medications — less likely to affect liquid-based thin-layer cytology (clean cervix with a large cotton swab to remove the obscuring blood/discharge/lubricants before taking the sample).
3. **No data are available** for douching, tampon use, barrier contraception and vaginal intercourse.

Specimen Adequacy/Unsatisfactory Pap Smear

- *Adequate smears* have an adequate number of well-preserved squamous cells and endocervical cells.
- *Unsatisfactory specimens include* inadequate squamous cells obscured by blood and inflammation — unreliable for detecting cervical epithelial cell abnormalities.

Follow-Up Management of Pap Smears

1. *Normal* — repeat smear in 3 years as per the routine screening
2. *Inflammatory* — treat any infection or atrophy. Repeat smear in 6 months — refer for colposcopy after three consecutive inflammatory smears 6 months apart
3. Presence of normal cytologically *benign appearing endometrial cells*
   - Check the age and risk factors for endometrial hyperplasia or malignancy, e.g., abnormal uterine bleeding, anovulatory cycles and family history of uterine cancer.
   - Check the last menstrual period: endometrial cells can be seen up to the 12th day of the menstrual cycle.
   - Refer to an **OBGYN** if endometrial cells are seen in ≥45 years old or <45 years old but with any of the above risk factors. An ultrasound scan of the pelvis and endometrial biopsy may be indicated to rule out endometrial pathology.
4. *No endocervical cells seen* — routine screening
5. *Atrophic smear* — routine screening
6. *Mild dyskaryosis* — colposcopy
7. *Moderate dyskaryosis* — colposcopy (50–75% CIN II–III)
8. *Severe dyskaryosis* — colposcopy (80–90% CIN II-III)
9. *Invasion suspected* — urgent colposcopy
10. *AGC, site not specified* — urgent colposcopy. If atypical endometrial cells — urgent referral to an **OBGYN**.

Follow-Up Management of hr-HPV Test Results

1. *Normal* — repeat the HPV test in 5 years as per the routine screening.
2. hr-HPV 16/18 positive — colposcopy.
3. hr-HPV non 16/18 positive or type unknown positive — perform reflex Pap smear testing.
   a. If the Pap smear is normal — repeat the HPV test in 1 year.
   If repeat hr-HPV is positive (16/18/non-16/18 subtypes), refer for colposcopy.
   If repeat HPV is negative, continue routine screening.
   b. If the Pap smear is ≥ASCUS — refer for colposcopy.

Follow-Up Management of Pap Smears

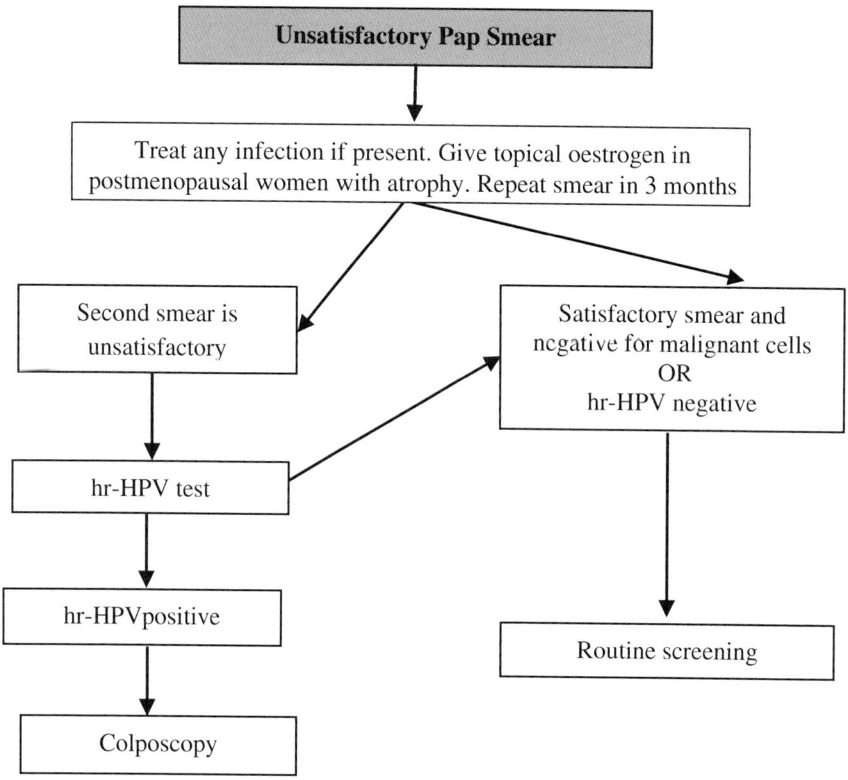

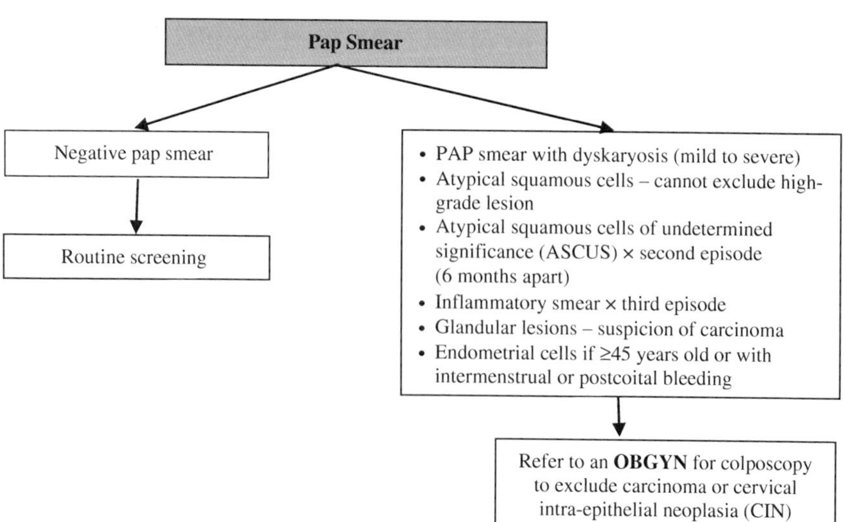

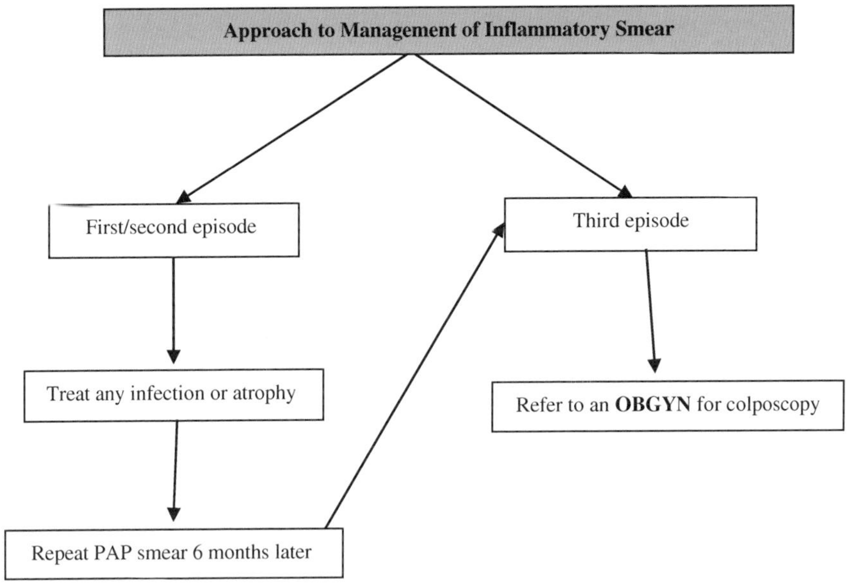

*The alternative management of an inflammatory smear is to add on an HPV test. If the HPV test is negative → return to routine cervical cancer screening.

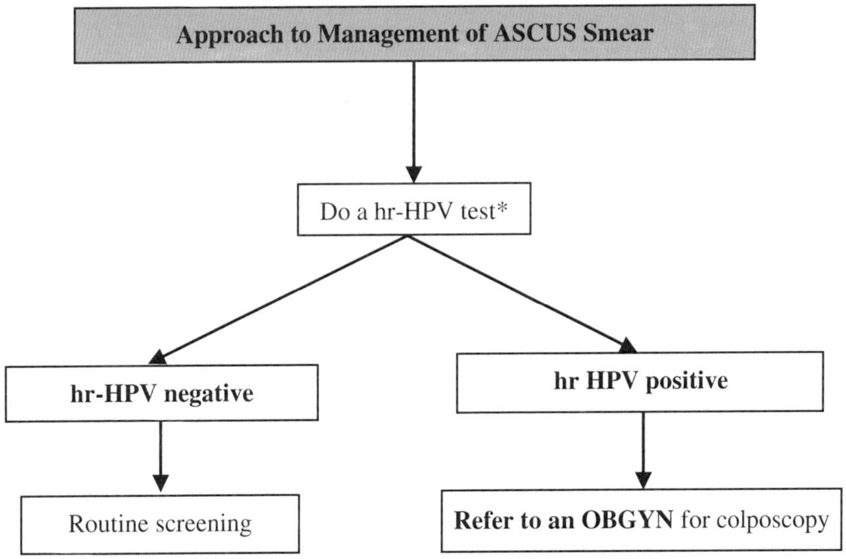

*If <30 years old, repeat Pap smear in 6 months instead. If persistent ASCUS, refer for colposcopy. If smear is negative, follow routine screening.

Approach to Management of Endometrial Cells on PAP Smear

↓

Correlate with age, last menstrual period (LMP) and risk factors for endometrial hyperplasia/cancer, e.g., high bodymass index (BMI), abnormal uterine bleeding, anovulatory cycles, family history of cancer

↓

- Age ≥45 years or <45 years with risk factors for endometrial hyperplasia/malignancy
- History of intermenstrual or post-coital bleeding
- PAP smear taken >12 days of LMP

↓

Refer to an OBGYN for endometrial evaluation

Approach to Management of Atrophic Smear

↓ If symptomatic (post-menopausal bleeding and cancer have been excluded)

Vagifem pessary every night for 2 weeks, then weekly for 3 months

↓

If asymptomatic, for routine screening

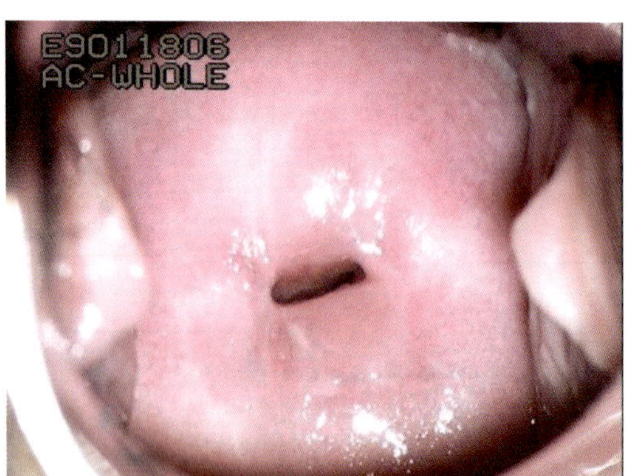

Fig. 38.10 Atrophic cervix, showing the squamocolumnar junction retracted into the endocervix.

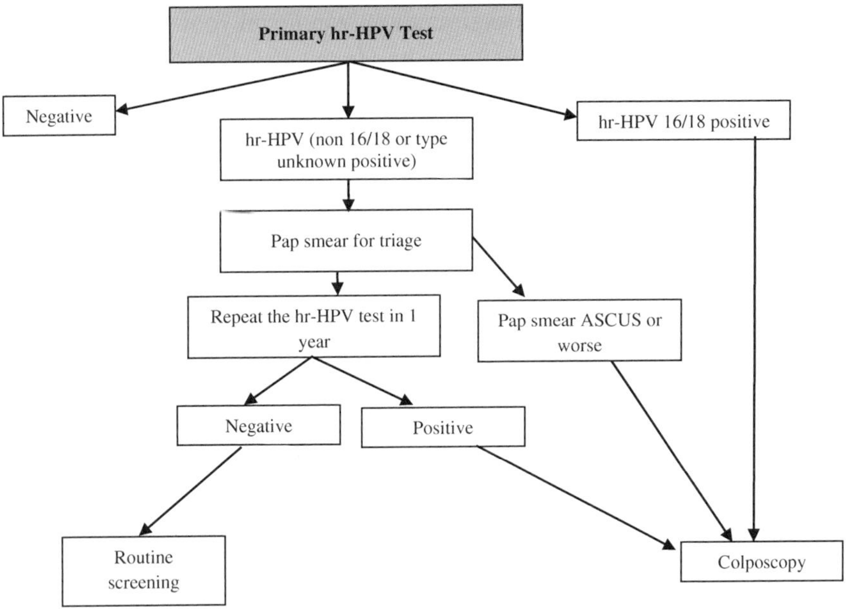

Referral Criteria for Colposcopy

- Any single smear showing mild/moderate/severe dyskaryosis
- Any smear suggestive of glandular abnormality
- hr-HPV positive with the second unsatisfactory smear
- Three consecutive inflammatory smears
- Two consecutive ASCUS smears or one ASCUS smear with hr-HPV positive
- Any positive smear suggestive of malignancy
- History of postcoital bleeding
- Abnormal looking cervix
- HPV 16/18 positive
- Others hr-HPV positive with Pap smear ≥ ASCUS
- Persistent other hr-HPV types positive with a normal Pap smear

What is Colposcopy? How to Explain It to Our Patients?

- It is a simple outpatient procedure.
- A colposcope is an instrument that shines a beam of light on the neck of the womb (cervix) and magnifies the view.

- At the beginning of the examination, you lie on your back and place your feet in the stirrups as you would for a Pap smear. Next, the doctor inserts a speculum into your vagina and opens it to visualise your cervix.
- Then, the doctor applies a vinegar solution (acetic acid) to the cervix and vagina with a cotton ball. The vinegar will make abnormal tissues white so that the doctor can identify the abnormal areas that may need further evaluation.
- If the doctor detects areas of abnormal tissue, he or she will perform a biopsy.
- A specialist doctor called a pathologist will then examine these samples.

Management of CIN

- Patients with low-grade CIN have options of close observation or treatment.
- Patients with high-grade CIN are usually treated.

Management of CIN 1

Counselling on the natural history of the disease

- Low pre-malignant potential
- Virtually all women with LSIL have a HPV infection
- 70% revert to normal after 1 year
- ~10% progress to carcinoma-in-situ
- 1% progress to malignancy
- Lesions less likely to regress in immunocompromised patients
- *Management* — either observation or treatment
- *Treatment* — excision/ablation

Management of CIN 2 or CIN 3

- At least 30–50% progression to malignancy after 10 years.
- The optimal treatment for CIN 2 in young women under 25 years old is controversial. Their spontaneous regression rate is higher, about 50–60%, within 3 years. Hence, observation is a possible option.

Overview of Treatment Options for CIN

CIN can be treated by the following methods, as appropriate:

(a) Ablation of the Cervix

- Laser vaporisation of the cervix
- Cryotherapy
- After treatment, there are limited data regarding the optimal duration before the patient should try to conceive. Generally, it is advised to wait for 3–6 months before trying to conceive.
- **Total hysterectomy for CIN** can be performed if there is co-existing gynaecological pathology, e.g., symptomatic uterine fibroids and endometrial hyperplasia, or for women who declined follow-up, ablative or excisional treatment.
- AIS or suspected AIS is a precursor to cervical adenocarcinoma.
- If AIS is diagnosed on a cervical biopsy, an excisional procedure is required to rule out any invasive disease. This is usually performed via a cold knife cone biopsy rather than a LEEP to avoid cautery effects affecting the margins and obscuring the diagnosis.
- **Total hysterectomy is the preferred treatment for AIS** if the patient does not want fertility.

  For patients who wish to conserve fertility, it depends on the margins of the cone specimen. However, they should be counselled on the need for compliance with long-term follow-up, the risk of recurrence of AIS and progression to adenocarcinoma.

(b) Excision of the Cervix

- LEEP/LLETZ — loop electrosurgical excision procedure/large loop excision of the TZ
- Laser cone biopsy
- Knife cone biopsy
- Needle cone biopsy

(c) Hysterectomy

- Indicated in women with positive margins post-excision of the cervix who are postmenopausal/do not desire future fertility

- In women with CIN and co-existing gynaecological pathology who require a hysterectomy

Summary of Treatment Methods for CIN

(a) Loop Electrosurgical Excision Procedure/Large Loop Excision of TZ (LEEP/LLETZ)

- TZ excised, depth depends on the type of TZ
  - *Type 1 TZ*: depth of 7–10 mm
  - *Type 2 TZ*: depth of 10–15 mm
  - *Type 3 TZ*: depth of 15–25 mm
- Provides tissue diagnosis
- Easy to perform, done in the outpatient setting
- Well tolerated by patients, low morbidity, high patient acceptability
- Success rates: 90–96%

Procedure

- Excise TZ with high current using a thin electrode.
- The size and shape of the loop should be tailored to the size and extent of TZ and extension to the endocervical canal.

Complications of LEEP/LLETZ

- Intraoperative and postoperative bleeding, vaginal discharge, infection
- Uterine perforation
- Injury to surrounding structures, e.g., bladder, ureters, bowels, vagina
- Cervical stenosis (1–8%)
- Cervical incompetence: increases the risk of subsequent miscarriage, especially second-trimester pregnancy loss, preterm labour (PTL), premature rupture of membranes (PROM) and low-birth-weight (LBW) infants. The risk increases with a depth of more than 15 mm.

Contraindications of LEEP

- Active cervical, vaginal and pelvic infection
- Pregnancy unless there is suspicion of invasive malignancy
- Suspected adenocarcinoma *in situ*, microinvasive or malignancy due to risk of thermal artefacts (relative contraindication)

(b) Cone Biopsy

Indications

- Cytologic abnormality *not* consistent with histological diagnosis
- Unsatisfactory colposcopy
- Microinvasion on biopsy, to rule out invasive cancer
- AIS

Methods:

- Cold knife cone biopsy
- Laser cone biopsy
- Needle cone biopsy

Complications of Cone Biopsy

- Intraoperative and postoperative bleeding, vaginal discharge, infection
- Uterine perforation
- Injury to surrounding structures, e.g., bladder, ureters, bowels, vagina
- Cervical stenosis (1–8%)
- Cervical incompetence: increases the risk of subsequent miscarriage, especially second-trimester pregnancy loss, PTL, PROM and LBW infants. The risk increases with a depth of more than 15 mm.

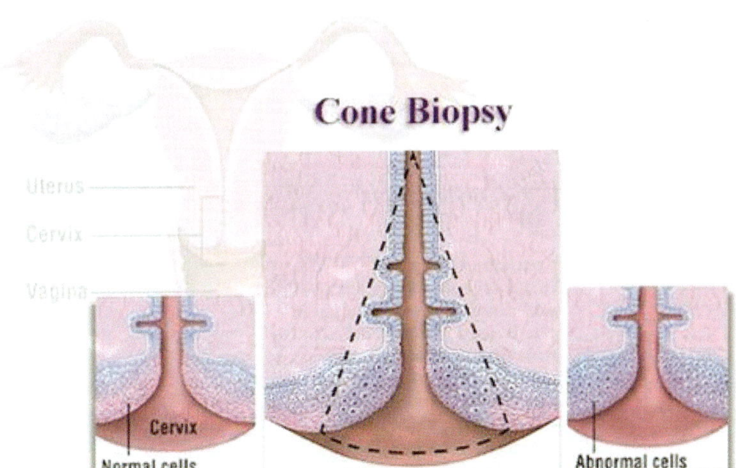

Fig. 38.11 Cone biopsy of the cervix.

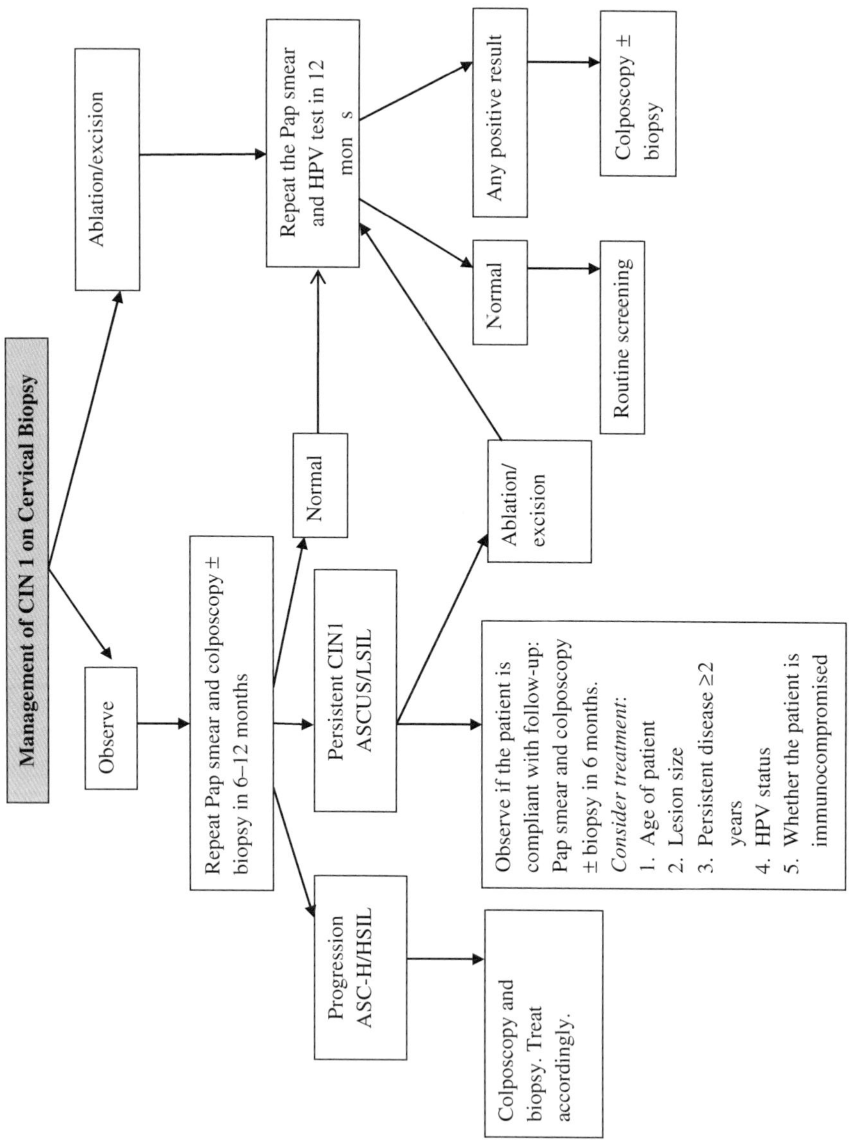
Management of CIN 1 on Cervical Biopsy
Ablation/excision
Observe
Repeat Pap smear and colposcopy ± biopsy in 6–12 months
Normal
Persistent CIN1 ASCUS/LSIL
Progression ASC-H/HSIL
Repeat the Pap smear and HPV test in 12 mon s
Ablation/ excision
Colposcopy and biopsy. Treat accordingly.
Observe if the patient is compliant with follow-up: Pap smear and colposcopy ± biopsy in 6 months.
Consider treatment:
1. Age of patient
2. Lesion size
3. Persistent disease ≥2 years
4. HPV status
5. Whether the patient is immunocompromised
Normal
Any positive result
Routine screening
Colposcopy ± biopsy

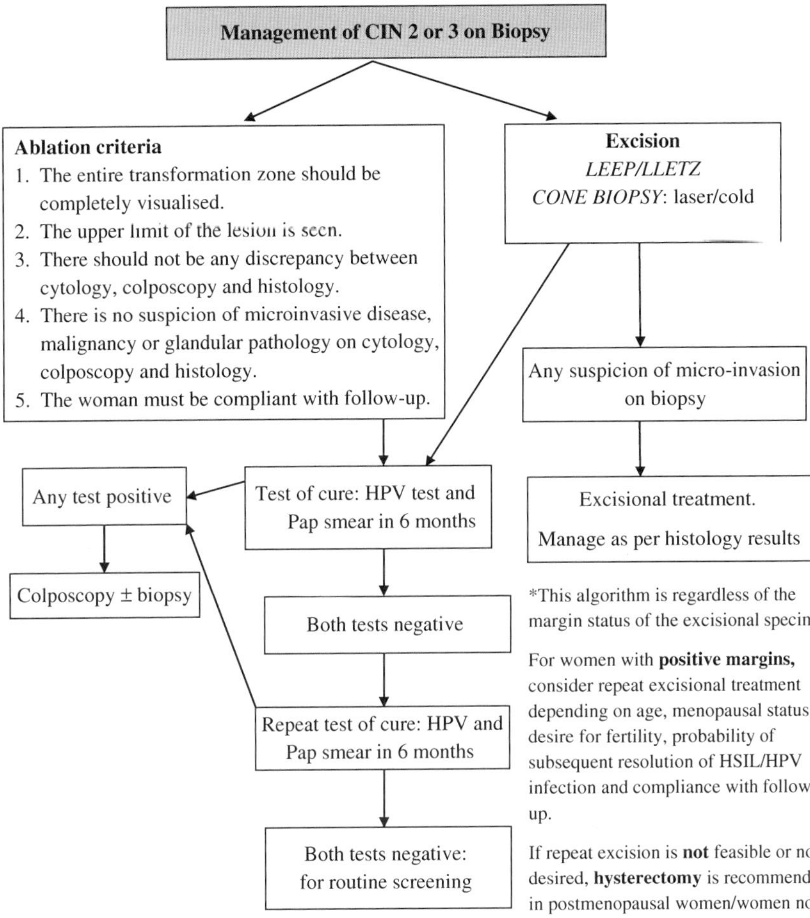

*This algorithm is regardless of the margin status of the excisional specimen.

For women with **positive margins,** consider repeat excisional treatment depending on age, menopausal status, desire for fertility, probability of subsequent resolution of HSIL/HPV infection and compliance with follow-up.

If repeat excision is **not** feasible or not desired, **hysterectomy** is recommended in postmenopausal women/women not desiring fertility.

Atypical Glandular Cells (AGC)

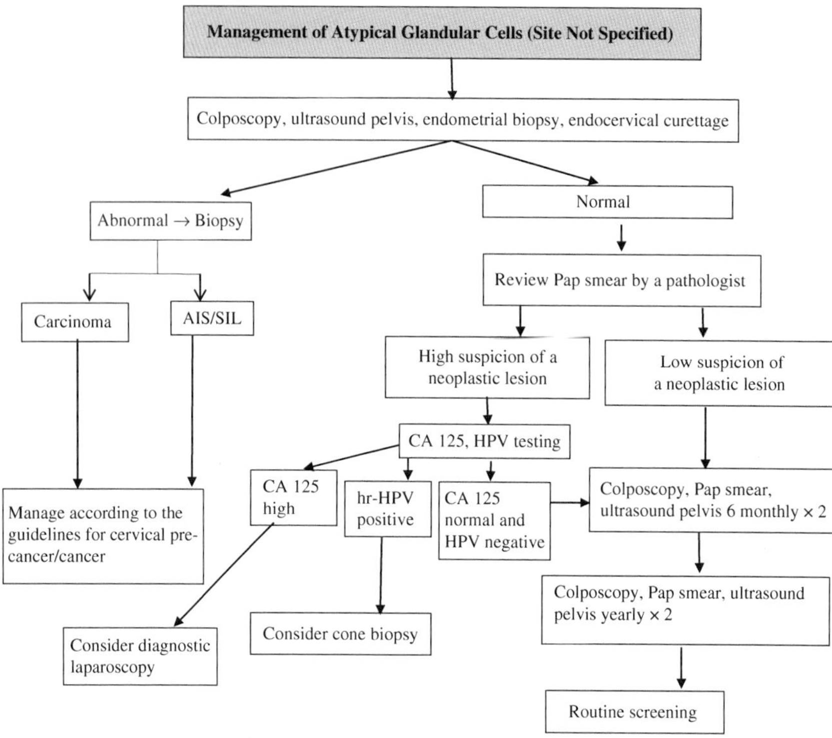

AGUS – Atypical glandular cells of undetermined significance
AIS – Adenocarcinoma *in situ*
ECC – Endocervical curettings
SIL – Squamous intra-epithelial lesion

Adenocarcinoma *in situ* (AIS)

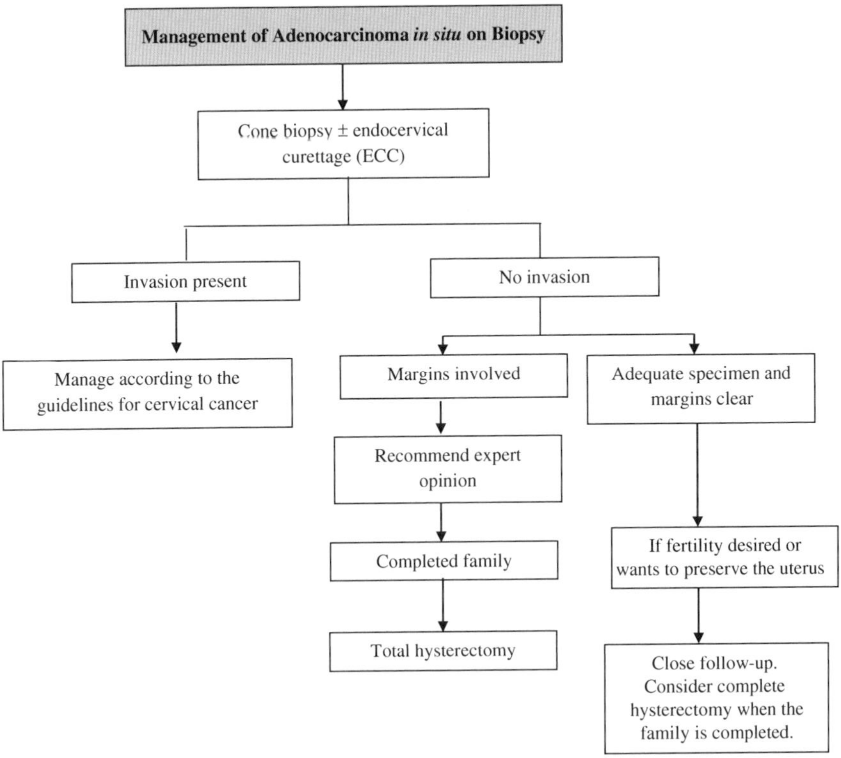

Note: For excisional biopsy for adenocarcinoma *in situ*, a single large specimen with clear margins is necessary for adequate histopathological interpretation. A cold knife cone under anaesthesia was preferred over LEEP because of the concern that a cautery defect could obscure the diagnosis. However, a meta-analysis showed no difference in residual disease or recurrence risk. The American Society for Colposcopy and Cervical Pathology (ASCCP) guidance is that diagnostic excision can be performed using any modality as long as the specimen is a single, intact specimen to ensure margins are interpretable and to avoid fragmentation of the specimen. The depth of excision should be at least 10 mm, increasing to 18–20 mm for patients *not* keen on future fertility.

CHAPTER 39

Postcoital Bleeding (PCB)

Causes of Postcoital Bleeding (PCB)

Benign Causes

- Cervical ectropion/polyps
- Infection: cervicitis (Figure 39.1), e.g., chlamydia (most common), bacterial vaginosis, pelvic inflammatory disease, endometritis
- Atrophic vaginitis
- Genital prolapse — secondary to ulceration
- Benign vascular neoplasms e.g., haemangioma/arteriovenous malformation
- Trauma/lacerations
- Granulation tissues at the site of previous injuries/surgery
- Vulvar dermatitis/inflammatory conditions, e.g., lichen sclerosus, lichen planus

Premalignant/Malignant Causes

- Cervical cancer (Figures 39.2 and 39.3)/cervical intra-epithelial neoplasia (CIN)
- Endometrial cancer/hyperplasia
- Vulvar/vaginal intra-epithelial neoplasia (VIN/VAIN)/malignancy

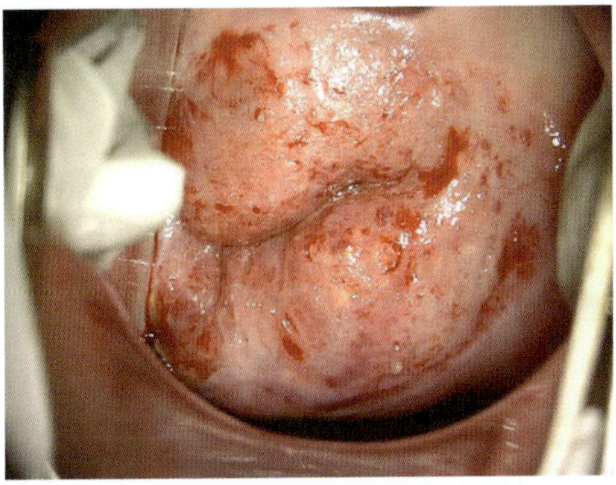

Fig. 39.1 Atrophic cervicitis, showing petechial haemorrhages and contact bleeding.

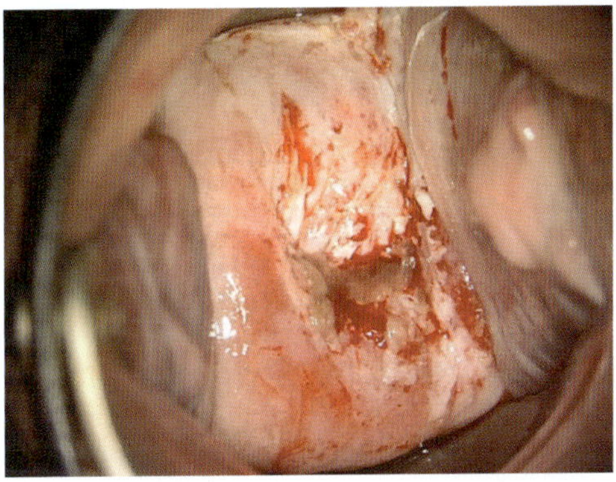

Fig. 39.2 Early cancer of the cervix. Note the eroded surface and contact bleeding.

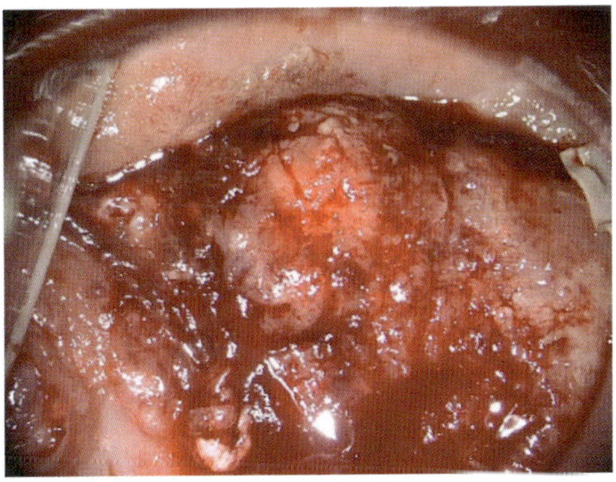

Fig. 39.3 Advanced cancer of the cervix occupying the entire cervix and extending to the vagina.

Approach to Management of Postcoital Bleeding

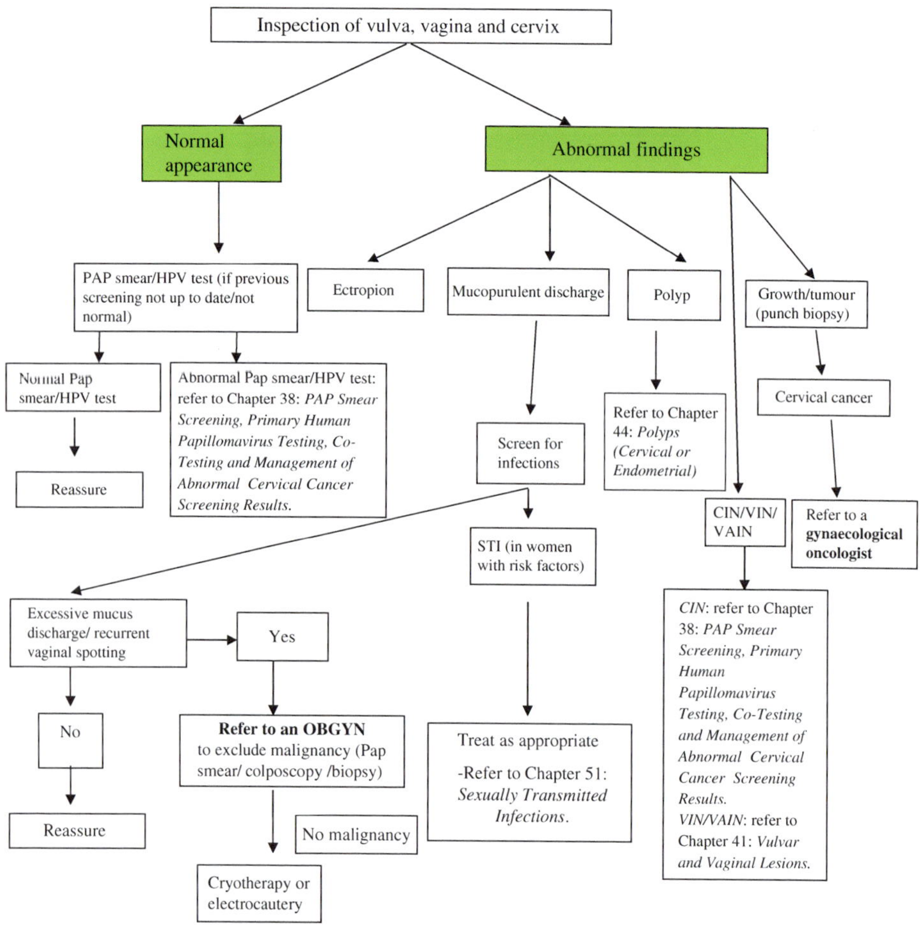

Note: If PCB is persistent, refer for colposcopy and evaluation of the endometrium.

CHAPTER 40

Human Papillomavirus Vaccines

Human Papillomavirus (HPV) Vaccination (Inactivated Vaccine)

- Two brands of HPV vaccines are available in Singapore: Cervarix® and Gardasil®.
- The two types of Gardasil vaccines available are Gardasil® 4 and Gardasil® 9.
- The latest HPV vaccine currently available is Gardasil® 9.
- Both Cervarix® and Gardasil® vaccines protect against high-risk HPV (hr-HPV) 16 and 18.
- They are prophylactic and *not* therapeutic vaccines. They are indicated for the prevention of premalignant and malignant cervical, vaginal, vulvar and anal conditions caused by the hr-HPV strains.

  The following are the differences between the two brands of HPV vaccines:
  1. Cervarix® contains a proprietor adjuvant, ASO4, which induces greater immunogenic responses, resulting in higher antibody titres against HPV 16 and 18. However, it is unsure whether higher antibody titres affect the degree and duration of protection.
  2. Both Gardasil® vaccines protect against HPV 6 and 11, which are responsible for 90% of genital warts.
  3. Gardasil® 9 provides the widest protection against nine HPV strains, i.e., HPV types 6, 11, 16, 18, 31, 33, 45, 52 and 58.
- *Dosages of vaccines*
  - *For ≥15 years old*: both vaccines are given in three doses.
  - *For 9–14 years old*: both vaccines are given in two doses.
  - *Cervarix®*: **Three doses** at 0, 1 and 6 months, **two doses** at 5–13 months apart.

- *Gardasil® 4 and 9*: **Three doses** at 0, 2 and 6 months, **two doses**: 6–12 months apart.

- The vaccines have very good safety profiles.
- *Common side effects* include pain, swelling, itch, redness at the injection site, fever, headache, muscle ache, joint pain, nausea and abdominal pain.
- *Severe side effects* such as allergic reactions or anaphylaxis are rare.
- Under the National School-based HPV programme, the Health Promotion Board offers fully subsidised HPV vaccination to all Secondary 1 female students between 12 and 13 years old.

  The vaccine used is Cervarix® and consists of two doses for this group of students.

Common Guidelines for Vaccination of Women

- HPV vaccines are most effective when given before the onset of sexual activity.
- They are recommended between 9 and 26 years of age.
- Vaccinated women should continue with routine cervical cancer screening.
- Women 27 years old and above have been shown to exhibit strong immune serological responses and demonstrated vaccine efficacy against HPV-related infection or CIN.
- HPV vaccines are licensed for use up to 45 years old.
- Those who are sexually active and may have been exposed to some strains of HPV may still benefit from the vaccines. They prevent infection with other types of HPV that the person has *not* had and prevent reinfection with the same type if the person already has an HPV infection.
- Likewise, women with current or prior HPV infection or CIN can also benefit from the vaccines against any of the HPV types with which they are *not* currently infected.
- The HPV vaccine is made of viral-like protein. It does *not* contain any HPV virion or DNA.
- There is *no evidence* for re-vaccination or booster doses.

- Women who are immunocompromised, e.g., those who are on steroids or have HIV infection, may be vaccinated, but their immune response to the vaccine may be poorer.

Missed doses

- There is *no need* to restart the entire vaccination schedule, regardless of any length of time, but there *should not* be a delay of more than 12 months between the second and third doses.
- The same vaccine should be used to complete the series. However, if the initial HPV vaccine used is not available or unknown, a different HPV vaccine can be used to complete the series.

Vaccination of Males

- Males can be vaccinated on request.
- Vaccination of males protects them against cancers caused by hr-HPV, such as anal, oropharyngeal or penile cancers. Gardasil® vaccines also protect them against genital warts.
- Male vaccination can induce herd immunity, and vaccinating both men and women have been shown to be more effective in reducing HPV infections and disease.
- The Advisory Committee on Immunisation Practices (ACIP) in the United States recommends HPV vaccination for males between 9 and 26 years old.
- In the United Kingdom, the HPV vaccine is available for males 12–25 years old and men who have sex with men (MSM) up to 45 years old.

CHAPTER 41

Vulvar and Vaginal Lesions

Vulvar Disorders

General Principles of Evaluation and Management of Vulvar Disorders

Evaluation of Vulva Disorders

1. ***Detailed history***
   Address the ideas, concerns and expectations of the patient.
   Address anxiety/psychosexual dysfunction/fear of malignancy/fear of sexually transmitted infections (STIs).
2. ***Examination***
   Proper positioning and exposure: Exaggerated lithotomy position to expose the perineum.
   Good illumination and magnification.
   Naked-eye inspection and inspection under magnification.
   Examination of the extragenital skin, perianal area and natal cleft, vagina and cervix.
   Palpation: Feel for induration. Perform a digital rectal examination.
   Photo documentation.
3. ***Investigations***
   Swabs, smears, serology and histology.
4. ***Patient education and information***

Management Principles

- Control secondary infection by oral antibiotics.
- Oral antifungals when necessary.
- Reduce irritation on the vulva (do not prescribe multiple creams).
- Night sedation for pruritic vulvar conditions.

- Topical oestrogens for atrophy.
- Follow up for flares and side effects of medication.
- Persistent Bartholin cysts, even if asymptomatic in postmenopausal women, warrant removal as the risk of malignancy is higher.
- Pigmented lesions — perform excision biopsy with at least a 2–3 mm margin.
- Remove all vulvar lumps with clear margins as they are potentially malignant; mesenchymal tumours may look benign.
- Patients with severe pain and burning sensation at the introitus and vestibule will need a prompt referral to the vulva clinic to exclude erosive vulvar disease.
- All pigmented lesions, including crusty white lesions (hyperkeratosis) of the vulva, should be biopsied.

***Topical corticosteroids*:**

- The mainstay of treatment for dermatoses.
- Ointments are stronger than cream, are less irritating, have fewer allergens and have a longer duration of action.
- Steroids are anti-inflammatory and control symptoms.
- Maintenance steroids always have low potency and are for intermittent use.
- Vulvar mucous membrane (vulvar trigone and inner labia minora) is steroid resistant. Inter-labial sulcus, labiocrural folds and thighs will thin easily and develop striae.
- Ultra-potent steroids should be used under close supervision for a shorter duration.
- Prescribe systemic steroids rather than topical steroids for painful ulcers and erosions as initial treatment when indicated.

***Side effects of corticosteroids*:**

- Hypertension.
- May worsen diabetic control.
- Secondary infection — candidiasis.
- Glaucoma.
- Atrophy/striae.
- Caution — systemic absorption from the vagina is high.

Alternatives to Corticosteroids

Calcineurin inhibitors:

- The main use is for maintenance of steroid-responsive dermatoses.
- They are topical immunosuppressants, are non-steroidal and do not cause atrophy.
- Pimecrolimus (Elidel) 1% cream: Equivalent to a mild topical steroid.
- Tacrolimus (Protopic) 0.03% and 0.1% ointment: Equivalent to a moderate to strong topical steroid.

***Side effects of calcineurin inhibitors*:**

- Burning, stinging sensation.
- Worsening of herpes simplex virus (HSV), human papillomavirus (HPV) and tinea infections.

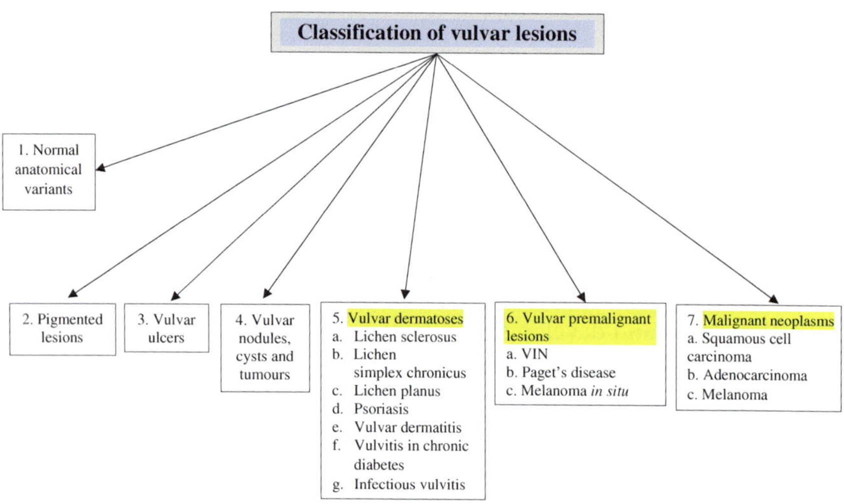

Vulvar Conditions

Normal Anatomical Variants

No treatment required.

(a) ***Vestibular papillomatosis*:**

30% of women.

Few to hundreds of lesions.

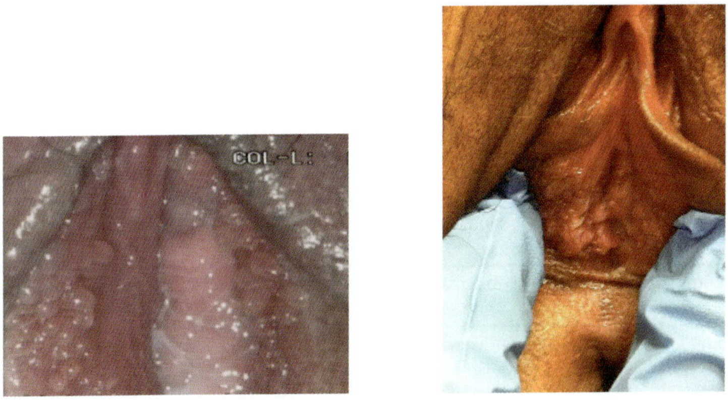

Fig. 41.1 Vestibular papillomatosis.

Asymptomatic, 2–10 mm lesions.
Homogeneous, skin-coloured, separate base.
Dome-shaped, cobblestone-like.

(b) ***Sebaceous gland hyperplasia*:**
Fordyce spots.
Enlarged ectopic sebaceous glands.
Inner labia minora.
Yellowish white.
Asymptomatic, 1–2 mm lesions.

Vulvar Pigmented Lesions

Genital tissue has a higher density of melanocytes than the rest of the body and is hormone-dependent. Hormone levels change during pregnancy and with contraceptive use.

Condition	Location and description of the lesion	Treatment
Physiological pigmentation	Posterior introitus, the tips of the labia minora, labia majora, perineum and proximal medial thighs. Macular and symmetric, no change in texture from the normal skin. Asymptomatic.	Reassurance.
Acanthosis nigricans	Genitocrural folds and the upper inner aspect of the thighs. Dark and velvety thickening of the skin.	Treat the primary cause, e.g., diabetes, obesity.

(Continued)

(*Continued*)

Condition	Location and description of the lesion	Treatment
Pigmented basal cell carcinoma (BCC)	Common on labia majora. Ulcer, nodule or plaque. Brown/black.	Wide local excision (WLE).
Pigmented condylomata acuminata (anogenital warts)	Anywhere on the vulva. A biopsy is required to exclude vulvar intraepithelial neoplasia (VIN) if warts appear atypical.	– Excision. – Laser vaporisation. – Liquid nitrogen. – Imiquimod.
Post-inflammatory hyperpigmentation	Labia majora secondary to scratching and excoriation.	Treat the primary cause.
Melanoma 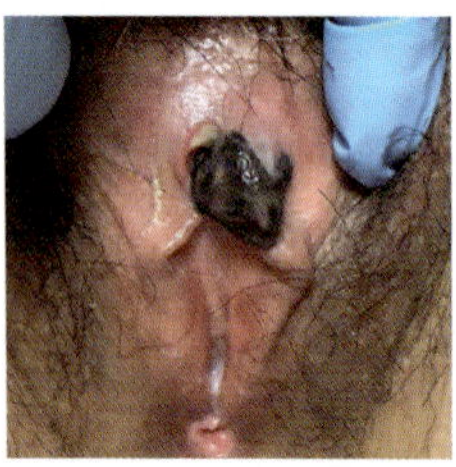	Anywhere on the vulva. Malignant neoplasm of melanocytes. Pigmented papule or nodule with asymmetry in colour or variability, border irregularity, surface ulceration or bleeding. The photo shows a nodular melanoma with variegated colour, blue-black, with ulceration and necrosis.	**Refer to a gynaecological oncologist.**
Seborrhoeic keratoses 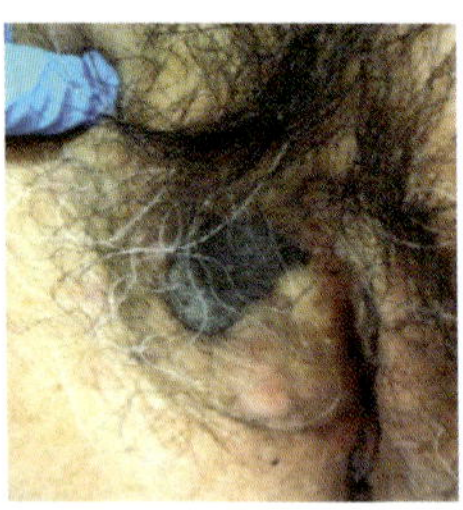	Hair-bearing areas, labia minora very common. They are benign, warty-surfaced pigmented growths. They can be flat-topped, sharply demarcated, brown or dark brown lesions with a stuck-on appearance.	No treatment is required if asymptomatic. Excision biopsy if the diagnosis is uncertain.
Vulvar melanosis/ lentiginosis	Brown-black, patchy hyperpigmentation.	No treatment required. Biopsy if the diagnosis is uncertain.
Melanocytic naevus 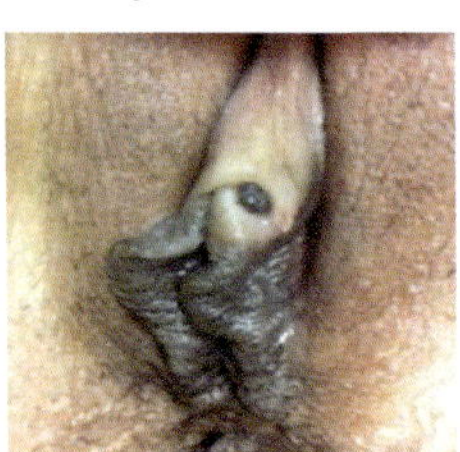	A small, circumscribed, pigmented papule made up of nests of melanocytic cells. It is a benign lesion.	No treatment required.

(*Continued*)

Condition	Location and description of the lesion	Treatment
Vulvar Intraepithelial neoplasia (VIN) 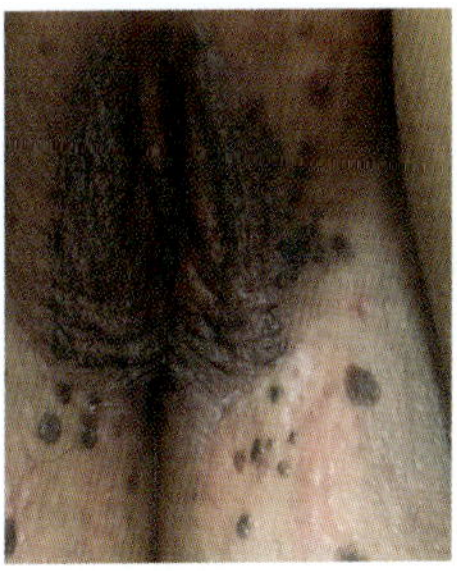 Bowenoid papulosis	Any area on the vulva and perianal area. Red, brown or white flat-topped papules and plaques. Bowenoid papulosis represents vulvar hSIL related to the oncogenic high-risk HPV. The lesion appears as multiple bilateral pigmented papules.	*VIN1* — no treatment is required. *VIN2 and VIN3* — refer to a gynae for management of VIN 2–3.

Vulvar Ulcers

Diagnostic challenge.

Ulcers should be differentiated from erosions.

1. *Erosions* involve the loss of the epidermis only — appear deep red, weeping. E.g., HSV, contact dermatitis, excoriated eczema.
2. *Ulcers* involve the loss of the epidermis and dermis. They are deeper and have a yellowish base. E.g., aphthous ulcer.

Common Causes of Vulvar Ulcers

Infective	Inflammatory	Neoplastic	Traumatic
STI — refer to Chapter 51: *Sexually Transmitted Infections*. Mycoplasma Herpes ***Non-STI*** Hand, foot and mouth disease Candida Staphylococcus Streptococcus Tuberculosis Actinomycosis	Aphthous ulcers Behcet's disease Crohn's disease Pemphigus vulgaris Pemphigoid *Drug reactions*, e.g., toxic epidermal necrolysis and erythema multiforme	VIN BCC SCC Extramammary Paget disease Melanoma Lymphoma Leukaemia	Female genital mutilation (FGM) Excoriations, fissures, ulceration secondary to itchy skin conditions

Management of Vulvar Ulcers

***History*:**

Sexual history.
Ulcer location.
Pain and severity.
Ulcer development (vesicle–erosion–ulcer).
Are there any associated skin, oral or ocular lesions?
Is the lesion primary or recurrent?
Any tender groin nodes or vaginal discharge?
History of viral infections and fever.
Systemic symptoms (fever, headache, gastrointestinal tract, respiratory, myalgia).
History of autoimmune disorders.

***Examination*:**

Skin, oral mucosa, eyes.
Lymphadenopathy (cervical/inguinal/femoral).
Size, shape, location of vulvar ulcer(s).
Examination of the vagina and cervix.

***Laboratory evaluation*:**

***All vulvar ulcers need HSV PCR on the first visit regardless of sexual history*:**

- Full blood count.
- Bacterial culture.
- Serology for HIV, syphilis.
- Serology for EBV, CMV, mycoplasma, antistreptolysin O titres (ASO) (based on the clinical situation).
- If the STI screen is negative and the patient still has recurrent vulvar ulcers, perform:
  - ANA (autoimmune workup).
  - Gastrointestinal tract (GIT) investigations for inflammatory conditions (based on the clinical situation).

***General principles of treatment of vulvar ulcers*:**

- General vulvar hygiene — educate the patient.
- Sitz bath with warm water.
- Zinc oxide barrier cream.

- Topical anaesthetics.
- Oral analgesics (NSAIDs) for mild pain.
- Opioids for severe pain.
- Oral fluconazole for secondary yeast infection.
- Antibiotics for secondary bacterial infection.

***Specific treatment of vulvar ulcers*:**

Antiviral: Acyclovir if HSV is the likely diagnosis.

Steroids: Consider topical corticosteroids for aphthous ulcers.

Antibiotics: If bacterial infection suspected.

Treatment of STIs (CDC guidelines — refer to Chapter 51: *Sexually Transmitted Infections*).

Immunosuppressants: (Behcet disease, inflammatory bowel disease and other suspected rheumatological conditions) in consultation with the relevant specialists.

Aphthous ulcers (Fig. 41.2) — Diagnosis of exclusion.
Painful, deep ulcers.
History of recurrence.

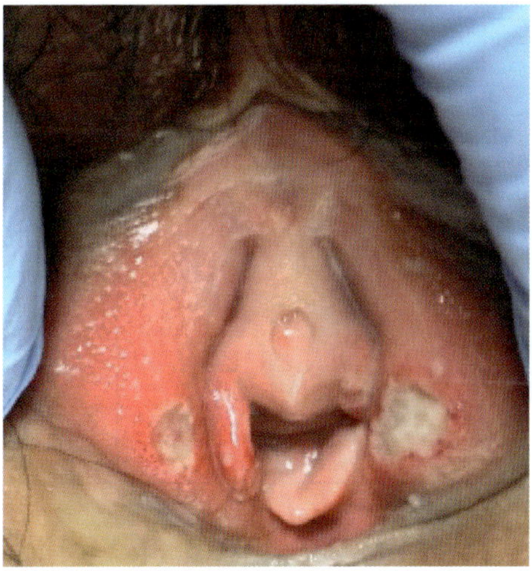

Fig. 41.2 Aphthous ulcers of the vulva: Sudden onset punched-out, shallow, well-defined acute painful ulcers.

Single or multiple.
Culture negative.
Biopsies are non-specific.
Test for HIV — **Note:** in HIV patients with genital ulcers — 60% of genital ulcers are due to aphthous ulcers and 40% due to HSV.

Treatment of aphthous ulcers:
Steroids: Topical, intralesional or oral.
Acute onset and painful lesions — prednisolone 40–60 mg daily for 3–5 days and taper depending on the response.
Pain relief.

Recurrent and recalcitrant ulcers (under specialist supervision):
Colchicine 0.6 mg BD to TDS.
Dapsone 50–150 mg per day.
Colchicine + dapsone together.
Thalidomide 100–150 mg per day.

Vulvar Nodules, Cysts or Tumours

Condyloma acuminatum (HPV 6, 11)	Warty surface, variable size, shape and location. Colposcopy. Examine the vagina and cervix. Do a Pap smear.	Imiquimod. Excision, laser vaporisation, liquid nitrogen.
Molluscum contagiosum (pox virus)	Umbilicated papules. Commonly multiple and in children.	Self-limiting. Local excision, electrocautery, cryotherapy or laser therapy.
Keratinocyte tumour: Epidermal inclusion cyst, sebaceous cyst 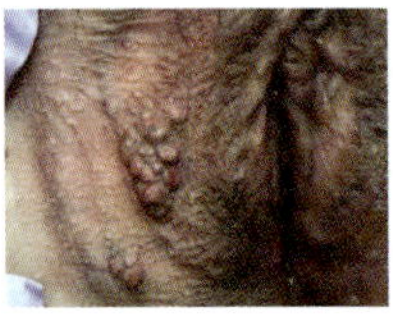 *Epidermal cysts*	Labia majora and minora. Other hair-bearing areas, yellowish papules with a visible opening. 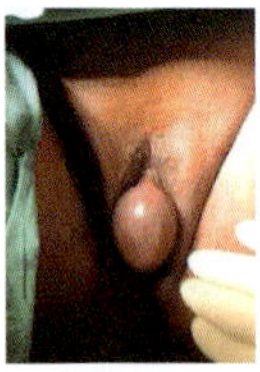 *Epidermal cyst*	Excision if symptomatic.

(*Continued*)

Keratinocyte tumour: Angiokeratoma	Purplish blue spots, bleeds on scratching.	Excision/laser vaporisation if symptomatic. All pigmented lesions need a biopsy if the clinical diagnosis is uncertain.
Keratinocyte tumour: Seborrhoeic keratoses	Brown to black, warty stuck-on appearance. **Location:** Labia majora and minora.	No treatment is required. All pigmented lesions need a biopsy if the diagnosis is uncertain.
Vulvar oedema	Lymphoedema or angioedema.	Treatment directed towards the cause.
***Mesenchymal cell origin*:** Lipoma, leiomyoma, fibroma, granular cell tumour, granular cell myoblastoma	Variable size and consistency.	Complete excision is required with a 10 mm margin.
Bartholin cyst 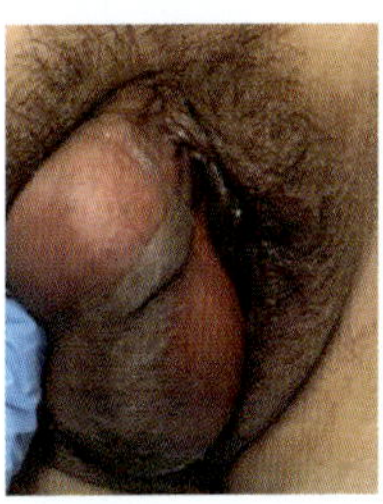	Within the posterior vestibule. Variable size. Labia minora always crosses the cyst.	Marsupialisation of cyst. Excision of the gland for recurrences. Indurated cysts in postmenopausal women need excision even if asymptomatic. *Histology* must be performed to exclude carcinoma.
Vulvar endometriosis	Biopsy of the lesion to confirm histology. Ultrasound of the pelvis to exclude endometriosis. Evaluate the menstrual history.	Offer the excision of endometriosis if symptomatic.
Fibroepithelial polyp	Pelvic examination.	If asymptomatic and <1 cm, offer conservative management. If symptomatic or ≥1 cm, offer excision.

Vulvar Dermatoses

Lesion	Presentation	Investigation	Management
Lichen sclerosus (LS) 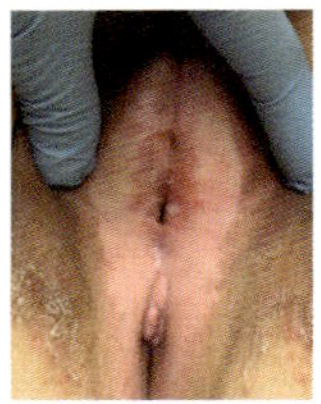 *Involves the modified mucous membrane of the vulva, usually starting in the periclitoral area, spreading to involve the entire labia minora and interlabial sulcus, and then extending down through the perineum and the perianal area, forming the typical figure-of-8 pattern.* Occurs in 1 in 300–1,000 women. Incidence peaks in pre-pubertal (3–5 years old) and postmenopausal women. Aetiology is multifactorial – 12% have a family history of LS.	**Symptoms:** Long-standing intense pruritus. Dyspareunia. Vulval soreness. 10–15% extragenital lesion on sites of friction. **Signs:** ***C****olour change*: Ivory white plaques/ hypopigmentation. ***T****exture change*: Cigarette paper-like crinkled texture, purpura and petechial haemorrhages. ***A****rchitectural loss* due to scarring and adhesions. ***I****ntegrity loss* — fissuring, excoriations, ulcers. Ecchymosis can be present. ***Classification of adhesions*** 1. Periclitoral adhesions cause the burying of the clitoris. 2. Anterior adhesions below the clitoris. 3. Posterior adhesions — posterior fourchette. Posterior band formation. 4. Lateral adhesions — adhesions between labia majora and minora, resorption of labia minora. *Is the area of the vulva involved?* Modified mucous membrane in the majority of cases. Hair-bearing skin and vulvar	Clinical diagnosis. Keyes punch biopsy. Investigations required to screen for autoimmune conditions: – Diabetes mellitus. – Thyroid dysfunction. – Pernicious anaemia. General skin examination. **When do you suspect VIN (differentiated VIN)?** – Nodule, ulceration or hyperkeratotic (dense white or leukoplakia) areas need an urgent biopsy. – ***Note:*** Differentiated VIN is associated with SCC. – Progression is very rapid. – Take multiple biopsies or wedge biopsies when differentiated VIN is suspected.	Use one fingertip unit. ***Ultra-potent steroid ointment:*** Topical clobetasol propionate 0.05% ointment daily for 1 month, alternate days for 1 month, then twice weekly for 1 month. Review in 3 months. ***Maintenance therapy*** with topical betamethasone valerate 0.05–0.1% twice or thrice a week is recommended indefinitely. Topical calcineurin inhibitors can be used as an alternative for maintenance. Night sedation. Vulva hygiene. Soap substitute/emollient as a barrier. Asymptomatic patients also need treatment (maintenance treatment should be regular regardless of symptoms rather than as-and-when-necessary basis). ***Complications:*** – Loss of sexual function. – Urinary problems due to midline fusion. – ***Vulvodynia:*** Neuropathic pain modulators may be required. – 5% risk of malignant transformation to SCC. – Loss of self-esteem/body image. If there is scarring, surgery may be required. Need to continue steroid use and dilators post-surgery.

(Continued)

Lesion	Presentation	Investigation	Management
Lichen sclerosus (LS) – Association with HLA (DQ7, A29, EYB 44). – 20% have other autoimmune conditions, e.g., vitiligo, thyroid disease, alopecia, pernicious anaemia.	vestibule are rarely involved. LS does ***not*** affect the vagina. *How is the LS distributed?* A figure-of-8 or keyhole distribution. Periclitoral perianal involvement.		**Lifelong follow-up due to the risk of malignancy (SCC) — 5%.** 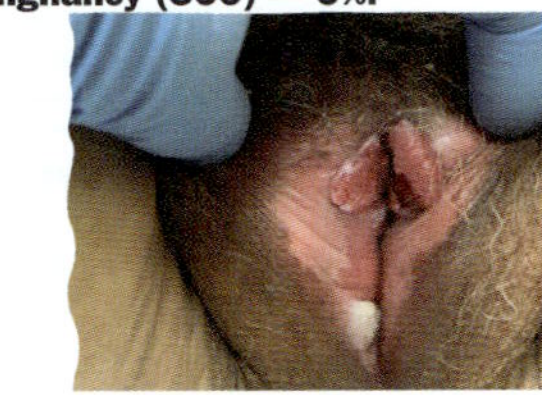 *Squamous cell carcinoma arising in the background of LS.*
Lichen simplex chronicus (LSC) 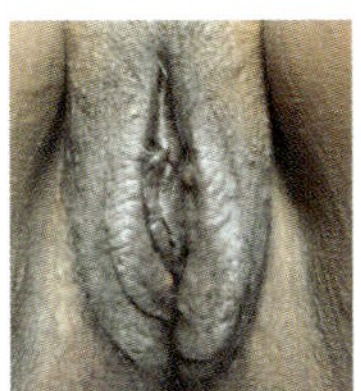 *LSC is the end stage of the itch–scratch–itch cycle. Hyperpigmented lichenified skin of labia majora.*	End-stage disorder due to the chronic itch–scratch cycle. Relentless pruritus symmetric, variable pigmentation. Leathery or coarse texture. Labia majora is commonly involved. Unilateral or bilateral.	Detailed history. Vulva biopsy to determine the underlying problem (often more than one cause). Heat, stress and menstruation worsen LSC. *Common underlying causes* are atopic and contact eczema. *Less common causes*: LS, VIN, psoriasis, candida, diabetes.	Mid- to high-potency steroids. Night sedation. Break the itch–scratch cycle. Stop irritation. Oral steroids may be required. Treat concurrent bacterial and fungal infections with oral medication. Sitz bath for inflamed and excoriated lesions.

(Continued)

(Continued)

Lesion	Presentation	Investigation	Management
Lichen planus (LP) 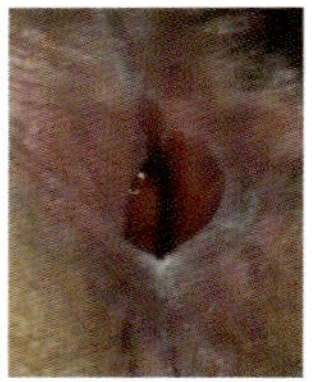 ***Erosive LP*** *of the vulva involves the vulvar vestibule causing pain, burning and irritation, resulting in scarring and loss of architecture.* 1–2% of the general population. Peak incidence in perimenopausal and postmenopausal women, very rarely in children.	Affects any mucous membranes. ***Types of LP:*** **1. *Classical cutaneous LP*** – White reticulations, violaceous papules without erosions. Usually will resolve spontaneously. – 10–15% with genital LP have cutaneous LP (wrist and ankles). **2. *Erosive LP*** – Mucous membrane LP is erosive; more commonly, the vagina (75%) and vestibule are involved. – Glossy red erosions and scarring, purulent vaginal discharge, bleeding. – Severe burning pain is predominant rather than itch. – Oral mucosa, scalp, skin, nails and eyes may be affected. **3. *Hypertrophic type*** – Thick watery plaques can become ulcerated, infected and painful. – Can be difficult to differentiate from VIN or SCC of the vulva.	Refer to the vulva clinic as it s challenging to treat and cure. Look at mouth and skin for LP. Rule out drug-induced erosions, bullous diseases such as pemphigus vulgaris and pemphigoid. Biopsy immunofluorescence if bullous diseases suspected. Refer to a gastroenterologist if the patient has gastrointestinal symptoms.	Emollients. Vaginal steroids for vaginal involvement. Vaginal dilatation for adhesions. Treatment of oral ulcers with topical steroids. *Erosive LP*: Super-potent corticosteroids. *Resistant cases need systemic steroids* (prednisone 40–60 mg/day, taper dose accordingly). Immunosuppressants are an option → patients to be followed-up by dermatologists and have close monitoring. ***Types of immunosuppressants:*** – Topical tacrolimus 0.1% or 0.03%. – Systemic: ▪ Methotrexate 7.5–15 mg PO or ▪ SC cyclosporine 3–4 mg/kg/day ▪ ***Others:*** Adalimumab, azathioprine ▪ Acitretin for hyperkeratosis. Pregnancy must be avoided for 2–3 years after acitretin. Surgery for scarring in selected cases. **Long-term follow-up for erosive vulval LP — the risk of malignancy 2–4%.**
Vulvar dermatitis *Types*: – Atopic dermatitis. – Irritant contact dermatitis. – Allergic contact dermatitis	Convex surfaces, e.g., labia majora and mons pubis, are involved. Erythema, oedema, blisters, scaling, excoriations. Search other crural folds, scalp, umbilicus, extremities.	Examine skin surfaces. Biopsy to exclude Paget disease.	Avoid allergens and irritants. Steroid ointments and emollients. Oral antihistamines to relieve pruritus. Vulva hygiene.

(Continued)

Lesion	Presentation	Investigation	Management
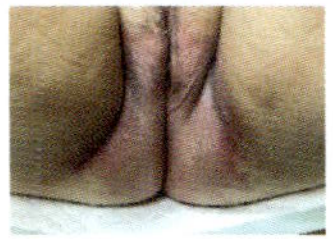 *Vulvar eczema with candidiasis in a woman with poorly controlled diabetes.*	Symmetric and extending into areas of "irritant" contact.		
Psoriasis 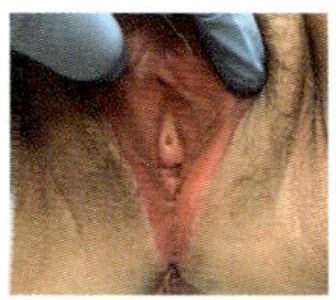	Erythema with silvery scales and well-defined margins. Scalp, nails and flexures of the body may be involved.	Biopsy elbows and knees (often affected), with greater scaling in extragenital regions. In moist flexural areas, the typical scaling of plaque psoriasis is lacking. There may be fissuring and secondary bacterial or yeast infection.	*Multidisciplinary (MDT) team care*: Refer to the vulva clinic, involving a dermatologist.
Vulvitis in chronic diabetic patients	Macerated vulva. Vulvovaginal candidiasis, folliculitis.	Biopsy suspicious lesions.	Optimise diabetes control. Vulva hygiene. Use steroids with caution.
Infectious vulvitis	Commonly candida. Consider dermatophytes (tinea cruris).	• VP3 (swab for candida, trichomonas, gardnerella). • Culture for resistant strains.	Refer to Chapter 49: *Vaginal Discharge, Vulvovaginal Candidiasis, Bacterial Vaginosis and Atrophic Vaginitis*.
Genitourinary syndrome of menopause (GSM) — previously called atrophic vaginitis, vulvovaginal atrophy or urogenital atrophy. 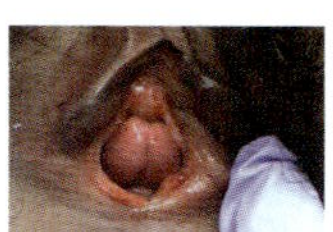	Dry, atrophic vulva/vagina. Itch.	Nil.	Topical oestrogen. Moisturisers. Perineal hygiene.

(Continued)

Vulvar Premalignant Lesions

a) VIN.
b) Paget disease.
c) Melanoma *in situ.*

Vulvar Intraepithelial Neoplasia (VIN)

2015 Nomenclature

The 2015 International Society for the Study of Vulvovaginal Disease terminology of vulvar squamous intraepithelial lesions re-classifies SIL into three main groups:

(1) Low-grade SIL of the vulva (vulvar LSIL, flat condyloma or HPV effect).
(2) High-grade SIL of the vulva (vulvar HSIL, VIN usual type).
(3) VIN, differentiated type, dVIN.

VIN usual type/HSIL	VIN differentiated type/dVIN
>90% of VIN, increasing incidence	5% of VIN
Multifocal/multicentric (HPV 16, 18, 31)	Unifocal lesions, HPV negative
Low risk of progression to SCC (5%)	High and rapid progression to SCC (>50%)
Young women	Postmenopausal women
Associated with immunosuppression, cigarette smoking	Associated with lichen sclerosus
Synchronous VAIN, CIN common	Often seen adjacent to SCC

Symptoms of VIN:
Burning and itch/irritation.
May be asymptomatic.

Signs of vulvar HSIL or usual VIN:
No specific morphology.
Papules, plaques, erosions, ulcers and warty lesions.
Can be red, white, grey-brown or black.

Differential diagnosis of VIN:
In total, 80–90% of cases are associated with LS.

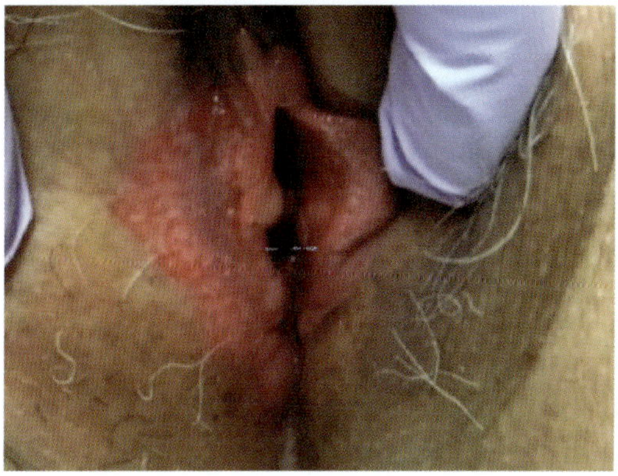

Fig. 41.3 Erythematous plaque of usual or HPV-related vulvar HSIL.

Any abnormal area in the background of LS, such as an ulcer, nodule or dense white plaque of hyperkeratosis, needs an *immediate biopsy.* Multiple biopsies or wedge biopsy is recommended as a histological diagnosis is challenging.

<u>*Diagnosis of VIN*</u> → *VIN is a histological diagnosis*:
Physical examination. Clinical suspicion and histological correlation.

Suspicious features: Hyperkeratosis, bleeding lesions, non-healing ulcers, colour change, fissures, erosions → biopsy if suspicious.
Vaginal examination.
Systematic examination of the vulva and perianal region.
Cytology, HPV testing.
Colposcopy where there is abnormal cytology to exclude VAIN and CIN.

<u>*Management of VIN*:</u>
General advice — healthy lifestyle and diet. Stop smoking.
Regular screening.
HPV vaccination.
(1) <u>***Usual VIN:***</u>
Excision

- Ablation with LASER.
    - Laser vaporisation (for multifocal and extensive lesions): 3 mm depth in hair bearing areas, 2 mm depth in non-hair-bearing areas.
- Liquid nitrogen and diathermy ablation for small lesions.

- 5% imiquimod.
- Cidofovir anti-viral.

(2) ***Differentiated VIN:***

- Wide local excision (WLE) with a 1 cm margin.
- Skinning vulvectomy.

Life-long follow-up is needed for VIN.

Extramammary Paget Disease (EMPD)

EMPD is a *rare* intraepithelial adenocarcinoma that frequently presents in areas where apocrine sweat glands are abundant.

Most commonly affects the vulva and perineum in females.

Proposed classification of EMPD vulva (Wilkinson et al.)

Primary cutaneous EMPD:

Intra-epithelial EMPD with no invasion.
Intra-epithelial EMPD with invasion.
EMPD with underlying primary adenocarcinoma of a skin appendage.

Secondary vulvar Paget disease:

EMPD secondary to anal or rectal adenocarcinoma.
EMPD secondary to urothelial neoplasm.
EMPD secondary to tumours of other sites.

Symptoms of EMPD:

Pruritus.
Soreness.
Bleeding.
Eczematous lesions *not* responding to topical steroids.
Itch is usually longer duration, from a few months to a few years.

Signs of EMPD:

Eczematous, erythematous plaques with a variable degree of scaling and a sharply demarcated border.
Any area on the vulva, groin and perianal area is involved.

Tip:

Red and white lesions.
Red sea with white islands (areas of erosions and hyperkeratosis).

Diagnosis — Keyes punch biopsy at least 4 mm deep.
Note: Always take a biopsy from nodular areas. Take more than one biopsy. Keyes punch biopsies cannot rule out early dermal invasion as multiple different foci of invasion are common.

Management of EMPD:

1. *Investigations* to detect associated adenocarcinoma (location dependent).
   Pap smear/mammogram.
   Staging computer tomography scan of the thorax, abdomen and pelvis (CTTAP).
   Urine cytology and cystoscopy if the lesion is close to the urethra.
   Colonoscopy in all perianal EMPD.

2. *Treatment of* ***EMPD.***
   A. Surgery
   WLE with full-thickness skin to the subcutaneous fat. There should be a 2–3 cm margin (traditional).
   More conservative excision to avoid mutilating surgery is advised.
   Margin positivity >50%.
   B. Medications
   5% imiquimod cream 2–3 times a week for ≥16 weeks for patients who are *not* suitable for surgery.
   No internationally agreed-upon guidelines are available.
   C. Radiation therapy
   For selected cases where surgery is *not* feasible and resistant to imiquimod.

3. Regular lifelong follow-up. Continue cancer screening as per guidelines.

Vulvar Pain

2015 ISSVD Consensus Terminology and Classification of Persistent Vulvar Pain.

A. Vulvar pain caused by a specific disorder*:

Infectious (e.g., recurrent candidiasis, herpes).
Inflammatory (e.g., LS, LP, immunobullous disorders).
Neoplastic (e.g., Paget disease, squamous cell carcinoma).

Neurologic (e.g., post-herpetic neuralgia, nerve compression or injury, neuroma).
Trauma (e.g., female genital mutilation, obstetrical).
Iatrogenic (e.g., post-operative, chemotherapy, radiation).
Hormonal deficiencies, e.g., genito-urinary syndrome of menopause (previously known as vulvo-vaginal atrophy), lactational amenorrhoea.

B. Vulvodynia — *vulvar pain of at least 3 months duration,* ***without*** *a clearly identifiable cause, which may have potential associated factors.*

Descriptors:

- *Localised (e.g., vestibulodynia, clitorodynia) or generalised or mixed (localised and generalised).*
- *Provoked (e.g., insertional, contact) or spontaneous or mixed (provoked and spontaneous).*
- *Onset (primary or secondary).*
- *Temporal pattern (intermittent, persistent, constant, immediate, delayed).*

**Women may have both a specific disorder (e.g., LS) and vulvodynia.*

Management (it is often difficult and requires a multidisciplinary team approach).

1. General measures:

Educate about vulvar pain.
Information leaflets, website referrals and local support groups.
Manage patients' expectations.
Stop offending irritant activities on the vulva. Discourage over-washing.
Sitz bath followed by application of petroleum as a moisturiser to seal the moisture.
Cool gel packs wrapped in a soft towel help in pain management.

2. Identify and eliminate any possible pain triggers:

Lubricant for sexual intercourse. Topical anaesthetic before sexual intercourse.
Diagnose and suppress any vaginitis: Candida, trichomonas, inflammatory vaginitis.
Identify and eliminate any possible pain triggers.

Identify and treat premalignant lesions.
Suppress herpes if active.
Marsupialise recurrent/persistent inflamed Bartholin cysts.
Provide adequate local oestrogen if there is atrophy.
Diagnose and treat lesions of dermatitis and dermatosis.
Recognise systemic diseases such as drug reactions.
Consider issues such as painful bladder syndrome and pelvic floor dysfunction.
Refer to a physiotherapist to evaluate and treat vaginismus and musculoskeletal problems possibly affecting the pelvic floor and pudendal nerve.
Rule out underlying endometriosis and painful bladder syndrome.
Desensitise with self-massage and topical anaesthetic ointment.

3. Medications for pain control:
Topical medications — emollients, anaesthetics and corticosteroids.
Local steroid injections.
Intralesional and trigger point injections using triamcinolone.
Oral medications — tricyclic antidepressants, neuromodulating agents such as gabapentin.

4. Other modalities of therapy:
Biofeedback/physical therapy.
Pelvic floor exercises.
A low-oxalate diet and calcium and citrate supplementation are suggested.
Cognitive behavioural therapy (CBT).
Sexual counselling.
Acupuncture.
Hypnotherapy.

5. Surgical excision — vestibulectomy:
Considerations for vestibulectomy for local provoked vulvodynia.
No unprovoked element.
Pain localised to the posterior vestibule.
No psychosexual issues.
Responds to topical anaesthetic medications before surgery.

Pudendal neuralgia:

***Symptoms*:** Unilateral pain, pain distribution corresponds to the area innervated by the pudendal nerve, worse with sitting, relieved with supine position, may have swelling within the vagina.

Hypertonic pelvic floor on examination.

Consider a magnetic resonance imaging (MRI) scan of the pelvis to rule out nerve compression.

***Management*:**

- o Physiotherapy.
- o Gabapentin/pregabalin.
- o Avoid exacerbating factors, e.g., constipation, trauma.
- o Nerve blockade — refer to the pain team.

Common Vaginal Lesions

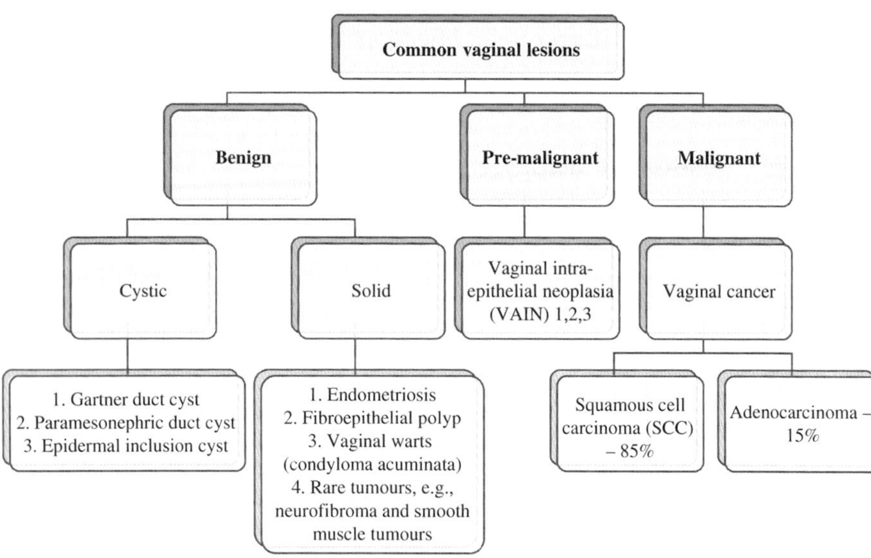

Lesion	Investigations	Management
Gartner duct cyst Remnant of mesonephric ducts. Usually asymptomatic <1 cm but can enlarge.	Pelvic examination. Biopsy of suspicious cysts to exclude malignancy. Imaging to localise large cysts.	If asymptomatic, offer conservative management with routine examination to follow up cysts. If symptomatic, offer excision of the cyst.
Paramesonephric duct cyst	Pelvic examination. Biopsy of suspicious cysts to exclude malignancy.	Asymptomatic cysts can be monitored.
Inclusion cyst	Pelvic examination. Biopsy of suspicious cysts to exclude malignancy.	Treatment involves excision of the intact cyst and approximation of normal epithelium.
Vaginal endometriosis	Biopsy of the lesion to confirm histology. Ultrasound scan of the pelvis to exclude pelvic endometriosis Evaluate menstrual history.	Small, symptomatic lesions are treated by excision or laser vaporisation. Large lesions arising in the posterior cul-de-sac and extending into the posterior vaginal fornix need laparoscopy and treatment.
Vagina fibroepithelial polyp	Pelvic examination.	Excision if large and symptomatic.
Vaginal warts (condyloma acuminata)	*Colposcopy*: To exclude warts affecting the cervix and vagina. Ensure a Pap smear is done if not up to date.	Depending on the number, size and location of warts. *To offer*: • Excision. • Laser vaporisation. • Topical imiquimod.
Vaginal intraepithelial neoplasia (VAIN) The prevalence of HPV in VAIN 2/3 is 92.6%. HPV 16 is most commonly involved. <u>Risk factors:</u> History of prior pelvic radiation or hysterectomy for lower genital tract neoplasia or high-grade CIN.	VAIN is a histological diagnosis, typically based on the colposcopic assessment and biopsy of the vagina. HPV-associated lesions are often multifocal and multicentric. Need to assess the entire vagina and cervix.	<u>VAIN 1:</u> Offer expectant management with repeat colposcopy in 6 months. Vaginal oestrogens in menopausal women. <u>VAIN 2–3:</u> Depending on the number/size and location of lesions. <u>*To offer:*</u> Excision. CO_2 laser vaporisation. Topical imiquimod. Topical 5FU.

(*Continued*)

(*Continued*)

Lesion	Investigations	Management
History of CIN or VIN. All risk factors associated with persistent HPV infection such as immunosuppression and smoking.		**For recalcitrant cases** — brachytherapy and vaginectomy.
Vaginal cancer (rare) SCC Adenocarcinoma	Colposcopy. Biopsy of the vaginal tumour for histology. CT scan of the thorax/ abdomen and MRI pelvis. PET-CT scan.	Refer to a gynae-oncologist. Refer to Chapter 37: *Approach to Gynaecological Cancers*.

CHAPTER 42

Postmenopausal Bleeding (PMB)

Definition of Postmenopausal Bleeding

Menopause is diagnosed after one year of amenorrhoea from the last menstrual period (in the absence of hormonal contraception or any other treatment that may account for amenorrhoea). PMB is vaginal bleeding that occurs after menopause.

Any uterine bleeding in a menopausal woman should be investigated, including:

1. Any breakthrough/unpredictable bleeding, bleeding not occurring at the expected time or heavy bleeding in women on cyclical hormone replacement therapy (HRT)/menopausal hormone therapy (MHT).
2. Persistent bleeding while receiving continuous combined MHT/tibolone after the first 6 months of treatment or after full amenorrhoea has been established.

Ensure that other sources of bleeding (e.g., urinary or gastrointestinal tract) have been ruled out.

Important Information on PMB

9 in 10 women with PMB do not have cancer, but the priority is to exclude malignancy.
1 in 10 women with PMB may have endometrial malignancy.
The most common cause of PMB is genital tract atrophy.

Causes of PMB

- Atrophic endometritis/vaginitis (most common cause)
- Polyps/fibroids (endometrial/endocervical/cervical)

- Endometritis [e.g., sexually transmitted infections (STIs), endometrial tuberculosis]
- Endometrial hyperplasia
- Carcinoma: endometrium/cervix/vagina/vulva/fallopian tube/ovary (oestrogen-secreting tumours, e.g., granulosa cell tumour)
- Foreign body (e.g., pessary)
- Hydrometra, pyometra, haematometra
- Bleeding disorders
- Trauma
- Iatrogenic (drug-induced), e.g., MHT, anticoagulants, antiplatelets

Incidence of Different Causes of PMB

Causes of PMB	Incidence (%)
Atrophic endometritis/vaginitis	60–80
Exogenous oestrogens	15–25
Endometrial carcinoma	10
Endometrial hyperplasia	5–10
Endometrial/cervical polyps	2–12

Management of Women With PMB

History:

- Screen for risk factors for endometrial cancer
- Cervical cancer screening — human papillomavirus (HPV) testing or Pap smear
- *Medications*: anticoagulants, antiplatelets, MHT, tamoxifen use

Physical examination:

- BMI
- Abdominal, speculum and vaginal examination

Investigation:

- Transabdominal ultrasound (TAUS)/transvaginal ultrasound (TVUS) scan to determine endometrial thickness (ET) and to exclude uterine/ovarian pathology

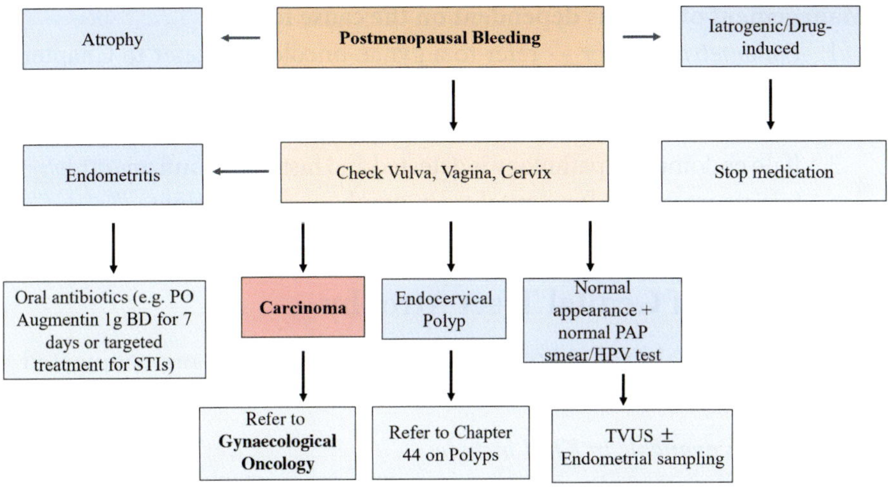

ET via TVUS scan (mm)	Sensitivity for detection of endometrial cancer (%)	Specificity for detection of endometrial cancer (%)
4	96	53
5	96	61

Ultrasound measurement of ET alone *cannot* be used reliably to exclude endometrial cancer.

A thin ET on ultrasound does **not** reliably exclude type 2 endometrial cancer (e.g., uterine papillary serous or clear cell carcinoma).

If ET is <4 mm, the risk of endometrial cancer is <1%.

Endometrial biopsy methods:

1. Pipelle*
2. Explora*
3. Hysteroscopy and endometrial sampling/dilatation and curettage (gold standard)

******Note*: Pipelle and Explora devices are bedside endometrial sampling techniques for obtaining an adequate and representative endometrial sample. Any failure to obtain an adequate endometrial sample using Pipelle/Explora would necessitate hysteroscopy, dilatation and curettage.

Management of PMB is dependent on the cause found

1. *Endometrial cancer* — refer to a gynae-oncologist. Refer to Chapter 37: *Approach to Gynaecological Cancers.*
2. *Endometrial hyperplasia* — refer to Chapter 43: *Thickened Endometrium.*
3. If no endometrial pathology is detected and histology confirms *atrophy*: initiate treatment for *genital tract atrophy* as stated below.

Treatment of Genital Tract Atrophy

Low-dose vaginal oestrogen (≤50 μg oestradiol or ≤0.3 mg conjugated oestrogen).

Preparations available in KKH include:

1) *Vaginal oestradiol pessary* (Vagifem®) — 10 μg daily ON × 2 weeks, then once weekly for maintenance
2) *Premarin®/Ovestin-oestriol cream* — 1 mg/g one application ON × 3 weeks, then once weekly for maintenance

PMB and Tamoxifen Use

Tamoxifen users have a 3–6-fold increased incidence of endometrial cancer because of its weak oestrogenic effect on the endometrium, resulting in tamoxifen-induced subepithelial stromal hypertrophy.

Tamoxifen use is associated with increased risks of endometrial proliferation, polyps, endometrial hyperplasia, cancer and uterine sarcomas.

Refer to a **gynae** for urgent assessment of the endometrium in patients on tamoxifen with abnormal uterine bleeding (AUB) or PMB.

Routine ultrasound surveillance for asymptomatic women on tamoxifen is <u>*not*</u> recommended because of the low specificity and low positive predictive value. Endometrium evaluation should be reserved for women with AUB.

Refer to Chapter 43: *Thickened Endometrium* for more information on the use of tamoxifen.

Further Treatment for Women With Recurrent PMB

If the woman has recurrent PMB despite no cause found 3–6 months after initial investigations and treatment, consider repeating investigations or offer definitive surgical treatment (hysterectomy and bilateral salpingo-oophorectomy) for symptomatic relief and histological evaluation.

CHAPTER 43

Thickened Endometrium

- Management should depend on clinical symptoms.
- If increased endometrial thickness (ET) is persistent or the patient is symptomatic, refer to an **OBGYN** for further evaluation.

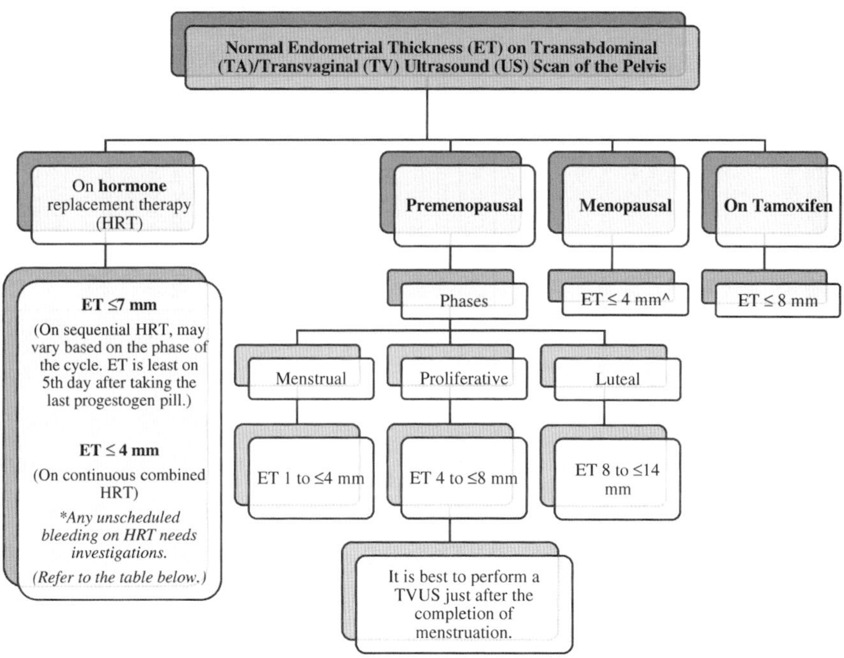

^For women who present with postmenopausal bleeding:
ET ≥ 4 mm: sensitivity 96% and specificity 53% for the detection of endometrial cancer.
ET ≥ 5 mm: sensitivity 96% and specificity 61% for the detection of endometrial cancer.
There is no consensus regarding the cut-off for ET for asymptomatic postmenopausal women.
Assess the risk factors for CA endometrium and investigate accordingly.

Causes of increased ET on US scan of the pelvis	Investigation	Management
1. Luteal phase	Ensure a normal menstrual history Repeat ultrasound (TA/TVUS) on days 4–6 of menses	Reassure if repeat ET is normal
2. Early pregnancy	Urine pregnancy test (UPT)	If UPT positive, offer a dating/viability ultrasound scan. If no intra-uterine pregnancy is visualised, do serum βHCG and trend in 48 hours if indicated.
3. Early-pregnancy complications: **(a) Miscarriage**	Serum βHCG if no intrauterine pregnancy is seen – >50% drop in βHCG over 48 hours indicates a failing pregnancy. TVUS to confirm the fetal heart activity is negative (if the crown-rump length is ≥7 mm)	*Expectant*: ~50% will have spontaneous expulsion. Review in 3 weeks with a UPT. *Medical*: ~80–90% success rate. Various protocols exist — either oral mifepristone followed by vaginal misoprostol or oral/buccal/vaginal misoprostol 600–800 μg. Review in 3 weeks with a UPT. Routine antibiotic prophylaxis is *not* required. *Surgical*: If symptomatic with heavy vaginal bleeding or abdominal pain — offer evacuation of the uterus by suction curettage.
(b) Ectopic pregnancy	Serum βHCG and TVUS	Refer to Chapter 8: *Approach to Ectopic Pregnancy*.
(c) Molar pregnancy	Serum βHCG FBC, T&S, U/E/Cr, LFT, PT/PTT, thyroid function test (TFT), chest X-ray, ECG Histology of products of conception (POC) — definitive diagnosis of molar pregnancy via histology.	Refer to Chapter 9: *Approach to Gestational Trophoblastic Disease*. Evacuation of the uterus by suction curettage, under US guidance, by an experienced clinician. Cervical priming is safe. Follow-up βHCG trending until it normalises and another 6 months either from the βHCG normalisation date or from the date of evacuation of the uterus. **Follow-up of complete mole:** If βHCG normalises within 56 days of evacuation of the uterus, continue follow-up for 6 months from the date of evacuation of the uterus. If βHCG normalises >56 days after evacuation of the uterus, continue follow-up for 6 months from the date of βHCG normalisation. **Follow-up of partial mole:** Follow-up is concluded once βHCG has returned to normal on two samples at least 4 weeks apart (RCOG 2020). Advise **not** to get pregnant until the follow-up is complete. Discuss contraception — all contraception except intrauterine contraceptive devices (IUCDs) can be used during the follow-up. IUCD can only be used when βHCG has normalised. Anti-D is needed for rhesus-negative patients with rhesus-positive partners.

(Continued)

Causes of increased ET on US scan of the pelvis	Investigation	Management
4. Retained POC (RPOC) (a) Incomplete miscarriage (b) Post-termination of pregnancy (c) Postnatal	ET ≥15 mm hyperechoic/hypoechoic with vascularity. Irregular interface between the endometrium and myometrium	If **symptomatic** (vaginal bleeding, abdominal pain, fever), either medical treatment or evacuation of the uterus by suction curettage. If **asymptomatic,** can offer expectant management. Follow-up in 1–2 weeks to review symptoms.
5. Endometrial polyp	If the polyp is <1 cm and the woman is asymptomatic, offer repeat TA/TVUS in 3–6 months (on days 2–5 of menses) to follow-up If the polyp is ≥1 cm, refer to Chapter 44: *Polyps (Cervical or Endometrial)*.	Diagnostic hysteroscopy, dilatation and curettage, polypectomy. Incidence of polyp recurrence: 2.5–43.6%.
6. Submucosal fibroid	If asymptomatic, offer repeat TA/TVUS for follow-up	If the *fibroid is ≤5 cm and symptomatic*, treatment options: 1. Tranexamic acid PRN for heavy menses. 2. Hormonal methods, e.g., Mirena® IUCD. 3. Transcervical resection of myoma (TCRM). If the *fibroid is >5 cm*, offer Gonadotrophin-releasing hormone (GnRH) agonist for 2–3 months to reduce the size before TCRM. The success rate of TCRM is approximately 80%. **Complications of TCRM** (a) Bleeding (b) Infection (c) Cervical trauma (d) Uterine perforation 1–2 in 1,000, with possible bowel/bladder/ureteric injury (e) Fluid overload in 1–5% (pulmonary oedema, hyponatraemia, hypo-osmolarity, cerebral oedema) (f) Intrauterine adhesions/Asherman syndrome (g) Recurrence of fibroids Incidence of fibroid recurrence post-TCRM: 15–30% over 10 years • 50% of those with incomplete resection will require repeat surgery within 2 years

(Continued)

(*Continued*)

Causes of increased ET on US scan of the pelvis	Investigation	Management
7. Endometrial hyperplasia ***Risk factors:*** • Older age >35 years old • Obesity • Nulliparity • Anovulatory cycles (e.g., PCOS) • Unopposed oestrogen exposure • Tamoxifen use • Early menarche, late menopause • Smoking • Diabetes mellitus • Genetic syndromes — e.g., Lynch or Cowden syndrome	*Endometrial biopsy for histology* 1. Bedside endometrial sampling • Sensitivity for atypical hyperplasia is 80% • Specificity >90% 2. Hysteroscopy, dilatation and curettage (outpatient/GA) – Gold standard	➢ Correct reversible factors **Endometrial hyperplasia without atypia** ➢ Risk of progression to malignancy (5% over 20 years) ➢ *First line*: medical treatment ➢ Mirena® IUCD ➢ Oral progestogens, e.g., norethisterone, Provera (continuous/cyclical) – Repeat endometrial biopsy *6 months* post-treatment. – Advise surgery if persistent/progression of the disease. ➢ *Second line*: surgical treatment — total hysterectomy, bilateral salpingectomy ± oophorectomy (THBS ± O) *Consider surgery for patients with:* ➢ Contraindications to medical therapy ➢ Concomitant gynaecological pathology, e.g., fibroids, adenomyosis ➢ Patient's preference/inability to follow up ➢ Postmenopausal patient ➢ Failed medical treatment **Endometrial hyperplasia with atypia** – The risk of progression to malignancy is 25%, and up to 40% risk of concomitant endometrial cancer – *First line*: surgical treatment — THBS ± O – *Second line*: medical treatment ➢ High-dose progestogens, e.g., Megace (megestrol acetate) ➢ Mirena® IUCD – *For patients who*: ➢ Are poor surgical candidates ➢ Declined surgery ➢ Desire fertility ➢ Are compliant with the follow-up – Repeat endometrial biopsy *3 months* post-treatment. – Advise surgery if persistent/progression of the disease. *Side effects of progesterone:* bloatedness, headache, breast pain, weight gain, mood disturbances, acne, drowsiness and irregular vaginal spotting. The most severe side effect is venous thromboembolism (VTE).

(Continued)

Causes of increased ET on US scan of the pelvis	Investigation	Management
8. Endometrial cancer ***Risk factors*:** • Older age >35 years old • Obesity • Nulliparity • Anovulatory cycles (e.g., PCOS) • Unopposed oestrogen exposure • Tamoxifen use • Early menarche, late menopause • Smoking • Diabetes mellitus • Genetic syndromes — e.g., Lynch or Cowden Syndrome	Endometrial biopsy for histology 1. Bedside endometrial sampling • Sensitivity for atypical hyperplasia is 80% • Specificity >90% 2. Hysteroscopy, dilatation and curettage (outpatient/under general anaesthesia) – Gold standard	Refer to Chapter 37: *Approach to Gynaecological Cancers.* Refer to a gynaecological oncologist. Discuss at the multidisciplinary tumour board meeting Preoperative work-up: – CT scan of the thorax/abdomen, CT or MRI pelvis – FBC, U/E/Cr, LFT, PT/PTT, T&S ± CA-125 (if indicated by atypical presentation or histology) **Staging surgery:** THBS ± O, sentinel lymph node biopsy or pelvic lymph node dissection. Depending on the stage/grade/histology of the disease, the patient may require adjuvant therapy (i.e., radiotherapy, chemotherapy) or hormonal treatment. **Fertility-sparing surgery** approach for patients keen on fertility and stage 1A grade 1 endometrioid adenocarcinoma of the endometrium. Refer to a fertility specialist.
9. On tamoxifen Tamoxifen increases the risk of endometrial cancer 2–3 times. 1.26 per 1,000 patient-years. • Premenopausal women on tamoxifen have <u>no</u> known increased risk of uterine cancer. • Postmenopausal women on tamoxifen have an increased risk. Tamoxifen also increases the risk of endometrial proliferation, endometrial hyperplasia and uterine sarcomas.	Assess for any abnormal bleeding or postmenopausal bleeding Assess for risk factors for endometrial cancer (as stated above) *If <u>symptomatic</u>* (abnormal vaginal bleeding/postmenopausal bleeding): – TA/TVUS – Endometrial biopsy: bedside sampling or hysteroscopy, D&C *If <u>asymptomatic</u>*: – No role for routine screening as it has not been shown to be effective in the early detection of endometrial cancer – If high risk for endometrial cancer/ET >8 mm, refer to a gynaecologist for further evaluation Consider pre-treatment screening in postmenopausal women before starting tamoxifen treatment.	– Treat any abnormal histology *If diagnosed with endometrial hyperplasia*: – Assess the need for tamoxifen. To discuss with her breast surgeon – Manage with a breast surgeon/medical oncologist – Consider surgical management: hysterectomy

(Continued)

(Continued)

Causes of increased ET on US scan of the pelvis	Investigation	Management
10. On hormone replacement therapy (HRT)	Exclude poor compliance, drug interactions, malabsorption Assess for any unscheduled bleeding for >6 months after starting on HRT, defined as: a) <u>*On sequential HRT*</u>: – Heavy bleeding or prolonged bleeding near the end of the progestogen phase or after it – Breakthrough bleeding at any time during the cycle b) <u>*On continuous combined HRT*</u>: – Bleeding after 6 months of starting HRT – Bleeding after a period of amenorrhoea Assess for risk factors of endometrial cancer (as stated above)	Reinforce compliance If any risk factors or unscheduled bleeding >6 months after HRT initiation: – TA/TV US to exclude other intrauterine pathology, e.g., fibroids – Endometrial biopsy (bedside sampling/D&C hysteroscopy) Once endometrial pathology has been excluded: a) <u>*On sequential HRT*</u>: – If withdrawal bleeding is heavy/prolonged: increase the dose of progestogen, change the type of progestogen or reduce the oestrogen dose – If spotting occurs before withdrawal bleed: increase the oestrogen dose – If irregular bleeding: change the regimen or increase the progestogen dose – If painful bleeding: change the type of progestogen b) <u>*On continuous combined HRT*</u>: – Increase the dose of progestogen or change the type of progestogen, e.g., change to a 52 mg levonorgestrel-releasing intrauterine system – Change to sequential HRT

CHAPTER 44

Polyps (Cervical or Endometrial)

Cervical Polyps

Ensure cervical cancer screening (HPV testing or Pap smear) is normal and up to date.

<u>Presentation of cervical polyps</u>:
Incidental finding during cervical cancer screening or symptoms such as abnormal uterine bleeding (AUB), e.g., intermenstrual bleeding (IMB), postcoital bleeding (PCB), postmenopausal bleeding (PMB) or vaginal discharge.

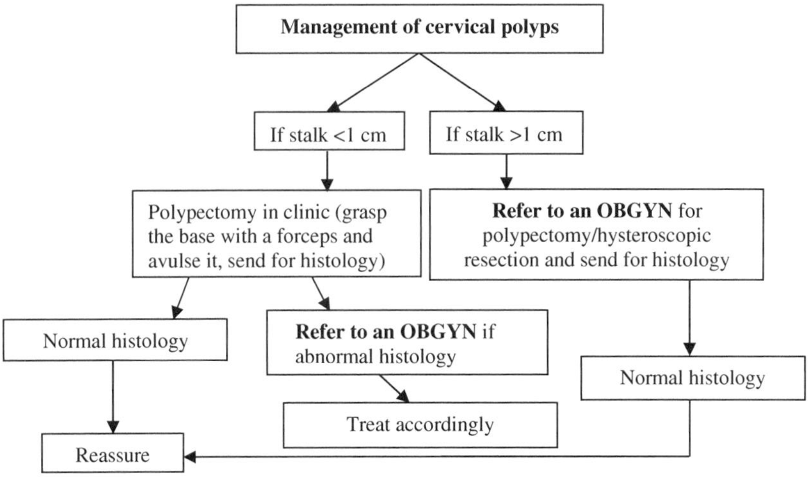

***If needed, apply Monsel's solution to secure haemostasis after cervical polypectomy.**

Management of Endocervical/Cervical Polyps in Pregnancy

Asymptomatic polyps — conservative management is preferred.
Reassess and remove the polyp after delivery if it is still present.

Polypectomy is usually **not** performed in pregnancy unless there is

- Suspicion of malignancy.
- Recurrent heavy vaginal bleeding ± anaemia.
- Heavy bleeding that is not controlled with Monsel's solution.

Cervical Polyps (Figures 44.1 and 44.2)

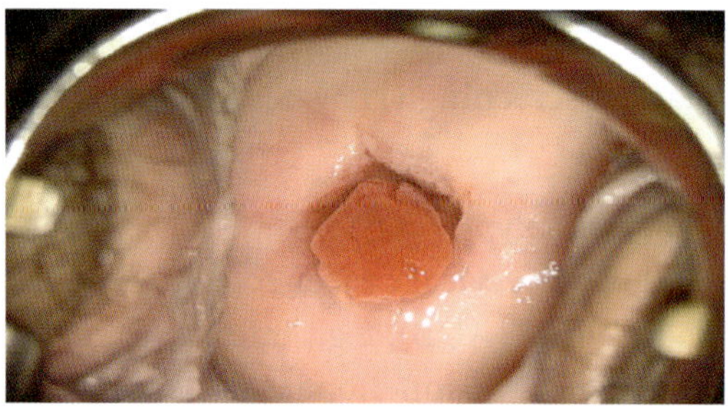

Fig. 44.1 Pedunculated cervical polyp.

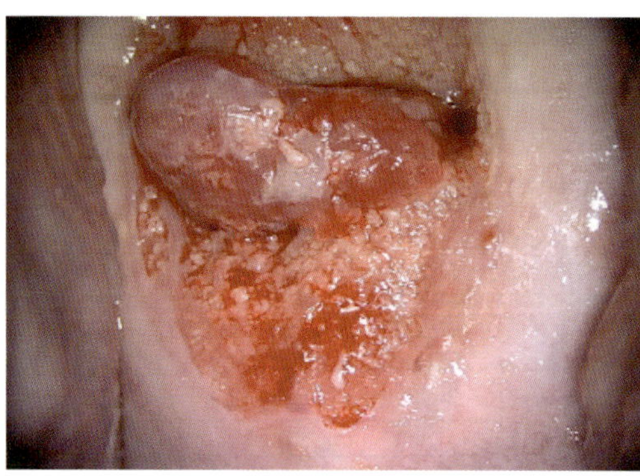

Fig. 44.2 Broad-based cervical polyp.

Endometrial Polyps (Figure 44.3)

They are hyperplastic overgrowth of endometrial glands and stroma from the endometrium. 95% of polyps are benign. They can be sessile or pedunculated. Polyps are more likely to be malignant in postmenopausal women who present with bleeding.

Risk factors of endometrial polyps include:
Older age.
Chronic tamoxifen use.
Hormone therapy (oestrogen ± progestogen).
Hypertension.
Obesity.
PCOS.

Clinical presentation of endometrial polyps:
Discovered incidentally on ultrasound, during hysteroscopy or during speculum examination (may prolapse at the external cervical os).

AUB — polyps are found in up to 40% of women with AUB.

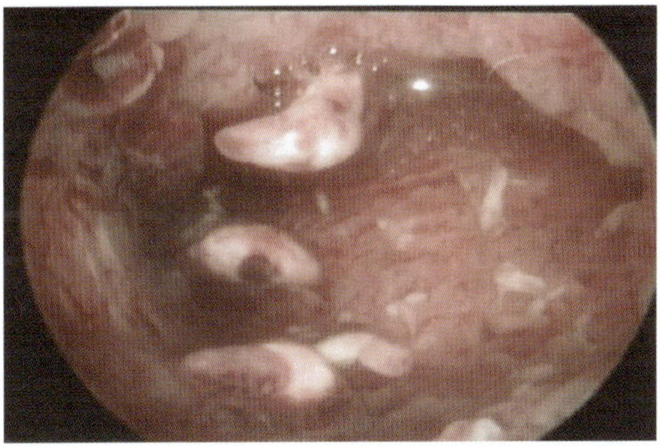

Fig. 44.3 Hysteroscopic image of endometrial polyps.

Diagnosis of Endometrial Polyps

Transabdominal/transvaginal ultrasound scan (TA/TVUS) — most accurate if done in the proliferative phase; either polyp seen or thickened endometrium present.

Saline infusion sonogram (SIS).

Diagnostic hysteroscopy.

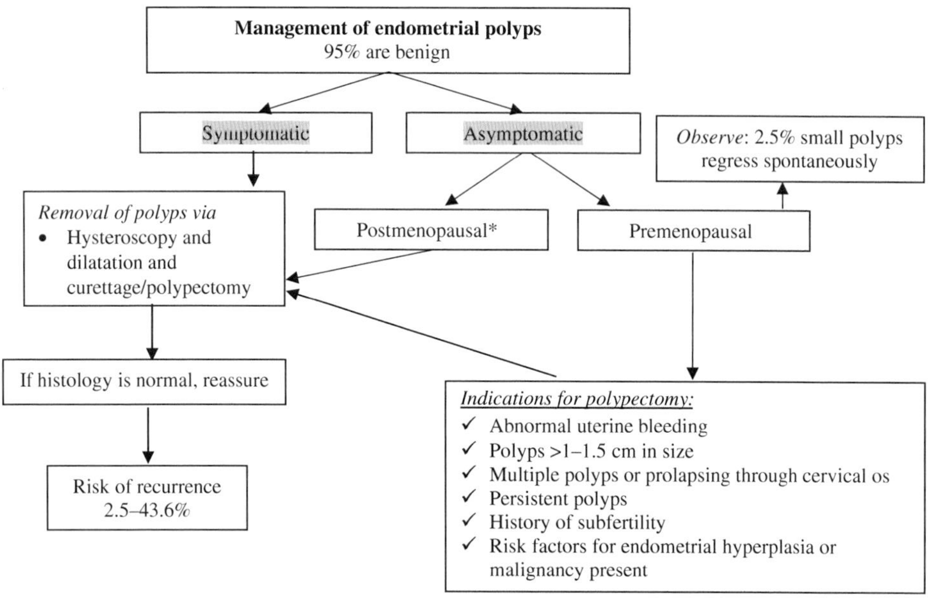

*Removal of endometrial polyps is recommended in all **postmenopausal women** as their risk of malignancy is high.

Differential diagnoses of endometrial polyp(s):

1) Submucosal fibroid, adenomyoma
2) Endometrial hyperplasia/cancer
3) Uterine sarcomas
4) Retained products of conception or blood clots

CHAPTER 45

Fibroids, Fibroids in Pregnancy, Fibroid Variants and Leiomyosarcoma

Fibroids are benign smooth muscle tumours of the uterus and are present in 30% of women in the reproductive age group. They grow in response to oestrogen and progesterone and may even shrink after menopause.

The risk of malignancy for uterine fibroids is very low, with a prevalence of leiomyosarcoma being 1 in 400 or 0.25% of women who had surgery for fibroids.

The exact aetiology of fibroids is *not* clearly understood.

Risk Factors for Uterine Fibroids

Black women have a 2–3-fold increased risk compared to white women.
Early menarche: <10 years old.
Older age >40 years old.
Nulliparity.
Obesity.
Polycystic ovarian syndrome (PCOS).
Hypertension/diabetes mellitus.
Family history of fibroids.

Location of Fibroids (Figures 45.1 and 45.2)

1. Intramural
2. Submucosal/fibroid polyp
3. Subserosal/pedunculated
4. Cervical
5. Broad ligament

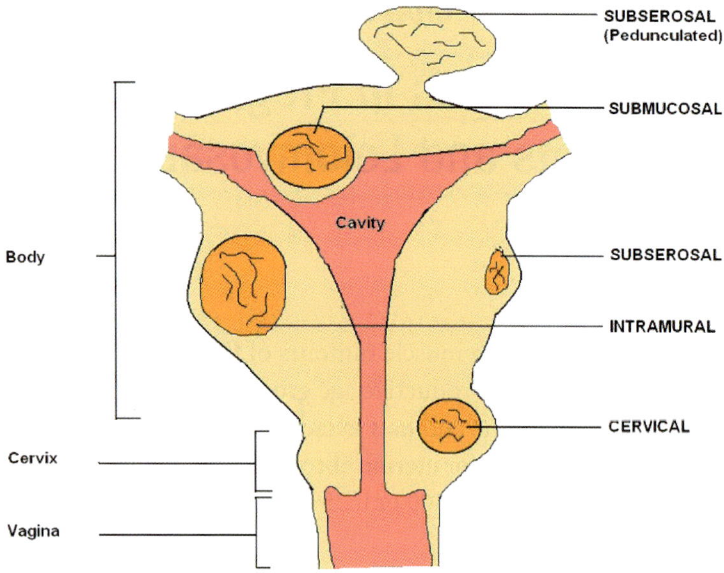

Fig. 45.1 Different locations of uterine fibroids.

Leiomyoma Subclassification System

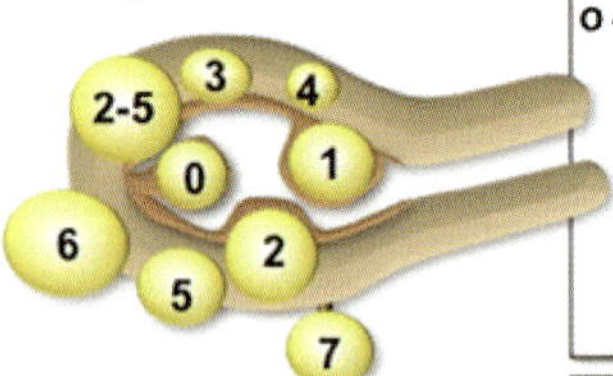

SM- Submucosal	0	Pedunculated Intracavitary
	1	<50% Intramural
	2	≥50% Intramural
O - Other	3	Contacts endometrium; 100% Intramural
	4	Intramural
	5	Subserosal ≥50% Intramural
	6	Subserosal <50% Intramural
	7	Subserosal Pedunculated
	8	Other (specify e.g. cervical, parasitic)
Hybrid Leiomyomas (impact both endometrium and serosa)	Two numbers are listed separated by a hyphen. By convention, the first refers to the relationship with the endometrium while the second refers to the relationship to the serosa. One example is below	
	2-5	Submucosal and subserosal, each with less than half the diameter in the endometrial and peritoneal cavities, respectively.

Fig. 45.2 The International Federation of Gynecology and Obstetrics (FIGO) classification system for fibroids.

Symptoms of Fibroids

Fibroids can be asymptomatic (majority) or symptomatic.

Symptoms include:

1) Heavy menstrual bleeding (HMB) leading to anaemia.
2) *Pain* — dysmenorrhoea, dyspareunia or low back pain.

   Usually due to fibroid "red degeneration", torsion or associated adenomyosis.

   Dysmenorrhoea is usually associated with adenomyosis, heavy menstrual flow or passage of blood clots.
3) Pelvic pressure and pain.

   Urinary frequency, difficulty passing urine or acute retention of urine, causing direct pressure on the bladder/bladder outlet.

   Obstructive uropathy (hydronephrosis/hydroureter) can occur with obstruction of the distal ureter.

   Constipation can occur with external pressure on the rectum.

   Rarely, venous thromboembolism (VTE) can occur because of venous compression.
4) Pelvi-abdominal mass and abdominal bloatedness caused by large fibroids (Fig. 45.3).
5) Vaginal mass due to a prolapsed fibroid.
6) *Reproductive and obstetric outcomes.*

   Difficulty in conceiving and higher risk of miscarriage (particularly second-trimester miscarriages in patients with submucosal fibroids or intramural fibroids with a submucosal component distorting the endometrial cavity).

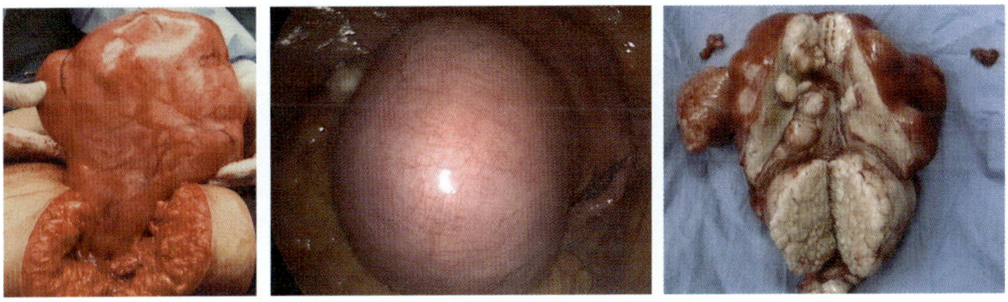

Fig. 45.3 Large uterine fibroids seen intraoperatively and a cut section of the uterus.

Risk of acute fibroid degeneration during pregnancy, especially with fibroids >5 cm and in the second or third trimesters.

Possible adverse pregnancy outcomes: Miscarriage, abruptio placentae, placenta praevia, preterm labour, malpresentation, labour dystocia, increased risk of caesarean section and postpartum haemorrhage (PPH).

Risk of uterine rupture after myomectomy ~0.5 to 1%.

There have been case reports of fetal anomalies in women with large submucosal fibroids, e.g., dolichocephaly and torticollis.

Physical examination:

For small fibroids, the uterus size may be normal.

There can be an enlarged, palpable uterus per abdomen or bimanual palpation for large fibroids.

Size is usually described in weeks, corresponding to uterine size in pregnancy.

Investigations:

1. **Full blood count** to check for anaemia.
2. **Transabdominal/transvaginal ultrasound scan of pelvis (TA/TVUS) (Fig. 45.4):**
   - Preferred imaging modality — highly sensitive to detect fibroids.
   - However, the US is limited in precisely localising fibroids in a large uterus or multiple fibroids.
3. **Magnetic resonance imaging (MRI) pelvis (Fig. 45.5):**
   - Indicated if suspicious of leiomyosarcoma or if precise localisation of a fibroid is required.

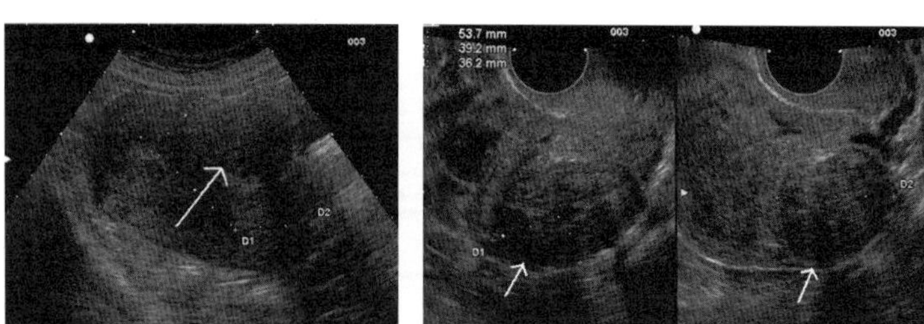

Fig. 45.4 Ultrasound images of fibroids.

- Can differentiate between fibroids, adenomyosis and adenomyomas.
- Can be done as part of preoperative planning for complex surgeries.

4. **Saline infusion sonography:**
   - Can identify submucosal and intramural fibroids that protrude into the uterine cavity.
   - Useful if the patient requires workup for subfertility or to plan hysteroscopic resection of a fibroid.
5. **Diagnostic hysteroscopy (Fig. 45.6):**
   - Allows us to differentiate between type 0 and type 1 fibroids and endometrial polyps. Usually done in the same setting as that of hysteroscopic myomectomy.

Management of Uterine Fibroids

It is important to exclude an underlying endometrial pathology in women with abnormal uterine bleeding (AUB) before treatment, especially before surgery. Perform an endometrial biopsy to rule out endometrial hyperplasia/malignancy if there are risk factors.

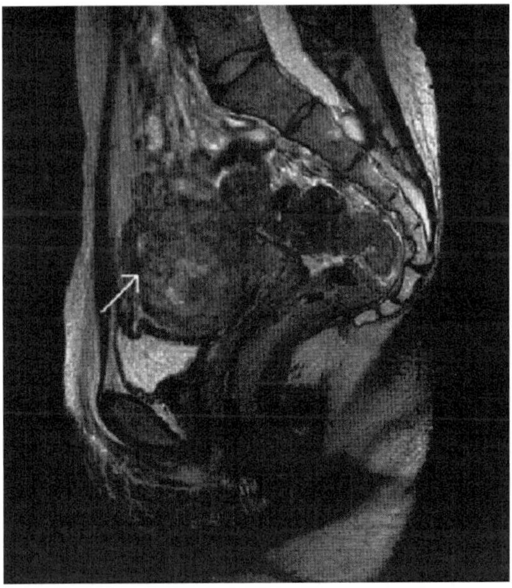

Fig. 45.5 MRI image of a large intramural fibroid.

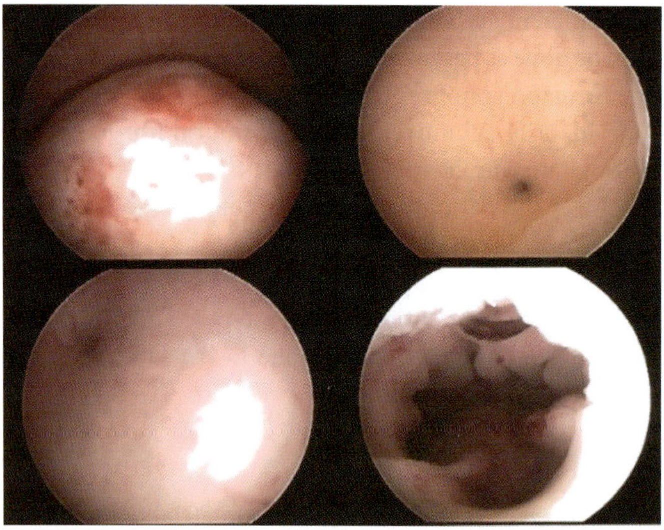

Fig. 45.6 Hysteroscopic image of a submucosal fibroid.

***Factors to consider in the management of fibroids*:**

1) Size and location of fibroids
2) Age of the patient
3) Desire for fertility
4) Symptoms
5) Types of treatment available
6) Surgeon's expertise

Expectant

Fibroids are benign tumours. They can be managed expectantly if the woman is asymptomatic. To do surveillance with follow-up ultrasound scans.

Medical Therapy

A. **Levonorgestrel (LNG) intrauterine devices (Mirena®)** should be considered a first-line treatment for women with HMB with fibroids <3 cm in diameter that do not distort the uterine cavity.
B. **Tranexamic acid (TxA) and non-steroidal anti-inflammatory drugs (NSAIDs)** decrease menstrual blood flow. Tranexamic acid is an

anti-fibrinolytic. NSAIDs act by reducing prostaglandin production. NSAIDs also reduce pain. The most effective NSAID is mefenamic acid. Before starting treatment, the woman should be informed of side effects such as diarrhoea and indigestion. It is essential to give anti-gastric medications with NSAIDs, e.g., antacids, famotidine or omeprazole.

C. **Hormonal therapy, e.g., combined oral contraception pills** (COCPs) and **progesterone-only pills** (POPs), can reduce menstrual flow and dysmenorrhoea.

D. **GnRH agonists** induce a menopausal state and are very effective for short-term relief of symptoms and preoperative preparation. They cause fibroids to shrink by up to 50% of their volume within 3 months, but re-growth usually occurs within 12 weeks of stopping treatment. Their use should <u>*not*</u> be continued for more than 6 months as there are concerns about reduced bone mineral density. For women who require long-term GnRH agonist treatment for more than 12 months, hormonal add-back therapy should be considered to reduce the side effects.

<u>Surgery</u>

A. ***Myomectomy*** is ideal for patients who desire fertility or wish to retain their uterus. There is a risk of uterine rupture in subsequent pregnancies following myomectomy. Patients should wait at least 6 *months* after a myomectomy before trying to conceive. There is also a 15–33% recurrence rate for fibroids following myomectomy. In total, 10% of women who have had a myomectomy, may need a hysterectomy within the next 5–10 years.

A. ***Myomectomy***
Various approaches for myomectomy:
(Laparotomy, laparoscopy, vaginal and hysteroscopy.)

i. ***Hysteroscopic myomectomy/transcervical resection of myoma (TCRM):***
   - Indicated for submucosal fibroids FIGO type 0, 1 and some type 2.
   - The maximum fibroid size deemed suitable for TCRM depends on the type of fibroid, location and surgeon's expertise. The larger the fibroid, the higher the risk of complications and the possible need to be done under laparoscopic guidance or as a staged procedure.

- Generally, if the fibroid is ≥5 cm, consider a GnRH agonist pre-operatively to decrease the size before TCRM.
- Another classification can be used to assess the feasibility of submucosal fibroids for hysteroscopic myomectomy. The ***STEP-W submucosal fibroid classification*** considers and scores five characteristics of fibroids. This classification is more accurate in predicting the difficulty of TCRM and the likelihood of complete resection.

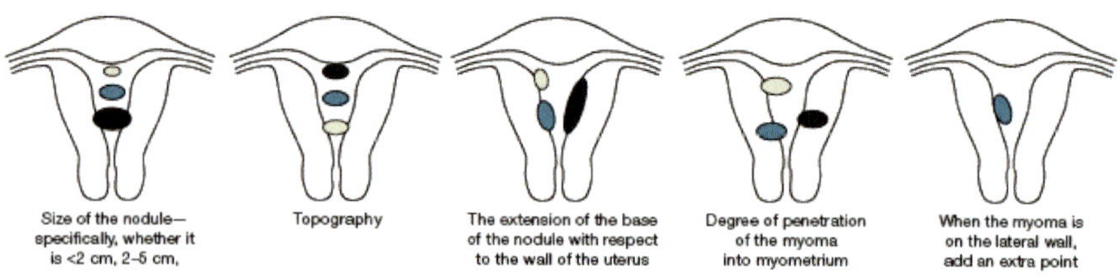

STEP-W Submucosal Fibroid Classification

Score	**Size (cm)**	**Topography (relation to the uterine cavity)**	**Extension of the base**	**Penetration**	**Lateral wall**
0	<2	Lower third	<1/3	0	+1
1	>2 to 5	Middle third	>1/3 to 2/3	<50%	
2	>5	Upper third	>2/3	>50%	
Total score	**Group**	**Complexity and therapeutic options**			
0–4	I	Low-complexity hysteroscopic myomectomy.			
5–6	II	High-complexity hysteroscopic myomectomy. Consider GnRH use. Consider a two-step hysteroscopic myomectomy.			
7–9	III	Consider alternatives to the hysteroscopic technique.			

Source: https://cdn.mdedge.com/files/s3fs-public/images/RTEmagicC_OBG_0215_Bradley_fig2.jpg.jpg.

- The recurrence rate of AUB or fibroids following hysteroscopic myomectomy is about 20% after 3 years.

ii. ***Vaginal myomectomy*** can be performed for prolapsed fibroids (Fig. 45.7).

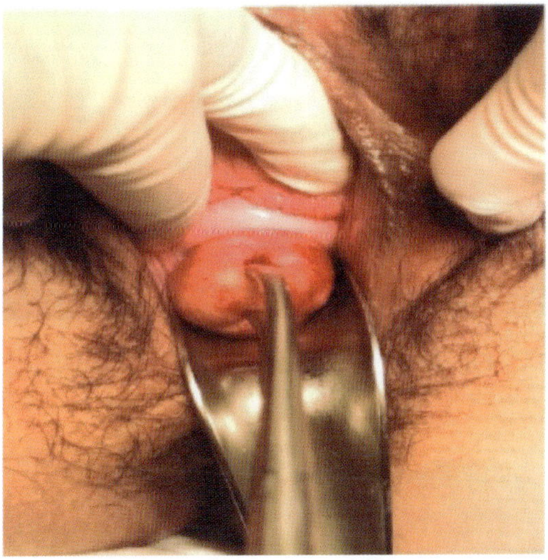

Fig. 45.7 Fibroid prolapsing through the cervical os.

iii. ***Laparoscopic Myomectomy*** **(Figures 45.8 and 45.9)**

- Preferred over laparotomy for intramural/subserosal fibroids because of less pain, faster recovery post-operatively and lower morbidity.
- However, not all women are suitable for laparoscopic myomectomy. For example, in women with large fibroids, multiple fibroids or previous surgery, it may be technically challenging, and a laparotomy may be more suitable.
- *Morcellation of fibroids* performed during a laparoscopic surgery should be *contained within a morcellation-safe bag* to reduce risks of recurrence and dissemination of fibroids, which can result in parasitic fibroids or dissemination of malignancy, which can upstage the cancer and worsen prognosis.

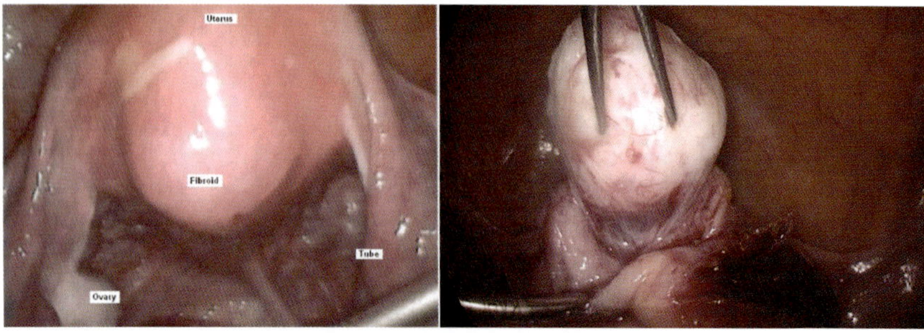

Fig. 45.8 Laparoscopic myomectomy.

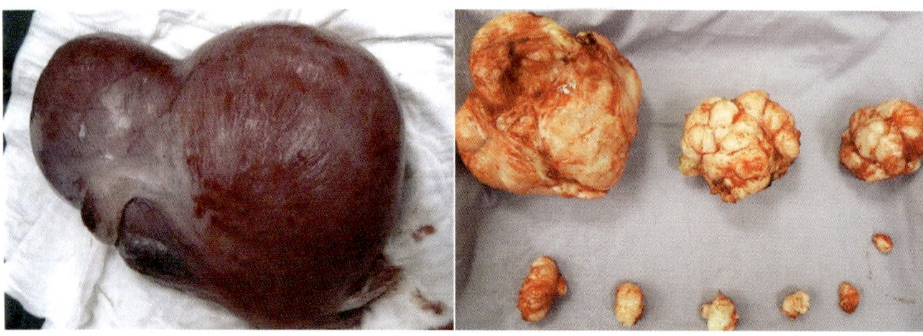

Fig. 45.9 Uterus enlarged with multiple fibroids (left) and fibroid specimens from myomectomy (right).

iv. ***Laparotomy or open myomectomy***
It is indicated in women with large fibroids, with dense adhesions from previous surgeries or suspicious of leiomyosarcoma.

B. ***Hysterectomy*** is a *definitive treatment for* fibroids in women who *do not* desire fertility (routes — abdominal, vaginal or laparoscopic). Another method is vNOTES hysterectomy (vaginal natural orifice transluminal endoscopic surgery) — which combines advanced laparoscopic and vaginal approaches in gynaecological surgery.

Uterine Artery Embolisation (UAE)

UAE is a minimally invasive interventional radiology technique where a catheter is passed via the femoral artery. As a result, the blood supply to the fibroids is diminished, decreasing the size and providing symptomatic relief.

Side effects of UAE include:

- *Postembolisation syndrome*: Occurs in the first 72 hours. There can be pain, nausea, vomiting, fever and vaginal discharge.
- *Infection*: Due to ischaemia and necrosis, especially if tissue is retained.
- Primary ovarian insufficiency (POI).
- Bleeding due to fibroid necrosis.
- *May need future intervention*. In a study of 2,112 women who underwent UAE, 15% had a hysterectomy or myomectomy within 3 years of UAE. As there are inadequate data on the impact of UAE on fertility, patients who desire fertility should consider alternative treatment modalities.
- *Local site reactions*: Groin haematoma, infection, arterial dissection, contrast allergy/reaction, vascular dissection/rupture.

Fibroids and Fertility

Fibroids account for only 1–2% of patients with subfertility. Hence, other causes should be excluded before considering fibroids as the cause of subfertility.

Submucosal and intramural fibroids with an intracavitary component that distort the endometrial cavity or compress the fallopian tubes can affect fertility. Women with such fibroids have decreased spontaneous and IVF pregnancy rates and an increased risk of spontaneous miscarriages, usually in the second trimester.

Subserosal fibroids do *not* affect fertility.

Myomectomy improved pregnancy rates by 2-fold in women with submucosal fibroids.

Fibroids in Pregnancy

Most pregnant women with fibroids do *not* have any major fibroid-related complications. Complications are more common in women with large fibroids, i.e., >5 cm, or submucosal fibroids.

Potential complications of fibroids in pregnancy include:

1) Pain
   - Most common complication, usually due to red degeneration.
   - Another cause is torsion of a pedunculated fibroid.

2) Pregnancy loss/miscarriage
   - Fibroids may interfere with the circulation to the placenta, causing pregnancy loss or affecting implantation.
3) Increase in size
   - 20–30% of fibroids increase in size during pregnancy, especially large fibroids (>5 cm). It usually occurs in the first trimester.
4) Antepartum haemorrhage (APH)/placental abnormalities
   - Placental abruption and praevia/accreta may be more common.
5) Preterm labour (PTL) and preterm premature rupture of membranes (PPROM)
6) Malpresentation — may cause breech presentation/transverse lie
7) Intrauterine growth restriction (IUGR)
8) Labour dystocia
9) Caesarean delivery — occurs more commonly if fibroids are in the lower uterine segment
10) PPH — usually due to uterine atony

Myomectomy in Pregnancy

Myomectomy is generally *contraindicated* during pregnancy because of the risk of severe haemorrhage and pregnancy loss.

Women who have undergone myomectomy have a higher chance of uterine rupture in subsequent pregnancies. However, those who have undergone open myomectomy are thought to have a lower risk of uterine rupture than those who have undergone laparoscopic myomectomy. This is due to better myometrial defect suturing and closure during open surgery.

No high-quality data are available that compare the rates of uterine rupture in open versus laparoscopic myomectomy. Based on small case series, the risk of pre-labour uterine rupture is very low (0.002%) in women with open surgery. On the other hand, there are case reports of uterine rupture in women as early as 17 weeks of gestation who have had a previous laparoscopic myomectomy. In one of the largest studies following pregnancies after laparoscopic myomectomies, only one uterine rupture was reported in 386 pregnancies. Thus, the risk of uterine rupture is highly dependent on the surgeon's technique. The surgeon should counsel women post-myomectomy on the possibility of a trial of vaginal delivery or whether an elective caesarean section is indicated.

If the endometrial cavity was breached during myomectomy, there is a higher chance of uterine rupture, so an elective caesarean section should be performed for subsequent pregnancies.

Some Rare Fibroid Variants

1) Disseminated peritoneal leiomyomatosis.
2) Benign metastasising leiomyoma (BML) (Fig. 45.10). Commonly metastasises to the lungs. May mimic a metastatic gynaecological malignancy. Responds to anti-oestrogen therapy.
3) Intravenous leiomyomatosis.
4) Leiomyomas can be associated with genetic disorders, e.g., fumarate-hydrase-deficient leiomyoma, Alport syndrome with diffuse leiomyomatosis.
   - Refer to a genetic counsellor for risk evaluation of hereditary leiomyomatosis in family members and screening for other related conditions, e.g., renal cell carcinoma.

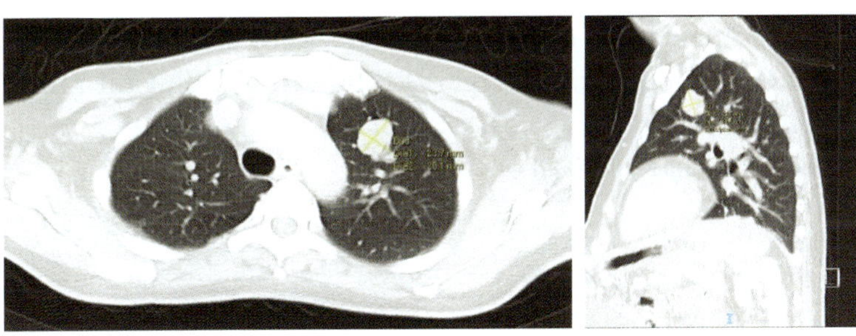

Fig. 45.10 CT images of benign metastasising leiomyomas with lung involvement.

Uterine Leiomyosarcoma

It is a rare tumour with an extremely poor prognosis. It is difficult to differentiate between leiomyoma and sarcoma clinically *without* histopathology. Sarcomas are generally thought to arise *de novo* and not from a sarcomatous change in leiomyomas. The mean age of diagnosis is 60.

***Risk factors*:**
Age, postmenopausal status, pelvic irradiation, long-term tamoxifen use, childhood retinoblastoma, hereditary leiomyomatosis and renal cell carcinoma syndrome.

Symptoms of Uterine Sarcoma

AUB, pelvic pain, pelvic mass, foul-smelling vaginal discharge.

Warning sign: A rapidly enlarging uterine mass in a postmenopausal woman is a red flag.

MRI imaging can help differentiate leiomyoma from leiomyosarcoma. Some features specific to leiomyosarcoma are the absence of calcifications and ill-defined margins.

The diagnosis of leiomyosarcoma is ultimately based on histopathology and immunohistochemistry.

Rapid growth in a fibroid may *not* indicate a sarcomatous change in the fibroid.

Treatment of Uterine Sarcoma

Staging laparotomy (total abdominal hysterectomy and bilateral salpingo-oophorectomy ± debulking surgery) followed by adjuvant radiation/chemotherapy.

Refer to a gynaecological oncologist.

Table 45.1 Comparison Between Benign Leiomyoma and Uterine Leiomyosarcoma

		Benign leiomyoma	Uterine leiomyosarcoma
Lifetime risk		7 to 8/10	3 to 7/100,000
Risk factors		Early menarche Nulliparity Obesity Family history of fibroids	Increasing age Postmenopausal Tamoxifen Pelvic irradiation Hereditary conditions, e.g., hereditary leiomyomatosis and renal cell carcinoma syndrome
Radiological features	Pelvic ultrasound	Hypoechoic Cystic areas of necrosis or degeneration Calcification	Mixed echogenicity Central necrosis Irregular vessels on colour Doppler
	MRI with gadolinium contrast	Hypointense/isointense on T1- and T2-weighted images Dark and homogenous in T2-weighted images No restricted diffusion	Heterogeneous/hyperintense on T1- and T2-weighted images No calcifications Ill-defined margins, irregular Infiltrating, often solitary Intralesional haemorrhage Restricted diffusion present
	Computer tomography (CT)/positron emission tomography-CT (PET-CT)/ CT with FDG	Absent/low FDG uptake	Generally high FDG uptake (variable for different tumours)
Gross features		Whorled appearance Well circumscribed White Firm	Loss of whorled appearance Ill-defined margins Yellow Soft Homogenous texture
Microscopic features	Mitotic index	Low	High
	Cellular atypia	Absent	Present
	Necrosis	Absent	Present
	Cellularity	Low	High
	Vascularity	Absent	Present
Immunohistochemical stains	*SMA, desmin, caldesmon, calponin*	Positive	Positive
	Ki-67, P16, P53	Negative	Positive
	ER, PR	Positive	Variable
	miR-221	Negative	Positive
Cytogenetics	*Terminal deletions in 19q, 22q*	Present in 3% of fibroids Present in most BML lesions	Absent
Prognosis		Good	Poor

CHAPTER 46

Endometriosis and Adenomyosis

Endometriosis

- Endometriosis is the presence and growth of endometrial-like epithelium or stroma outside the uterus and is usually associated with an inflammatory rcaction.
- It affects up to 10% of reproductive-age women and up to 50% of women with subfertility.

  <u>*Three types of endometriosis*:</u>
  1. Superficial peritoneal endometriosis
  2. Ovarian endometriosis (Fig. 46.1)
  3. Deep endometriosis

  Implications:
  - Associated with subfertility
  - Increased risk of cardiovascular diseases
  - 2.5% risk of ovarian cancer, 13.3% risk of breast cancer and 1.8% of thyroid cancer (compared to the background risk of 1.3% of ovarian cancer, 12.8% of breast cancer and 1.8% of thyroid cancer)

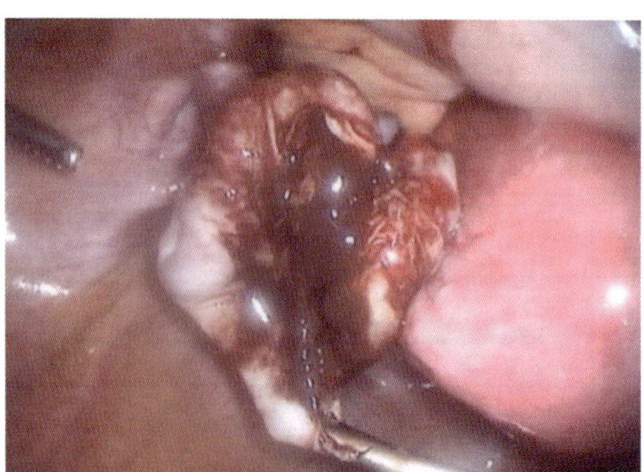

Fig. 46.1 Endometriotic cyst of the ovary.

Risk factors for endometriosis:

- Family history of endometriosis
- Obstructive genital malformations
- Early menarche
- Short menstrual cycle

Symptoms of Endometriosis

Can be cyclical or non-cyclical. Enquire regarding the impact on the quality of life, sexual intercourse and mood.

Consider a symptom diary to aid in the diagnosis of endometriosis.

- Dysmenorrhoea
- Deep dyspareunia
- Chronic pelvic pain (CPP)
- Cyclical or perimenstrual symptoms, such as bowel or bladder symptoms
    - Dyschezia/constipation/painful rectal bleeding/bloating/diarrhoea
    - Dysuria/haematuria
    - Shoulder tip pain
    - Catamenial pneumothorax (a spontaneous pneumothorax that recurs with menstruation, occurring within 72 hours before or after the onset of a menstrual cycle)
    - Cyclical cough/haemoptysis/chest pain
    - Cyclical scar pain/swelling
- Subfertility
- Low back pain
- Fatigue

Pregnancy does *not* always improve symptoms or reduce disease progression.

Signs of Endometriosis

On vaginal examination:

- Pelvic tenderness/fixed, retroverted uterus/tender uterosacral ligaments
- Endometriotic ovarian cysts

The diagnosis is more certain if deeply infiltrating nodules are palpated on the uterosacral ligaments or in the pouch of Douglas or if visible lesions are seen in the vagina or cervix.

Investigations for Endometriosis

1. ***Imaging studies***
   - Similar or slightly higher sensitivity and specificity for ovarian and deep endometriosis when compared to surgery.
   - Non-invasive.
   - Lack of adequate resolution for visualising adhesions and superficial peritoneal/ovarian implants.
     A. *Transabdominal (TA)/transvaginal ultrasound scan of the pelvis (TVUS)*:
       - Useful in diagnosing ovarian endometriomas and may help diagnose rectovaginal disease.
       - Transrectal ultrasound may be done if a transvaginal route is *not* possible.

     B. *Magnetic resonance imaging (MRI)*:
       - Good sensitivity and specificity for ovarian endometriomas.
       - Useful for deep infiltrating endometriosis, to assess any involvement of the bladder/ureters/bowels.
       - Pre-operative imaging before endometriosis surgery.

2. ***Laparoscopy***
   - *No longer* the gold standard for diagnosis.
   - Indicated in women with negative imaging results and/or *not* responding to empirical treatment.
   - *Appearance of lesions on laparoscopy.*
     - o Superficial powder-burn or gunshot lesions on the ovaries, serosal surfaces and peritoneum, especially the posterior cul-de-sac, uterosacral ligaments and ovarian fossa. The lesions are black, dark brown or bluish, puckered lesions, nodules or small cysts containing old haemorrhage surrounded by a variable extent of fibrosis.
     - o Lesions can have a variety of shapes and colours, including clear, red, blue-black, yellow, brown, white or mixed. In addition, the lesions may be microscopic or macroscopic or appear as a peritoneal window.

  - Endometriomas typically contain thick fluid and are densely adherent to the surrounding structures, e.g., peritoneum, tubes and bowel. Deeply infiltrating endometriotic nodules extend >5 mm beneath the peritoneum and may involve the uterosacral ligaments, vagina, bowel, bladder or ureters.
- Positive histology confirms the diagnosis of endometriosis. However, negative histology does not exclude it.
- Visual inspection is usually adequate, but histological confirmation of at least one lesion is ideal. In cases of ovarian endometrioma and deeply infiltrating disease, histological diagnosis should be obtained to identify endometriosis and exclude malignancy (endometriosis is associated with ovarian endometrioid or clear cell carcinoma). Some studies quote a risk of 1.9%, as opposed to the background lifetime risk of ovarian cancer of 1.4%.

3. ***Serum CA125 — usually elevated (>35 U/ml)***
   - Serum CA125 is *not* a specific marker of endometriosis (refer to Chapter 60: *Tumour Markers in Gynaecology and Pregnancy*) and should *not* be used to diagnose endometriosis.

Differential diagnosis of endometriosis:
- Pelvic inflammatory disease.
- Adenomyosis.
- Ovarian neoplasms.
- Irritable bowel syndrome.
- Bladder pain syndrome (previously known as interstitial cystitis)

Management of endometriosis:
- Counsel the patient on diagnosis, implications and possible complications.
- Individualise treatment, taking into account:
  - Patient's age.
  - Fertility wishes.
  - Association with pain or subfertility.
  - Side effects of treatment.
  - Patient's preferences.
  - Costs.
- Goals of management.

(1) Endometriosis-associated pain.
(2) Endometriosis-associated subfertility.

1. Endometriosis-associated pain

- Can start empirical treatment in suspected endometriosis
- ***Medical treatment:***

First-line

A. Analgesics: Paracetamol, non-steroidal anti-inflammatory drugs (NSAIDs), etc.

B. Visanne® (2 mg dienogest — fourth-generation progestin).
- Inhibits gonadotrophin secretion, which, when given continuously, leads to a hypo-oestrogenic state and initial decidualisation of endometrial tissue, followed by atrophy of endometriotic lesions. Inhibits the proliferation of endometrium-like tissue directly.
- Effectively reduces painful symptoms of endometriosis.
- Efficacy in pain reduction comparable to that of gonadotrophin-releasing hormone agonists (GnRHa).
- It can start on any day of the menstrual cycle and must be continuous regardless of vaginal bleeding/spotting.

C. Progestogens:
- Oral progestins, e.g., Provera, norethisterone.
- Injections, e.g., Depo-Provera.
- Levonorgestrel-releasing intrauterine system LNG-IUS: Mirena®.
- Implants: Implanon®.

D. Combined oral contraceptive pills (COCPs)
- Reduce endometriosis-associated dysmenorrhoea, dyspareunia and non-menstrual pain.
- Can be cyclical or continuous use.

Second-line

E. GnRHa
- Associated with menopausal side effects.
- Duration of use is usually up to 6 months as prolonged use is associated with a risk of bone mineral density (BMD) loss/osteoporosis.

- Add-back therapy is recommended to reduce the side effects of GnRHa. The type of add-back therapy includes norethisterone/norethindrone acetate and tibolone.
- Limited evidence regarding the duration and dosage of GnRHa.

<u>*Third-line*</u>

F. **Letrozole** (ESHRE 2022 guidelines)
   - Indicated only if the woman's pain is refractory to medical treatment or surgery.
   - May be used in combination with COCP, progestogens or GnRHa.
   - Side effects: vaginal dryness, hot flushes, reduced BMD.

G. **Danazol**
   - A synthetic steroid derived from ethinyl testosterone.
   - Should **no longer be used** unless there is no other medical treatment possible because of its severe side effects.
   - Has virilising side effects, e.g., acne, *irreversible* deepening of the voice, facial hair growth, oedema, weight gain.

- ***Surgery***
  - o <u>*Indications for surgery*:</u>
    a. Severe acute symptoms.
    b. No response to medical treatment.
    c. Suspicious of malignancy.
    d. To diagnose and remove endometriosis surgically.
  - o *Classify the severity of endometriosis.* There are various classifications available.
  - o A commonly used one is the revised American Society for Reproductive Medicine (ASRM) classification:
    - *Four stages*: **Stage I** (minimal, score 1–5), **Stage II** (mild, score 6–15), **Stage III** (moderate, score 16–40) and **Stage IV** (severe, score >40).
  - o A *laparoscopic approach* is preferred as it is associated with lesser pain, shorter hospitalisation, faster recovery and better cosmesis.
  - o Complete excision of visible endometriosis may reduce the risk of ovarian cancer.
  - o *Consider pre-operative hormonal treatment*, e.g., GnRHa, to facilitate surgery or treat the woman's pain while waiting for surgery.

PERITONEUM	ENDOMETRIOSIS	<1cm	1.3cm	>3cm
	Superficial	1	2	4
	Deep	2	4	6
OVARY	R Superficial	1	2	4
	Deep	4	16	20
	L Superficial	1	2	4
	Deep	4	16	20
	POSTERIOR CULDESAC OBLITERATION	Partial		Complete
		4		40
OVARY	ADHESIONS	< 1/3 Enclosure	1/3–2/3 Enclosure	> 2/3 Enclosure
	R Filmy	1	2	4
	Dense	4	8	16
	L Filmy	1	2	4
	Dense	4	8	16
TUBE	R Filmy	1	2	4
	Dense	4*	8*	16
	L Filmy	1	2	4
	Dense	4*	8*	16

Fig. 46.2 ASRM classification. If the fimbriated end of the fallopian tube is completely enclosed, change the point assignment to 16. Denote the appearance of superficial implant types as red [(R), red-pink, flame-like, vesicular blobs, clear vesicles], white [(W), opacifications, peritoneal defects, yellow-brown] or black [(B), black, hemosiderin deposits, blue]. Denote the percent of the total described as R percent, W percent and B percent. The total should equal 100%.

Source: Revised American Society for Reproductive Medicine classification of endometriosis: 1996. *Fertil Steril*. 1997; 67(5):817–821. doi:10.1016/s0015-0282(97)81391-x.

- o *Offer post-operative hormonal treatment* to improve the surgical outcome for endometriosis-associated pain if the woman does not desire fertility immediately.
  - E.g., Mirena® or COCP for at least 18–24 months to prevent endometriosis-associated dysmenorrhoea.
  - Long-term hormonal treatment can reduce the risk of recurrence of endometriomas and symptoms.

<u>*Types of surgery*</u>

- o Excise rather than ablate endometriosis to reduce endometriosis-associated pain.
- o **Ovarian endometriomas.**
  - Usually recommended if >5 cm.
  - Clinicians should discuss the impact on ovarian reserve before surgery.

- Ovarian endometriomas are associated with a small increased risk of ovarian cancers such as clear cell or endometrioid carcinoma. Some studies quote a risk of 1.9%, as opposed to the background lifetime risk of ovarian cancer of 1.4%.
- Do cystectomy instead of drainage and coagulation as it reduces the risk of recurrence and endometriosis-associated pain, dyspareunia and non-menstrual pelvic pain.
- Avoid excessive diathermy. Consider suturing or haemostatic agents for haemostasis. This minimises damage to normal ovarian tissues as cystectomy can reduce ovarian reserve and affect fertility.
- If the cysts are suspicious of ovarian malignancy, refer to a gynaecological oncologist and manage as for a suspicious ovarian neoplasm.

o **Deep endometriosis**
- Refer to a multidisciplinary team: a gynaecologist with expertise in endometriosis, a colorectal surgeon and a urologist.
- Excise deep endometriosis as it may reduce endometriosis-associated pain and improve the quality of life.

o **Total hysterectomy ± bilateral salpingo-oophorectomy**
- All visible endometriotic tissues should be removed at the same time.
- Conserving ovaries has a higher risk of recurrence of pain and the need for a second surgery in the future. The risk of recurrence of endometriosis can be as high as 40–50% over 5 years.
- Bilateral oophorectomy can result in early menopause (depending on the woman's age at surgery), and the patient may subsequently need hormone replacement therapy (HRT), e.g., combined oestrogen/progestogen therapy or tibolone.
- Avoid oestrogen-only HRT for treating vasomotor symptoms as it is associated with a higher risk of malignant transformation.

• ***<u>Others</u>***

o **Presacral neurectomy (PSN)** — requires expertise.
- For endometriosis-associated midline pain.
- *<u>Side effects</u>:* Bleeding, constipation, urinary urgency, painless first stage of labour.

- **Laparoscopic uterosacral nerve ablation (LUNA)** — *not* beneficial.

- ***Complementary therapies***, e.g., acupuncture and traditional Chinese medicine, have *unclear* benefits and harms.

<u>2. Endometriosis-associated subfertility</u>

- Refer to a fertility specialist to discuss management options.
- Discuss the pros and cons of fertility preservation in women with extensive endometriosis.
- Suppression of ovarian function does **not** improve fertility in subfertile women with endometriosis.
- *Operative laparoscopy*:
  - May increase the chance of natural pregnancy.
  - ASRM Stage I/II endometriosis — does improve the rate of ongoing pregnancy.
  - Deep endometriosis — **no** strong evidence that it improves fertility.
  - Consider using the endometriosis fertility index (EFI) to predict the pregnancy rate in patients with surgically documented endometriosis who underwent *in vitro* fertilisation (IVF).

Assisted reproductive technology (ART) in endometriosis:

- The is **no** increased recurrence risk of endometriosis with ART.
- **Do not** routinely operate on ovarian endometriomas before ART as it does **not** have a benefit and can negatively impact the ovarian reserve.

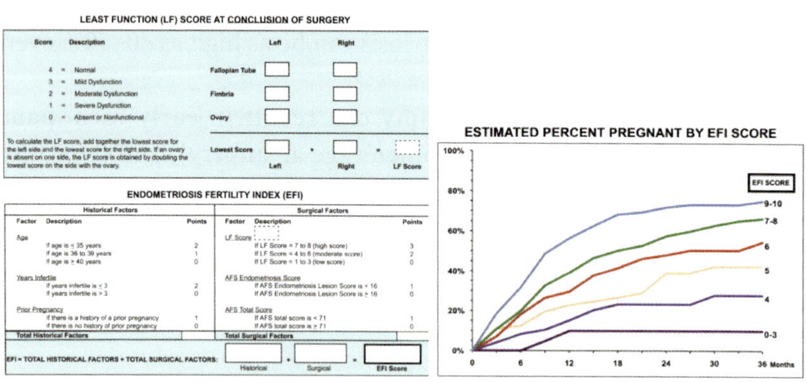

Fig. 46.3 EFI surgery form.

Source: Adamson GD, Pasta DJ. (2010) Endometriosis fertility index: the new, validated endometriosis staging system. *Fertil Steril* 94(5):1609–1615. doi:10.1016/j.fertnstert.2009.09.035.

Indications for surgery:

- ✓ To improve endometriosis-associated pain or access to follicles
- ✓ Rapid growth
- ✓ Suspicious of malignancy

Pros and Cons of Surgery versus Expectant Management for Endometriomas

	Pros	Cons
Endometrioma surgery pre ART	• Obtains histological diagnosis • Treats symptoms of pain • Avoids cyst complications during pregnancy • Improves access to follicles • Reduces infection risk during oocyte retrieval	• Reduces ovarian reserve • Risk of primary ovarian insufficiency with repeated surgeries • Causes adhesions • Recurrence risk • Risks of surgery
Expectant management for endometriomas	• Does not impact the ovarian reserve • Avoids risks of surgery	• Increase in size • Risk of cyst accidents/ torsion • Risk of malignancy • Infection during oocyte retrieval • Hinders access to follicles • Risk of follicular fluid contamination with endometrioma

1. **Treatment with SO-IUI (superovulation intrauterine insemination).**
   - Increases the pregnancy rate in women with minimal to mild endometriosis.
2. **IVF** is an appropriate treatment, especially if the tubal function is compromised or there is associated male factor infertility, low endometriosis fertility index (EFI) or other failed treatment.
   - Both GnRH agonist and antagonist protocols can be offered as there is no difference in pregnancy or live birth rates.
   - Uncertain benefit of giving extended GnRH agonists before ART to improve the live birth rates.

- May give antibiotics at the time of oocyte retrieval in women with endometriomas, although the risk of ovarian abscess is low post-procedure.

***Endometriosis and pregnancy*:**

- May have an increased risk of first-trimester miscarriage and ectopic pregnancy.
- Endometriomas can change in appearance. Therefore, there should be follow-up ultrasound scans of the endometriomas during pregnancy. If the scan shows atypical endometriomas or suspicious of malignancy, refer to a multidisciplinary team involving a gynaecological oncology specialist and a maternal–fetal medicine specialist.
- Complications are rare: these include ovarian accidents, e.g., infection, rupture and spontaneous gastrointestinal perforation.

***Extra-pelvic endometriosis*:**

- Surgical treatment is preferred. If not, hormonal treatment is an option.

Adenomyosis (Fig. 46.4)

***Definition of adenomyosis*:**

- Adenomyosis is a benign, common gynaecological condition defined histologically by the presence of endometrial-like glands and stroma in the myometrium (usually on a hysterectomy specimen).
- Adenomyosis may co-exist with other gynaecological conditions, such as endometriosis and fibroids, in 15–57% of patients.

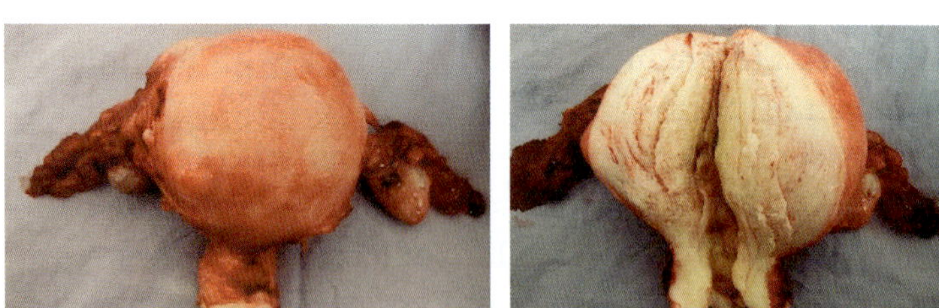

Fig. 46.4 Adenomyotic uterus and the cut section of the uterus.

Symptoms and complications of adenomyosis:

- Patients with adenomyosis may be asymptomatic or symptomatic.
- Heavy menstrual bleeding (HMB).
- Dysmenorrhoea.
- Infertility.
- Dyspareunia.
- Chronic pelvic pain (CPP).

Risks of adenomyosis in pregnancy:

- Miscarriage.
- Preterm premature rupture of membranes.
- Preterm delivery.
- Fetal growth restriction.
- Fetal malpresentation.
- Postpartum haemorrhage (PPH).

Differential diagnosis of adenomyosis:

- Uterine fibroids, endometriosis and HMB due to ovulatory or endometrial dysregulation.

Investigations for Adenomyosis

1. ***TA/TVUS ultrasound pelvis— 70% sensitivity/specificity.***

Criteria used — enlarged globular, regular uterus with no fibroids, myometrial cystic areas and decreased myometrial echogenicity.

2. ***MRI pelvis — 85% sensitivity/specificity.***

Higher diagnostic capability, irrespective of the presence or absence of uterine fibroids.

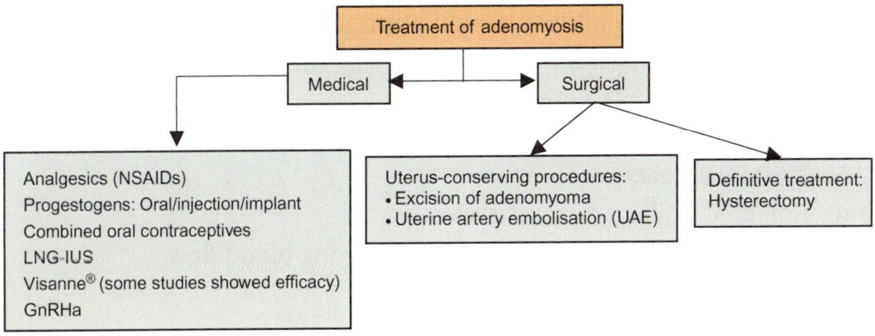

CHAPTER 47

Ovarian Cysts and Borderline Ovarian Tumours

Types of Adnexal Masses

Ovarian mass	Extra-ovarian mass
Benign ovarian cysts, e.g., simple cyst, haemorrhagic cyst, follicular cyst, corpus luteal cyst, theca lutein cyst (Fig. 47.1)	Tubal — ectopic pregnancy, hydrosalpinx/pyosalpinx/haematosalpinx/tubo-ovarian abscess, fallopian tube cancer
Endometriomas	Para-ovarian/para-tubal cysts
Benign cystadenomas, e.g., serous or mucinous cystadenoma	Uterine — pedunculated/broad ligament/cervical fibroid
Dermoid cysts	Bowel pathology — diverticular abscess, appendicular tumour/abscess, malignancy
Fibroma (Fig. 47.2)	Pelvic kidney
Borderline ovarian tumours	Peritoneal inclusion cyst
Primary neoplasms of the ovary	Retroperitoneal masses (benign/malignant)
Metastatic ovarian cancer (from gastric, colon, breast, endometrium)	

Ultrasound (US) findings suspicious of malignancy:

1. Irregular solid/multilocular-solid tumour
2. Solid components/at least four papillary structures
3. Thick septations (>2–3 mm)
4. Ascites
5. Peritoneal masses
6. Enlarged nodes
7. Colour Doppler demonstrating very strong blood flow
8. Bilateral tumours
9. Large tumours (≥10 cm)

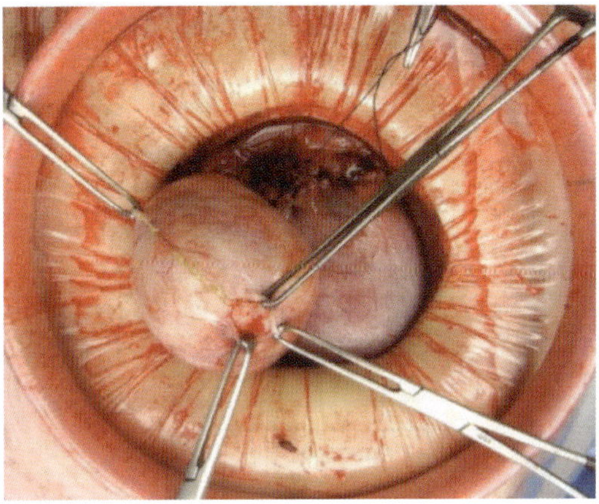

Fig. 47.1 Ovarian cyst.

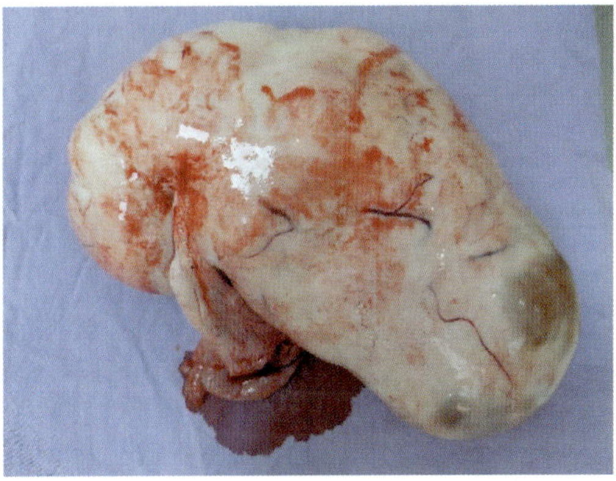

Fig. 47.2 Ovarian fibroma (benign).

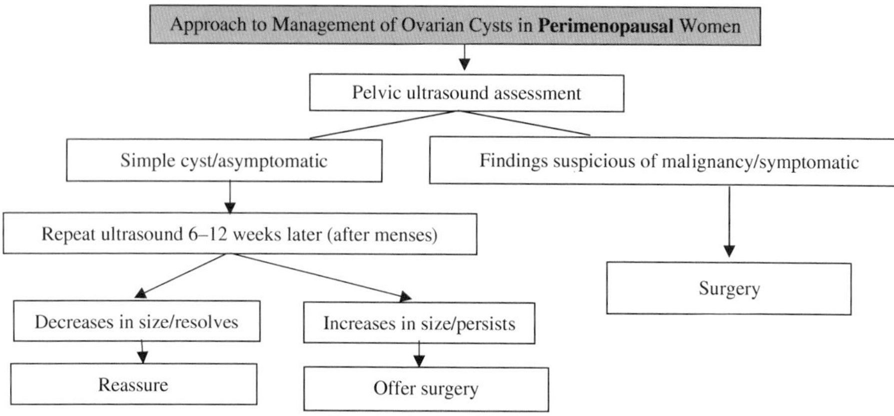

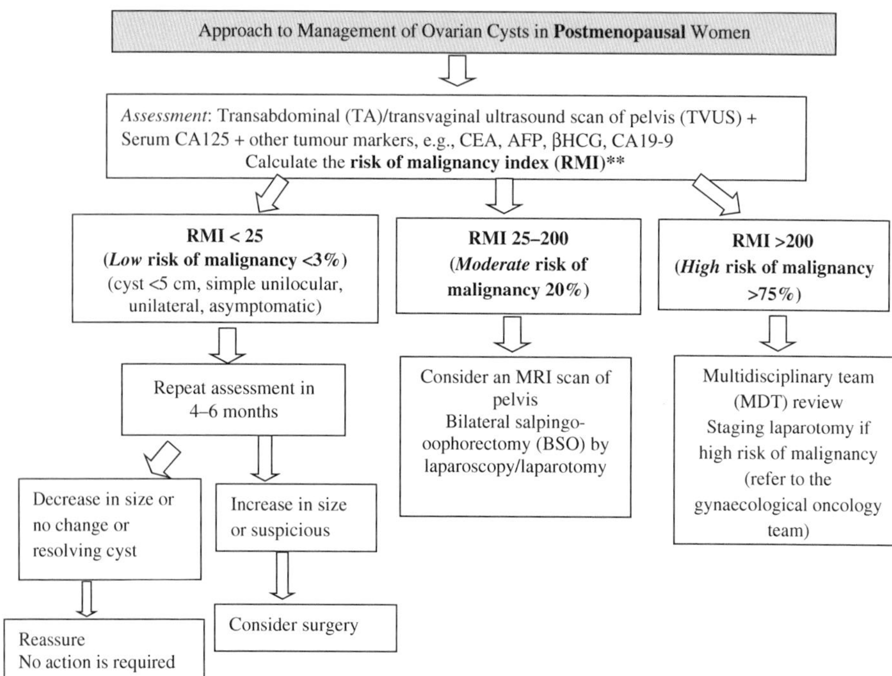

****Calculating the risk of malignancy index (RMI) = $U \times M \times CA125$**
U = 0 (for US score of 0); **U** = 1 (for US score of 1); **U** = 3 (for US score of 2–5)
US scans are scored one point for each of the following characteristics: multilocular cyst, evidence of solid areas, evidence of metastases, the presence of ascites, bilateral lesions.
M = 3 for all postmenopausal women dealt with by this guideline. ***CA125*** is serum CA125 measurement in μ/ml. At RMI >200: Sensitivity 78% and specificity 87% for ovarian cancer

Other Models to Investigate the Risk of Malignancy of Ovarian Masses Pre-Operatively

(a) International Ovarian Tumour Analysis (IOTA) Simple Rules

- It can be used to diagnose the risk of ovarian cancer pre-operatively in women with ovarian/para-ovarian/tubal mass.
- Sensitivity is 93%, specificity is 90%.
- Consists of five features typical of benign tumours (B-features) and five features typical of malignant tumours (M-features).
- Tumours are classified as *benign* (only has B-features), *malignant* (only has M-features) or *inconclusive* (no features apply or both B- and M-features are present).

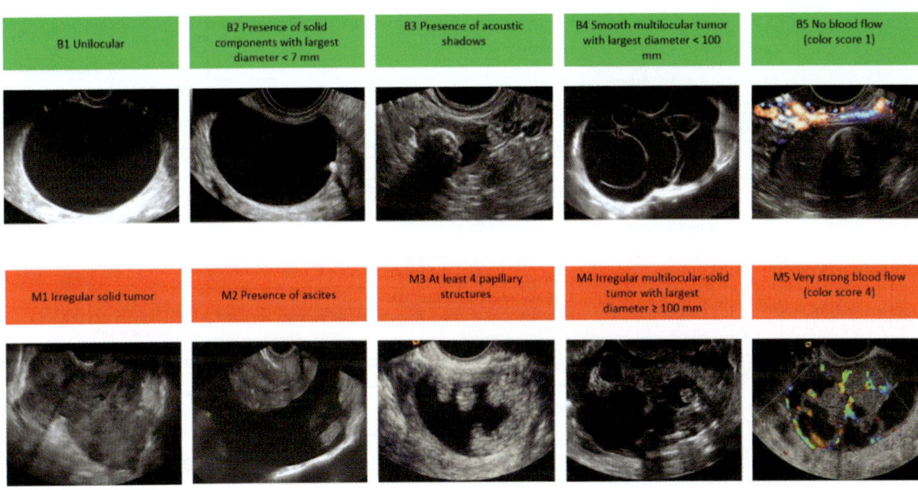

Source: https://www.iotagroup.org/research/iota-models-software/iota-simple-rules-and-srrisk-calculator-diagnose-ovarian-cancer and Timmerman D, Ameye L, Fischerova D, *et al*. Simple ultrasound rules to distinguish between benign and malignant adnexal masses before surgery: prospective validation by IOTA group. *BMJ*. 2010;341:c6839. Published 2010 Dec 14. doi:10.1136/bmj.c6839.

(b) Ovarian-Adnexal Reporting and Data System (O-RADS) Scoring — Used in KKH

- It uses US features to stratify risk and determine the management of ovarian/tubal masses. In addition, it can be used for pelvic masses of which the origin is indeterminate but suspected to be ovarian/tubal/paraovarian in origin or peritoneal inclusion cyst.

- There are *six categories*: O-RADS 0–5, which range from normal to high risk of malignancy. Characterise each lesion separately for multiple or bilateral lesions and manage based on the highest O-RADS score.

O-RADS Score	Risk Category [IOTA Model]	Lexicon Descriptors		Management: Pre-menopausal	Management: Post-menopausal
0	Incomplete Evaluation [N/A]	N/A		Repeat study or alternate study	
1	Normal Ovary [N/A]	Follicle defined as a simple cyst ≤ 3 cm		None	N/A
		Corpus Luteum ≤ 3cm			
2	Almost Certainly Benign [< 1%]	Simple cyst	≤ 3 cm	N/A	None
			> 3 cm to 5 cm	None	Follow up in 1 year. *
			> 5 cm but < 10 cm	Follow up in 8 - 12 weeks	
		Classic Benign Lesions	See **Figure 3** for separate descriptors	See **Figure 3** for management strategies	
		Non-simple unilocular cyst, smooth inner margin	≤ 3 cm	None	Follow up in 1 year * If concerning, US specialist or MRI
			> 3 cm but < 10 cm	Follow-up in 8 - 12 weeks If concerning, US specialist	US specialist or MRI
3	Low Risk Malignancy [1-<10%]	Unilocular cyst ≥ 10 cm (simple or non-simple)		US specialist or MRI Management by gynecologist	
		Typical dermoid cysts, endometriomas, hemorrhagic cysts ≥ 10 cm			
		Unilocular cyst, any size with irregular inner wall <3 mm height			
		Multilocular cyst < 10 cm, smooth inner wall, CS = 1-3			
		Solid smooth, any size, CS = 1			
4	Intermediate Risk [10- < 50%]	Multilocular cyst, no solid component	≥ 10 cm, smooth inner wall, CS = 1-3	US specialist or MRI Management by gynecologist with GYN-oncologist consultation or solely by GYN-oncologist	
			Any size, smooth inner wall, CS = 4		
			Any size, irregular inner wall and/or irregular septation, any color score		
		Unilocular cyst with solid component	Any size, 0-3 papillary projections, CS = any		
		Multilocular cyst with solid component	Any size, CS = 1-2		
		Solid	Smooth, any size, CS = 2-3		
5	High Risk [≥ 50%]	Unilocular cyst, any size, ≥ 4 papillary projections, CS = any		GYN-oncologist	
		Multilocular cyst with solid component, any size, CS = 3-4			
		Solid smooth, any size, CS = 4			
		Solid irregular, any size, CS = any			
		Ascites and/or peritoneal nodules**			

Source: Andreotti RF, Timmerman D, Strachowski LM, *et al*. O-RADS US Risk Stratification and Management System: A Consensus Guideline from the ACR Ovarian-Adnexal Reporting and Data System Committee. *Radiology*. 2020;294(1):168-185. doi:10.1148/radiol.2019191150.

Assessment of Different Neoplasias in the adneXa (ADNEX) Model

- It can be used for patients with adnexal masses planned for surgery → the ADNEX model gives the percentage risk of malignancy.
- Sensitivity varies across studies, ranging from >80–90%; specificity 60–70%.
- Model to differentiate between benign, borderline, stage 1 invasive cancer, stage 2–4 invasive cancer or secondary metastatic cancer.
- Consists of three clinical parameters (age, serum CA 125 level and type of gynaecological centre: gynaecological oncology centre versus other hospitals) and six US predictors (maximum diameter of the lesion in mm, percentage proportion of solid tissue, number of papillary projections, presence of more than 10 cyst locules, presence of acoustic shadows and presence of ascites).

Types of ovarian masses:

1. **Benign ovarian masses**
2. **Ovarian malignancy** — refer to Chapter 37: *Approach to Gynaecological Cancers*.
3. **Borderline ovarian tumours — previously known as ovarian tumours of low malignant potential**

   Definition of borderline ovarian tumours
   - They are ovarian tumours defined by the *absence* of stromal invasion and the *presence* of atypical epithelial proliferation.
   - They are distinct from ovarian carcinoma and are *not* considered ovarian malignancy.

   Risk factors
   - Possible association with assisted reproductive technique (ART) treatment
   - Generally not associated with BRCA carriers

   Symptoms and signs
   - Similar to how patients present with ovarian malignancy
   - **Asymptomatic** — incidental finding on imaging scans OR **Symptomatic** — abdominal mass, abdominal bloatedness/pain, early satiety
   - Signs — abdominal distension

Diagnosis of borderline ovarian tumour

- Requires histological diagnosis
- Investigations are similar to those for ovarian malignancy
  - Ovarian tumour markers, e.g., CA125, CEA, CA 19-9 — most have normal levels
  - *Imaging scans*: US scan of the pelvis, computer tomography (CT) scan of the thorax, abdomen and pelvis (CTTAP), magnetic resonance imaging (MRI) scan of the pelvis

Histological subtypes

Most common subtypes:

- ***Serous*** (65–70%)
  - Most (~70%) are diagnosed with stage 1 disease
  - Up to 50% are bilateral
  - 10–20% have invasive implants
  - *Serous borderline tumour with micropapillary subtype*: This is a subtype of serous ovarian tumour that is associated with adverse prognostic outcomes, i.e., associated with a higher risk of invasive implants and a higher recurrence risk of ~25%.
- ***Mucinous*** (~20–30%)
  - >80% are diagnosed with stage 1 disease
  - >90% are unilateral
  - It can be associated with intraepithelial carcinoma and microinvasion.
  - Higher malignant potential

Others (rare)

- Seromucinous — frequently associated with endometriosis
- Endometrioid
- Clear cell
- Brenner tumour

Borderline ovarian tumours can be associated with the presence of implants.

- **Types:** non-invasive and invasive

Management of borderline ovarian tumours

- Multidisciplinary team (MDT) care. Refer to a gynaecological oncologist.

- Management depends on the patient's age and desire for fertility
  - Intraoperative frozen section may *not* be accurate for borderline ovarian tumours. About 10% of borderline ovarian tumours diagnosed on the frozen section will be invasive carcinoma on the final histology.
  - *Staging surgery* includes intraperitoneal survey, peritoneal washings, omentectomy and biopsy of any suspicious areas ± appendicectomy (for mucinous borderline ovarian tumour). Lymph node dissection is not required.
  - The type of surgical approach is individualised — laparoscopy versus laparotomy.

If a borderline ovarian tumour is <u>suspected pre-operatively</u>:

- *If the patient has completed family* → advise total hysterectomy, bilateral salpingo-oophorectomy (THBSO) and staging surgery
- *If the patient is keen on fertility* → discuss fertility-sparing surgery
  - It is important to discuss with the patient pre-operatively the option for cystectomy versus salpingo-oophorectomy, especially in young women who desire fertility or have bilateral ovarian tumours.
  - Refer to a dedicated **oncofertility clinic** to discuss fertility-sparing surgery and fertility-preservation methods.
  - **For unilateral ovarian tumour:** option of cystectomy versus unilateral salpingo-oophorectomy.
  - **For bilateral ovarian tumours:** bilateral ovarian cystectomy versus unilateral wedge resection of the ovary/salpingo-oophorectomy + ovarian cystectomy.
  - The recurrence risk of borderline ovarian tumours is higher with cystectomy (~30%) versus with salpingo-oophorectomy (~15%). However, some newer studies suggest that the type of surgery does **not** affect the recurrence rate.
  - The risk of invasive recurrence is ~<5%.
  - The recurrence risk of borderline *mucinous* ovarian tumours is *lower* than that of borderline serous tumours. However, when borderline mucinous ovarian tumours recur, they are more likely to recur as invasive carcinoma.

- Post-surgery pregnancy has *not* been shown to impact survival adversely.
- **For <u>post-operative diagnosis</u> of borderline ovarian tumours:**
  - Discuss at a MDT tumour board meeting.
  - If THBSO has been done → continue surveillance.
  - If fertility-sparing surgery has been done → close surveillance with a US scan of the pelvis and ovarian tumour markers.
  - Chemotherapy is *rarely* required for borderline ovarian tumours.
  - Consider chemotherapy for borderline ovarian tumours with invasive implants.
- **Management of recurrence:** usually surgical resection.

<u>Prognosis of borderline ovarian tumours</u>

- Stage of borderline ovarian tumours:
  The staging follows the same FIGO staging for ovarian cancer — refer to Chapter 37: *Approach to Gynaecological Cancers.*
- Good prognosis.
- 5-year survival is 99% for stage 1 disease, 98% for stage 2, 96% for stage 3 and 75% for stage 4.
- The prognosis worsens if there is the *presence* of invasive implants.

<u>Refer to gynaecological oncology:</u>

- If there are other characteristics suspicious of malignancy in premenopausal/postmenopausal women with ovarian cysts, such as:
  - *Physical examination* revealed a pelvic mass, fixed uterus, groin or cervical lymphadenopathy and ascites.
  - *Investigations* suggestive of metastatic cancer.
  - Hereditary breast/ovarian cancer syndrome or history of ovarian cancer in a first-degree relative.
  - Atypical glandular cells (AGC) on cervical cytology in a woman with negative findings on evaluation of the cervix and endometrium.
- Histology showed borderline or malignant ovarian tumours.

Pregnancy With an Adnexal Mass

- The incidence of adnexal masses in pregnancy varies from 0.05 to 9%.
- The incidence of ovarian cancer in pregnancy is 1 in 1,500–32,000 pregnancies.

- Most are diagnosed via incidental findings during routine antenatal US scans.

Causes of Adnexal Masses in Women With an Intrauterine Pregnancy (IUP)

Benign	Borderline/Malignant
a) *Ovarian* – Simple/follicular cyst – Corpus luteal cyst – Haemorrhagic cyst – Endometrioma – Dermoid cyst – Benign cystadenoma (serous/ mucinous) *Related to pregnancy* – Hyperstimulated ovaries following fertility treatment – Hyperreactio luteinalis – Theca lutein cysts – Luteoma of pregnancy b) *Tubal* – Heterotopic pregnancy – Hydrosalpinx/haematosalpinx – Pyosalpinx/tubo-ovarian abscesses c) *Uterine* – Leiomyoma (pedunculated) d) *Non-gynaecological* – Appendicular/diverticular mass – Mesenteric cyst – Pelvic kidney	a) *Ovarian* – Borderline ovarian tumours (serous/ mucinous) – Epithelial tumours – Germ cell tumours – Sex cord-stromal tumours b) *Tubal* – Tubal malignancies c) *Metastatic (Krukenburg tumour)* – Breast – Gastrointestinal (gastric, colon)

Role of ovarian tumour markers in pregnancy

(Refer to Chapter 60: *Tumour Markers in Gynaecology and Pregnancy.*)

Tumour markers can be *difficult to interpret*, as a normal pregnancy can result in raised tumour markers.

- **CA125** peaks in the first trimester and after delivery. It may be useful as a marker from 16 weeks of gestation onwards. Very high levels, e.g., ≥1,000, are suspicious of malignancy.

  Values between 75 and 150 could be related to pregnancy. It can be done as a baseline test.
- **Lactate dehydrogenase (LDH)** is **not** elevated in normal pregnancies unless there is pre-eclampsia/HELLP syndrome. It can be used reliably as a tumour marker for ovarian dysgerminoma.
- **Alpha-fetoprotein (AFP)** rises during pregnancy and is part of the second-trimester maternal serum screening for Down syndrome or fetal neural tube defects.

  AFP levels associated with ovarian cancer are much higher than those associated with fetal neural tube defects, usually ≥9 multiples of median (MoM).
- **Beta-human chorionic gonadotrophin (*β*HCG)** is *not* recommended as it is elevated in pregnancy.
- **Inhibin A** is a component of the second-trimester maternal serum screening for Down syndrome. Levels are raised in pregnancy and may **not** be useful as a tumour marker.
- **Human epididymis protein 4 (HE4)** can be used in pregnancy as levels are *not* raised.

Imaging modalities that are safe in pregnancy — no ionising radiation risk to the fetus

- Transabdominal/transvaginal US (TA/TVUS) scan of the pelvis
- Chest X-ray (CXR) with abdominal shield
- MRI scan of the abdomen/pelvis

Complications of adnexal mass in pregnancy

- Asymptomatic
- Cyst accidents, e.g., rupture (<1%), bleeding, infection
- Torsion (~5% or up to 20% if ovarian cyst >6 cm) → tubal/ovarian necrosis, need for emergency surgery/salpingo-oophorectomy

- Progression in size → pressure symptoms
- Obstructed labour
- Fetal malpresentation
- Risk of malignancy and progression of the disease

Management of Adnexal Mass in Pregnancy

Expectant Management

- Up to 70% of adnexal masses resolve during pregnancy.
- Most functional cysts resolve spontaneously by the 16th week of pregnancy.
- *Corpus luteal cysts* usually regress by the 8th week of pregnancy. They are highly vascular and can bleed. If they are removed before the 8th week of pregnancy, progesterone supplementation is required till the 10th week of gestation, when the placenta is developed and is the source of progesterone (luteo-placental shift).
- *Risk factors for persistence*: cyst size >5 cm, complex morphology on TA/TVUS.
- More than 60% of ovarian torsions occur most frequently in the first trimester, occasionally in the second trimester up to the 17th week of gestation and rarely in the third trimester.
- The reported rate of complications with expectant management is <2%.

Suspected Malignant Masses

- Approximately 10% of adnexal masses that persist during pregnancy are malignant.
- Most are borderline ovarian tumours or early-stage ovarian cancers, which have a good prognosis.
- Refer to a gynaecological oncologist, a maternal–fetal medicine specialist, an anaesthetist ± neonatologist and a medical social worker.
- Discuss at a multidisciplinary tumour board meeting.
- May need staging scans, e.g., MRI abdomen/pelvis, CXR with an abdominal shield.

- Consider fertility-sparing surgery, e.g., cystectomy/unilateral salpingo-oophorectomy, peritoneal washings, omentectomy, intraperitoneal survey, peritoneal biopsies ± lymph node dissection.

  Re-staging for lymph node assessment may be required post-delivery if *not* done during the primary surgery.
- If the diagnosis was made in the *first trimester*, discuss with the patient regarding continuing the pregnancy versus termination of pregnancy (especially in advanced disease).

  In addition, inform the patient of the background risk of a miscarriage of 15–20% in the first trimester.
- If the diagnosis was made in the *second or third trimester*, discuss with the patient regarding surgery. Some may require early delivery via caesarean section. Hence, patients should be informed about the risks of prematurity to the fetus.
- Certain chemotherapy drugs are safe in the second and third trimesters.

Surgical Management

Indications for surgery include:
- Suspected malignancy.
- Acute abdomen from complications, e.g., torsion or rupture.
- Cyst >10 cm due to the risk of obstructed labour.
- Rapidly enlarging masses (>20% increase in size).
  - Surgeries are usually planned during the second trimester of the pregnancy unless it is an emergency.
  - For benign cysts, surgical removal can be performed at the same time as a caesarean section (if indicated for obstetric reasons) or performed at least 6 weeks postpartum via laparoscopy/laparotomy (depending on the size and characteristics of the ovarian cyst).
  - **Laparoscopy** is safe in pregnancy and can be performed in any trimester.
    - **Benefits:** faster recovery, lesser pain, lower risk of venous thromboembolism, wound infection or post-operative ileus. It also decreases maternal hypoventilation and has a lower risk of neonatal respiratory distress because of maternal opioid use.

- No increased risk of preterm labour, fetal malformations or stillbirth.
- As there is an increased risk of uterine injury during the insertion of ports, consider alternative port sites, Hasson's technique or Palmer's point entry.

- **Laparotomy** may be advisable in cases suspicious of malignancy to avoid intraperitoneal spillage, dissemination of malignancy and port site metastases.
- <u>*Factors affecting the choice of surgical approach*</u>: laparoscopy versus laparotomy are:
  - Gestational age
  - Size of mass
  - Possibility of malignancy
  - Surgical expertise
  - Patient's preference

CHAPTER 48

Urogynaecology

Urinary Incontinence

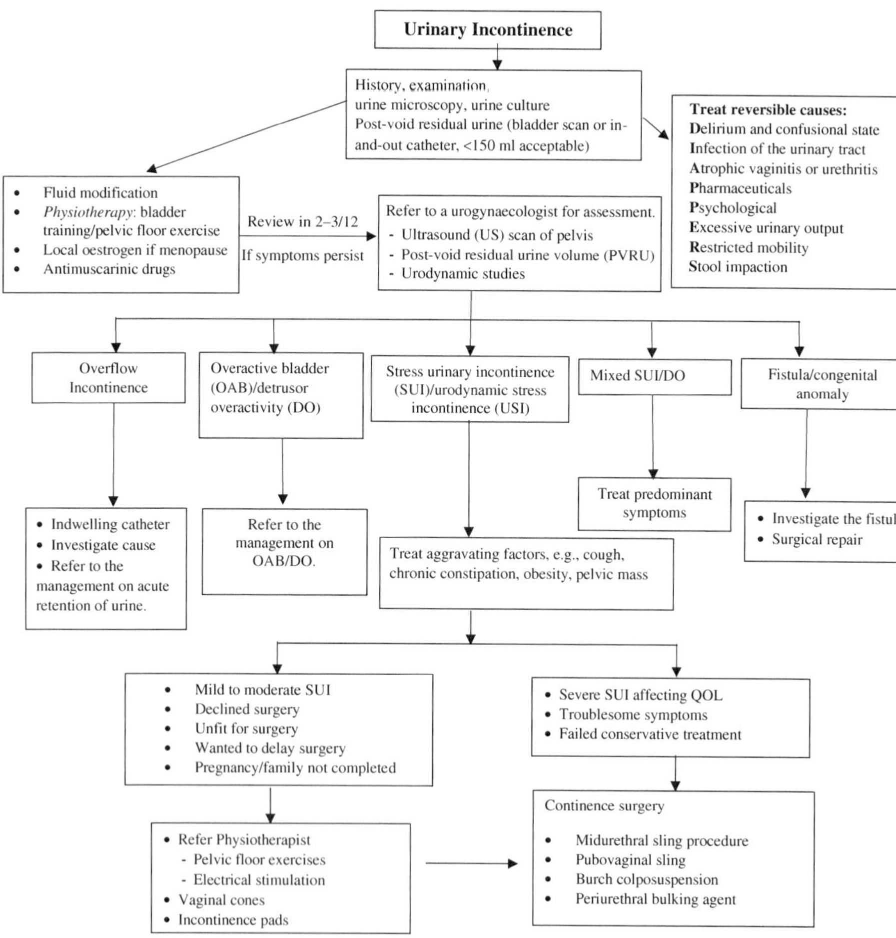

Overactive Bladder (OAB)/Detrusor Overactivity (DO)

Management of OAB/DO

1. Lifestyle modification
Weight loss if obese

2. Fluid modification
Restrict fluid intake (<2 L/day)
Reduce caffeine intake

3. Refer to a physiotherapist
Bladder training/pelvic floor exercise

4. Medications (at least for 6–8 weeks)

- Vaginal oestrogen if menopausal

OAB/DO:
Anticholinergics:
- **Contraindications**: glaucoma, elderly with cognitive impairment

- Oxybutynin (Ditropan) – 2.5 mg BD to 5 mg BD (cheapest but more side effects)
- Tolterodine (Detrusitol) – 2 mg BD or tolterodine SR 4 mg OM (cheaper but a higher side effect profile)
- Solifenacin (Vesicare) – 5mg OM (better side effects profile, cheaper if use generic formulation)

Nocturia (exclude OSA):
- Anticholinergics
- Imipramine 25mg to 50mg ON: especially if there is insomnia
  - *Side effects*: Drowsiness which can increase the risk of falls
- Desmopressin 200µg ON: use for nocturnal polyuria
  - *Side effect*: Hyponatraemia. Be cautious when prescribing, especially in elderly patients. Need to monitor the renal panel/electrolytes

↓

Any improvement in symptoms OR tolerable side effects → Yes → Continue treatment

↓ No

1. Refer to a urogynaecologist
2. *Change medication*:
- Solifenacin (Vesicare) 5 mg OM
- Dariferacin 7.5 mg OM

If no response in 2 months
1. Increase the dose of solifenacin/dariferacin
2. Change medication to mirabegron 25–50 mg OM – need to monitor BP, LFT/renal panel
- *Contraindications*: uncontrolled hypertension, liver or renal impairment, ischaemic heart disease

↓

- Still no improvement in symptoms
- Medications contraindicated

↓

Investigation:
- Cystoscopy ± biopsy if suspecting bladder pain syndrome/interstitial cystitis
- Urodynamic studies

↓

Treatment for refractory OAB
(failure of or intolerable to at least two medications)

→ Intravesical injection Botulinum toxin A
→ Percutaneous tibial nerve stimulation (PTNS)
→ Sacral nerve stimulation (SNS)

↓ If no response

Terminal management
→ Bladder augmentation
→ Urinary diversion
→ Detrusor myomectomy

Overactive Bladder (OAB)/Nocturia

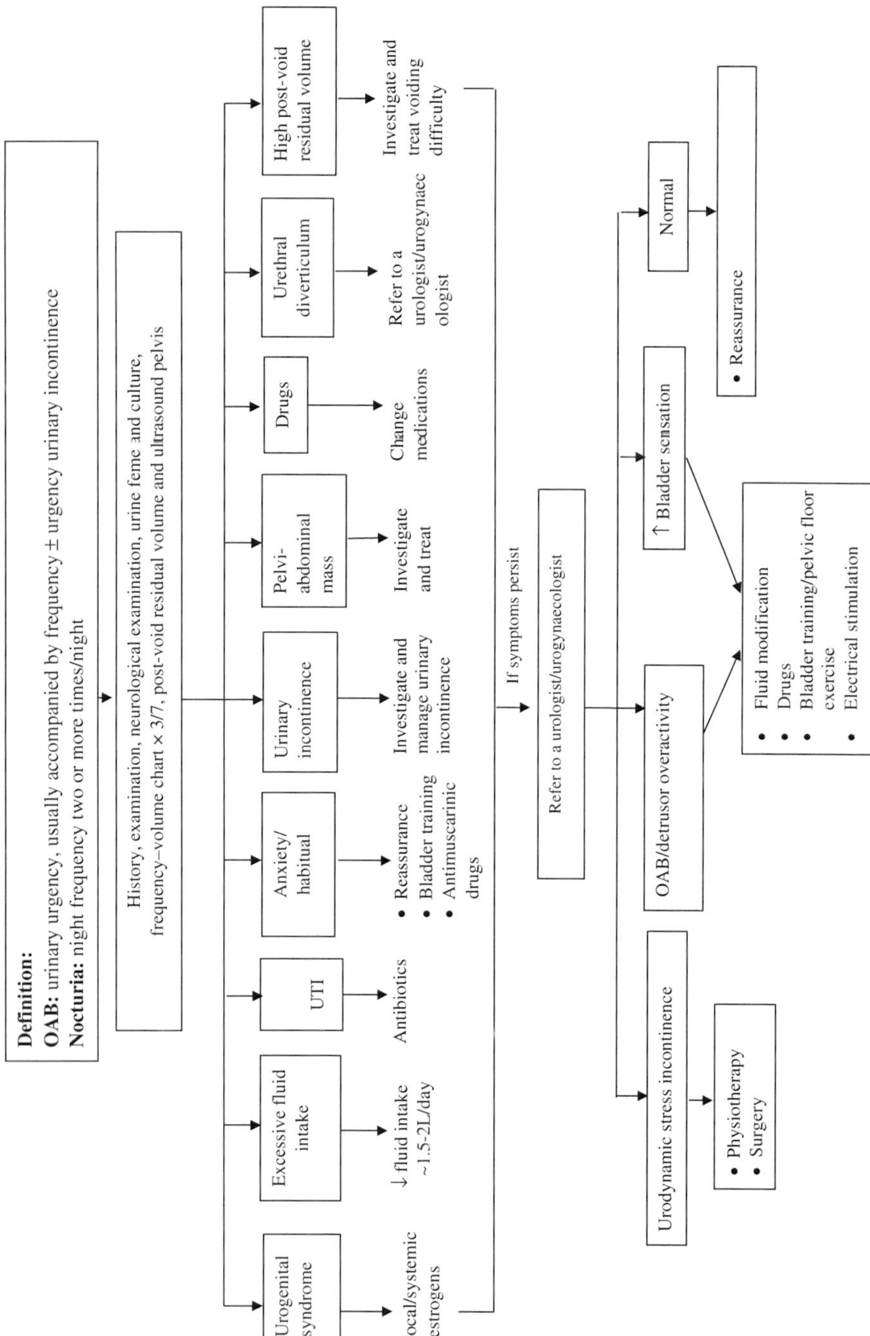

Pelvic Organ Prolapse (POP)

Lump at Introitus

1. History:

- Vaginal bulge/heaviness, lump at the introitus
- Urine — voiding difficulty especially after standing, any need for manually reducing the bulge to improve urinary flow, OAB/SUI symptoms
- Bowel — straining or needing to splint/digitate to evacuate bowel
- Sexual — dyspareunia/coital continence
- *Complications of prolapse* — ulcer, pain, infection, bleeding
- *Risk factors for POP* — chronic cough or constipation, carrying heavy weights, pelvic mass

2. Examination:

- Body mass index (BMI).
- Assessment of the extent of POP in the supine position. If unclear of the extent of POP, need to examine in the erect position.
- Perform POP-Q assessment to quantify the degree of prolapse.
- Exclude any co-existent pathology, any prolapse decubitus ulceration or infection, any pelvic or adnexal mass
- Local examination for any urogenital atrophy
- Digital rectal examination to evaluate anal sphincter tone and presence of rectal prolapse if bowel symptoms are present.

3. Investigation:

- Post-void residual urine (PVRU)
- UFEME and culture

First-line management

1. **Lifestyle modification:**
   - Weight reduction if obese.
   - Smoking cessation.
   - Treat risk factors, e.g., chronic cough and constipation. Avoid carrying heavy weights.
2. **Physiotherapy referral** for supervised pelvic floor muscle therapy.
3. **Topical vaginal oestrogen** in menopausal women if no contraindications.
4. **Conservative management** if mild POP.

If keen on conservative treatment

- Vaginal ring pessary: risk of ulceration, bleeding, infection
- Review in every 4–6 months

If failed conservative treatment →

If keen on surgery

Refer to a urogynaecologist

Do nothing

Non-surgical treatment

Surgical treatment

Types of Pelvic Organ Prolapse (POP) Surgery

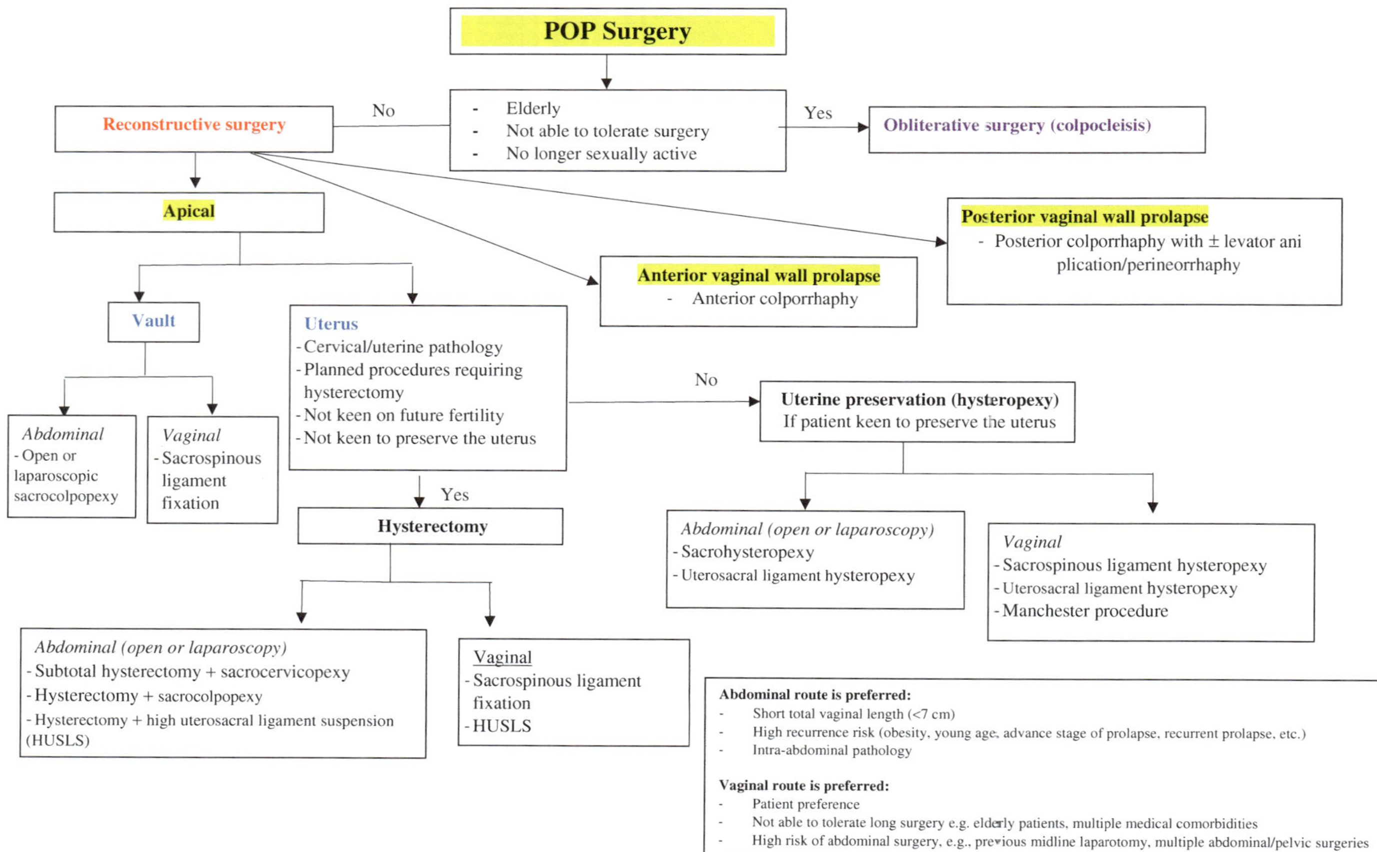

POP and Urinary Incontinence

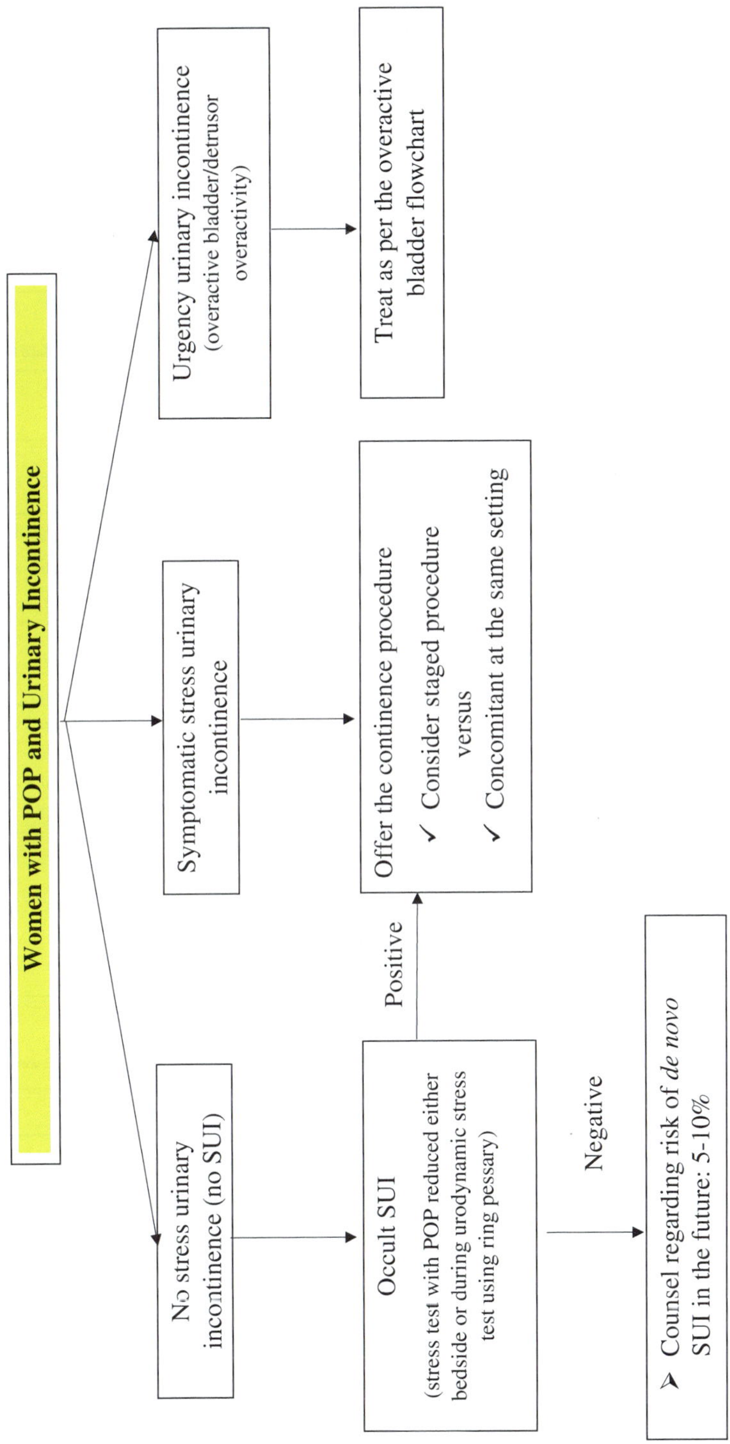

Uncomplicated Urinary Tract Infection (UTI)

Also known as cystitis or *lower* UTI

Typical symptoms presented are:
Urinary frequency, urgency, hesitancy, dysuria and suprapubic discomfort, haematuria

Absence of:
Fever, flank pain, vomiting or other suspicion of pyelonephritis
Absence of vaginal discharge and irritation

↓

Urine microscopy (UFEME)/urine culture
Midstream clean catch specimen in non-obese patients
May need in-out catheterised sample in obese women to avoid contamination from genital surface flora

Negative

↓

Symptomatic treatment

↓

Look for other causes, e.g., urethritis – urethral culture for mycoplasma/gonococcus/chlamydia, and treat accordingly

Positive

↓

First line (depending on availability, tolerability and allergy history)

1. PO nitrofurantoin 50–100 mg QDS ×5 days (avoid if early pyelonephritis suspected and G6PD deficiency) OR
2. PO trimethoprim-sulfamethoxazole (Bactrim) 160mg/800 mg BD × 5 days (be aware that resistance prevalence can be >20% in some populations/avoid if used for UTI in last 3 months) OR
3. PO fosfomycin 3 g single dose (avoid if early pyelonephritis suspected)
4. PO Cephalexin 500 mg TDS x 5 days

Alternative therapy:

1. PO Ciprofloxacin 500mg BD x 5 days (be aware that resistance prevalence high is some population/Avoid in pregnancy)
2. PO Amoxycillin-clavulanate (Augmentin) 1gm BD x 5 days
3. Avoid ampicillin or amoxicillin as lower efficacy and high prevalence of resistance
4. Choose antibiotics according to culture and sensitivity results

↓

Is test of cure required?

No

If symptoms resolved

↓

Routine follow-up

Yes

- If symptoms do not resolve by end of treatment or
- Those whose symptoms resolve but recur within 2 weeks

↓

Repeat treatment with another antimicrobial agent with a 7 days' regime

↓

Symptoms resolved

No → Routine follow-up

Yes → Investigate and treat as for recurrent UTI

Recurrent UTI

Recurrent UTI is defined as two or more UTI episodes in the last 6 months or three UTI episodes during the last 12 months.

History and physical examination
1. Previous UTI diagnoses
2. UFEME and urine culture
3. Pelvic examination

↓

Two culture-proven episodes of UTI within 6 months or three episodes within 1 year

→

Look for high risk factors and treat accordingly
- Immunocompromised patients
- Diabetic patients
- Patients on steroids
- Cancer patients
- Advanced age
- Inefficient bladder emptying (e.g., neuropathic bladder, post operation, drug-induced voiding difficulties)
- Indwelling catheter
- Recurrent vulvovaginitis
- Post menopause

↓

Investigations:
- Post-void residual urine (PVRU)
- US KUB
- *Cystoscopy*: if bladder pain syndrome, bladder calculi or urothelial cancer suspected

↓

Urine culture positive

↓

Acute/episodic treatment

1st Line: Nitrofurantoin, Fosfomycin, Bactrim, Cephalexin
2nd Line: Ciprofloxacin, Augmentin
Duration: as short a duration as possible (≤ 7 days)
1. Culture directed
2. Depending on local antibiogram
3. Test of cure *not* required

Urine culture negative → **Prophylaxis**

↓

Vaginal oestrogen – for peri- and postmenopausal women *without* contraindications

Non-antibiotic prophylaxis
1. Cranberry
2. Behavioural modifications such as wiping from front to back after defaecation, double voiding
3. Immediate post-coital voiding
4. Perineal hygiene education
5. Increased fluid intake

Low-dose antibiotic prophylaxis

Continuous:
- No longer than 12 months with periodic assessment and monitoring

Intermittent:
- Single-dose antibiotic used for exposure to UTI-predisposing conditions such as post-coital exposure during menses

Commonly used antibiotic regimens include:
- Nitrofurantoin 50 mg/100 mg once daily
- Cephalexin 250 mg once daily
- Trimethoprim 100 mg once daily
- TMP-SMX 40 mg/200 mg once daily
- Fosfomycin 3 g every 10 days

- **Refer to a urologist:**
  If *upper tract abnormality* such as calculi or a tumour is suspected.
- **Refer to a urogynaecologist/urologist:**
  If *lower tract abnormality* suspected.

Acute Retention of Urine (ARU)

Acute Retention of Urine

↓

- Inability to pass urine for >6 hours
- Inability to pass >50% of normal bladder capacity [400–600 ml or if post-void residual urine (PVR) >150 ml]

↓

History: small voided volumes, urinary frequency, bladder pain/discomfort, need to strain, poor stream, urinary incontinence (overflow)
Examination: abdominal distension with normal bowel sounds, stony dull percussable bladder
Investigation: bladder scan or in-and-out catheter

↓

Urine microscopy and culture
Indwelling catheter for 24–48 hours, then trial-off catheter (TOC)
Look for causes of ARU and treat if any cause is found

Causes of ARU	Management
Drugs (e.g., anticholinergics)	Stop or change medication
Post-operative ARU, epidural and spinal anaesthesia	Adequate analgesia and continuous drainage for 1–2 days
Obstetric cause, e.g., prolonged labour/prolonged second stage, instrumental delivery, perineal trauma	Adequate analgesia and continuous drainage for 1–2 days If a vaginal pack was inserted, remove it before TOC (trial off catheter).
Neurological (e.g., spinal injury)	Refer to a neurosurgeon/neurologist.
Gynaecological (e.g., uterine prolapse, fibroids or cystocele)	**Refer to a UROGYN** for assessment/ surgery.
UTI	Treat with antibiotics
Constipation	Treat with laxatives
Urethral stricture	Refer to a urologist for urethral dilatation.
Urethritis/herpes infection	Antibiotics, analgesics, acyclovir

↓

If failed TOC:
- Inability to pass urine for >6 hours
- Inability to pass >50% of normal bladder capacity
- If PVR urine >150 ml (with voided volume >150 ml)

↓

Reinsert the catheter and repeat TOC after 1 week.

Passed TOC →

Encourage PU 2–3 hours
Double voiding

Poor prognosis with PVR >700 ml
CISC: If PVR consistently <100 ml then can stop
May need investigation if persistent voiding dysfunction beyond 1 month
- ➢ Urodynamic studies and uroflowmetry
- ➢ Cystoscopy to assess any urethral stricture or trauma

No evidence on role of medication such as distigmine or bethanechol

Failed TOC →

Indwelling catheter × 2 weeks or
Clean intermittent self-catheterisation (CISC)

Refer to a urologist/urogynaecologist.
Surgical options:
- Urethral dilatation for suspected urethral stenosis
- Sacral nerve stimulation (SNS)
- Turbine valve (*not* widely used)

Asymptomatic Microscopic Haematuria (AMH)

Defined as ≥3 red blood cells per high-power field (RBC/HPF) on UFEME

UFEME
≥3 RBC/HPF

→ Exclude transient causes, e.g., UTI, menses, recent sexual intercourse, exercise

↓

Send urine culture
(if not done yet)

→ **If positive urine culture:**
Treat UTI and repeat UFEME
3 weeks later

↓

If negative urine culture:
Repeat UFEME
Give vaginal oestrogen for 4-6 weeks if atrophic vaginitis is suspected before repeating UFEME

If second UFEME for RBC is negative: discharge

If second UFEME is positive for RBC:
1) Check BP (to exclude renal causes of HPT)
2) Blood test for serum creatinine
3) Urine for urine phase contrast for dysmorphic RBCs/red cell casts/acanthocytes (ring)/proteinuria

↓

If positive urine phase contrast:
Refer to a nephrologist and assess for risk factors for renal tract malignancy.

↓

- **Patients with risk factors for renal tract malignancy***
  Do urine cytology and cystoscopy and take a CT urogram
- **If low risk of renal tract malignancy**
  (age <40, RBC 3–10/HPF, non-smoker, no other high-risk factors)
  - Do US KUB/cystoscopy
  - If patient not keen on further investigations, then repeat UFEME 6/12 later. Do US KUB/cystoscopy if persistent RBCs are present

↓

Follow-Up: yearly UFEME
If UFEME is negative ⇒ discharge the patient
If UFEME remains positive for RBCs ⇒ continue yearly follow-up for 3–5 years
If worsening AMH (RBC ↑) or persistent AMH beyond 3–5 years after full workup ⇒ consider re-evaluation

*** Risk factors for malignancy**
- *Age > 40 years*
- *RBC > 10/HPF*
- *Past/current smoking*
- *Irritative voiding symptoms (urgency/frequency/nocturia/incomplete voiding sensation)*
- *Chronic UTI*
- *Chronic indwelling catheter*
- *Pelvic irradiation*
- *Exposure to alkylating chemotherapy/known carcinogenic agents such as rubber, petrochemicals and dyes.*

Non-contrast computer tomography (CT) scan of kidneys, ureters and bladder (KUB) if
- Contraindication to CT urogram (e.g., impaired renal function)
- Allergy to contrast
- Magnetic resonance imaging (MRI) urography not available where CT urography contraindicated

Ultrasound (US) scan of KUB only if
- Low risk of malignancy
- Cost is an issue for patients with high risk factors for malignancy
- Important to explain to the patient that the sensitivity of US KUB is only ~50% for upper renal tract malignancies

CHAPTER 49

Vaginal Discharge, Vulvovaginal Candidiasis, Bacterial Vaginosis and Atrophic Vaginitis/Genitourinary Syndrome of Menopause (GSM)

Causes of vaginal discharge

1. **Physiological** — periods when there are fluctuating levels of oestrogen and progesterone, such as ovulation and pregnancy
2. **Pathological:**
   - **Infections** — bacterial vaginosis (BV), candidiasis, trichomoniasis, *Chlamydia trachomatis, Neisseria gonorrhoea,* endometritis, pelvic inflammatory disease (PID)
   - **Cancer** — endometrial, cervical, vaginal, vulval, ovarian, fallopian tube
   - **Atrophic vaginitis**
   - **Local causes** — intrauterine contraceptive devices (IUCDs), polyps, fistulas, foreign bodies, e.g., a retained tampon
   - **Dermatitis**, e.g., due to a change in soap

Causes, Symptoms and Signs of Vaginitis

		Clinical symptoms			Clinical signs	
Type	**Aetiology**	**Discharge**	**Pain**	**Pruritus**	**Vagina**	**Vulva**
Bacterial vaginosis (BV)	Gardnerella vaginalis, Mycoplasma hominis, *anaerobic bacteria*: *Prevotella* species, *Mobiluncus* species	Malodorous; homogeneous; clear, white, or grey: fishy odour	Not primary symptom	Not primary symptom	No signs of inflammation	Unaffected
Trichomoniasis	*Trichomonas vaginalis*	Green-yellow, frothy	Pain with sexual intercourse, vaginal soreness, dysuria	Not primary symptom	Signs of inflammation ("strawberry cervix")	Vestibular erythema may be present
Vulvovaginal candidiasis (VVC)	*Candida albicans*, *Candida krusei*, *Candida glabrata*	White, thick, lack of odour	Burning, dysuria, dyspareunia	Frequent	Signs of inflammation, oedema	Excoriations/Fissures
Atrophic vaginitis	Oestrogen deficiency	Yellow, greenish, lack of odour	Vaginal dryness, pain with sexual intercourse	Rare	Vagina mildly erythematous, easily traumatised	Vestibule thin and dry; labia majora lose their subcutaneous fat; labia minora irritated and friable
Erosive lichen planus	Aetiology is unknown	Yellow or grey	Intense pain, dyspareunia, postcoital bleeding	Intense	Erythema with friable epithelium	Erosions, white plaques
Irritant or allergic contact dermatitis	Contact irritation or allergic reaction with episodic flares	Minimal	Burning on acute contact, soreness	More likely in allergic reactions	Vulvar erythema possible	Erythema with or without oedema; vesicles or bullae rare

Source: Table adapted from https://www.aafp.org/afp/2011/0401/p807.html.

When should investigations be done for vaginal discharge?
If the patient:

- Is at high risk of sexually transmitted infections (i.e., <25 years old, change of sexual partner or has more than one sexual partner in the last year)
- Has fever or abdominal pain suggestive of PID (refer to Chapter 50: *Pelvic Inflammatory Disease*)
- Has failed medical treatment
- Is postnatal, post-abortal or has had a recent miscarriage
- History of recent IUCD insertion in the last 2 months

It is reasonable to treat the patient with vaginal discharge empirically *without investigations* if a thorough sexual history and physical examination revealed that she is at *low risk of STI*, has no signs to suggest PID and can return for follow-up if her symptoms do not resolve.

Investigations

VP3 test: vaginal swab to screen for *Candida*, *Gardnerella vaginalis* and *Trichomonas vaginalis*.

STI screening tests (in patients at high risk of STIs): vaginal, urethral, rectal swabs or urine samples for chlamydia and gonorrhoea.

In most cases, the symptoms and clinical appearance of the vaginal discharge are variable and may *not* accurately suggest the causative organism (s) involved.

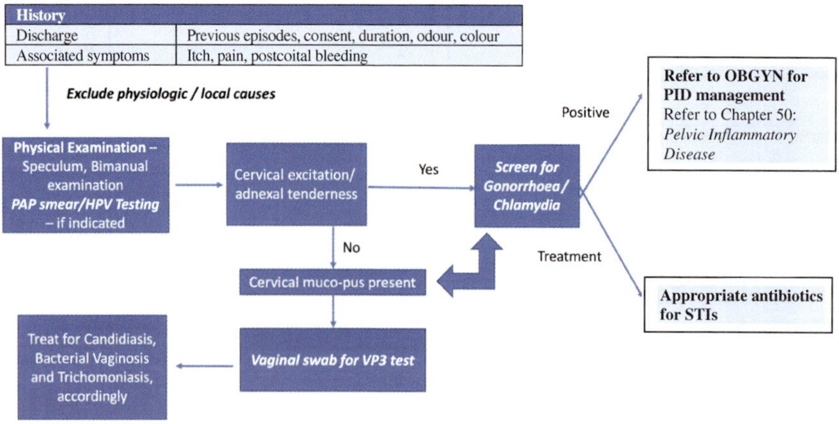

Management of Vaginal Discharge

- Take a medical and sexual history and assess risk factors for STIs
- Perform a physical examination, including abdominal and pelvic examination, to assess for PID, other surgical conditions or pregnancy. External vulvovaginal examination to visualise any lesions, overt genital discharge, vulval erythema or excoriations

Speculum/vaginal examination:
- Assess for cervical tenderness or pain on palpation of the pelvic area to exclude PID
- Presence of vaginal discharge, its colour and consistency
- Offer human immunodeficiency virus (HIV) and syphilis screening

General advice
- Educate and counsel on perineal hygiene
- Avoidance of triggers, use of soaps instead of feminine wash

(a) Vulvovaginal Candidiasis (VVC) — Main Causative Organism: *Candida Albicans (90% of Cases)* (Figure 49.1)

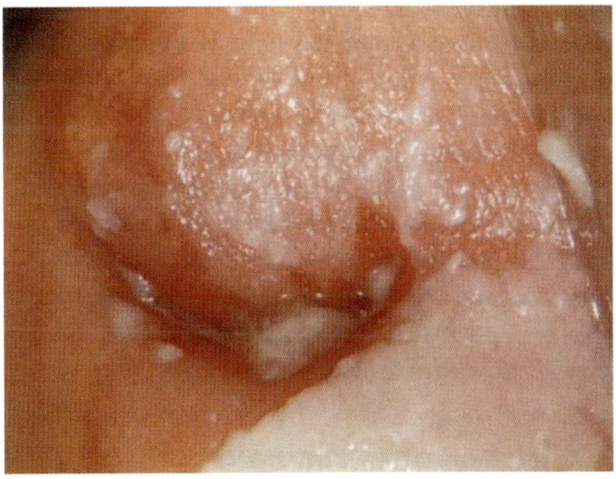

Fig. 49.1 Cervico-vaginal *Candidiasis*.

Types of Vulvovaginal Candidiasis (VVC)

Uncomplicated acute VVC	**Complicated** acute VVC
• Sporadic or infrequent • Mild–moderate infection • *Candida albicans* • Immunocompetent host	• Recurrent infection • Severe infection • Non-*Candida albicans* • Immunocompromised, e.g., diabetes mellitus (DM), HIV, immunodeficiency syndromes or on immunosuppressants

Treatment of Uncomplicated Acute VVC

Vaginal pessary	**Oral antifungals** (avoid in pregnancy because of the risk of miscarriage and teratogenicity)
Isoconazole 600 mg once OR	
Clotrimazole 100 mg every night (ON) × 6 days OR 500 mg ON × 1 day OR 200 mg ON × 3 days	PO fluconazole 150 mg once OR PO itraconazole 200 mg once In pregnancy, use *topical azoles* instead
Miconazole nitrate 200 mg ON × 3 days OR 100 mg ON × 7 days	
Nystatin 100,000 U daily × 7 days	

<u>**Recurrent (complicated) VVC**</u> — affects <5% of women

Definition:

- **BASHH guidelines:** Four episodes per 12 months with two episodes confirmed by microscopy or culture when symptomatic (≥1 must be confirmed by culture)
- **CDC guidelines:** ≥3 symptomatic episodes of VVC within 12 months

Treatment of Recurrent (Complicated) VVC

- **Initial treatment:** 7–14 days of topical therapy OR
  PO fluconazole (100 mg, 150 mg or 200 mg) every third day for 3 doses (on days 1, 4, 7)
- **Maintenance treatment:** PO fluconazole (100 mg, 150 mg or 200 mg) weekly × 6 months
- **Recurrent VVC in pregnancy:** Topical imidazole therapy × 10–14 days followed by clotrimazole vaginal pessary 500 mg weekly for maintenance therapy

(b) Bacterial Vaginosis (BV) — Most Common Cause of Lower Genital Tract Infection (LGTI)

- Main causative organism: *Gardnerella vaginalis.*
- *Investigation*: VP3 test.
- BV is associated with an increased risk of complications in pregnancy, e.g., preterm delivery (PTD), preterm premature rupture of the membranes (PPROM), chorioamnionitis, low-birth-weight babies and postpartum endometritis.

Treatment of BV in Non-Pregnant Females

- PO metronidazole 400–500 mg twice a day (BD) × 7 days OR
  2 g stat × 1 dose OR
- PO clindamycin 300 mg BD × 7 days OR
- PO tinidazole 2 g daily × 2 days OR
  PO tinidazole 1 g daily × 5 days OR
- PV metronidazole gel (0.75%) 5 g daily × 5 days OR
- PV clindamycin cream (2%) 5 g daily × 7 days OR
- Flagystatin vaginal pessary ON × 10 days

Treatment of BV in Pregnancy

- PO clindamycin 300 mg BD × 7 days OR
- PO metronidazole 400 mg BD × 7 days (conflicting guidelines regarding recommendations for metronidazole use in the first trimester. *CDC/BASHH guidelines*: It is safe to use metronidazole in pregnancy, including the first trimester. *In KKH*, we avoid the use of metronidazole in the first trimester.)

Treatment of BV in Breastfeeding Mothers

- Metronidazole is excreted in breast milk, but the doses that breastfeed infants receive are lower than those used to treat infants' infections. There have been *no* associated adverse outcomes in studies.
- Avoid *high-dose* regimens in breastfeeding mothers.
- As a precaution, advise deferring breastfeeding for 24 hours after an oral 2 g dose or for at least 3 hours after each dose if PO/IV metronidazole duration exceeds 7 days.

Treatment of Recurrent BV

- Repeat the course of PO metronidazole or clindamycin × 7 days.
- Consider suppressive therapy with 0.75% metronidazole vaginal gel twice per week for 4–6 months (not available in KKH).
- Probiotic treatment with *Lactobacillus* — however, *no data* regarding its efficacy.

Summary of Treatment Options for LGTI (WHO 2021)

Therapy for BV and trichomoniasis PLUS
Therapy for *Candida* if curd-like white discharge, vulvovaginal redness and itching are present

Infection	First-line option	Effective alternatives	***In pregnancy*: avoid metronidazole in the first trimester**
Bacterial Vaginosis (BV)	PO metronidazole 400 mg or 500 mg BD × 7 days **OR** PO metronidazole 2 g once	PO clindamycin 300 mg BD × 7 days **OR** PO metronidazole 2 g once	PO metronidazole 200 mg or 250 mg TDS × 7 days **OR** Metronidazole gel 0.75%, one full applicator (5 g) intravaginally, BD × 7 days **OR** PO clindamycin 300 mg BD × 7 days
Trichomonas vaginalis *For more details on trichomoniasis,* refer to Chapter 50: *Pelvic Inflammatory Disease*	PO metronidazole 2 g once **OR** PO metronidazole 400 mg or 500 mg BD × 7 days	PO tinidazole 2 g once **OR** PO tinidazole 500 mg BD × 5 days	PO metronidazole 200 mg or 250 mg TDS × 7 days **OR** Metronidazole gel 0.75%, one full applicator (5 g) intravaginally, BD × 7 days
Candida albicans	Miconazole vaginal pessary, 200 mg ON × 3 nights **OR** Clotrimazole vaginal pessary 100 mg ON × 7 nights	PO fluconazole 150 mg or 200 mg once **OR** Nystatin vaginal pessaries 200,000 units ON × 7 nights	Miconazole vaginal pessary, 200 mg ON × 3 nights **OR** Clotrimazole vaginal pessary 100 mg ON × 7 nights **OR** Nystatin vaginal pessaries 200,000 units ON × 7 nights

People taking metronidazole should be cautioned to avoid alcohol. Use of metronidazole in the first trimester of pregnancy is not recommended unless the benefits outweigh the potential risks.

(c) Atrophic Vaginitis/Vulvovaginal Atrophy

Now named "Genitourinary Syndrome of Menopause (GSM)"

- *Related to hypoestrogenic states*, e.g., natural or surgical menopause, primary ovarian insufficiency (POI), postpartum/lactation, hypothalamic amenorrhoea, anti-oestrogen medications, e.g., GnRH agonists, selective oestrogen receptor modulator (SERM) (e.g., tamoxifen), aromatase inhibitors.

Symptoms of GSM

Vaginal symptoms: dryness, burning, dyspareunia, loss of vaginal secretions, leukorrhoea, vulvar pruritus, a feeling of pressure and yellow malodorous discharge.

Urinary symptoms: urethral discomfort, frequency, haematuria, dysuria and stress incontinence.

Treatment of GSM

Local (hormonal/non-hormonal)	Systemic
Non-hormonal therapy *Vaginal moisturisers* (they are usually bio-adhesives) *Lubricants*: water-based, silicone-based or oil-based **Topical hormonal** therapy • Premarin cream (0.625 mg conjugated oestrogens/g) one application ON × 3 weeks followed by twice-weekly maintenance dose **OR** • Vagifem pessary 10 mcg daily ON × 2 weeks, then weekly for maintenance dose The duration of therapy should be individualised.	– Menopausal hormone therapy (MHT)/ Hormone replacement therapy (HRT) SERMs, e.g., ospemifene (to treat vulvovaginal atrophy)

CHAPTER 50

Pelvic Inflammatory Disease (PID)

Pelvic inflammatory disease (PID) refers to infection of the **upper** genital tract in a woman, involving any or all of the uterus, cervix, fallopian tubes and ovaries. It can be accompanied by the involvement of the neighbouring pelvic organs, resulting in endometritis, salpingitis, oophoritis, peritonitis, perihepatitis (Fitz-Hugh–Curtis syndrome) and tubo-ovarian abscess (TOA).

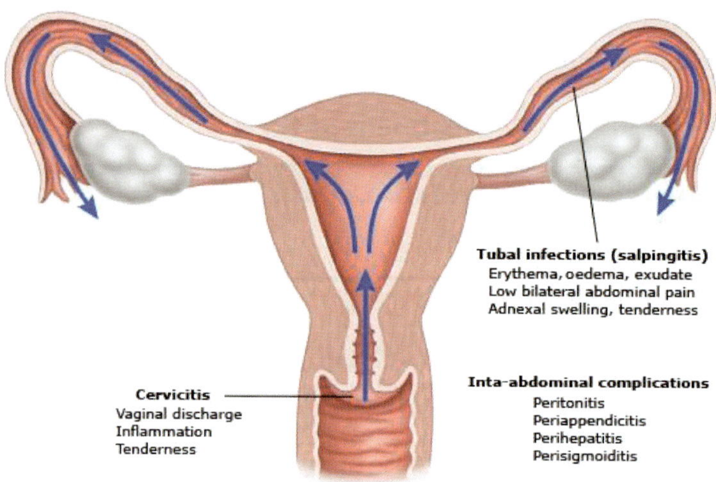

Risk factors for sexually transmitted infections (STIs) — Refer to Chapter 51: *Sexually Transmitted Infections*

Factors that potentially facilitate PID

- History of hydrosalpinx or PID
- Vaginal douching
- Bacterial vaginosis

- Intrauterine contraceptive device (IUCD) use — PID risk is <1%, usually within the first 20 days of insertion. PID risk with IUCD use is *not increased* compared to the background risk in low-risk women.
  - o Assess the risk of STIs before IUCD insertion.
  - o If the patient has a high risk of STIs, perform STI screening and ideally await results before IUCD insertion.
  - o If the woman is asymptomatic, IUCD can be inserted without antibiotic cover if she can be contacted for treatment later.
  - o If the woman is symptomatic, delay the IUCD insertion. If the insertion cannot be delayed, cover with antibiotics during the insertion.

Pathogenesis of PID

1. STIs: most common organisms are *Neisseria gonorrhoea, Chlamydia trachomatis* and *Mycoplasma genitalium* (account for 40% of cases)
2. Normal vaginal flora of healthy women: *Streptococci, Staphylococci*
3. Enterobacteriaceae (e.g., *Klebsiella, Escherichia coli, Proteus*) and anaerobes, e.g., bacterial vaginosis
4. Post-operative pelvic abscess
5. Pregnancy-related pelvic infection
6. Pelvic infection secondary to the spread of a primary infection, e.g., appendicitis, diverticulitis, tuberculosis (TB) peritonitis, actinomycosis
7. IUCD users — *actinomyces*

Clinical Features of PID

PID represents a spectrum of clinical diseases, which ranges from asymptomatic patients to fatal intra-abdominal sepsis.

Acute PID refers to inflammation of the uterus, fallopian tubes, ovaries and pelvis caused by an infection. If left untreated, it may cause long-term problems such as chronic pelvic pain or scarring of the fallopian tube resulting in hydrosalpinges, subfertility or increased risk of ectopic pregnancies.

Subclinical PID is common, so an index of suspicion for clinical diagnosis of PID should be high, especially in adolescent women — do STI screening swabs if necessary.

Pelvic Inflammatory Disease (PID)

Symptoms
- Bilateral lower abdominal pain
- Abnormal uterine bleeding (AUB)
- Intermenstrual bleeding (IMB)
- Postcoital bleeding (PCB)
- New-onset vaginal discharge
- Fever and chills (50%)
- Deep dyspareunia
- Urethritis

Signs
- Fever (>38°C), chills
- Rebound tenderness in the lower abdomen
- Right upper quadrant tenderness (possible Fitz-Hugh–Curtis in 10% of patients)
- Purulent endocervical discharge
- Cervical excitation
- Adnexal tenderness on bimanual examination ± adnexal mass

Differential Diagnoses of Lower Abdominal Pain in a Young Woman

Gynaecological causes	Non-gynaecological causes
• Ectopic pregnancy • Complications of ovarian or paraovarian cysts, e.g., torsion, rupture, infection • Endometriosis • Complications of tubal pathology, e.g., haematosalpinx, paratubal cyst accidents • Complications of uterine pathology, e.g., fibroid degeneration or torsion	• Acute appendicitis • Diverticulitis • Cystitis • Pyelonephritis • Irritable bowel syndrome • Functional pain

A low threshold for empirical treatment for PID is recommended as the potential consequences of untreated PID are serious.

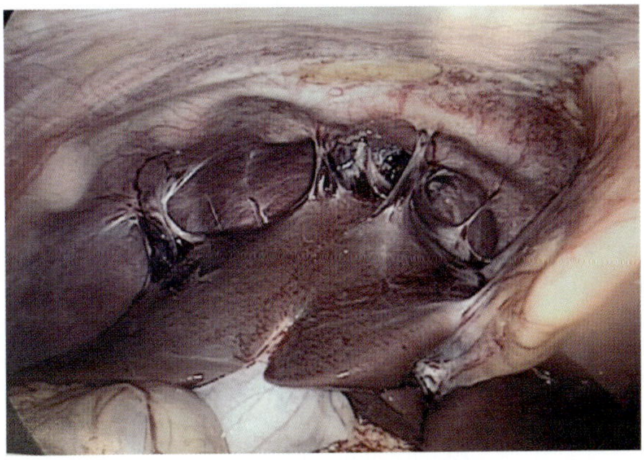

Fig. 50.1 Peri-hepatic adhesions (Fitz-Hugh–Curtis syndrome).

Fitz-Hugh–Curtis syndrome (Fig. 50.1)

- A form of peri-hepatitis associated with PID, usually caused by chlamydia or gonorrhoea.
- Results from infection of the liver capsule and peritoneal surfaces of the anterior right upper quadrant of the abdominal wall, with minimal stromal hepatic involvement.
- Presents with a sudden onset of severe right upper quadrant abdominal pain, with a distinct pleuritic component, and hence can mask the diagnosis of PID.
- May result in abnormal aminotransferases on the liver function test (LFT) in about 50% of patients.

Management of PID

History

↓

Sexual history
Abdominal pain with:
Fever (>38°C)
Abnormal vaginal discharge
Dyspareunia
Intermenstrual bleeding
Postcoital bleeding
Abnormal uterine bleeding

↓

Examination:
Vitals: fever, tachycardia, hypotension
Abdomen: right upper quadrant/lower abdominal tenderness
Speculum: strawberry cervix, mucopurulent discharge
Vaginal examination: cervical excitation, adnexal tenderness/mass

↓

Investigations:
Urine pregnancy test: to exclude ectopic pregnancy
Full blood count (FBC)/C-reactive protein **(CRP)**
Endocervical swabs to exclude chlamydia and gonorrhoea
High vaginal swab to exclude trichomonas, bacterial vaginosis and *Candida*
Ultrasound pelvis to look for tubo-ovarian abscess, pyosalpinx
Other STI testing: HIV, syphilis, hepatitis B
Cervical cancer screening (to do at a later date)

↓

Treatment:
Mild PID: outpatient management with oral antibiotics for 14 days
Moderate/severe PID: inpatient monitoring with intravenous antibiotics

Medical treatment: if not responding to antibiotics, may require drainage either radiologically or laparoscopically
Interventional radiology: US- versus CT-guided drainage of tubo-ovarian abscess
Surgery: Laparoscopy versus laparotomy drainage of abscess/unilateral or bilateral salpingo-oophorectomy or total hysterectomy and bilateral salpingo-oophorectomy

Investigations for PID

- **Urine:** urine pregnancy test (UPT) to exclude pregnancy, chlamydia and gonorrhoea testing, urine FEME, culture and sensitivity.
- **Blood:** FBC, C-reactive protein (CRP), STI screening (HIV, syphilis and hepatitis B).
- **Blood cultures and serum lactate** if the patient is **septic.**
- **Vulvovaginal/endocervical swabs** to exclude chlamydia and gonorrhoea.
- **Vaginal swab (VP3)** to exclude trichomonas, bacterial vaginosis, *Candida* and other bacteria.
- **Ultrasound scan of the pelvis** to look for other associated PID pathology, e.g., TOA and other genital tract pathology.
- **Other imaging modalities** include computer tomography (CT) scan or magnetic resonance imaging (MRI) scan of the abdomen and pelvis.
- **Interventional radiological procedures for drainage of abscess.**
- **Diagnostic laparoscopy:** 15–30% of cases may not have laparoscopic evidence of acute infection despite organisms being identified from swabs. May be converted to therapeutic laparoscopy for drainage of abscess if an abscess is seen during laparoscopy.
- **Pus for culture and sensitivity** from the TOA or pelvic collections.

Treatment of PID

Cover with broad-spectrum antibiotics.
Surgical management or interventional radiological procedures should be considered if the clinical condition is severe or deteriorates despite adequate antibiotic therapy, e.g., for a pelvic abscess.

Indications for inpatient management

- ➢ Lack of response or tolerance to oral medications
- ➢ Non-adherence to therapy
- ➢ Severe clinical illness, e.g., high fever, nausea, vomiting, severe abdominal pain
- ➢ Pregnancy
- ➢ Possibilities of requiring surgery or if the diagnosis is uncertain
- ➢ Large tubo-ovarian abscess (TOA) ≥5 cm.

(a) Treatment of Mild/Moderate PID

May be treated with intramuscular (IM) or oral (PO) regimens, e.g.

- IM ceftriaxone 500 mg once (use 1 g if body weight is ≥150 kg) with PO doxycycline 100 mg BD + PO metronidazole 400 mg BD × 14 days **OR**
- IM cefoxitin 2 g once + PO probenecid 1 g once with PO doxycycline 100 mg BD + PO metronidazole 400 mg BD × 14 days

Patients who do not respond to IM or oral therapy within 48–72 hours should be re-evaluated to confirm the diagnosis and to consider IV antibiotic therapy.

(b) Treatment of severe PID (usually inpatient with intravenous antibiotics)

- IV ceftriaxone 1 g every Q24H + IV/PO doxycycline 100 mg BD + IV/PO metroidazole 400 mg BD **OR**
- IV cefotetan 2 g Q12H + IV/PO doxycycline 100 mg BD **OR**
- IV cefoxitin 2 g Q6H + IV/PO doxycycline 100 mg BD **OR**
- IV clindamycin 900 mg Q8H + IV/IM gentamicin (2 mg/kg body weight), followed by a maintenance dose (1.5 mg/kg body weight) Q8H

After clinical improvement with IV antibiotics, convert to PO doxycycline 100 mg BD + PO metronidazole 400 mg BD to complete a total of 14 days of antibiotics

Summary of Antibiotic Treatment Options for PID

Severity of PID	Suggested therapy		Duration
	First line therapy	Alternative therapy	
Mild to moderate	IM ceftriaxone 500 mg once + PO doxycycline 100 mg BD + PO metronidazole 400 mg BD	PO levofloxacin 500 mg OD + PO metronidazole 400 mg BD	14 days
Severe	IV ceftriaxone 1 g OD + PO doxycycline 100 mg BD + PO metronidazole 400 mg BD *then convert to:* PO metronidazole 400 mg BD + PO doxycycline 100 mg BD	IV clindamycin 900 mg Q8H + IV gentamicin OM (3–5 mg/kg body weight) *then convert to:* PO clindamycin 450 mg QDS **OR** PO metronidazole 400 mg BD + PO doxycycline 100 mg BD	14 days Convert to oral therapy within 24–48 hours of clinical improvement
Pregnancy	IV cefoxitin 2 g QDS + PO azithromycin 1 g once **OR** IV cefotetan 2 g BD + PO azithromycin 1 g once	Consider referring to an infectious disease specialist for advice	

PID — complicated with pelvic abscess (including tubo-ovarian abscess)

- May need surgical/interventional radiological procedures or diagnostic exploration for alternative aetiology, e.g., appendicitis. If a non-gynaecological cause is found, refer to a general surgeon and consider further imaging with a CT scan of the abdomen and pelvis (CTAP).
- Close monitoring and counselling are crucial components in the management of PID.
- Should outpatient therapy be used, the patient should be reviewed within 24–48 hours to ensure clinical improvement.
- Educate the patient to ensure compliance with medications and follow-up.
- **Counselling** on the route of acquiring STIs, with concomitant partner treatment and safe sex practices. Possible long-term complications of PID should also be explained.
- Screening for other STIs should be offered (HIV, syphilis, hepatitis B and C).
- Contact tracing of all recent sexual partners.

Summary of Treatment Options for PID — WHO 2021

Treatment for uncomplicated *Neisseria gonorrhoeae, Chlamydia trachomatis*, anaerobic infections		
Infection	**First-line option**	**Effective alternatives**
In settings where local antimicrobial resistance data are unavailable, the WHO STI guidelines suggest **dual** therapy for gonorrhoea.		
Neisseria gonorrhoea	IM ceftriaxone 250 mg once + PO azithromycin 1 g once	PO cefixime 400 mg once + PO azithromycin 1 g once
Chlamydia trachomatis	PO doxycycline 100 mg BD × 14 days	PO erythromycin 500 mg, QDS × 14 days (to be given only if gonorrhoea treatment did not include azithromycin)
In settings where local antimicrobial resistance data reliably confirm the susceptibility of *Neisseria gonorrhoea* to the antimicrobial agent, **single therapy** may be given, as stated below.		
Neisseria gonorrhoea	IM ceftriaxone 250 mg once	PO cefixime 400 mg once
The treatment for anaerobes must be included in either treatment option stated above.		
Anaerobes	PO metronidazole 400 or 500 mg BD × 14 days	

Tubo-Ovarian Abscess (TOA)

- TOA is a gynaecological emergency with possible life-threatening complications.
- Septic patients will require admission to the high dependency unit (HDU) or intensive care unit (ICU). Multidisciplinary team (MDT) care is important.
- Occurs in about one-third of women who are hospitalised for PID.
- Requires aggressive medical, interventional radiological or surgical treatment.
- Overwhelming sepsis might ensue if TOA ruptures (15% of cases), which may lead to severe morbidity or even mortality.
- If the TOA has ruptured, immediate surgery is required.
- The approach depends on the patient's clinical status and the surgeon's expertise.
- It can be via diagnostic laparoscopy with the possibility of conversion to an open approach or exploratory laparotomy. For unruptured cases, laparoscopy is the preferred route of treatment.
- CTAP scan will be useful if the pathology is associated with the gastrointestinal tract.
- **Antibiotics** remain the mainstay of treatment for TOA.
    - Treatment with antibiotics alone or in combination with drainage of abscess or surgery is dependent on the clinical status and the characteristics of the abscess.
- For postmenopausal women with TOA, an underlying gynaecological malignancy should be considered.
- If surgery is required, the risks of visceral injury to organs such as the bowel, bladder and ureter are high. Therefore, patients need adequate counselling on the extent of surgery, as in a life-saving situation, total hysterectomy and bilateral salpingo-oophorectomy (THBSO) may be required.
- Surgery for TOA is usually complex and challenging. It may range from conservative (including drainage and wash out of pelvic abscess) to more extensive pelvic surgery (e.g., unilateral/bilateral salpingo-oophorectomy

or THBSO), depending on the clinical condition. The woman should be counselled on the impact on fertility and premature menopause in those requiring THBSO.

Tubo-Ovarian Abscess (TOA)

Mainstay of treatment: Antibiotics
- Haemodynamically stable (no signs of rupture of abscess)
- Adequate response to antibiotic therapy
- Pre-menopausal

Drainage of abscess
- Can be either under ultrasound or CT guidance
- Some reports have highlighted occasional onset of peritonitis and sepsis after drainage of TOA

Indications for surgery:
- Rupture of TOA
- New-onset or persistent fever
- Persistent or worsening abdomino-pelvic tenderness
- Enlarging pelvic mass
- Worsening leucocytosis
- Sepsis

Long-term complications of PID

Hydrosalpinx: secondary to tubal damage

Subfertility/infertility: secondary to tubal damage

Ectopic pregnancy: After 1, 2 and 3 episodes of PID, the risk of ectopic pregnancy is 5%, 15% and 30%, respectively.

Complications of recurrent PID

- **Chronic pelvic pain:** may affect up to one-third of patients with a history of PID secondary to scarring and adhesions from the inflammatory process
- **Ovarian cancer:** Nearly 2-fold increase in ovarian cancer risk, with the highest risk in women with multiple episodes of PID

Organisms causing PID

- *Neisseria gonorrhoea* and *Chlamydia trachomatis* — 30–40% of PID
- *Trichomonas vaginalis*
- *Mycoplasma genitalium*
- Gram-negative bacteria, e.g., *Escherichia coli, Colonic anaerobes*
- Others, e.g., *Mycobacterium tuberculosis, Haemophilus influenzae, Streptococcus pneumoniae*, actinomycosis
- Polymicrobial infection

Screening of sexually active young women (aged <25 years old)
Women at high risk of PID should be screened for chlamydia and gonorrhoea.

A. *Neisseria gonorrhoea* — first identified cause of PID

- Gram-negative diplococci
- Rapid decline in incidence with the introduction of penicillin
- 15% of women with endocervical gonorrhoea develop PID

Clinical manifestations of gonorrhoea

- May present as PID: abdominal pain, fever
- Cervicitis: 50% of infected women are asymptomatic
- Vaginal pruritus, mucopurulent discharge
- Abnormal uterine bleeding
- Dyspareunia
- *Urethritis*: dysuria, urgency, frequency of urination
- *Anorectal infection/proctitis*: usually asymptomatic
- *Oropharyngeal disease*: usually asymptomatic colonisation-increased risk in pregnant women
- Peri-hepatitis

Investigations for gonorrhoea

Culture: endocervical swab for culture. It can also be used to detect oropharyngeal, conjunctival or rectal infection.

Nucleic acid amplification test (NAAT): vaginal or endocervical swabs/urine sample.

Complications of gonorrhoea infection in pregnancy

- Miscarriage
- Preterm labour (PTL)
- Preterm premature rupture of membranes (PPROM)
- Chorioamnionitis
- Low birthweight babies (LBW)
- **Neonatal infections:** conjunctivitis, arthritis, pharyngitis

Treatment of *Neisseria gonorrhoea*

<table>
<tr><th>Non-pregnant women</th><th>Pregnant women</th></tr>
<tr><td rowspan="2">• IM ceftriaxone 500 mg once
OR
• PO azithromycin 2 g +
IM gentamicin 240 mg once
OR
• PO cefixime 800 mg once
OR
• IM spectinomycin 2 g once +
PO azithromycin 2 g once</td><td>• IM ceftriaxone 500 mg once OR
o Cephalosporins are safe and effective in pregnancy
• IM spectinomycin 2 g once
o Spectinomycin can be used if patients are unable to tolerate cephalosporins</td></tr>
<tr><td>Simultaneous treatment for chlamydia infection with PO azithromycin 1 g once if chlamydia status is unknown

Inform the neonatologist if the mother has gonorrhoea infection due to the risk of ophthalmia neonatorum.
• Prophylactic treatment with erythromycin 0.5% ophthalmic ointment can be administered <24 hours after birth</td></tr>
</table>

B. *Chlamydia trachomatis*

- Obligate intracellular parasite
- Fewer acute manifestations and more significant long-term complications than *Neisseria gonorrhoea*
- 15% of women with endocervical chlamydia develop PID

Clinical manifestations of chlamydia
- >70% of infected women are asymptomatic
- Cervicitis
- Abnormal uterine bleeding (AUB)
- Urethritis
- Fitz-Hugh–Curtis syndrome

Investigations for chlamydia

NAAT: most sensitive method

Vulvo-vaginal swabs are more sensitive than endocervical swabs

- *Alternative*: urine sample/urethral swabs or rectal/pharyngeal swabs can be taken for extra-genital sampling

Complications of chlamydia infection in pregnancy

- Preterm labour (PTL)
- Preterm premature rupture of membranes (PPROM)
- Chorioamnionitis
- Low birthweight babies (LBW)
- *Neonatal infections*: conjunctivitis, pneumonia

Treatment of Chlamydia trachomatis Infection

Non-pregnant women	Pregnant women
• PO doxycycline 100 mg BD × 7 days **OR** • PO azithromycin 1 g STAT **OR** • PO levofloxacin 500 mg OD × 7 days **OR** • PO erythromycin 500 mg BD × 10–14 days	• PO azithromycin 1 g × 1 dose • PO amoxicillin 500 mg TDS × 7 days • PO erythromycin 500 mg QDS × 7 days

Follow-Up After Initial Treatment of Chlamydia and Gonorrhoea — Test of Cure (TOC)

TOC	Non-pregnant	Pregnant
Chlamydia	No need unless: • Suspect non-compliance to treatment or • Symptoms persist or • Suspect reinfection Then check 4 weeks later	4 weeks
Gonorrhoea	No need unless • Suspect non-compliance to treatment or • Symptoms persist or • Suspect reinfection or • Pharyngeal gonorrhoea BASHH recommends TOC for all patients • Check at least 7–14 days after treatment either by culture or NAAT. If NAAT is used and is positive, a culture should be sent for confirmatory testing. All positive cultures for TOC should undergo antimicrobial sensitivity testing.	At least 7-14 days after treatment

Repeat tests for chlamydia and gonorrhoea 3 months post-treatment due to the high risk of re-infection, for all patients.

Refer for screening for other STIs, contact tracing, treatment and education.

All sexual partners within 60 days should be screened and treated for STIs.

Abstain from sexual intercourse until all sexual partners have been treated.

C. *Trichomoniasis*

Caused by a flagellated protozoan — *Trichomonas vaginalis*

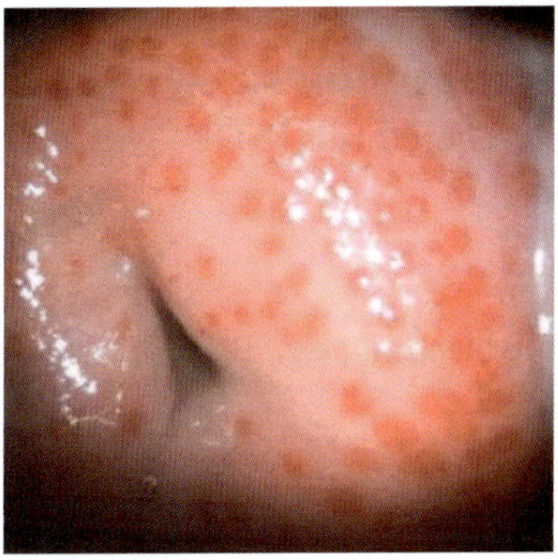

Fig. 50.2 Strawberry cervix.

Clinical manifestations:

- Asymptomatic carrier
- Frothy, purulent vaginal discharge
- Lower abdominal pain
- Dysuria
- Punctate haemorrhages on the cervix ("strawberry cervix") — Fig. 50.2

Investigations for Trichomonas vaginalis

- Wet-mount microscopy of vaginal discharge: look for mobile trichomonads
- VP3 swab for *Trichomonas vaginalis*

Complications of trichomoniasis in pregnancy

- Preterm labour (PTL)
- Preterm premature rupture of membranes (PPROM)
- Chorioamnionitis
- Low birthweight babies (LBW)

Treatment of Trichomoniasis

Non-pregnant women	Pregnant women
PO metronidazole 400–500 mg BD × 7 days or 2 g once o *Avoid alcohol during and 24 hours after treatment (possible disulfiram-like reaction)* **PO tinidazole 2 g once** o *To avoid alcohol during and 48 hours after treatment (possible disulfiram-like reaction)* o Sex partners should be screened and treated	**PO metronidazole 400–500 mg BD × 7 days** – Conflicting data regarding the safety of metronidazole use in pregnancy, use if benefits outweigh risks *Avoid the use of tinidazole in pregnancy, especially in first trimester — lack of safety data

D. *Mycoplasma genitalium* — strongly associated with non-gonococcal urethritis (NGU)

Clinical manifestations

- Asymptomatic
- Abnormal uterine bleeding, e.g., PCB, IMB
- Cervicitis
- Endometritis
- Infertility

Investigations for Mycoplasma genitalium

Culture: Not useful as it is a slow-growing bacterium
NAAT: Vaginal/endocervical swabs or urine sample

Complications of Mycoplasma genitalium in pregnancy

Miscarriage and preterm labour

Treatment of *Mycoplasma genitalium*

Non-pregnant women	Pregnant women
1. **Uncomplicated**, e.g., cervicitis PO doxycycline 100 mg BD × 7 days, then azithromycin 1 g once and then 500 mg daily × 3 days **OR** *If macrolide-resistant*: PO doxycycline 100 mg BD × 7 days then moxifloxacin 400 mg daily × 7–10 days 2. **Complicated**, e.g., PID PO moxifloxacin 400 mg daily × 14 days	• PO azithromycin — moxifloxacin is *contraindicated* in pregnancy *Limited options* if macrolide-resistant infection

No sexual intercourse till 14 days after the start of treatment and when symptoms have resolved.

Do a TOC 3–5 weeks after the start of treatment.

Summary of Treatment Options for Cervical Infection — WHO 2021

Treatment for uncomplicated *Neisseria gonorrhoea, Chlamydia trachomatis* and *Mycoplasma genitalium*			
Infection	**First-line options**	**Effective alternatives**	**Pregnancy/lactation**
In settings where local antimicrobial resistance data are unavailable, the WHO STI guidelines suggest dual therapy for gonorrhoea.			
Neisseria gonorrhoea	IM ceftriaxone 250 mg once + PO azithromycin 1 g once	PO cefixime 400 mg once + PO azithromycin 1 g once	IM ceftriaxone 250 mg once + PO azithromycin 1 g once OR PO cefixime 400 mg once + PO azithromycin 1 g once
Chlamydia trachomatis	PO doxycycline 100 mg BD × 7 days (to be given only if gonorrhoea treatment did not include azithromycin)	PO azithromycin 1 g once OR PO erythromycin 500 mg QDS × 7 days *or* PO ofloxacin 200–400 mg BD × 7 days (to be given only if gonorrhoea treatment did not include azithromycin)	PO erythromycin 500 mg QDS × 7 days OR PO azithromycin 1 g once (to be given only if gonorrhoea treatment did not include azithromycin)
Mycoplasma genitalium	PO azithromycin 500 mg on day 1, 250 mg daily on days 2–5 (in the absence of macrolide resistance)		PO azithromycin 500 mg on day 1, 250 mg daily on days 2–5 (in the absence of macrolide resistance)

Due to rising antimicrobial resistance to azithromycin in *Neisseria gonorrhoea* and *Mycoplasma genitalium* and reduced susceptibility of *Neisseria gonorrhoea* to cephalosporins, WHO is revising the current treatment recommendations.

CHAPTER 51

Sexually Transmitted Infections (STIs)

Objectives of Sexually Transmitted Infections (STIs) Management

- To provide treatment, cure and reduce the risk of developing complications of STIs.
- To reduce or prevent future risk-taking behaviour, including other bio-behavioural interventions, e.g., pre-exposure prophylaxis (PrEP) and voluntary male circumcision.
- To ensure all sexual partners are screened and treated.
- This requires that the person with an STI receive the following services:
  - Detailed medical and sexual history.
  - Correct diagnosis (whether syndromic or based on diagnostic tests).
  - Effective treatment for STI.
  - Health education and counselling on STI and risk reduction strategies.
  - Advice on the importance of compliance with treatment and follow-up.
  - Promotion and/or provision of barrier contraception, i.e., condoms.
  - Promotion and/or provision of PrEP.
  - Provision of other preventive measures, e.g., hepatitis A, B and HPV vaccination, voluntary male circumcision and offer screening for other STIs.
  - Contact tracing and ensuring all sexual partners are treated before resuming sexual activities.

Organism	STI	Causative agent
Bacteria	Chlamydia lymphogranuloma venereum (LGV)	*Chlamydia trachomatis*
	Gonorrhoea	*Neisseria gonorrhoea*
	Chancroid	*Hemophilus ducreyi*
	Granuloma inguinale (GI)	*Klebsiella granulomatis*
	Syphilis	*Treponema pallidum*
Virus	Genital herpes	*Herpes simplex virus (HSV 1 & 2)*
	Genital warts	*Human papillomavirus (HPV)*
	HIV/AIDS	*Human immunodeficiency virus (HIV)*
	Molluscum contagiosum	*Pox virus*
	Hepatitis B/ C	*Hepatitis virus*
Protozoan	Trichomoniasis	*Trichomonas vaginalis*

Hence, effective management of STIs involves not only antimicrobial therapy to achieve cure and reduce transmission but also thorough assessment and care of the patients' reproductive health and their sex partners. For adolescents, the approach must be appropriate and user-friendly so that the provision of STI services in primary healthcare settings can be accessible and non-judgemental as assessed by this vulnerable group of people — a view that they may carry with them into adulthood.

- ***<u>Four curable STIs:</u>*** *Gardnerella*, chlamydia, syphilis and trichomonas
- ***<u>Four incurable STIs:</u>*** Hepatitis B, HSV, HIV and human papillomavirus

For chlamydia/gonorrhoea/trichomonas infection — Refer to Chapter 50: *Pelvic Inflammatory Disease*

For hepatitis B and C infection — Refer to Chapter 15: *Infections in Pregnancy*

Risk factors for STI

Young age (15–24 years), unmarried, new sexual partners in the past 2 months, multiple sex partners, history of prior STI, illicit drug use, contact with sex workers.

Screening Approach for STI

1. **Offer** universal HIV screening to all patients being evaluated for STI.
2. **High risk (gonorrhoea/chlamydia)**
   Screen annually for gonorrhoea/chlamydia if risk factors for STI are present.
   Chlamydia is the most reported STI. Young women (aged 15–24) account for 43% of reported cases. They face the most severe consequences of undiagnosed infections.
3. **High-risk and pregnant**
   Screen for hepatitis B and C, syphilis, HIV, gonorrhoea and chlamydia.
4. **Antenatal screening for HSV infection**
   Screening is <u>not</u> recommended for asymptomatic women.
   However, type-specific serologic tests may be useful for identifying pregnant women at risk of HSV infection and guiding counselling on the risk of getting genital herpes in pregnancy.
5. **Consequences of STIs in women**
   - PID and infertility.
   - Adverse pregnancy outcomes, e.g., ectopic pregnancy.
   - Fetal complications, e.g., congenital infections or fetal anomalies.
   - Organ damage: e.g., peri-hepatitis.
   - Cancers, e.g., cervical cancer.
   - Mortality, e.g., acquired immunodeficiency syndrome (AIDs).
   - Psychological and social issues.
   - STIs (e.g., herpes, syphilis, chlamydia, gonorrhoea and chancroid) increase the risk of HIV acquisition.

Approach to Management of STI

History

a. Lesion history
b. Medical history
c. *Sexual history*: 5 "P"s (CDC) — partners (sexual), prevention of pregnancy/pregnancy, practices, protection from STIs, past history of STIs

Physical examination — differentials for genital ulcers

a. *STI-related genital ulcers*
- Genital herpes (HSV-1 or HSV-2)
- Primary syphilis
- Chancroid
- Granuloma inguinale (GI)
- Lymphogranuloma venereum (LGV)

b. *Non-STI-related genital ulcers/lesions*
Bullous dermatoses, non-bullous dermatoses, yeast, fixed drug eruption, trauma, psoriasis, malignancy, Behcet disease

Symptoms/signs of STI	Differential diagnoses based on symptoms
Urethral or vaginal discharge	Gonorrhoea, chlamydia, trichomonas, bacterial vaginosis *Candidiasis*, *Mycoplasma genitalium*, HSV (occasionally)
Genital ulcers in adolescents	HSV, primary syphilis, other STIs, e.g., HIV, gonorrhoea, chlamydia
Skin lesions/rash	HPV (warts), syphilis (primary and secondary), disseminated gonorrhoea, pediculosis pubis, scabies
Oral lesions/ulcers	Syphilis, gonorrhoea, HPV, HSV, LGV

STI-Related Genital Ulcers

Infection	Genital herpes	Primary syphilis	Chancroid	Granuloma Inguinale	Lympho-granuloma venereum
Infective organism	HSV 1 or 2	*Treponema pallidum*	*Hemophilus ducreyi*	*Klebsiella granulomatis*	*Chlamydia trachomatis*
Incubation period	2–14 days	10–90 days (average 21)	3–10 days (average 4–7)	50 days	5–21 days
Initial lesions	Papule — vesicle	Papule	Papule/pustule	Extensive progressive granulation-like tissue with "beefy" red ulcer	Small, painless blister or sore
Presenting lesion	Vesicles	Chancre	Ulcer/bubo	Papules/ulcer	
Number	Multiple/ coalesce Bilateral in primary Unilateral in recurrent	Usually, one	Single/multiple	Single	Multiple
Diameter	1–2 mm	5–15 mm	Variable	Extensive	Small
Edges	Erythematous	Sharply demarcated, elevated, round or oval	Undermined, ragged, irregular	Rolled	

Infection	Genital herpes	Primary syphilis	Chancroid	Granuloma Inguinale	Lympho-granuloma venereum
Depth	Superficial	Superficial deep	Excavated deep	Deep	Shallow
Base	Serous/ erythematous non-vascular	Smooth, clean Non-purulent Non-vascular	Necrotic Generally purulent, grey or yellow exudate Bleeds easily	"Beefy" red ulcer	
Pain	Common, often with a prodrome of tingling	Usually painless	Common Severe	Painless	Usually painless
Lymphadenopathy	*Present* in the primary episode *Absent* in recurrences	Firm, non-tender, bilateral	Tender Suppurative Unilateral Fluctuant buboes	Absent	Tender inguinal/femoral nodes (buboes–painful, fluctuant, suppurative nodes) ± sinuses ± strictures
Treatment	Systemic antivirals – Acyclovir – Valacyclovir – Famciclovir	Intramuscular (IM) Benzathine penicillin	PO azithromycin 1 g stat OR IM ceftriaxone 250 mg stat	PO azithromycin 1 g weekly OR 500 mg OM for >3 weeks and until all lesions have completely healed	PO Doxycycline 100 mg BD × 3 weeks PO Azithromycin 1 g weekly × 3 weeks PO Erythromycin 500 mg QDS × 3 weeks

Investigations for STI

- Send swab for herpes simplex virus PCR
- If chancroid or other diagnoses are suspected — Refer to the Department of STI
- Send 5 ml of blood in a plain tube for chemiluminescent microparticle immunoassay (CMIA) test to screen for syphilis → Venereal Disease Research Laboratory (VDRL)/*Treponema pallidum* particle agglutination (TPPA)
- Offer HIV testing
- Empirical treatment is recommended as 25% will have no laboratory-confirmed diagnosis
- Offer cervical cancer screening — Pap smear for 25–29 years old or HPV testing from 30 years old onwards

Investigations and Management for Specific STIs

(A) Genital Herpes (HSV) (Fig. 51.1)

Investigations for genital herpes

- Virus isolation in cell culture is sensitive and specific. Viral typing is possible.
- Type-specific serological tests (TSST) for HSV 1 and 2-based on recombinant type-specific glycoproteins G1 and G2 have good sensitivity and specificity.

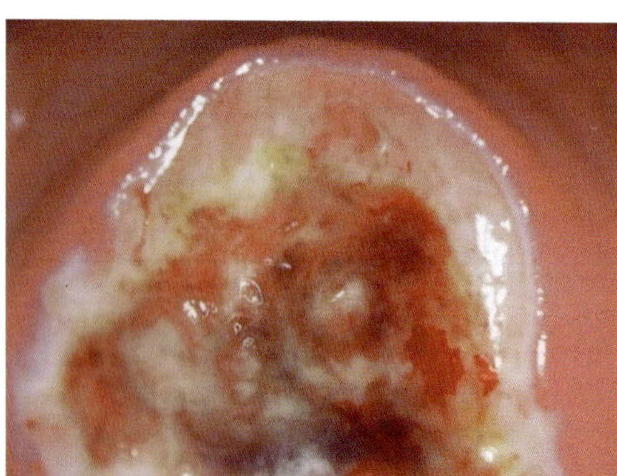

Fig. 51.1 Herpes simplex ulcer of the cervix.

  - o TSST is useful in certain clinical situations, e.g., confirming a clinical diagnosis of genital herpes, counselling sexual partners of infected persons and detecting infection.
- HSV antigen detection by direct fluorescent antibody (DFA) or enzyme immunoassay (EIA) techniques are economical and quick but insensitive; viral typing is *not* possible.
- PCR detection of viral nucleic acid has the highest sensitivity but is expensive and not widely available; viral typing is possible. It is available in KKH and is the preferred investigation.
- Tzanck test demonstrates giant cells from lesions but is not sensitive; only presumptive evidence of infection by a herpes virus.
- Women with genital herpes should be screened for HIV (2–3 fold increased risk of HIV).

Treatment of Primary Genital Herpes Infection

- PO acyclovir 400 mg TDS × 7–10 days OR
- PO valacyclovir 1 g BD × 7–10 days OR
- PO famciclovir 250 mg TDS × 7–10 days

Treatment should be started within 72 hours of the onset of lesions for optimal benefit, when new lesions continue to form or when symptoms and signs are severe. The duration of treatment depends on the clinical response. Treatment can be extended if healing is incomplete after 10 days of therapy.

Treatment of Recurrent Genital Herpes

Episodic treatment for recurrent genital herpes (CDC guidelines 2021)
Initiate during the prodrome or within 1 day of the attack

- PO acyclovir 800 mg BD × 5 days or 800 mg TDS × 2 days
- PO valacyclovir 500 mg BD × 3 days or 1 g daily × 5 days
- PO famciclovir 1 g BD × 1 day or 500 mg once, followed by 250 mg BD × 2 days or 125 mg BD × 5 days

Suppressive treatment for recurrent genital herpes (CDC guidelines 2021)
Reduces the number of recurrences by 70–80% and reduces transmission of HSV

- PO acyclovir 400 mg BD OR
- PO valacyclovir 500 mg or 1 g daily OR
- PO famciclovir 250 mg BD

Frequent recurrences = 10 or more episodes per year

For the management of genital herpes in pregnancy, refer to Chapter 15: *Infections in Pregnancy*

Management of sexual contacts of genital herpes

Sex partners of patients with genital herpes are likely to benefit from evaluation and counselling. They should be questioned on their history of typical and atypical genital lesions and encouraged to examine themselves for lesions and to seek medical attention promptly if lesions appear. TSST may be useful in counselling.

(B) Syphilis (*Treponema pallidum*)

Primary syphilis — painless ulcer or chancre.

Secondary syphilis — skin rash, mucocutaneous lesions, lymphadenopathy. *Primary and secondary syphilis are the most infectious stages of the disease.*

Tertiary syphilis — cardiac involvement, gummas, psychiatric manifestations (e.g., memory loss or personality changes).

Latent syphilis and late syphilis

- *Early latent syphilis:* syphilis of <2 years from acquiring infection.
- *Late latent syphilis:* syphilis of >2 years without clinical evidence of treponemal infection; gummatous, nervous system and cardiovascular syphilis.

Investigations for Syphilis

Dark-field microscopy — to demonstrate *Treponema pallidum* in the secretions from the primary chancre or moist lesions of secondary syphilis.

Serological tests

- **Non-treponemal tests** (VDRL[a] or RPR[b]) — screening tests, titres are useful for monitoring response to therapy
- **Treponemal tests** — TPHA[c], TPPA[d], FTA-Abs[e], LIA[f], EIA[g] and rapid diagnostic tests are specific tests
- *Screen with* CMIA (a chemiluminescent immunoassay) on Abbott Architect analyser — normal or abnormal (reactive) result
    - If reactive result, samples are tested for VDRL and TPPA[d] — these tests for *Treponema pallidum* antibodies as well

Interpretation and Management Guidelines of Tests for Syphilis

Result	VDRL positive	VDRL negative
TPPA positive	Active infection	Past infection
TPPA negative	False positive	No infection

[a]VDRL — Venereal Disease Research Laboratory
[b]RPR — rapid plasma reagin
[c]TPHA — *Treponema pallidum* haemagglutination assay
[d]TPPA — *Treponema pallidum* particle agglutination assay
[e]FTA-Abs — Fluorescent treponemal antibody absorption
[f]LIA — line immunoassay
[g]EIA — enzyme immunoassay

- If the second treponemal test is negative, but the patient has a high risk of syphilis, repeat serology in 4 weeks. If the serology remains the same, then syphilis infection is excluded.

Interpretation and Follow-Up of Reverse Screening Results

Patient history	Test and result			Interpretation	Follow up
	EIA/CMIA/MFI	RPR	TPPA		
Unknown history of syphilis	Non-reactive	N/A	N/A	No serological evidence of syphilis	None, unless clinically indicated (e.g., early syphilis)
Unknown history of syphilis	Reactive	Reactive	N/A	Untreated or recently treated syphilis	Treat as per CDC guidelines
Unknown history of syphilis	Reactive	Non-reactive	Non-reactive	Probable false-positive screening test	No follow-up testing, unless clinically indicated
Unknown history of syphilis	Reactive	Non-reactive	reactive	Possible syphilis (e.g., early or latent) OR previously treated syphilis	Historical or clinical evaluation required
Known history of syphilis	Reactive	Non-reactive	Reactive or N/A	Past, successfully treated syphilis	None

CMIA, chemiluminescence immunoassay; EIA, enzyme immunoassay; MFI, multiplex flow immunoassay; N/A, not applicable; RPR, rapid plasma reagin; TPPA, *Treponema pallidum* particle agglutination. http://www.cdc.gov/std/treatment/2010/.

Treatment of Syphilis

a. *Treatment of primary, secondary and early latent syphilis <2 years duration*
- IM benzathine penicillin G 2.4 million units once

For penicillin-allergic patients
- Try desensitisation and treat with benzathine penicillin (first-line treatment)
- Alternative treatments include PO tetracycline 500 mg QDS × 14 days **OR**

 PO doxycycline 100 mg BD × 14 days **OR**
 PO erythromycin 500 mg QDS × 14 days **OR**
 IM/IV ceftriaxone 1 g daily × 10 days/PO azithromycin 2 g once dose (limited data only)

b. *Treatment of late latent syphilis >2 years duration or of unknown duration, tertiary or cardiovascular syphilis*
- IM benzathine penicillin G 2.4 million units weekly × 3 doses **OR**
- IM aqueous procaine penicillin G 600,000 units daily × 14–21 days

For penicillin-allergic patients
PO tetracycline 500 mg QDS × 28 days **OR**
PO doxycycline 100 mg BD × 28 days **OR**
IM or IV ceftriaxone 2 g daily × 14 days **OR**
PO erythromycin 500 mg daily × 28 days

c. *Treatment of neurosyphilis, ocular syphilis and otosyphilis*
- Aqueous crystalline penicillin G 18–24 million units per day, administered at 3–4 million units IV every 4 hours or continuous infusion for 10–14 days **OR**
- Procaine penicillin G 2.4 million units IM once daily + PO probenecid 500 mg QDS — to give both drugs for 10–14 days

For penicillin-allergic patients
- RAST tests, skin testing and desensitisation should be done in consultation with an expert. Penicillin is the drug of choice unless truly contraindicated.
- *Alternatives:* PO tetracycline 500 mg QDS × 28 days **OR** PO doxycycline 100 mg BD × 28 days OR IM/IV ceftriaxone 2 g daily × 14 days OR PO erythromycin base or stearate 500 mg QDS × 28 days (least effective).

Follow-up of syphilis

- Refer to the Department of STI Control (DSC Clinic)
- At 3, 6, 12, 18 and 24 months
- If the VDRL titre increases/persistently high (>1:32) or develops symptoms and signs — it indicates treatment failure or re-infection

For syphilis in pregnancy – Refer to Chapter 15: *Infections in Pregnancy.*

Management of sexual contacts of patients with syphilis

- At-risk partners are those who have been exposed within 3 months of symptoms for primary syphilis, 6 months for secondary syphilis and 1 year for early latent syphilis.
- Treatment should be given to sexual contacts who were exposed 3 months before the diagnosis of primary, secondary or early latent syphilis or if follow-up is uncertain.
- Sexual partners of patients with late syphilis should be screened and evaluated for syphilis and treated based on these findings.

Summary of Treatment Options for Genital Ulcer Disease — Genital Herpes and Syphilis — WHO 2021

Multiple-dose treatment for HSV infection *plus*
Single-dose long-acting penicillin treatment or multi-dose treatment of alternatives

Infection	First-line options	Effective alternatives	In pregnancy/lactation and <16 years old
Genital herpes	**Primary infection** • PO acyclovir 400 mg TDS × 10 days OR • PO acyclovir 200 mg five times a day × 10 days	**Primary infection** • PO valaciclovir 500 mg BD × 10 days OR • PO famciclovir 250 mg TDS × 10 days	**Primary infection** Use acyclovir only when the benefits > risks. The dosage is the same as for primary infection in non-pregnant patients
	Recurrent infection — Episodic therapy • PO acyclovir 400 mg TDS × 5 days OR • PO acyclovir 800 mg BD × 5 days OR • PO acyclovir 800 mg TDS × 2 days	**Recurrent infection — episodic therapy** • PO valaciclovir 500 mg BD × 5 days OR • PO famciclovir 250 mg BD × 5 days	**Recurrent infection — episodic therapy** • PO acyclovir 400 mg TDS × 5 days OR • PO acyclovir 800 mg BD × 5 days OR • PO acyclovir 800 mg TDS × 2 days
	Suppressive therapy for recurrent herpes • PO acyclovir 400 mg BD OR • PO valaciclovir 500 mg once daily	**Suppressive therapy for recurrent herpes:** • PO famciclovir 250 mg BD	**Suppressive therapy for recurrent herpes** • PO acyclovir 400 mg BD OR • PO valaciclovir 500 mg once daily

(Continued)

Infection	First-line options	Effective alternatives	In pregnancy/lactation and <16 yr old
Early syphilis (primary, secondary, early latent syphilis)	IM benzathine penicillin 2.4 million units once	• PO doxycycline 100 mg BD × 14 days OR • PO erythromycin 500 mg QDS × 14 days	• IM benzathine penicillin 2.4 million units once OR • PO erythromycin 500 mg QDS × 14 days
Late syphilis (late latent and tertiary syphilis)	IM benzathine penicillin 2.4 million units weekly for three consecutive weeks	• IM procaine penicillin 1.2 million units daily × 20 consecutive days OR • PO doxycycline 100 mg BD × 30 days	PO erythromycin 500 mg QDS × 30 days

Suppressive therapy for recurrent herpes is recommended for individuals with 4–6 or more recurrent episodes per year, severe symptoms or episodes that cause distress. Increased dosages or duration of treatment are required for people living with HIV.

Although erythromycin is used to treat pregnant women, it does not cross the placental barrier completely, and the fetus is not treated. Thus, the newborn needs treatment immediately after delivery.

(C) Chancroid (*Hemophilus ducreyi*)

Investigations for chancroid

- Culture for *Hemophilus ducreyi* of smear from ulcer or aspirate from buboes
- Diagnosis is often based on typical clinical presentation and after excluding syphilis and HSV infection
- PCR detection

Treatment of chancroid

Treatment is typically given if chancroid is suspected clinically:

PO azithromycin 1 g once **OR** IM ceftriaxone 250 mg once **OR** PO ciprofloxacin 500 mg BD × 3 days (contraindicated in pregnancy and lactation)

Management of sexual contacts of chancroid

Sex partners should be screened and treated when indicated.

(D) Granuloma Inguinale (GI) — *Klebsiella Granulomatis*

Investigations for GI

- Tissue biopsy — "Donovan" bodies in tissue samples
- On Wright Giemsa stain, large mononuclear cells with intra-cytoplasmic cysts filled with deep purple Gram-negative Donovan bodies

Treatment of GI

PO azithromycin 1 g weekly or 500 mg daily for >3 weeks until all lesions have completely healed

Alternatives:

PO doxycycline 100 mg BD for at least 3 weeks until all lesions completely healed OR

PO erythromycin base 500 mg QDS for >3 weeks until all lesions completely healed OR

PO trimethoprim-sulfamethoxazole (160 mg/800 mg) 1 tab BD for >3 weeks until all lesions have completely healed

Management of sexual contacts of GI:

Contact tracing within 60 days before symptom onset and treatment of sexual contacts

Screen for other STIs, including HIV

(E) Lymphogranuloma Venereum (LGV) — *Chlamydia Trachomatis*

Investigations for LGV (difficult diagnosis)

- *NAAT*
- *Culture* — low yield from ulcers/lymph node aspirates
- *Serology* — complement fixation/microimmunofluorescence — should not be used routinely for diagnosis (use has *not* been established)

Treatment of LGV

PO doxycycline 100 mg BD × 3 weeks

Alternatives: PO azithromycin 1 g weekly × 3 weeks, PO erythromycin base 500 mg QDS × 3 weeks

Management of sexual contacts of LGV

Contact tracing and treatment of sexual contacts (within 60 days before symptom onset)

Screen for other STIs

(F) Genital Warts (*Human Papillomavirus*)

- The commonest cause of anogenital growths — ~50% get warts at least once in their lifetime.
- 90% of genital warts (Fig. 51.2) are caused by HPV types 6 or 11.
- Incubation period: 1–6 months.
- Transmission is approximately 60% between partners.
- Asymptomatic or itching, bleeding, dyspareunia.
- Painful, pruritic, papular genital lesions.
- Multifocal — usually 5–15; in areas of trauma during sex, about 1–10 mm diameter; may coalesce, especially in immunosuppressed or diabetics.
- Maybe co-infected with oncogenic "high-risk" HPV (e.g., types 16 and 18) — mostly give rise to subclinical lesions, intraepithelial neoplasia (IN) and anogenital cancer.

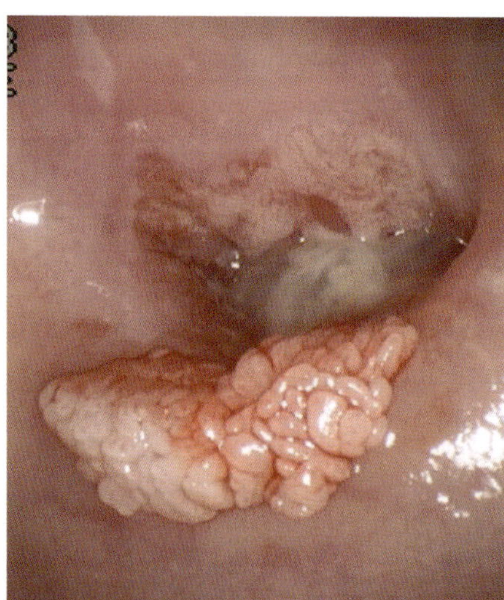

Fig. 51.2 Wart/condyloma on cervix.

- *Consider other differentials*: condylomata lata, seborrhoeic keratosis, squamous cell carcinoma, molluscum contagiosum and angiofibromas.
- *Skin biopsy* is indicated for atypical cases: Bowenoid papulosis, ulceration, dermal induration, pigmented lesions, cases *not* responding to treatment or worsening during treatment, immunocompromised and postmenopausal patients as immunosuppression increases the risk of malignant transformation.
- Subclinical mucosal warts can be identified as they turn white after the application of 5% acetic acid for 3 minutes.
- Regular cervical cancer screening as per guidelines (to exclude pre-cancer or cancer of the cervix).
- HPV DNA testing is not recommended as it does not alter management.
- Advise smoking cessation, condom use and screening of partners in the last 6 months.
- Asymptomatic or subclinical genital HPV is self-limiting.
- In the absence of lesions, treatment is *not* recommended.
- Pre-exposure HPV vaccination is recommended (Refer to Chapter 40: *Human Papillomavirus Vaccines*).
- Genital warts can have a psycho-sexual impact.

Treatment of Genital Warts

Vulval, perineal and peri-anal warts (up to 40% will resolve without any treatment)

Patient administered therapy

1. **Imiquimod** (5% cream), e.g., Aldara — 3 × a week at bedtime, wash off next morning, continue until clearance or for a maximum of 16 weeks
   - **No studies** on the safety of Aldara use in pregnancy
2. **Podophyllotoxin** (0.15% cream) BD × 3 days a week, rest for 4–7 days
   - *Contraindicated* in pregnancy (teratogenic)
   - Women of childbearing age must use contraception
   - Duration of treatment: 4–5 weeks

Provider-administered therapy or clinic-based therapy

1. Cryotherapy — weekly liquid nitrogen
2. Trichloroacetic acid (80–90%) weekly, one application for 8–10 weeks

3. Electrosurgery (1–6 sessions) or electrocautery
4. CO_2 laser vaporisation
5. Scissors excision (1–2 sessions)

Vaginal or cervical warts

1. Carbon dioxide laser vaporisation
2. Electrosurgery
3. Trichloroacetic acid

Dysplasia must be *excluded* before starting treatment
Cervical cytology and colposcopy (if necessary) are advised
Interferon alpha and beta as adjuvants to surgery in problematic cases

Adverse effects of treatment for genital warts

- Hypo/hyperpigmentation
- Depressed/hypertrophic scarring
- Chronic pain syndrome (hyperaesthesia/vulvodynia)
- Systemic effects from podophyllotoxin

For treatment of genital warts in pregnancy — Refer to Chapter 15: *Infections in Pregnancy*
Management of sexual contacts of women with genital warts
All regular sexual contacts should be examined and clinical warts treated.

Only surgical treatment has primary clearance rates of about 100%. Recurrence after all other therapies is often ≥20–30%.

Side effects of treatments — local skin reactions, pain, itch, burns or erosion.

Role of HPV vaccines for genital warts

- Effective for primary prevention of HPV infection (for coverage against HPV types 6 and 11, which cause genital warts — use Gardasil® 4 or 9) — Refer to Chapter 40: *Human Papillomavirus Vaccines*, for more information.
- HPV vaccination is not recommended for treating anogenital warts or preventing recurrent disease.

Algorithm for Management of Ano-Genital Warts

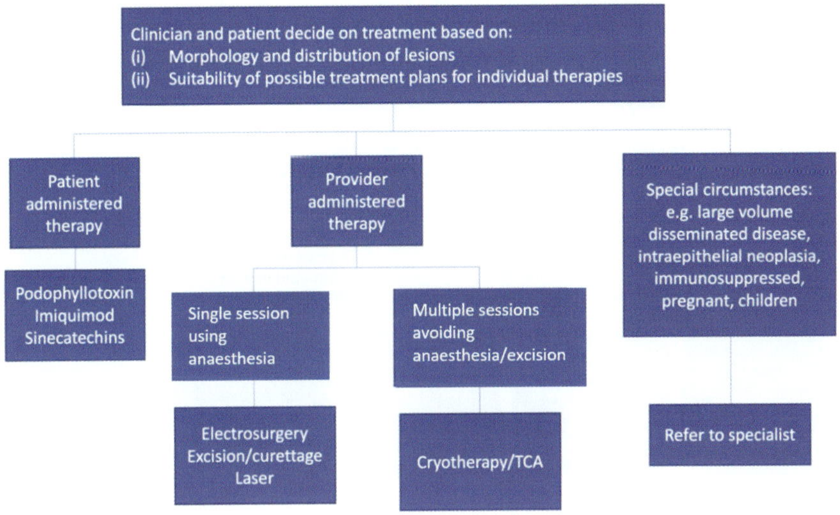

(G) HIV Infection

- There were 202 newly reported HIV infections in Singapore residents in 2022.
- This brings the total number of HIV-infected Singapore residents to 9,331 as of end 2022, of whom 2,362 had passed away.
- MOH and HPB urge individuals to protect themselves from HIV infection and its effects by following the principles of "ABCD." (A) Abstinence, (B) being faithful, (C) correct and consistent use of condoms, (D) early detection.
- HIV is transmitted through sexual intercourse with an infected person or through contaminated syringes and needles, transfusion of infected blood and blood products and from infected mothers to babies.
- HIV-1 accounts for almost all global infections except for a small number caused by HIV-2, which originates in West Africa.
- HIV-1 is divided into four groups: M, N, O and P. M is the most widespread worldwide. Within group M, there are at least nine subtypes of HIV, i.e., subtypes A–K.
- HIV-2 is less infectious and takes a longer time to develop into AIDs.

Signs and symptoms of acute HIV infection include

Fever, skin rash, myalgia, arthralgia, headache, lymphadenopathy, oral ulcers, leukopenia, thrombocytopenia or elevated transaminitis. Patients with untreated HIV infection may be symptomatic with life-threatening immune deficiency.

Clinical Features of HIV Infection

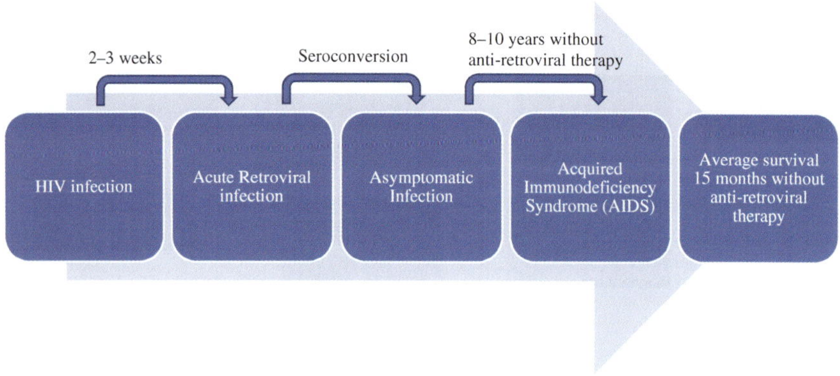

Opportunistic diseases associated with AIDS include

1. *Bacterial* diseases, e.g., tuberculosis
2. *Protozoal* diseases, e.g., *Pneumocystis carinii* pneumonia, toxoplasmosis
3. *Fungal* diseases, e.g., *Candidiasis*
4. *Viral* diseases, e.g., cytomegalovirus (CMV), herpes simplex and herpes zoster
5. HIV-associated cancers, e.g., Kaposi sarcoma, lymphoma and squamous cell carcinoma

Tests for HIV Infection

a. *Screening tests*

- **Rapid HIV testing** (results out within 20 minutes) — fourth generation tests detect both HIV antibodies and p24 antigens, unlike third generation tests, which can only detect HIV antibodies.
- **HIV ribonucleic acid (RNA)/deoxyribonucleic acid (DNA) polymerase chain reaction (PCR) test** — Recommended when the time of exposure is between 10 and 14 days.

b. *Confirmatory tests*

- **Western blot (WB) technique**
- **ELISA HIV antibody test** (ideal for exposure period >4 weeks)

Indeterminate HIV tests may be seen during seroconversion, late-stage HIV infection, cross-reacting antibodies, infection with the O strain or HIV-2 infection. Therefore, repeat testing is recommended after 3 months.

Using both ELISA and WB tests, the sensitivity and specificity >99.9%.

<u>*Treatment of HIV infection*</u>

Refer to the infection disease specialist for treatment.

Antiviral treatment should be started as soon as possible for patients with HIV infection regardless of the CD4 and T cell counts.

For treatment of women with HIV in pregnancy, refer to Chapter 15: *Infections in Pregnancy.*

<u>Prevention of STIs</u>

(i) Vaccination

- Immunisations are available for the prevention of hepatitis A, B and HPV.
- HPV vaccine — Gardasil 9 is useful for the prevention of warts and cervical cancer.
- No vaccines are presently available for HIV and hepatitis C.

(ii) Use of barrier contraception — condoms

Though the amount of protection provided is difficult to establish, condoms are recommended by CDC and WHO as an essential component in public health strategies to prevent STIs.

(iii) Counselling

- Behavioural interventions/partner notification/empiric therapy in victims of sexual assault (including HIV post-exposure prophylaxis)/ strategies to improve sexual health.
- Get tested and screened, abstain or be monogamous and limit the number of sexual partners.
- Do not douche the vagina. Do not abuse alcohol or other drugs. Advise male circumcision.

(iv) Suppressive therapy with antiviral therapy (Acyclovir) — e.g., for genital HSV infection

(v) Prevention of mother-to-child transmission (MTCT) of STI

- MTCT of STIs can result in fetal anomalies, low birth weight, stillbirth, neonatal death, sepsis, pneumonia and neonatal conjunctivitis.
- In women with hepatitis B infection:
  - o *Peripartum antiviral prophylaxis*: Women with a high viral load in the third trimester HBV DNA (≥200,000 IU/ml equivalent to ≥5.3 $\log_{10}$ IU/ml) should be started on antiviral treatment (Tenofovir) from 28 weeks to reduce viral load before pregnancy and to reduce risk of MTCT of hepatitis B.
  - o The risk of MTCT is low (0.04%) if the maternal hepatitis B DNA level is <5.3 $\log_{10}$ IU/ml or 200,000 IU/ml.
  - o *Neonatal passive immune prophylaxis consists of two components*:
    1. Hepatitis B vaccine: the first dose is administered to the neonate within 12 hours of the delivery. The second dose of the hepatitis vaccine is administered at 1 month and the third dose at 6 months. The baby is to complete the 3-dose hepatitis B vaccine series.
    2. Hepatitis B immunoglobulin (HBIg) is administered to the neonate within 12 hours of the delivery.
- Breastfeeding is ***contraindicated*** for HIV-positive mothers.
- <u>Caesarean section is recommended for:</u>
  a) *Primary genital herpes*
  Primary genital herpes at the time of labour or within 6 weeks of the expected date of delivery.
  The risk of transmission to the neonate is ~40% for **primary** genital herpes via vaginal delivery.
  b) *HIV infection*
  HIV pregnant women on Zidovudine monotherapy, on HAART with viral load >50 copies/ml or co-existent hepatitis C infection. With ART, the risk of MTCT is <2%. Without ART, the risk of MTCT transmission is ~30%.
  c) *Genital warts*
  If genital warts obstruct the pelvic outlet or if a vaginal delivery would result in excessive bleeding.
    - Screening, vaccinating and treating all neonates of women with STI.

CHAPTER 52

Contraception

Introduction

Contraception is a method used to prevent unintended pregnancies and their consequences. It also helps patients space their pregnancies and conceive only when they are ready. Contraception is useful for patients who need to optimise their medical disorders before conception for better pregnancy outcomes.

Factors to consider when prescribing contraception:

- Age, parity, sexual, obstetric, medical, surgical, drug, social history, religious beliefs and patient preference.
- Hormonal versus non-hormonal methods.
- Reversible versus non-reversible methods.
- Different types/routes — natural family planning, oral, injectables, rings, patch, intrauterine contraceptive device (IUCD, also known as intrauterine device), implant, surgery.
- Benefits, risks, failure rates and cost of each method.
  - ➢ The failure rate is defined as the percentage (%) of women with unintended pregnancies within the first year of use.
- Other non-contraceptive benefits for the patient based on her medical history.
- Whether she has completed her family or when she wants to conceive in the future.
- Emergency contraception (EC) and sexually transmitted infection (STI) prevention.

Ultimately, the patient will select the contraceptive method after counselling by the health care provider based on her clinical situation.

Summary of Contraceptive Methods

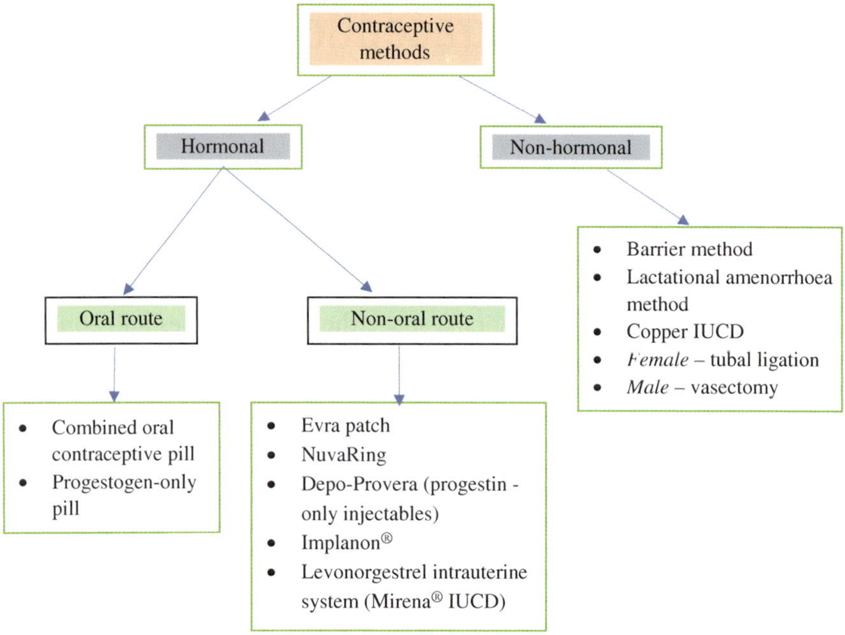

Oral Hormonal Contraception (OHC)

A) Combined oral contraceptive pill (COCP)
B) Progestogen-only pill (POP)

Combined Oral Contraceptive Pill (COCP)

Mode of action of COCP:

- Suppresses ovulation by abolishing the luteinising hormone (LH) surge
- Reduces sperm penetrability by thickening the cervical mucus
- Alters the endometrium and reduces the likelihood of implantation

COCP

Contraceptive usage

- Failure rate 0.3–9%
- Effectiveness of all COCP is similar

Non-contraceptive benefits

Alleviation of

- Abnormal uterine bleeding
- Heavy menstrual bleeding and dysmenorrhoea
- Chronic pelvic pain
- Hirsutism, acne and irregular menses in polycystic ovarian syndrome (PCOS)
- Acne (if contraception is also required)
- Premenstrual syndrome (PMS) and premenstrual dysphoric disorder (PMDD)
- Endometriosis (use continuous COCP post-surgery)
- Benign breast disease

***Reduction in*:**

- Risk of Colorectal Cancer
- Risk of Ovarian and Endometrial cancer that continues several decades after stopping COCP (50% reduction)
- ***Regulation*** of menstrual cycles
- ***Manipulation*** of timing of menstruation

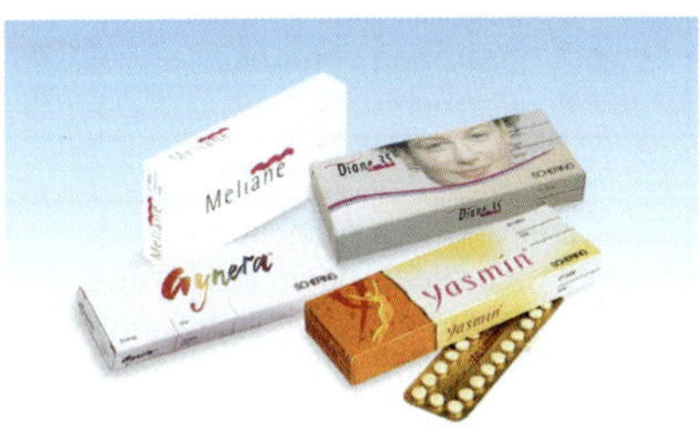

Various types of combined oral contraceptive pills.

Table 52.1 Different Types of COCPs

COCP		
Type	**Composition of each pill**	**Remarks**
A. Monophasic	A constant amount of oestrogen and progestin in each pill.	
First generation		
	E.g., COCP with progestogens such as: Norethisterone, norethindrone, ethynodiolacetate, lynestrenol.	No longer used.
Second generation		
Nordette/ Microgynon	Ethinyl estradiol 30 μg and levonorgestrel 150 μg.	Less thrombogenic side effects than third- or fourth-generation COCP.

(Continued)

(Continued)

COCP		
Type	**Composition of each pill**	**Remarks**
Third generation		
Meliane	Ethinyl estradiol 20 μg and 0.075 mg gestodene.	Less androgenic side effects. Lowest oestrogen content.
Gynera	Ethinyl estradiol 30 μg and 0.075 mg gestodene.	Less androgenic side effects.
Mercilon	Ethinyl estradiol 20 μg and 150 μg desogestrel.	Less androgenic side effects. Lowest oestrogen content.
Fourth generation		
Yasmin/Liza	Ethinyl estradiol 30 μg and 3 mg drospirenone.	Drospirenone is a progestogen with anti-mineralocorticoid properties. ■ No reported clinically significant changes in potassium concentration. ■ Counteracts water retention weight gain. Favourable effect on the skin. Reduces the severity of PMS.
Yaz/Liz	Ethinyl estradiol 20 μg and 3 mg drospirenone.	"24/4," i.e., 24 days of active pills and 4 days of placebo pills with shortened pill-free interval. Benefits of a lower daily oestrogen dose while maintaining a lower breakthrough bleeding pattern. Used for treatment of PMS/PMSS with significant improvements in physical, mood and behavioural symptoms. Treatment of moderate acne vulgaris.
Others		
Diane 35/ Estelle	Ethinyl estradiol 35 μg and 2 mg cyproterone acetate.	Has anti-androgenic properties. Used for treatment of acne/hirsutism in PCOS.
B. Multiphasic	The dose of oestrogen and/or progestin varies during the active pill phase.	Used to reduce hormone dose and side effects, e.g., unscheduled bleeding. However, studies do not show an advantage over monophasic pills. Contraceptive efficacy is similar to that of monophasic pills.
Qlaira	Estradiol valerate doses range from 1 to 3 mg and dienogest doses range from 2 to 3 mg.	26 days of active pill phase and 2 days of placebo pills.

Side effects of COCP:

- Breakthrough bleeding
- Amenorrhoea
- Leukorrhoea
- Nausea, vomiting, bloating
- Headache
- Melasma/mastalgia
- Gallstone formation

Risks associated with COCPs:

- Venous and arterial thromboembolism, i.e., deep vein thrombosis (DVT) and pulmonary embolism.
    - o COCPs containing desogestrel, gestodene and cyproterone are associated with higher thrombotic risk than those with levonorgestrel, norethisterone and norgestimate (third- and fourth-generation COCPs have higher thromboembolic risk than second-generation COCPs).

VTE risk of various progestins used in COCP		
First-generation progestin	Norethindrone Norethisterone	– Mildly androgenic – **Lowest** thrombotic risk
Second-generation progestin	Levonorgestrel Norgestrel	– Most androgenic – **Low** thrombotic risk 5–7/10,000
Third-generation progestin	Norgestimate Gestodene Desogestrel	– Less androgenic, longer half-life, less metabolic effects on carbohydrates and lipids – **Higher thrombotic risk of** 9–12/10,000 (except Norgestimate: ~5-7/10,000)
Newer/Other	Drospirenone Cyproterone acetate	– Less androgenic; low-risk acne/hirsutism – **Higher thrombotic risk of** 9–12/10,000

- A small increase in absolute risk of ischaemic stroke, breast and cervical cancer.
- Breast and cervical cancer risk decline after cessation, with a return to baseline risk after 10 years post-cessation.

Factors affecting the effectiveness of COCPs:

- Bariatric surgery
- *Enzyme-inducing drugs (EID):* Anti-epileptics, e.g., phenytoin, phenobarbitone, carbamazepine, antibiotics, e.g., rifampicin, lamotrigine
- Progesterone receptor modulators, e.g., ulipristal acetate (ELLA)
- Severe diarrhoea or vomiting

Contraindications to COCP use:

Absolute contraindications	Relative contraindications
• Cardiovascular disease with multiple risk factors (e.g., smoking, diabetes, hypertension, hyperlipidaemia, obesity) • Cerebrovascular disease (past and present) • VTE (past and present)	
• Family history of abnormal lipid profile or haemostatic profile and age <45 • Poorly controlled diabetes mellitus (DM) with complications, e.g., retinopathy • BP consistently ≥160/100 mmHg • Smoker, age ≥35, ≥15 cigarettes/day • BMI ≥35 • Migraine with aura-higher risk of ischaemic stroke	• Family history of abnormal lipid and haemostatic profiles and age >45 • Well-controlled, short-duration DM • BP > 140–159/90–99 mmHg • Smoker, age <35, <15 cigarettes/day • BMI 30–34 • Uncomplicated migraine
• Active liver disease • Recurrent cholestatic jaundice or cholestatic jaundice in pregnancy • Dubin–Johnson or Rotor syndrome • Liver adenoma/carcinoma • Gallstones • Porphyria	• Long-term partial immobilisation, e.g., wheelchair dependent women • Hyperprolactinaemia • Chronic systemic diseases **[refer to FSRH UK Medical Eligibility Criteria for Contraceptive Use (UKMEC) for guidance]**
• Medical conditions affected by sex steroids (e.g., chorea, pemphigoid gestationis)	• Very severe depression

• Pregnancy
• Postpartum
  o Breastfeeding (within 6 weeks)
  o Non-breastfeeding (within 3 weeks or 6 weeks if there are risk factors for VTE)
	• Some malabsorption conditions

• Undiagnosed genital tract bleeding	• Conditions requiring drug treatment that may interact with COCP use
• Oestrogen-dependent tumours, e.g., breast cancer	

Note: It takes **7** consecutive pills to ensure that ovulation has been suppressed. In some women, follicular activity may resume at the end of a 7-day break.

***Tailored combined hormonal contraception (CHC) regimens* can reduce the frequency of withdrawal bleeding and withdrawal symptoms associated with the hormone-free interval (HFI) compared to the *standard regime.* However, unscheduled bleeding is more common with tailored regimes. Thus, the woman should be counselled on both regimes to broaden her contraceptive choices (FSRH).**

Check BMI and BP before starting COCPs.
Can use COCPs till age 49 if medically eligible.
Stop COCPs 4 weeks before major surgery and restart 2 weeks after full mobilisation.

Management of missed pills:
Definition of missed pills:
A "missed pill" is defined as a pill that has been missed for >24 hours since the time the woman should have taken it. This is a common cause of contraceptive failure.

The following table is a guide for women on monophasic COCPs without placebo pills where the regimen is a 21-day cycle with a 7-day pill-free interval (i.e., HFI).

Scenario	Management
A: If the woman starts the new pack ≥9 days after the last active pill	Take the missed pill ASAP. Continue the rest of the pills as usual. Abstain from sex/use barrier method for contraception until the pills are taken for 7 consecutive days. Consider EC if unprotected sexual intercourse (UPSI) has occurred during or after the HFI. Consider a follow-up urine pregnancy test (UPT) 3 weeks after UPSI.
B: If the woman misses one pill, i.e., 48 to <72 hours since the last pill in the current cycle was taken	**If the missed pill is the first pill of the cycle,** – Refer to scenario A. **If the missed pill occurs in the first week after HFI,** – Take the missed pill ASAP. – Continue the rest of the pills as usual. – EC and additional contraception are *not* required if there is consistent and correct use in the first week and the 7 days before HFI. **If the missed pill occurs in the second or third week after HFI,** – Take the missed pill ASAP. – Continue the rest of the pills as usual. – EC and additional contraception are *not* required if there is consistent and correct use 7 days prior.

(Continued)

(Continued)

Scenario	Management
C: If the woman misses ≥2 pills, i.e., ≥72 hours since the last pill in the current cycle was taken	**If >7 consecutive pills were missed in ANY week** – Consider immediate UPT and EC. – If UPT is negative, start a new COCP packet or use another contraception method. – Abstain from sex/use barrier method for contraception until the pills/other method are taken for 7 consecutive days. – Follow-up UPT 3 weeks after UPSI. **If the 2–7 missed pills occur in the first week after HFI and the first pill of the pack is involved,** – Refer to scenario A. **If the 2–7 missed pills occur in the first week after HFI and the first pill of the pack is NOT involved,** – Take the missed pill ASAP. – Continue rest of the pills as usual. – Abstain from sex/use barrier method for contraception until the pills are taken for 7 consecutive days. – Consider EC if UPSI has occurred during or after the HFI. Consider follow-up UPT 3 weeks after UPSI. **If the 2–7 missed pills occur in the second and third weeks after HFI or any subsequent week in continuous pill-taking,** – Take the missed pill ASAP. – Continue rest of the pills as usual. – Abstain from sex/use barrier method for contraception until the pills are taken for 7 consecutive days. **If the 2–7 missed pills occur in the 7 days before HFI,** – Take the missed pill ASAP. – Continue rest of the pills as usual. – Abstain from sex/use barrier method for contraception until the pills are taken for 7 consecutive days. – Omit the HFI and continue the next COCP pack.

Source: FSRH CEU Guidance: Recommended Actions after Incorrect Use of Combined Hormonal Contraception (e.g., late or missed pills, ring and patch). Published March 2020, Amended 6 July 2021. Accessed 16 May 2022.

For users of 24/4 or 26/2 COCPs:

- If inactive pills are missed in week 4, the woman should discard the missed inactive pills and continue the usual pills as prescribed.
- If >7 pills are missed by the woman: Advise the woman to restart COCPs on day 2 of her next menses as if she had not used the pills before.
- If ≥2 pills are missed by the woman: Contraception failure is most likely when ≥2 pills (for 20 μg ethinyl estradiol pills) and 3 pills (for 30 μg ethinyl estradiol pills) are missed.
  REMEMBER: "2 for Twenty and 3 for Thirty".

- Advise additional contraceptive protection, such as condoms or abstinence, until the woman has taken her COCPs for 7 days in a row if contraception is unreliable.
- If the patient has had UPSI, consider EC.

Progestogen-Only Pill (POP)

- Useful for lactating mothers and older pre-menopausal women who wish to avoid risks from exogenous oestrogen.
- Pre-requisite: Motivated woman who can maintain reliable and timely pill-taking.
- Can start on day 1–2 of menses or the same day after abortion, miscarriage or immediately after childbirth.
- No pill-free interval.
- *Failure:* 0.3–9%.
- It can be used till age 55 years if medically eligible.

***Mode of action of POP*:**

- Decreases sperm permeability by altering the cervical mucus.
- Reduces endometrial receptivity to implantation.

***Benefits of POP*:**

- Lighter, shorter and less painful periods.
- No increased risk of VTE/stroke/myocardial infarction.

***Disadvantages of POP*:**

- Women may have an irregular bleeding pattern.
- *Side effects* include tender breasts, nausea, headache, dizziness, mood changes and weight gain.
- Although the overall risk of pregnancy is low, 10% may be ectopic pregnancy if pregnancy occurs.
  - Previous ectopic pregnancy is not a contraindication to POP use.
- Short effect of each pill which lasts only 24 hours.
- Requires the woman to take the pill at the same time every day.
- Consider it as missed pill if:
  - >3 hours late with traditional POPs.
  - >12 hours late with Desogestrel POP (Cerazette®)

- o >24 hours late with Drospirenone POP (SLINDA® 4 mg-in KKH,we use this POP). This is preferred as it has a longer 24-hour window for missed pills.
- o Extra protection is needed for the next 2 days for traditional and Desogestrel POP unless started on day 1 to 5 of a menstrual cycle, day 5 after abortion or day 21 after childbirth.
- o For Drospirenone POP, additional contraception is needed for 7 days unless it is started on day 1 of menstrual cycle, day 1 after abortion or by day 21 after childbirth.

Contraindications to POP:

- Present/past history of breast cancer.
- Sensitivity to progesterone.
- Unreliable pill taker.
- Pregnancy.
- Undiagnosed vaginal bleeding.
- Past/current history of ischaemic heart disease (IHD)/stroke: Consider the duration of use in relation to disease onset and consult a neurologist.
- Severe decompensated liver cirrhosis/hepatocellular adenoma/liver malignancy.

Management of Problematic Bleeding with POP

- Take history: correct use of method, associated symptoms, e.g. pain, discharge
- Exclude sexually transmitted infections
- Ensure cervical screening up to date
- Exclude pregnancy
- ± Ultrasound scan of the pelvis

Options:

1. Observe. Ensure correct and consistent use
2. NSAIDS for 5 days. (Mefenamic acid 500 mg BD/TDS or ibuprofen 400 mg TDS)
3. Tranexamic acid 1g TDS for 5 days
4. Try a different POP
5. Oestrogen supplementation — evidence does not support routine use
6. Change to a different contraception

Non-Oral Contraceptive Methods

Barrier Method

- Includes condom, femidom or diaphragm.
- Has the additional *benefit* of protection against STIs.
- Failure rate: 6–18%.
- *Disadvantages:*
    - Highly operator-dependent.
    - Disrupts sexual intercourse as condoms must be put on before penetration and removed immediately after ejaculation.
- The diaphragm must be left in place for 6 hours after intercourse, has a risk of infection (including toxic shock syndrome and UTI), needs an anatomically normal genital tract (not suitable for women with uterovaginal prolapse, shortened cervix), need to have a normal Pap smear before starting use.
- Spermicides can be used with condoms or a diaphragm to increase efficacy.

Combined Hormonal Vaginal Ring — NuvaRing

- Soft vaginal ring (~5 cm in diameter) that delivers 15 μg of ethinyl estradiol and 0.12 mg of etonogestrel a day.
- *Mode of action:* Inhibits ovulation.
- One NuvaRing is placed in the vagina for 3 weeks and removed for a break of one week.
- *Timing of insertion*:
    - Days 1–5 of the menstrual cycle
    - After first-trimester miscarriage or abortion — within 5 days.
    - After second-trimester miscarriage or abortion — >4 weeks.
- If the ring was accidentally removed within the 3 weeks — rinse with lukewarm water and re-insert within 3 hours.
- If the ring has been removed for >1 week, exclude pregnancy before insertion and use a barrier method or spermicide for 7 days following insertion.
- *Failure rate*: 0.3–9%.
- *Contraindications*: As per COCP.

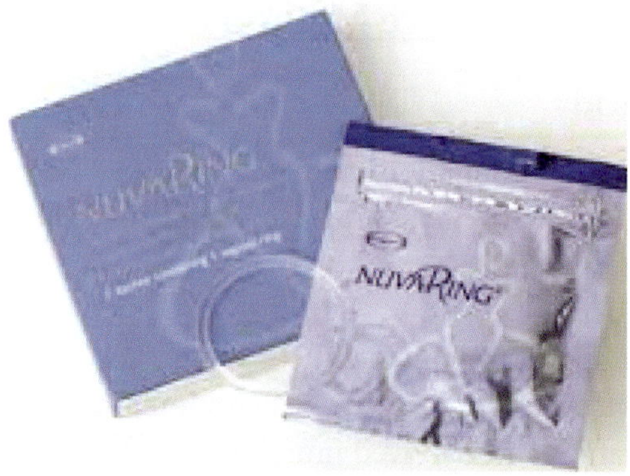

NuvaRing.

Source: https://onlinelibrary.wiley.com/doi/full/10.1002/tre.135.

- *Risks*: As per COCP. VTE, migraine, depression.
- *Side effects*: Headache, nausea, weight gain, mood changes, chloasma, breakthrough bleeding.

Combined Hormonal Transdermal Patch — Evra

- One patch (0.75 mg ethinylestradiol and 6 mg norelgestromin) apply weekly for 3 consecutive weeks, followed by a patch-free week.
- *Failure rate*: 0.3–9%.
- *Timing of application*:
  - If no hormonal contraception has been used in the past month — day 1 of menses/any other day of the cycle — use additional contraception, either spermicide or barrier contraception, for the next 7 days.
  - After first-trimester miscarriage or abortion — apply within the first 5 days.
  - After second-trimester miscarriage or abortion — apply 4 weeks later (to use spermicide or barrier for the next 7 days).
- ***If the Evra patch is detached***:
  - For <24 hours: Re-apply at the same place or apply a new patch.
  - For >24 hours or unsure when it dropped off: Start a new cycle by applying a new patch and use barrier contraception for the next 7 days.

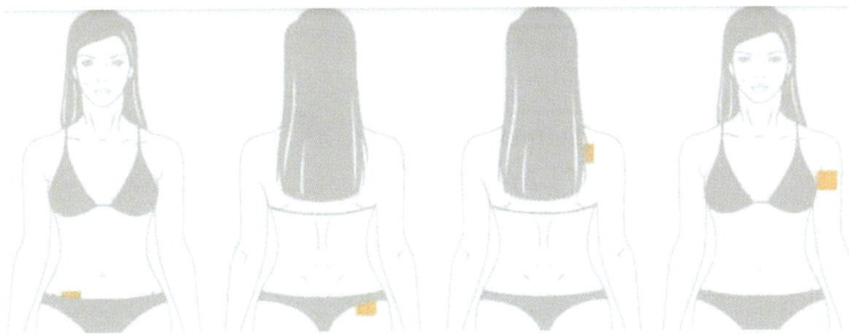

Different sites of Evra patch application.

Source: https://www.healthexpress.co.uk/evra.

- *Risks:* As per COCP (refer above).
- *Side effects:*
  - Unscheduled vaginal bleeding, headache, nausea, breast tenderness, mood changes or allergy/irritation to the patch.
  - A modest increased risk of VTE for Evra users compared to current COCP users.
- *Contraindications:* As per COCP (refer to the table above).
- *Special precaution:* Possible reduction in efficacy for women ≥90 kg or BMI ≥30.

Progestogen-Only Injectable — IM Depo-Provera

- Depot medroxyprogesterone acetate (DMPA) 150 mg intramuscular injection every 12 weeks.
- First injection on day 1–5 of menses or day of last COCP or at 6 weeks after childbirth.
- Adolescents ≥18 years old, obese and perimenopausal women are candidates for DMPA use.
- *Mode of action of DMPA:*
  a. Suppresses hypothalamic-pituitary axis to inhibit ovulation.
  b. Thickens cervical mucus and reduces tubal mobility — alters sperm penetration and inhibits fertilisation.
  c. Alters the normal growth of endometrium and reduces implantation.
- *Non-contraceptive benefits of DMPA:*
  - *Alleviation of:* Endometriosis, heavy menstrual bleeding and dysmenorrhoea.

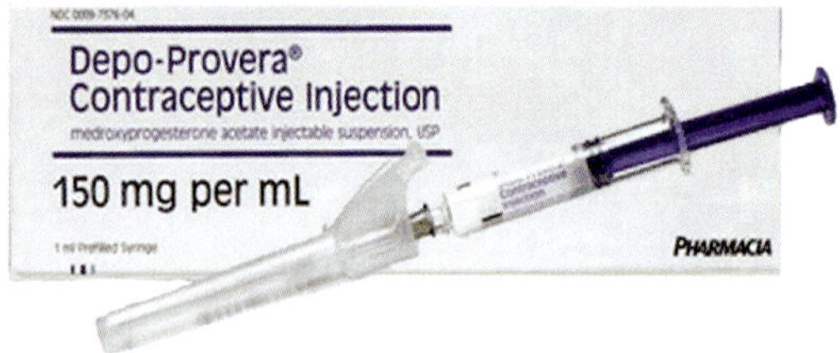

Depo-Provera®.

Source: https://www.obgynsupply.com/pfizer-pharmacia-depo-provera-contraceptive-injection-birth-control-shot-150mg-prefilled-syringe.html.

- ○ Decreased risk of pelvic inflammatory disease (PID) — due to changes in cervical mucus and decreased menstrual flow.
- ○ Prevention of haemorrhagic corpus luteal cysts in women on anti-coagulants.

- *Failure rate*: 0.2–6%.
- *Common side effects*: Irregular menstrual cycles, amenorrhoea (50% or more are amenorrheic at 12 months) headache, breast tenderness, mood changes and weight gain.
- *Long-term use*: Increases risk of osteoporosis (though it is reversible).
  - ○ **DMPA — use as second-line treatment in adolescents <18 years old.**
  - ○ **Assess osteoporosis risk every 2 years if the woman wishes to continue Depo-Provera.**
- *Delayed return of fertility*: May be delayed for up to 12–18 months after the last injection.
- *Contraindication*: Past/current breast cancer, unexplained vaginal bleeding.
- *Relative contraindication* if there are multiple risk factors for cardiovascular disease, hypertension with vascular disease, current or past history of IHD/stroke and severe decompensated liver cirrhosis/hepatocellular adenoma/malignancy.

Management of Problematic Bleeding with IM Depo-provera.

- Take history: correct use of method, associated symptoms, e.g. pain, discharge.
- Exclude sexually transmitted infections.

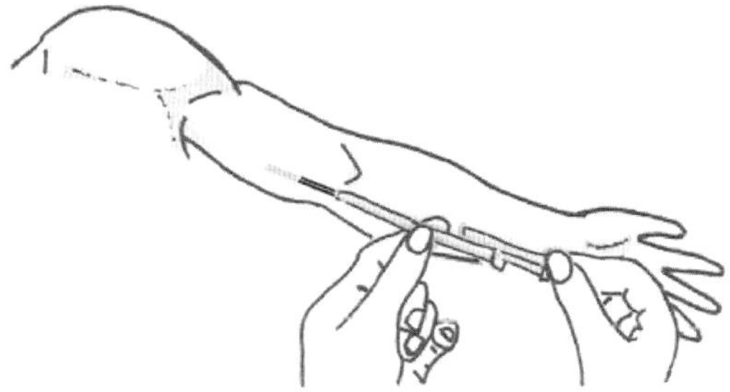

Implanon insertion.

- Ensure cervical screening up to date.
- Exclude pregnancy.
- ± Ultrasound scan of the pelvis.

Options

1. Observe
2. NSAIDS
   - mefenamic acid 500 mg BD/TDS for 5–7 days
   - ibuprofen 400 mg TDS for 5 days
3. Tranexamic acid 1g TDS for 5 days.
4. Hormonal treatment
   - COC (30–35 μg ethinylestradiol with levonorgestrel/noresthisterone) for up to 3 months: cyclical or continuous regimen.
5. Reduce interval between injection to 10 weeks
6. Change to a different contraception.

Progestogen-Only Implant (IMP) — Implanon®

- Single-rod subdermal contraceptive implant, biodegradable, radiopaque.
- Contains 68 mg etonogestrel.
- Long-acting reversible contraception (LARC): Provides effective reversible contraception for 3 years.
- FSRH supports the use of Implanon if medically eligible from menarche to age 55 years.
- *Mode of action*: Suppresses the hypothalamic-pituitary axis with inhibition of ovulation and change in cervical mucus and tubal motility.

- *Insertion:* It is placed subdermally in the medial aspect of the non-dominant upper arm under local anaesthesia.
- *Timing of insertion:*
  - o Days 1–5 of the menstrual cycle.
  - o After miscarriage or abortion — within 5 days.
  - o Postpartum (breastfeeding/non-breastfeeding) — within 21 days.
- *Failure rate:* 0.05%.
- *Benefit:* Most effective contraception, no oestrogen side effects.
- *Contraindication:* In breast cancer patients, unexplained vaginal bleeding.
- *Relative contraindication* if there is a current or past history of IHD/stroke and severe decompensated liver cirrhosis/hepatocellular adenoma/malignancy.
- *Common side effects:*
  - o Irregular menstrual cycles (30% infrequent bleeding, 20% prolonged bleeding, <10% frequent bleeding, 20% amenorrhoea), headache, breast tenderness, mood changes and weight gain.
  - o *Problems at insertion site:* Pain, irritation, infection, haematoma, scarring, migration, expulsion.
- *Problems with removal:* If the implant is deeply placed and not palpable under the skin, perform an X-ray/ultrasound to locate the implant before removal.
- Ovulation resumes shortly after Implanon removal.
- *Return of fertility:* >90% of women ovulate within 3–4 weeks of removal.
- Individuals on EID should be counselled that the contraceptive efficacy of Implanon could be reduced during enzyme inducer use and for 28 days after stopping the enzyme inducer.

Management of Problematic Bleeding with Implant

- Take history associated symptoms, e.g. pain, discharge
- Exclude sexually transmitted infections
- Ensure cervical screening up to date
- Exclude pregnancy
- ±Ultrasound scan of the pelvis

Options

1. Observe
2. NSAIDS
   - mefenamic acid 500 mg TDS for 5 days
   - ibuprofen 400 mg TDS for 5 days
3. Tranexamic acid 1g TDS for 5 days
4. Hormonal treatment
   - COC (30–35μg ethinylestradiol with levonorgestrel/noresthisterone) for up to 3 months: cyclical or continuous regimen
5. Change to a different contraception.

Intrauterine Contraceptive Device — Copper/Mirena® IUCD

Types of IUCD:

1. *Non-hormonal* = copper IUCDs (e.g., Nova T and Multi-Safe).
2. *Hormonal* = levonorgestrel-containing IUCD (Mirena® IUCD).

1. *Copper IUCD*

- *Mode of action*: Exact mechanism unknown. Proposed theories — inhibition of sperm transport/inhibition of fertilisation and implantation.
- *Benefits*:
  - o LARC: Provides 5 years of protection depending on the type of IUCD. Effective immediately after insertion. Any CU-IUCD with copper surface ≥ 300 mm^2 inserted at ≥ 40 years old can be used for contraception until menopause.
  - o **Copper IUCD is an effective** emergency contraceptive (EC) if inserted within 5 days of UPSI or up to 5 days after the earliest estimated ovulation date.
  - o Copper IUCD has **no** hormonal side effects.
- *Timing of insertion*:
  - o Days 1–5 of the menstrual cycle.
  - o After miscarriage or abortion: Within 5 days.
  - o Postpartum (breastfeeding/bon-breastfeeding): Within 0–48 hours or >4 weeks after childbirth.

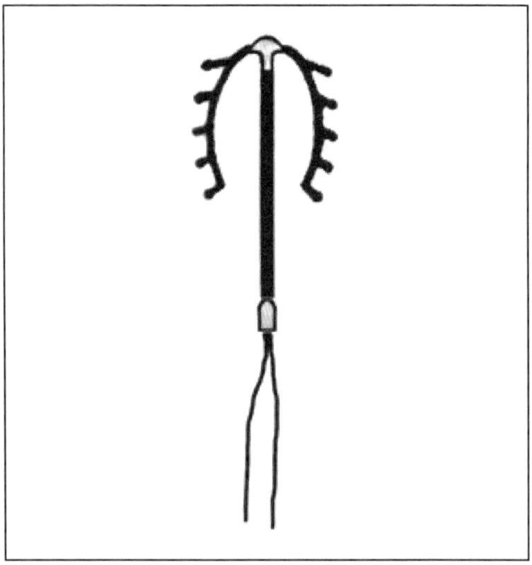

Multiload copper IUCD.

- *Failure rate:* 0.6–0.8%.
- *Contraindications to IUCD use*
  - o Pregnancy.
  - o Severe distortion of the uterine cavity due to fibroids/uterine anomaly.
  - o Acute/recurrent pelvic infection. Post abortion sepsis
  - o Known copper allergy or Wilson's disease (for copper IUCDs).
  - o Unexplained vaginal bleeding or heavy, painful menses with anaemia.
  - o ***Malignancy*:** Cervical, endometrial cancer.
  - o Gestational trophoblastic disease (GTD): Can only be inserted when βHCG has normalised.
- *Removal:* On expiry at any time during the menstrual cycle or at menopause. It can also be removed 1 year after final menstrual period if this occurs after 50 years old.
- *Immediate risk:* Uterine perforation 1–2 in 1000, vasovagal response, expulsion risk 1 in 20.
- *Common side effects:* Pelvic infection <1% (usually within the first 3 weeks of insertion), heavier menses and pelvic pain.

- *Problems:* Refer to the section *IUCD and its problems.*
- *Follow up:* After 1–3 months or earlier if symptoms like severe abdominal pain/fever/heavy menstrual bleeding/foul-smelling vaginal discharge/suspected expulsion or pregnancy.

2. ***Levonorgestrel-containing IUCD (Mirena® IUCD)***
   - *Mode of action*: Contraceptive effect by achieving endometrial glandular and stromal atrophy.
   - Contains 52 mg reservoir of levonorgestrel (LNG) in Nova T-shaped device.
   - It releases 20 μg of LNG daily with a low systemic circulation of hormones.
   - ***Benefits:***
     - LARC: Can be used for up to 8 years (As per FDA 2022). Effective 7 days after insertion.
     - Extended use in perimenopausal women: If inserted at ≥45 years old, it can be left till menopause or 55 years old. However, if Mirena® is used for endometrial protection, it needs to be changed every 4 years.
     - No oestrogen side effects.
     - Causes lighter, irregular menses, especially in the first 3–6 months.
     - ***Other indications for MIRENA IUCD:***
       - Heavy menstrual bleeding (HMB): Can be used for up to 5 years
       - Dysmenorrhoea.

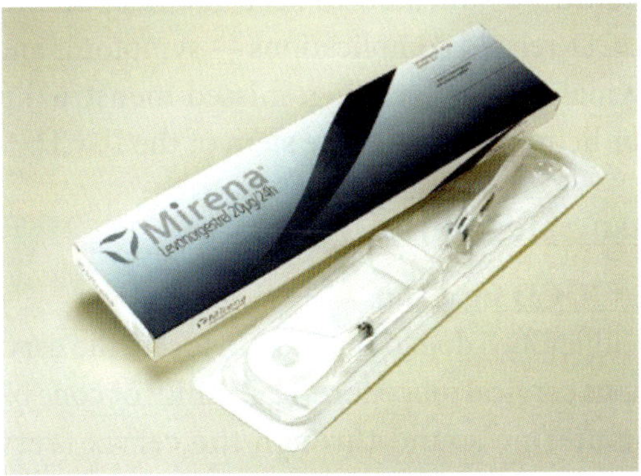

Mirena® IUCD.

    - Endometriosis.
    - Adenomyosis.
    - Treatment for endometrial hyperplasia.
    - Fertility-sparing management for endometrial cancer.
    - Endometrial protection as part of menopausal hormonal therapy to prevent endometrial hyperplasia: Can be used for 4 years (as per Bayer's recommendation 2023)
- *Timing of insertion/contraindications/removal:*
  - Similar to copper IUCD.
  - Mirena® should be removed in patients who are subsequently diagnosed with hormone receptor-positive breast cancer. Consult the medical oncologist.
- *Failure rate:* 0.2%
- *Common side effects:*
  - 20% of women have intermittent vaginal spotting in first 6 months. 90% decrease in menstrual blood loss by 12 months.
  - 20% of women are amenorrhoeic after 1 year.
  - 5–10% may experience headaches, migraine or depressed moods due to systemic hormonal effects.

IUCD and Its Problems

IUCD is a commonly used method of LARC. It is cost-effective and does not require patient compliance to ensure its effectiveness.

Women should be educated to seek medical attention if they are experiencing IUCD-related complications — symptoms and signs of pelvic infection, abnormal uterine bleeding, missed menstrual period, missing IUCD threads or being able to feel the stem of the IUCD.

Problems Associated with IUCD

1. At the time of IUCD insertion

- Insertion difficulties due to inability to locate the cervical os (women with previous cervical procedures, e.g., LEEP or cone biopsy), difficulty in passing uterine sound through the cervix (cervical stenosis), vasovagal reaction.
- Uterine cavity size <6 cm (small) or >9 cm (large).
  Small cavity: Higher risk of IUCD misplacement/migration.

Large cavity: Lower efficacy of copper IUCD → consider hormonal IUCD or subdermal contraceptive implant.
- _Signs of pelvic infection:_ Cervicitis, mucopurulent discharge, cervical motion tenderness → test and treat PID first and delay IUCD insertion till the patient is asymptomatic.
- Uterine perforation (1–2 in 1000 insertions, 6-fold increased risk in breastfeeding women).

2. **Immediately post-insertion 0–7 days**
   - Post-insertion bleeding: This can be common from minor trauma during insertion. The amount of bleeding should _not_ exceed that of a normal menstrual period.
   - Uterine cramps.
   - Endometritis, PID: The risk of infection is <1%.
3. **Early post-insertion 0–3 months**
   - Irregular vaginal bleeding/abdominal cramps.
   - Endometritis or PID: The risk of infection is <1%.
     - ***Symptomatic PID*** — start antibiotics. Remove IUCD after 48–72 hours of antibiotics if there is *no* clinical improvement and prescribe alternative contraception.
     - ***Symptomatic PID + actinomyces*** — remove IUCD, send IUCD for culture and obtain an ultrasound (US) scan of the pelvis to evaluate for abscess. If actinomyces are cultured from the IUCD, manage the patient with an infectious disease specialist. Prolonged

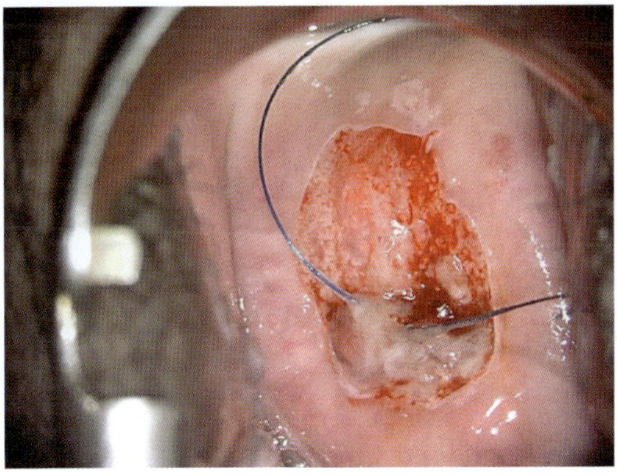

Ectropion with IUCD thread seen protruding from cervical os.

antibiotics are required, usually treated with penicillin in addition to standard PID treatment. Exclude other causes of pelvic pain.

- ***Asymptomatic PID (laboratory evidence of gonorrhoea or chlamydia)*** — start antibiotic treatment for PID without IUCD removal. Assess appropriateness for continued IUCD use and follow up after starting antibiotics. IUCD should be removed if there is no response to treatment after about 48–72 hours.
- ***Asymptomatic + actinomyces seen on Pap smear*** — colonised by actinomyces and *not* infected; there is *no* need for antibiotic treatment or IUCD removal.

– **Non-palpable threads** → perform a speculum examination to visualise IUCD threads. If threads are *not* visible, possibilities are as stated below (from most to least common):
  - IUCD is *in situ*, but the thread has curled and retracted into the endocervical canal or uterine cavity, or the thread is broken. Uterine enlargement secondary to fibroids or pregnancy or rotation of the IUCD can also cause retraction of threads.
  - IUCD has been expelled.

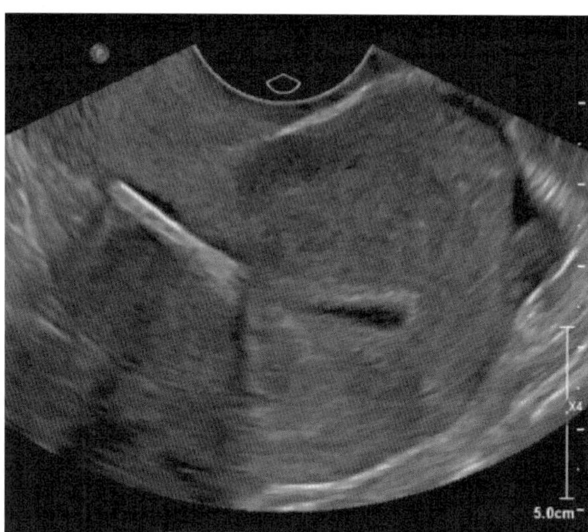

Malpositioned IUCD — in the lower endometrial cavity.

  - o IUCD has perforated the uterus and is in the myometrium or abdomen.

4. **Anytime post-insertion**
   - Bleeding Problems with IUCD: Ongoing vaginal bleeding, abdominal cramps or new-onset bleeding in a woman with long-standing IUCD → to exclude IUCD malposition/expulsion, pregnancy, infection and cervical dysplasia. Once these complications are excluded, *consider medical therapy*.
     - o NSAIDs for abdominal pain/bleeding (mefenamic acid 500 mg tds for 5 days).
     - o Tranexamic acid 1g TDS for 5 days.
     - o Combined oral contraceptive pills for irregular bleeding — can try continuous or cyclical therapy for 3 months.
     - o Heavy bleeding with copper IUCD — can try NSAIDs/tranexamic acid.
   - IUCD **malposition** (≥2 cm from fundus in a normal uterus).
     - o Remove IUCD if the patient is symptomatic or if IUCD is *below* the level of the internal os (fully/partially) or >2 cm from the fundus.
     - o Can consider keeping IUCD if asymptomatic, IUCD is *above* the internal os and woman would *not* replace it or choose another highly effective contraceptive method.
   - IUCD **expulsion** (1:20 risk, most common in first year, especially within the first 3 months of insertion).
   - Pregnancy (<1% risk) — perform an ultrasound scan to assess if it is an intrauterine or ectopic pregnancy. If pregnancy does occur, there is a higher risk of ectopic pregnancy among IUCD users. However, the overall risk of ectopic pregnancy is still lower than in women *not* on contraception.
   - ***Hormonal side effects*** (5–10%) in women using Mirena IUCD include acne, breast tenderness, headache and mood changes. They are common (incidence ≥1/100 to <1/10), and symptoms often settle with time.
   - **Functional ovarian cysts** are common and asymptomatic in women using Mirena IUCD. They are often managed conservatively — usually resolve spontaneously in 2–3 months.

Management of Missing IUCD

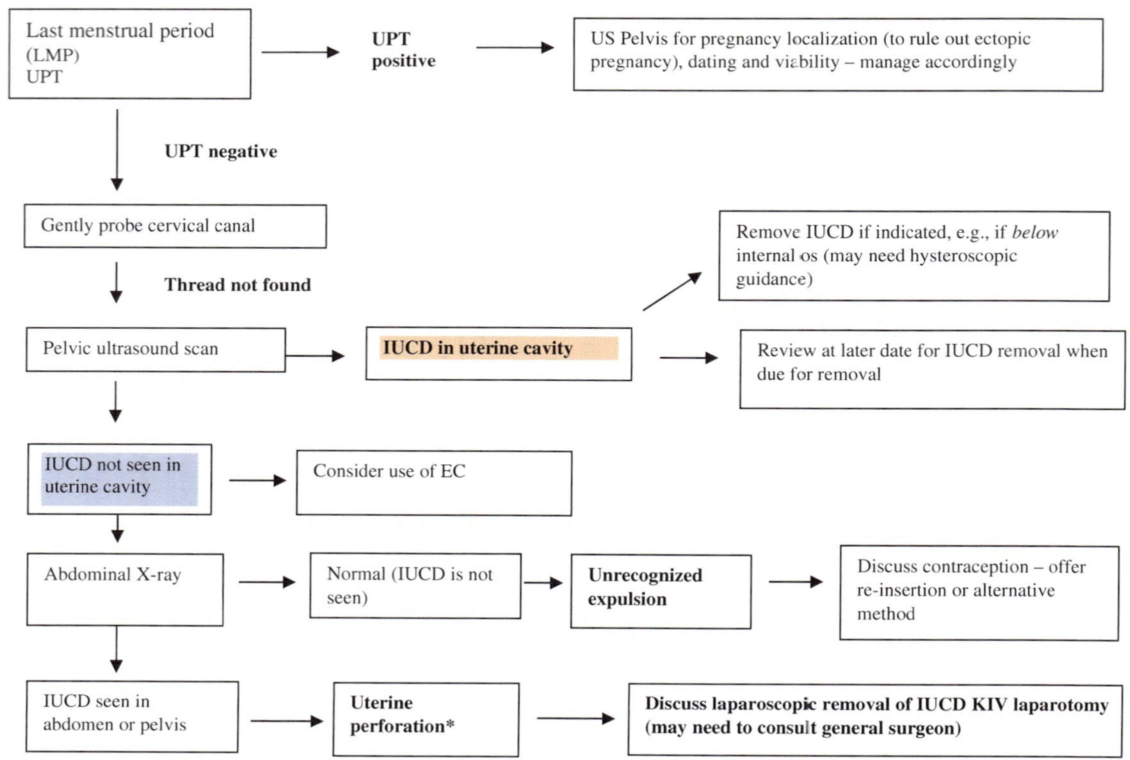

***Signs and symptoms of uterine perforation** include lower abdominal pain, missing threads, changes in bleeding pattern (with Mirena IUCD), history of severe pain during IUCD insertion.

Although serious complications following uterine perforation are rare, any perforated IUCD should be removed unless the surgical risk is very high. The risks associated with uterine perforation are adhesion formation and perforation into the intestines, bladder or blood vessels.

If the IUCD is in the abdomen or perforating through the myometrium, laparoscopy is the preferred method of removal. It can be performed electively in asymptomatic patients and is usually successful. Conversion to laparotomy may be required if there are extensive adhesions.

If the IUCD is embedded in the myometrium, therapeutic hysteroscopy may be required for removal. An intra-operative X-ray can help to localise the IUCD.

After surgical removal of the perforated IUCD, another IUCD may be offered in the future but recommended to wait at least 4 weeks after the initial surgery.

Management of pregnancy with IUCD *in situ*

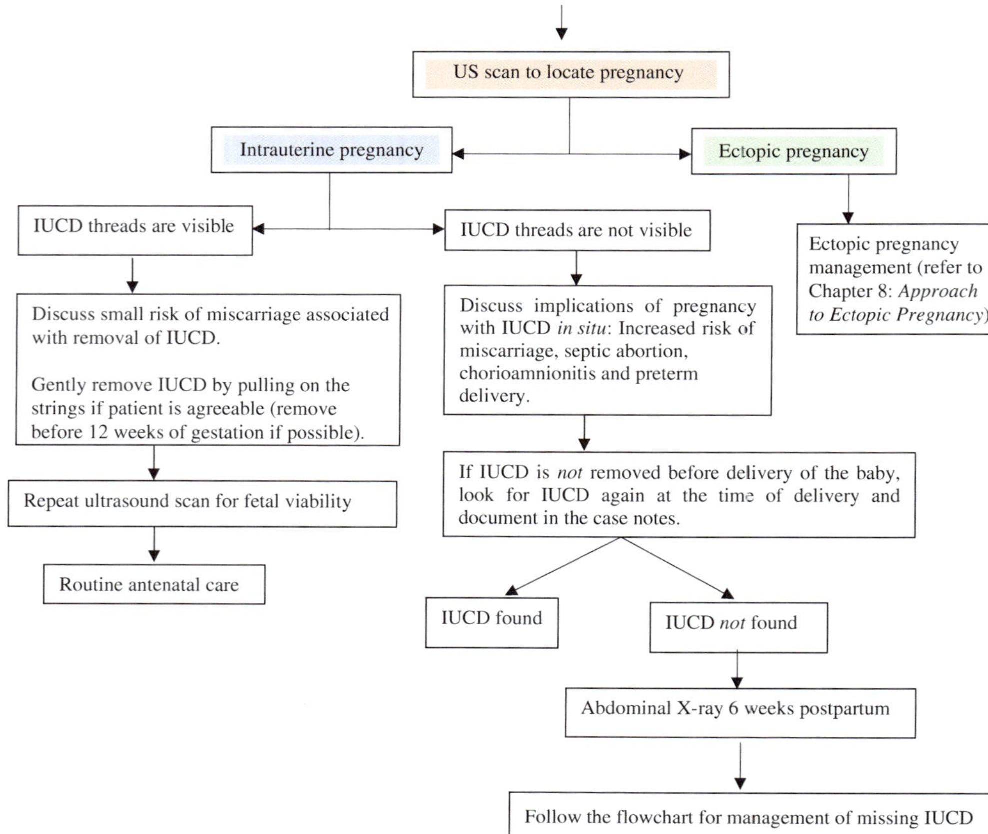

Permanent Sterilisation-Female Tubal Ligation/Male Vasectomy

1) *Female Tubal ligation*

- Sterilisation is a permanent method of contraception for women who have completed their families. Hence, we need to counsel women on the surgical risks, permanent nature of sterilisation, risk of regret, low

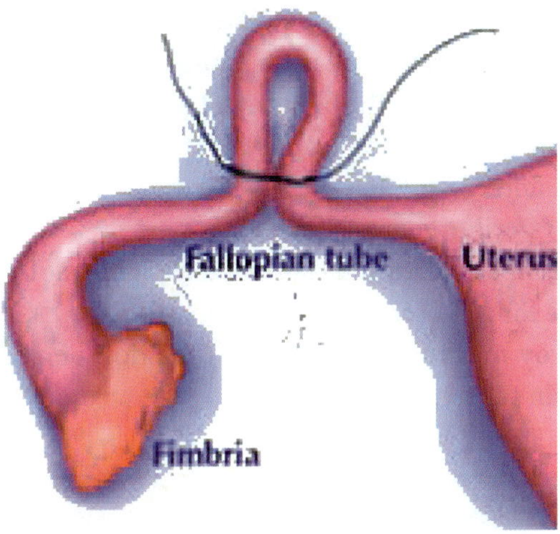

Female sterilisation using Pomeroy method — resected tubes are sent for histological confirmation.

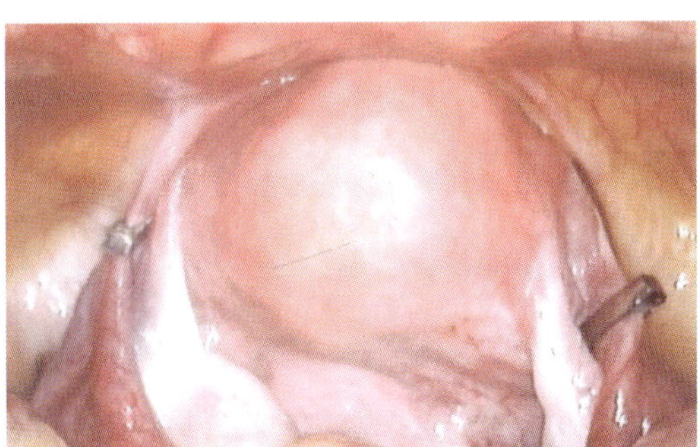

Laparoscopic ligation of both fallopian tubes with Filshie clips.

success rate for reversal of sterilisation, the need for *in vitro* fertilisation (IVF) if they are keen to pursue pregnancy in the future and the risk of ectopic pregnancy if failure of ligation occurs.

- To offer options of LARC and male sterilisation (vasectomy) to patients.
- *Timing*: Postpartum, post-abortion, or interval ligation of both fallopian tubes. Tubal ligation can be done any time during the menstrual cycle, provided the woman has a negative urine pregnancy test and has not had UPSI in the preceding 3 weeks. If there has been UPSI in the prior 3 weeks, there is a possibility of a luteal phase pregnancy. Proceeding with tubal ligation can result in an iatrogenic ectopic pregnancy as the tube is occluded before the blastocyst has passed the site of occlusion. Hence, postpone the procedure, use contraception until at least 3 weeks after UPSI and ensure that UPT is negative.
- *Methods of sterilisation*:
  - **Filshie clips application** (Filshie® clips are made of titanium, hence are safe for MRI scans up to 3T).
  - **Pomeroy method** (ligation and resection of a segment of both fallopian tubes).

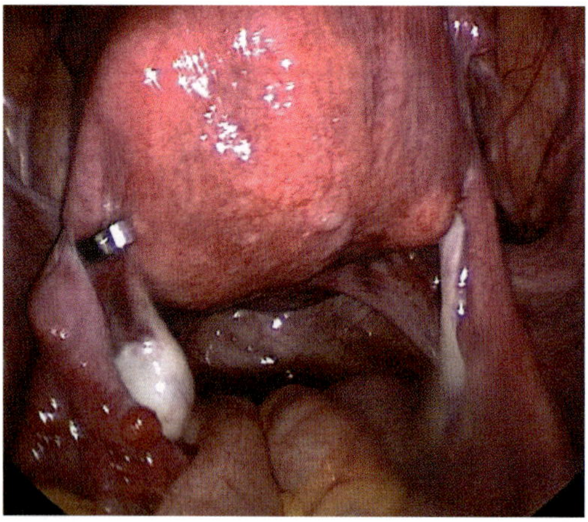

The right Filshie clip was missing as it had migrated but the right tube remained occluded.

  - o **Bilateral salpingectomy.**
    The benefit of bilateral salpingectomy and clipping of fallopian tubes is a 65% and 28% reduction in ovarian cancer risk, respectively.
  - o Tubal ligation can be done laparoscopically for interval ligation or via a mini-laparotomy (sub-umbilical incision) for postpartum sterilization. For patients who deliver via caesarean, postpartum sterilisation is usually done at the time of the caesarean section.
- *Failure rate:* 0.5%.
- *Long-term risks:*
  - o Device migration with Filshie clips — migration of the Filshie clips can occur in up to 25% of patients. It would remain effective as long as the tube was obstructed from the previous clip ligation. Migrated clips are usually not associated with significant morbidity. If the patient is asymptomatic, these displaced Filshie clips do not need to be removed. Rarely, up to 0.1–0.6% of patients with migrated Filshie clips may experience symptoms, e.g., chronic abdominal pain or chronic groin sinus. There are also case reports of the clips being expelled via the vagina, bladder or rectum.
  - o Little or no association with change in menstrual symptoms.
  - o No evidence that it results in significant changes in hormone levels.

2) ***Vasectomy:***
- This is a permanent method of contraception for men.
- Involves a surgery performed by the urologist where the vas deferens are cut or tied so that the sperms are *not* released during ejaculation.
- It can be done under local anaesthesia.
- No hormonal side effects
- *Failure rate:* 0.1–0.15%.
- Not effective immediately. Post-vasectomy semen analysis is needed 3 months after surgery to ensure that azoospermia has been confirmed.

Contraceptive Choice Based on Personal Characteristics and Reproductive History

Many factors determine the method of contraception a woman selects to use. Contraception should be used correctly and safely for maximum efficacy.

The FSRH in the UK categorised contraception risk into four categories and published guidelines for using different contraceptive methods in various medical conditions.

It is important to use the UKMEC table to relate the safety of contraception with particular personal characteristics.

UKMEC	Definition of category
Category 1	A condition for which there is no restriction for the use of the method.
Category 2	A condition where the advantages of using the method generally outweigh the theoretical or proven risks.
Category 3	A condition where the **theoretical or proven risks usually outweigh the advantages** of using the method. The provision of a method requires expert clinical judgement and/or referral to a specialist contraceptive provider since the use of the method is not usually recommended unless other more appropriate methods are not available or not acceptable.
Category 4	A condition that represents an **unacceptable health risk** if the method is used.

Key for terms used in UKMEC:

CHC-combined hormonal contraception, e.g., oral contraceptive pill/patch/vaginal ring, POP, DMPA, IMP, copper intrauterine device (Cu-IUD), levonorgestrel intrauterine device (LNG-IUD), barrier methods (CD), e.g., condom/diaphragm/spermicide.

There are *no* specific contraindications to sterilisation/surgical ligation. However, fitness for surgery and anaesthesia must be considered. It is only recommended for women >30 years old and who have completed family as the likelihood of young women regretting their choice of sterilisation is high.

Personal characteristics and reproductive history	Best choice *UKMEC 1*	Alternative *UKMEC 2*	Not recommended *UKMEC 3 and 4*	Additional information
Age	POP, IMP, CHC in patients <40 years old. DPMA in patients 18–45 years old. Cu-IUD and LNG-IUD in patients >20 years old. Barrier method – All ages.	CHC in patients ≥40 years old. DPMA in patients <18 and >45 years old. Cu-IUD and LNG-IUD in patients ≤20 years old. – Concern about the risk for expulsion from nulliparity and STIs from sexual behaviour in younger age groups.		The risk for cardiovascular disease increases with age and might increase with CHC use. Without other adverse clinical conditions, CHCs can be used until menopause. Women lose BMD while using DMPA but regain BMD after discontinuation.
Past ectopic pregnancy	All methods can be used.		None.	All methods protect against pregnancy in general, including ectopic pregnancy.
Post abortion First trimester	All methods.			Women who started taking combined oral contraceptives (COCs) immediately after a first-trimester abortion did not experience more side effects/adverse vaginal bleeding outcomes/clinically significant changes in coagulation profile than those who used a placebo/IUD/non-hormonal contraceptive method or delayed COC initiation.
Second trimester	CHC, POP, DMPA, IMP, CD.	Cu-IUD and LNG-IUD.		
Post abortion sepsis	CHC, POP, DMPA, IMP, CD.	Expulsion was greater when an IUD was inserted after a second-trimester abortion than when inserted after a first-trimester abortion. Safety or expulsion for post-abortion insertion of an LNG-IUD did *not* differ from that of a Cu-IUD.	Cu-IUD and LNG-IUD.	
Obesity BMI >30–34	POP, DMPA, IMP, Cu-IUD, LNG-IUD, CD.	CHC.		Obese women who use CHC are more likely than non-users to experience VTE. The effectiveness of the patch decreased among women who weighed >90 kg.
BMI ≥35	POP, DMPA, IMP, Cu-IUD, LNG-IUD, CD.		CHC not advised.	
Smoking WHO study showed significantly increased risks of myocardial infarction in women >35 years old who smoke and use the CHC	POP, DMPA, IMP, Cu-IUD, LNG-IUD, CD.	CHC can be used in patients <35 years old or ex-smokers who have stopped for at least 1 year.	CHC should be denied to smokers ≥35 years old.	

Contraception in Women With Medical Conditions and Drug Interactions

Medical conditions and drug interactions may affect the efficacy of contraception. Therefore, it is important to obtain a detailed history from this group of women, provide accurate information on possible contraception that they are medically eligible for and help them to decide on the option that suits them best. UKMEC provide a safe guide in delivering effective and reliable contraception.

Medical condition	Best choice *UKMEC 1*	Alternative *UKMEC 2*	Not recommended *UKMEC 3 and 4*	Additional information
Hypertension BP >140/90 mmHg. Known risk factors for cardiovascular disease and cerebrovascular accidents.	POP, IMP, Cu-IUD, LNG-IUD, CD.	DPMA.	CHC (users are at higher risk than non-users for stroke, acute myocardial infarction, and peripheral arterial disease).	DPMA is associated with a slight increased risk of cardiovascular events. Use of all hormone-related contraception is not recommended if there is existing vascular disease.
DM Good glycemic control is important to minimise complications during pregnancy. Effective contraception is crucial to preventing unplanned pregnancy. Monitoring BP, BMI, fasting lipids and investigations to exclude retinopathy, vascular and renal complications should be performed regularly.	Cu-IUD (no increased pelvic infection rates compared to non-diabetics), CD.	*Well-controlled diabetes* with no systemic complications: CHC, POP, IMP, DMPA, LNG-IUD.	Diabetes with underlying renal or vascular disease: Avoid CHC and DMPA.	POP and DMPA increase insulin resistance and progestogen implants have minimal effect. Oestrogen has *no* effect on insulin resistance.
Thrombophilia/VTE ***Thrombophilia* include thrombogenic mutations like factor V Leiden, prothrombin mutation, protein C, protein S and antithrombin deficiencies.** ***VTE risk assessment*:** – Personal history. – Family history. – Surgery. – Prolonged immobilisation.	Cu-IUD, CD.	POP, DMPA, IMP, LNG-IUD (progestogen-containing contraceptives are UKMEC 2 in women with a history of VTE, current VTE on anti-coagulants, with known thrombogenic mutations or undergoing major surgery with prolonged immobilisation).	CHC (CHC increases the VTE risk through the effect of oestrogen on clotting factors. Third-generation progestogen is associated with a 2-fold increase compared to a second-generation progestogen).	Among women with thrombogenic mutations, CHC users had a 2–20-fold higher risk of thrombosis than non-users. All methods may be used in women with superficial venous thrombosis, e.g., varicose veins. All methods except CHC can be used in women with immobility *not* related to surgery.

(*Continued*)

(Continued)

Medical condition	Best choice *UKMEC 1*	Alternative *UKMEC 2*	Not recommended *UKMEC 3 and 4*	Additional information
Current and history of IHD and stroke	Cu-IUD, CD.	POP, IMP and LNG-IUD can be initiated in never-before users. New users are advised to stop if patient develops IHD or stroke while on the above methods.	CHC, DMPA.	
Hyperlipidaemia	Cu-IUD, CD.	POP, DMPA, IMP, LNG-IUD, CHC.		
Valvular heart disease (VHD) and congenital heart disease **Uncomplicated.**	POP, DMPA, IMP, Cu-IUD, LNG-IUD, CD.	CHC.		CHC use may further increase the risk of arterial thrombosis in women with VHD. Prophylactic antibiotics to prevent endocarditis are not recommended for inserting or removing IUDs.
Complicated (pulmonary hypertension, atrial fibrillation, history of subacute bacterial endocarditis).	POP, DMPA, IMP, CD.	Cu-IUD, LNG-IUD.	CHC.	
Headaches **Non-migrainous.**	All methods.			Women with migraine with aura had a higher risk of stroke than those without aura. Women with a history of migraine who use CHC are about 2–4 times as likely to have an ischaemic stroke as non-users.
Migraine without aura.	Cu-IUD, CD.	POP, DMPA, IMP, LNG-IUD. CHC may be initiated but should be advised to stop if migraine develops while on the CHC.		
Migraine with aura.	Cu-IUD, CD.	POP, DMPA, IMP, LNG-IUD.	CHC.	

Medical condition	Best choice *UKMEC 1*	Alternative *UKMEC 2*	Not recommended *UKMEC 3 and 4*	Additional information
Epilepsy Anti-epileptic drugs (AEDs) are associated with an increased risk of congenital malformations (fetal hydantoin syndrome, congenital cardiac and limb defects, cleft lip/palate, and neural tube defects). Hence, effective contraception is crucial to preventing unplanned pregnancies.	All contraceptive methods can be used in epileptic patients with no restrictions. *First-line*: Cu-IUCD (metabolic neutrality, lack of drug interaction and high efficacy).			EID (phenytoin, primidone, carbamazepine and phenobarbitone) *induces* the hepatic microsomal oxidase system, which accelerates the metabolism of CHC and POP. *Special precautions*: – Use a CHC with a higher oestrogen dose (50 mcg) or – Double dosage of CHC with a lower oestrogen content (30 mcg). – Double the normal dose of POP. DMPA and LNG-IUD are **not** affected by EIA. No change in the dosage is needed.
Gallbladder disease	Cu-IUD, CD.	POP, DMPA, IMP, LNG-IUD. CHC may be used in asymptomatic or women who had cholecystectomy.	CHC is not recommended in medically treated or current symptomatic gallbladder disease.	CHC might cause a small increased risk of gallbladder disease and might worsen existing gallbladder disease.
History of cholestasis • **Pregnancy-related.**	POP, DMPA, IMP, CU-IUD, LNG-IUD, CD.	CHC.		History of pregnancy-related cholestasis might predict an increased risk of COC-related cholestasis.
• **Past CHC-related.**	CU-IUD, CD.	POP, DMPA, IMP, LNG-IUD.	CHC.	
Viral hepatitis	POP, DMPA, IMP, Cu-IUD, LNG-IUD, CD.		Initiation of CHC is contraindicated in acute hepatitis/flares. However, it may be safely used in carrier/chronic hepatitis.	COC use does not worsen current cirrhotic fibrosis nor increase the risk of hepatocellular carcinoma in chronic hepatitis. COC use does *not* appear to trigger liver failure or severe dysfunction in carriers.

(*Continued*)

(*Continued*)

Medical condition	Best choice *UKMEC 1*	Alternative *UKMEC 2*	Not recommended *UKMEC 3 and 4*	Additional information
Cirrhosis • **Mild (compensated without complications).**	All methods can be used.			
• **Severe (decompensated).**	Cu-IUD, CD.		CHC, POP, DMPA, IMP, LNG-IUD.	
Liver tumours	CU-IUD, CD.	CHC, POP, DMPA, IMP and LNG-IUD may be used in focal nodular hyperplasia (no influence on either progression or regression).	CHC, POP, DMFA, IMP and LNG-IUD are <u>*not*</u> advised in hepatocel ular adenoma or malignant liver tumours.	COC use in healthy women is associated with the development and growth of hepatocellular adenoma. Whether other hormonal contraceptives have similar effects is *not* known.
Inflammatory bowel disease (IBD)	DMPA, IMP, Cu-IUD, LNG-IUD, CD.	CHC, POP.		Absorption might be reduced if the woman has severe disease or small bowel surgery.
Systemic lupus erythematosus (SLE) Women with SLE are at an increased risk of IHD, stroke and VTE.	Cu-IUD and CD are the only methods for women *with* positive antiphospholipid antibodies (APS).	POP, DMPA, IMP, LNG-IUD may be used in women *with* and *without* APS. CHC may be used in women *without* APS.	CHC (women with positive APS).	APS is associated with a higher risk of both arterial and venous thrombosis.
Thyroid disease	All methods can be used.			

Medical condition	Best choice *UKMEC 1*	Alternative *UKMEC 2*	Not recommended *UKMEC 3 and 4*	Additional information
HIV/AIDS Condom use is highly effective in preventing HIV infection in heterosexual couples in which one partner is infected and reduces transmission of other STIs. STIs can increase the risk of HIV seroconversion.	CD and CHC, POP, DMPA, IMP.	Cu-IUD and LNG-IUD.	Repeated and high-dose use of the spermicide nonoxynol-9 was associated with an increased risk of genital lesions, which might increase the risk of HIV infection.	Hormonal contraception does not interfere with antiviral drug effectiveness. The efficacy of CHC and POP is not affected by the administration of non-ritonavir boosted atazanavir or indinavir. DMPA may be safe to administer with efavirenz, nevirapine and nelfinavir.
Anatomical abnormalities/ uterine fibroids that distort the endometrial cavity	CHC, POP, DMPA, IMP, CD.		Cu-IUD and LNG-IUD.	
Breast disease	All methods can be used in patients with benign breast disease or a family history of cancer. Cu-IUD and CD are the only methods for patients with a current or history of breast cancer.	POP, DMPA, IMP, LNG-IUD (may be used for an undiagnosed breast lump and carriers of known gene mutations, e.g., BRCA 1).	CHC (women who have breast cancer, are gene mutation carriers or have an undiagnosed breast lump).	Breast cancer is a hormonally sensitive tumour. The prognosis for women with current or recent breast cancer might worsen with hormonal contraceptive use.

Contraceptive Advice for Women Using Enzyme Inducing Drugs (EID)

Contraceptive method	Short-term use of EID (<2 months)	Long-term use of EID (>2 months) or difficulty using additional contraceptive precautions
CHC 1. COC 2. Combined transdermal patch 3. Combined vaginal ring	***Recommended option*** Change to an alternative method unaffected by EID. This could include temporarily stopping COC and having a one-off DMPA injection to cover the short-term treatment and 28 days after.	Change to an alternative method unaffected by EID.
	Alternatives Use one COC pill daily [at least 30 μg ethinylestradiol (EE)], one patch weekly or one ring 3-weekly and use an extended or tricycling regimen with a HFI of 4 days **Plus** Additional contraceptive precautions (e.g., condoms) while taking and for 28 days after stopping the enzyme-inducing drug **Or** Use 2 COC pills as per long-term treatment (see opposite). *Not* recommended if using the potent EID rifampicin or rifabutin.	Use COC pills containing at least 50 μg EE (e.g., 20 and 30 μg COCs). Use an extended or tricycling regimen with a pill-free interval of 4 days ***Note:*** Not recommended if using the potent EID rfampicin or rifabutin.
Progestogen-only contraception POPs IMP	**Recommended option** Change to an alternative method unaffected by EID (including one dose of IMP to cover the period of risk and 28 days after stopping the EID).	Change to an alternative method unaffected by EID.
	Alternative option Continue use of POP or IMP. **Plus** Additional contraceptive precautions (e.g., condoms) while taking and for 28 days after stopping the EID.	No alternative change is advised.

Contraceptive method	Any change in contraception needed for women using enzyme inducing drugs (EID)
Progestogen-only injectable (DMPA) Levonorgestrel-releasing intrauterine system (LNG-IUS)	**No change is required** Efficacy of DMPA and LNG-IUS unaffected by EID and women can continue with the usual dose and dosing/replacement interval of 12 weeks or 5 years, respectively.
Non-hormonal methods Cu-IUD, barrier methods	**No change is required** Efficacy is unaffected.
Emergency contraception (EC) 1) Cu-IUD 2) LNG 3) Ulipristal acetate	1) Efficacy unaffected. Unless contraindicated, offer to all women (between 0 and 120 hours of UPSI or within 5 days of expected ovulation) taking or within 28 days of stopping EID. 2) Can use double dose, i.e., LNG 3 mg (2 × 1.5 mg tablet) as a single dose within <72 hours of UPSI if Cu-IUD is declined or unsuitable. The effectiveness of 3 mg LNG is unknown in this situation. 3) Double dose of ulipristal is <u>not</u> recommended.

Drugs That Increase Contraceptive Hormone Levels (Enzyme Inhibitors)

Drug type	Drug	Interaction	Clinical significance
Antibacterial	Erythromycin	Enzyme inhibitor	Modest to marked increases in estradiol and dienogest levels. The clinical significance is not known, but increased adverse events might be anticipated.
Antifungal	Fluconazole Itraconazole Ketoconazole	Enzyme inhibitor	Modest increases EE and progestogen. Breakthrough bleeding was noted in studies. Evidence in relation to fluconazole has been broadly reassuring in relation to contraceptive efficacy.
Antiretroviral	Atazanavir (upboosted)	Enzyme inhibitor	Modest to marked increases in EE when atazanavir is used unboosted. Concomitant use of combined methods is not advisable. When atazanavir is boosted with ritonavir, the net effect is a reduction in EE levels.
Immunosuppressant	Tacrolimus	Enzyme inhibitor	Theoretically inhibits the metabolism of oestrogens and progestogens, leading to increased levels. The clinical significance is unknown, but the increase is likely to be small.
Non-steroidal anti-inflammatory	Etoricoxib	Enzyme inhibitor	Doses of etoricoxib ≥60 mg raise EE levels by approximately ≥40%. The potential risk of oestrogen-related adverse events.
Statins	Atorvastatin Rosuvastatin	Enzyme inhibitor	Minor to a modest increase in EE and progestogens leading to increased levels. The clinical significance is not known but is likely to be small.

Drugs That Are Affected by Contraceptive Hormones

Drug type	Clinical effect
Anti-epileptics	***Decreased* levels or clinical effect** EE reduces plasma concentrations of lamotrigine. Possible increased risk of seizures. Consider increasing the dose of lamotrigine monotherapy. To avoid toxicity in the pill-free week, consider an extended regimen. EE may also modestly reduce valproate levels.
Anti-hypertensives	CHC may antagonise the hypotensive effect. Monitor effect.
Antidiabetics	Oestrogens and progestogens antagonise the hypoglycaemic effect of antidiabetics. Monitor effect.
Diuretics	Oestrogens may antagonise the diuretic effect.
Thyroid hormones	Oestrogens may increase the requirements for thyroid hormones in hypothyroidism. Monitor thyroid function.
Bronchodilators	Oestrogens reduce the excretion of theophylline, resulting in increased plasma concentrations. Therefore, a reduction of the theophylline dosage is recommended.
Dopaminergics	Oestrogens increase plasma concentrations of ropinirole. Defined by British National Formulary (BNF) as non-hazardous (i.e., does not usually have serious complications). Oestrogens and progestogens increase plasma concentrations of selegiline. Increased risk of toxicity. Concomitant use should be avoided.
Immuno-suppressants	Plasma levels of tacrolimus possibly increased by EE and gestodene. Monitor tacrolimus levels. cyclosporin levels could be increased by oestrogens and progestogens (interaction unconfirmed and uncertain clinical significance).
Muscle relaxants	Oestrogens and progestogens possibly increase plasma concentration of tizanidine, potentially leading to toxicity.
Potassium-sparing diuretics and aldosterone antagonists	Theoretical risk of hyperkalaemia when administered with drospirenone, but COCs containing drospirenone are not usually used in hypertensive patients.
Retinoids	The adverse effects of oral contraceptives on lipids may be additive with those of isotretinoin. As retinoids are teratogenic, the benefits of COC use may outweigh the risk and lipids should be monitored routinely during retinoid treatment.
Triptans	*COCs appear to modestly raise the level of frovatriptan, naratriptan, zolmitriptan and slightly increased levels of sumatriptan. Before prescribing triptans in CHC users with migraine, health professionals should refer to UKMEC as CHC may be contraindicated in some women with a history of migraine.*

How to Start or Switch Contraceptive Method

Starting a Contraceptive Method

Method	When?	Need for additional contraception?
CHC DMPA IMP	Start D1–5 of the menstrual cycle	No need.
	Start from D6 of the menstrual cycle	**If no UPSI** since the last menstrual period (LMP), abstain from sex/use condoms for 7 days. **If UPSI has occurred** since LMP, do a UPT first before starting. If UPT is negative, start the method and repeat UPT 3 weeks later. Consider EC if indicated.
POP	Start D1–5 of the menstrual cycle	No need.
	Start from D6 of the menstrual cycle	**If no UPSI** since the last LMP, abstain/use condoms for 2 days. **If UPSI has occurred** since LMP, do a UPT first before starting. If UPT is negative, start POP and repeat UPT 3 weeks later. Consider EC if indicated.
LNG-IUD (e.g., Mirena®)	Start D1–5 of the menstrual cycle	No need.
	Start from D6 of the menstrual cycle	**If no UPSI** since last LMP, abstain/use condoms for 7 days. **If UPSI has** occurred since LMP, do a UPT first. If UPT is negative, do **NOT** use LNG-IUD. Use a different method and repeat UPT 3 weeks later.
Copper IUCD (Cu-IUD	Start D1–5 of the menstrual cycle	No need.
	Start from D6 of the menstrual cycle	**If no UPSI** since the last LMP, **NO** need to abstain from sex/use additional contraception. **If UPSI has occurred** since LMP, do a UPT first. If UPT is negative, check if all UPSI is in the last 5 days OR if today is at least ≤5 days after the earliest ovulation date. If YES → proceed with Cu-IUD insertion. If NO → DO **NOT** use Cu-IUD. Use a different method. Repeat UPT 3 weeks later.

Switching Contraceptive Method

This assumes that the patient has been taking the current contraception correctly.

	Switch to					
Current method	**CHC**	**POP**	**DMPA**	**Implant**	**LNG-IUD**	**Cu-IUD**
CHC On week 1 of the pill	Start method. Abstain from sex/use condoms for 7 days.	Start method. Abstain from sex/use condoms for 2 days.	Start method. Abstain from sex/use condoms for 7 days.			Start method. No need to abstain from sex/use condoms.
On week 2–3 of the pill	Start method. No need to abstain from sex/use condoms.					
On D1–2 of HFI, i.e., pill-free interval	Start method. No need to abstain from sex/use condoms.				Start method. No need to abstain from sex/use condoms. If start on D2 of HFI, abstain from sex/use condoms for 7 days.	Start method. No need to abstain from sex/use condoms.
On D3–7 of HFI + **no** UPSI since HFI	Start method. Abstain from sex/use condoms for 7 days.	Start method. Abstain from sex/use condoms for 2 days.	Start method. Abstain from sex/use condoms for 7 days.			Start method. No need to abstain from sex/use condoms.
On D3–7 of HFI + UPSI has occurred since HFI	Continue the current CHC for 7 consecutive days, then change the method. No need to abstain from sex/use condoms.					Start method. No need to abstain from sex/use condoms.

(Continued)

(*Continued*)

	Switch to					
Current method	**CHC**	**POP**	**DMPA**	**Implant**	**LNG-IUD**	**Cu-IUD**
POP						
Traditional POP	Start method. Abstain from sex/use condoms for 7 days.	Start method. No need to abstain from sex/use condoms.	Start method. Abstain from sex/use condoms for 7 days.			Start method. No need to abstain from sex/use condoms.
Desogestrel POP	Start method. No need to abstain from sex/use condoms.					
Implant						
Implant *in situ* ≤3 yr	Start method. No need to abstain from sex/use condoms.					
Implant *in situ* >3 and ≤4 years + no UPSI for >3 weeks	Check UPT. If negative, start method. Abstain from sex/use condoms for 7 days.	Check UPT. If negative, start method. Abstain from sex/use condoms for 2 days.	Check UPT. If negative, start method. Abstain from sex/use condoms for 7 days.			Check UPT. If negative, start method. No need to abstain from sex/use condoms.
Implant *in situ* >3 years and ≤4 years + UPSI in the last 3 weeks	Check UPT. If negative, start method. Abstain from sex/use condoms for 7 days. Repeat UPT 3 weeks later.	Check UPT. If negative, start method. Abstain from sex/use condoms for 2 days. Repeat UPT 3 weeks later.	Check UPT. If negative, start method. Abstain from sex/use condoms for 7 days. Repeat UPT 3 weeks later.			Check UPT. If negative, start method. No need to abstain from sex/use condoms. Repeat UPT 3 weeks later.
DMPA						
DMPA ≤14 weeks since last injection	Start method. No need to abstain from sex/use condoms.					

	Switch to					
Current method	**CHC**	**POP**	**DMPA**	**Implant**	**LNG-IUD**	**Cu-IUD**
DMPA >14 weeks since last injection + **no UPSI** since 14 weeks post-injection	Start method. Abstain from sex/use condoms for 7 days.	Start method. Abstain from sex/use condoms for 2 days.	Start method. Abstain from sex/use condoms for 7 days.			Start method. No need to abstain from sex/use condoms.
DMPA >14 weeks since last injection + UPSI since 14 weeks post-injection	Check UPT. If negative, start method. Abstain from sex/use condoms for 7 days. Repeat UPT 3 weeks later.	Check UPT. If negative, start method. Abstain from sex/use condoms for 2 days. Repeat UPT 3 weeks later.	Check UPT. If negative, start method. Abstain from sex/use condoms for 7 days. Repeat UPT 3 weeks later.		**DO NO USE** unless able to exclude pregnancy.	If the only UPSI was in the last 5 days, start method. No need to abstain from sex/use condoms. If UPSI was >5 days ago and unable to exclude pregnancy, **DO NOT USE.**
LNG-IUD						
LNG-IUD *in situ* + no UPSI in last 7 days	Start method. Abstain from sex/use condoms for 7 days.	Start method. Abstain from sex/use condoms for 2 days.	Start method. Abstain from sex/use condoms for 7 days.		Start method. No need to abstain from sex/use condoms.	
LNG-IUD *in situ* + UPSI in last 7 days	Start method but keep current LNG-IUD for 7 days after starting new method before removing.				Abstain from sex for 7 days before changing method in case the new device cannot be inserted.	
Cu-IUD						
CU-IUD *in situ* + D1–5 of menses	Start method. No need to abstain from sex/use condoms.					

(*Continued*)

(*Continued*)

	Switch to					
Current method	**CHC**	**POP**	**DMPA**	**Implant**	**LNG-IUD**	**Cu-IUD**
CU-IUD *in situ* ≥D6 of menses + **no** UPSI in last 7 days	Start method. Abstain from sex/use condoms for 7 days.	Start method. Abstain from sex/use condoms for 2 days.	Start method. Abstain from sex/use condoms for 7 days.			Start method. No need to abstain from sex/use condoms.
CU-IUD *in situ* ≥D6 of menses + UPSI in last 7 days	Start method but keep current Cu-IUD for 7 days after starting new method before removing.				Abstain from sex for 7 days before changing, then use condoms/abstain from sex for 7 days.	Abstain from sex for 7 days before changing in case the new device cannot be inserted.
EC						
Immediately after ulipristal acetate EC (UPA-EC)	DO NOT start any hormonal contraception for 5 days after UPA-EC.				DO NOT USE.	If all UPSI within last 5 days or if today is ≤5 days after earliest likely ovulation date, start method. No need to abstain from sex/use condoms. If NOT → DO NOT USE.
5 days after UPA-EC	Start method. Abstain from sex/use condoms for 7 days. Check UPT 3 weeks later.	Start method. Abstain from sex/use condoms for 2 days. Check UPT 3 weeks later.	Start method. Abstain from sex/use condoms for 7 days. Check UPT 3 weeks later.			
Levonorgestrel 1.5 mg						

Source: Faculty of Sexual & Reproductive Healthcare, FSRH Guidance: Switching or Starting Methods of Contraception. Published February 2017 (Amended March 2021). Accessed 21 May 2022.

Contraception for Postpartum Women

The earliest time reported for ovulation in non-lactating women is 25 days, with the average varying from 45 to 94 days (UpToDate).

Types of Contraceptive Methods:
For mothers who are fully breastfeeding:

1. ***Lactational amenorrhoea method.***
   - For it to be effective, it has to fulfil the following criteria:
     - Exclusively or nearly full breastfeeding 24 hours daily — no other liquids to be given or only water/juice/vitamins given infrequently in addition to breastmilk AND
     - No long intervals between feeds day or night (e.g., >4 hours during the day and >6 hours at night) AND
     - Amenorrhoea (no bleeding after 56 days postnatal)
     - This lasts for up to 6 months
   - *Mode of action*: Breastfeeding inhibits the LH pulsatile release from the anterior pituitary.
   - *Failure rate:* 1–2%.
2. *Barrier method.*
3. *POP/progestogen-only injectables/IMP* — can start immediately postpartum. No significant negative effect of progestogen-only contraception on breastfeeding performance.
4. *MIRENA IUCD* — within 0–48 hours or >4 weeks after childbirth. Do not insert during postpartum sepsis.
5. *Copper IUCD* — within 0–48 hours or >4 weeks after childbirth. Do not insert during postpartum sepsis.
6. *Tubal ligation-female sterilization* — immediately postpartum or 6 weeks postpartum.
7. *Vasectomy-male sterilization* — performed by urologist.
8. *COCP* — should only be started at least 6 weeks postpartum. Theoretical concerns about the effects of CHCs on breast milk production are greater in the early postpartum period when milk flow is being established.

For mothers who are not breastfeeding:

1. Barrier method.
2. *POP/progestogen-only injectables/IMP* — can start immediately postpartum.
3. *Mirena®/copper IUCD* — within 0–48 hours or >4 weeks after childbirth. Do not insert during postpartum sepsis.
4. *Tubal ligation-female sterilization* — immediately postpartum or 6 weeks postpartum.
5. *Vasectomy-male sterilisation* — performed by urologist.
6. *COCP* — should **NOT** be started earlier than 21 days postpartum due to the increased risk of VTE.
   - If there are no risk factors for VTE, COCP can be started at least 21 days postpartum.
   - If there are risk factors for VTE, COCP can only be started at least 6 weeks postpartum or consider an alternative method.

Emergency Contraception (EC)

EC refers to products that prevent pregnancy from occurring after an episode of UPSI. It works by disrupting the timing of ovulation or preventing the fertilisation of an ovulated egg. It is not meant to be a form of regular contraception. EC can be used for all patients, including adolescents and breastfeeding women.

The ***absolute contraindication* for EC** is *pregnancy.*

Indications for *EC* include UPSI, imperfect use of current contraception or women who have unconsented sexual intercourse (sexual assault victims).

Currently, **three types of EC** are used in Singapore: Copper IUCD, oral LNG and UPA. *Copper IUCD* is the *most effective EC.* However, if copper IUCD is not acceptable or the criteria for IUCD insertion are *not* met, then consider oral EC.

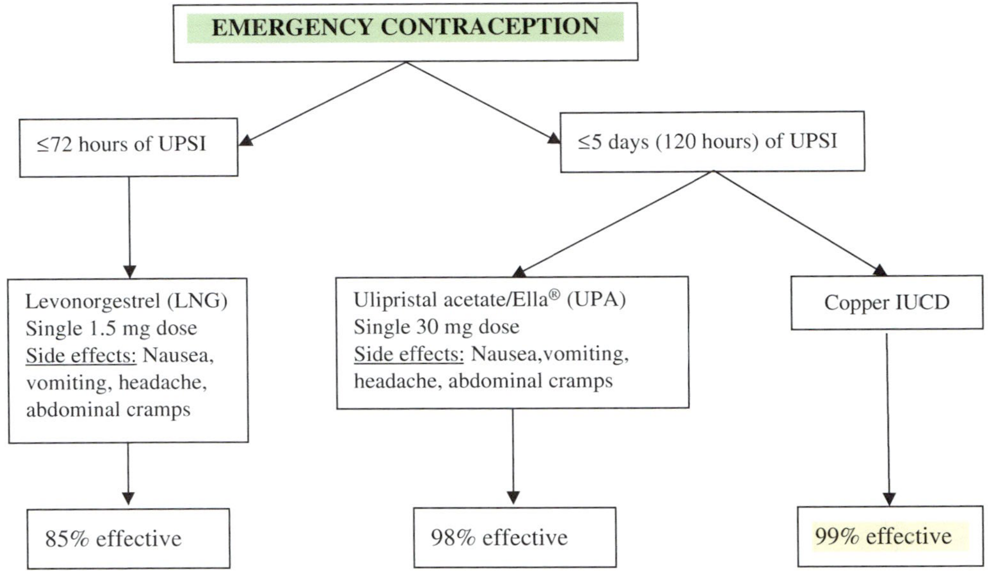

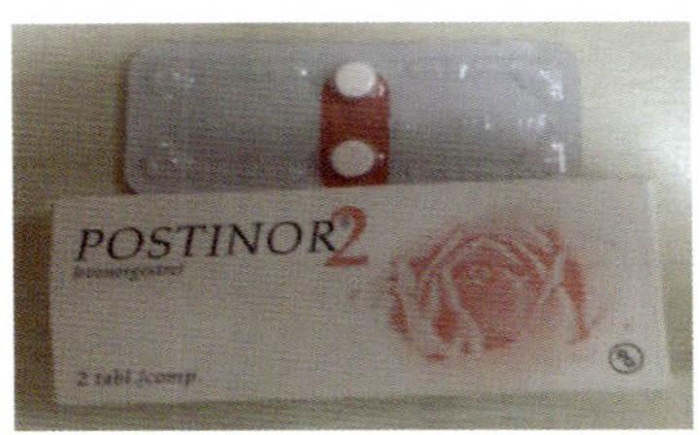

Levonorgestrel (Postinor 2)

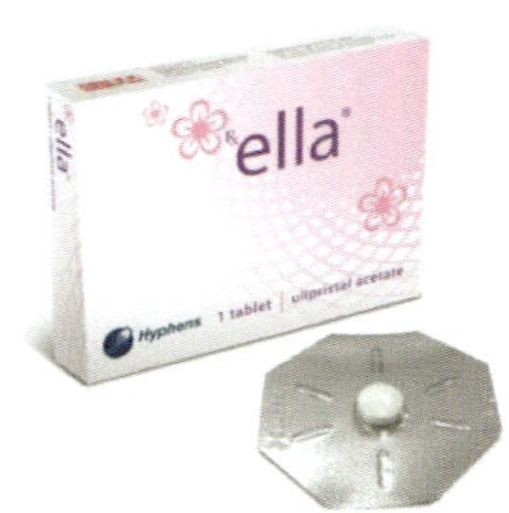

Ulipristal acetate (UPA)

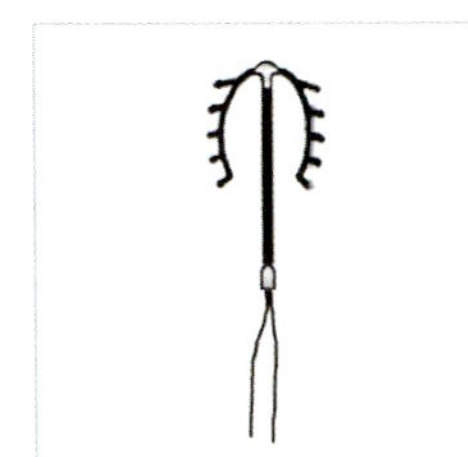

Multiload copper IUCD

Comparison of the different types of EC

<table>
<tr><th></th><th>LNG</th><th>UPA</th><th>Copper IUCD</th></tr>
<tr><td>Duration from last UPSI</td><td>72 hours</td><td>120 hours</td><td>120 hours</td></tr>
<tr><td>Components</td><td>Second-generation progestogen</td><td>Selective progestin receptor modulator — anti-progestin</td><td>Copper</td></tr>
<tr><td>Mechanism of action</td><td>Delays and inhibits ovulation</td><td>Delays ovulation, even after the start of LH surge</td><td>Copper is toxic to sperm/egg, prevents fertilisation and implantation</td></tr>
<tr><td>Efficacy</td><td>85%</td><td>98%</td><td>99%</td></tr>
<tr><td>Pros</td><td colspan="2">• Oral route.
• Can be offered to a woman who has had UPSI earlier in the same cycle and within the last 3 days (LNG) or last 5 days (UPA).
• Does not disrupt an existing pregnancy and is not associated with a fetal anomaly.
• Each can be used more than once in the same cycle if indicated.
*If the woman has already taken UPA in the same cycle: LNG should <u>not</u> be taken in the next 5 days.
*If the woman has already taken LNG: UPA should <u>not</u> be taken in the next 7 days.</td><td>• Most effective EC.
• The only method that is effective even after ovulation has occurred.
• It can be inserted up to 5 days from the last UPSI in a natural menstrual cycle or up to 5 days after the earliest likely date of ovulation (whichever is later). Estimated likely ovulation date = date of start of LMP + no of days in the shortest cycle - 14.
• Not affected by EID, or patient's bodyweight.</td></tr>
<tr><td rowspan="2">Cons</td><td>Need to double the dose (3 mg) if weight >70 kg, BMI >26 or on EID.
Not effective after the start of LH surge.
Can interfere with warfarin — check INR within 48 hours of taking it.</td><td>Reduced efficacy if progestogen was taken within 7 days prior or patient on EID.
Double dose UPA is not recommended.</td><td rowspan="2">• Pain/bleeding during IUCD insertion.
• Risk of uterine perforation/migration/expulsion
• For other complications, refer to the section IUCD and its problems.</td></tr>
<tr><td colspan="2">Special note: Oral EC is ineffective if taken after ovulation.
10% have side effects of headache, nausea and dysmenorrhoea. If vomiting occurs within 3 hours of dose → repeat dose.</td></tr>
</table>

(Continued)

(*Continued*)

	LNG	UPA	Copper IUCD
Future contraception	• Can start hormonal contraception immediately. • Need condoms for additional 7 days from the start of hormonal contraceptive.	• Start hormonal contraceptive **5** days after UPA ingestion. • Need condoms for additional 7 days from the start of hormonal contraceptive.	Form of effective LARC.
Contra-indication		Severe asthma on oral glucocorticoids.	Similar to routine IUCD insertion.
Breastfeeding women	Continue breastfeeding as limited data do *not* show any adverse effects on breastfeeding or the infants.	Advised *not* to breastfeed. Express and discard milk for a week after UPA.	Continue breastfeeding.

Post-EC advice:

- Advise regular contraception, except if copper IUCD is used for EC.
- Expect the return of the menstrual cycle within three weeks of taking oral EC.
- If there is *no return* of the menstrual cycle, do a urine pregnancy test (UPT).
- If UPT is positive after taking EC, the woman should be informed that oral EC (LNG or UPA) does *not* disrupt an existing pregnancy and is *not* associated with fetal anomalies.

CHAPTER 53

Menopause and Primary Ovarian Insufficiency (POI)

Menopause

Definition — Menopause is a clinical diagnosis made retrospectively after 1 year of amenorrhoea, to which there are no obvious physiological or pathological causes, e.g.,

1. Use of hormonal contraception, e.g., LNG-IUS/Mirena®, Depo-Provera or Implanon®
2. Pregnancy.

Primary ovarian insufficiency (POI) — menopause before age 40 years.
Early menopause (EM) — menopause between ages 40 and 45 years.
Surgical menopause — bilateral oophorectomy before natural menopause.

Mean Age of Menopause (Table 53.1)

It differs across different regions and ranges from 48 to 51 years old.

Table 53.1 Mean Age of Menopause

Region	Mean age
Asia	48.75 (48.08–49.42)
Australia	51.25 (49.75–52.76)
Africa	48.38 (48.12–48.65)
Europe	50.54 (50.04–51.05)
Latin America	47.24 (45.88–48.60)
Middle East	47.37 (46.91–47.84)
USA	49.11 (48.78–49.43)

Adapted from Schoenaker DA, Jackson CA, Rowlands JV, Mishra GD. (2014) Socio-economic position, lifestyle factors and age at natural menopause: A systematic review and meta-analyses of studies across six continents. *Int J Epidemiol* 43(5):1542–1562. doi:10.1093/ije/dyu094.

***Factors associated with earlier menopause*:**

- *Genetics*: e.g., Turner's syndrome, Fragile X syndrome and other X-linked and autosomal mutations (refer to the section: *Primary Ovarian Insufficiency*)
- Family history of early menopause (EM)
- Early menarche
- Low body weight
- Emotional stress at a young age, lower socio-economic status
- Adverse life events
- Smoking
- Nulliparity

Symptoms of menopause

- **Menstrual cycle** disturbances (Fig. 53.1).
- **Vasomotor symptoms (hot flushes)** are usually short-lived, lasting seconds to minutes, and involve the upper part of the trunk and head. They can start several years before the last menstrual period and are more common during early post-menopause (Fig. 53.1).
- **Sleep disturbances** are usually due to the frequent arousals caused by vasomotor symptoms.
- **Mood disorders** such as **depression** and **anxiety** are **NOT** caused by menopause, but women with a previous history are prone to relapse. Hence, a history of mood disorders should be obtained.
- **Body aches and joint pains** appear to be commonly reported in Asians.
- **Genitourinary Syndrome of Menopause (GSM) — vulvovaginal atrophy and dryness** tend to occur in late menopause because of the lack of oestrogen. This can result in dyspareunia, vaginal discharge, urinary tract infections, incontinence and urethral caruncle.
- **Breast pain and tenderness** usually occur in the early menopausal transition.

***Long-term consequences of menopause*:**

- Bone loss and osteoporosis
- Cardiovascular disease
- Skin changes

Last Menstrual Period (LMP)

Terminology	Menopause transition		Postmenopause		
	Early	Late	Early		Late
	Perimenopause				
Duration	Variable	1–3 years	2 years (1+1)	3–6 years	Remaining lifespan
Menstrual cycle	Variable length; persistent ≥7-day difference in length of consecutive cycles	An interval of amenorrhoea of ≥60 days			
Symptoms		Vasomotor symptoms — *likely*	Vasomotor symptoms — *most likely*		Increasing symptoms of urogenital atrophy

Fig. 53.1 Adapted from STRAW+10. The stages of the reproductive ageing workshop + 10 staging system for reproductive ageing in women.

Menopause Assessment

History:

- Clinical diagnosis: 12 months of amenorrhoea
- Perimenopausal symptoms (as described above)
- Past medical history of mood disorders
- Holistic assessment of family history, especially cardiovascular risk (which increases after menopause) and cancers

Examination:

- Vital signs include BMI and BP
- Heart and lung examination
- Abdominal examination
- Speculum and vaginal examination for GSM

Investigations:

- Not recommended in natural menopause as serum FSH levels will fluctuate during the transition.
- Perform investigations when evaluating for causes of early menopause/POI or when secondary amenorrhoea is suspected.

1. **FSH** — definition of POI = FSH >25 IU/L on two occasions >4 weeks apart.
    - o Women >50 years old, on progestogen-only implant, progestogen-only pill or Mirena IUCD and wish to stop contraception, to check the FSH level first.
        - If FSH is >30 IU/L, stop the contraception after 1 year.
        - If FSH is still within the premenopausal range, continue with the method and re-check FSH 1 year later.
2. **Thyroid function test (TFT)** to exclude hyperthyroidism.
3. **Prolactin.**
4. **Screening for cardiovascular risk** as part of holistic care — screen for diabetes and hyperlipidaemia.
5. **Mammogram** if not done, especially if considering menopausal hormone therapy (MHT) or hormone replacement therapy (HRT).
6. **Cervical cancer screening.**

Management of Menopause Symptoms

Vasomotor symptoms:

Severity	Symptoms	Management
Mild	Sensation of heat without sweating	Lifestyle management.
Moderate	Sensation of heat with sweating, able to continue activity	Trial of lifestyle management. Hormone therapy if lifestyle measures fail.
Severe	Sensation of heat with sweating, causing cessation of activity	Lifestyle management and consider hormone therapy after weighing the risks and benefits.

Source: ***Menopause:*** *An important milestone in women's health. SB Ang, CH How — SMJ 2013.*

Lifestyle management should be tried in cases of mild to moderate symptoms.

- Reducing core body temperature.
- Regular exercise and stress reduction with mind–body exercises.
- Maintaining a healthy weight.
- Smoking cessation.

- Avoiding triggers such as alcohol, caffeine and spicy food.
- Wearing light clothing.

Non-hormonal:

- Low-dose paroxetine is the only FDA-approved non-hormonal treatment for vasomotor symptoms.
- SSRIs, SNRIs and gabapentin have been studied to help with symptom control (off-label use).

Complementary/alternative therapies such as cimicifugae extract (black cohosh), soy or isoflavone (phytoestrogens) or vitamin E are commonly used, but benefits over placebo have not been consistent across studies.

Menopausal hormone therapy — MHT [refer to Chapter 54: *Menopausal Hormone Therapy (Also Known as Hormone Replacement Therapy)*].

MHT is still most effective for symptomatic relief, especially when symptoms adversely affect the quality of life of women. The lowest effective dose should be used for the shortest period necessary.

Vaginal dryness:

- Advise on regular foreplay during sexual intercourse and topical vaginal moisturiser/lubricant
- Topical oestrogen therapy if severe dryness, e.g., Vagifem pessaries

Sleep disturbances:

- Advise on sleep hygiene
- Treat hot flushes if they cause frequent wakening
- Consider treatment of mood disorders if contributing to sleep disturbances

Mood swings:

- Exercise
- Cognitive behavioural therapy (CBT)
- MHT
- Anti-depressants for depression

Consider using the consult for menopause to promote holistic health for midlife women:

	To screen for	Screening test	Screening frequency
Individuals ≥18 years old	Obesity	BMI, waist circumference	Yearly
	Hypertension	BP	2 yearly or more frequently, as advised by your doctor
Individuals ≥40 years old	Diabetes mellitus	Fasting blood glucose, HbA1c	3 yearly or more frequently, as advised by your doctor
	Hyperlipidaemia	Fasting lipids, Non-fasting lipids	
Individuals ≥50 years old	Colorectal cancer	Faecal immunochemical test (to test for blood in stools) OR Colonoscopy	Stool test for occult blood — yearly Colonoscopy — once every 10 years
Women aged 25–69 years who have had sexual intercourse	Cervical cancer	Pap smear (25–29 years old)	3 yearly
		HPV testing (≥30 years old)	5 yearly
Women aged 40–69 years	Breast cancer	Mammogram	Yearly: **40–49 years old** 2 yearly: **≥50 years old**

Primary Ovarian Insufficiency (POI)

Definition:

- **POI** is a clinical syndrome defined by loss of ovarian activity before the age of 40.
- Amenorrhoea or oligomenorrhoea.
- Raised gonadotrophins and low oestradiol.
- **EM** is defined as menopause between the age of 40 and 45 years.

Prevalence of POI — 1% of women.

Factors Associated with Early Menopause (EM)

Genetics:

- o Up to 30% have a family history of early menopause.
- o 21% have a karyotypic abnormality in primary amenorrhoea.

- o 11% have a karyotypic abnormality in secondary amenorrhoea.
- o X-linked chromosomal abnormalities.
  - ▪ Turner syndrome — the most common genetic cause of POI.
  - ▪ Fragile X syndrome.
  - ▪ Others, e.g., BMP-15, DIAPH2.
- o Autosomal mutations: Defects in genes such as GDF9, ESR 1, NOBOX, FSHR, LHR, FSH, inhibin A, etc.

Autoimmune — either isolated or part of polyglandular autoimmune syndrome — most commonly adrenal and thyroid auto-immunity.

- o Adrenal insufficiency.
- o Hashimoto's thyroiditis.
- o Type 1 diabetes mellitus.
- o Coeliac disease.
- o Polyglandular autoimmune syndromes (type I and type II).

Infections: Mumps, CMV, HIV, tuberculosis, malaria, varicella.
Toxins: Cigarette smoking.
Metabolic: Galactosaemia.
Iatrogenic:

- o Chemotherapy: Especially alkylating agents, e.g., cyclophosphamide, chlorambucil, busulphan and nitrogen mustard.
- o Radiotherapy.
- o Surgical: Bilateral oophorectomy, repeated cystectomies for recurrent ovarian tumours or endometriomas, hysterectomy, uterine artery embolisation.

Idiopathic — the most common cause of spontaneous POI.

Evaluating POI

History:

- o Genetic abnormalities
- o Family history of premature or early menopause
- o Multiple pregnancies
- o Early menarche
- o Nulliparity/low parity
- o Cigarette smoking (dose–response effect)
- o Underweight

Symptoms:

- o Secondary amenorrhoea/oligomenorrhoea
- o Subfertility
- o Oestrogen-deficiency syndromes
- o Some may be asymptomatic except for amenorrhoea

Initial investigations:

- Urine pregnancy test (UPT).
- FSH, LH and oestradiol — done on days 2–3 of the cycle if menses are still present.
  - o POI is diagnosed with two elevated FSH levels (≥25 IU) done 4–6 weeks apart and oligomenorrhoea/amenorrhoea of at least 4 months.
  - o Oestradiol will be low.
- Serum prolactin.
- Thyroid function test (TFT).
- Ultrasound scan of the pelvis.

Additional investigations — if clinically indicated.

- o Karyotype and FMR1 gene testing (for early POI <30 years old).
- o Anti-thyroid autoantibodies, i.e., thyroid peroxidase antibody (TPOAb).
- o Anti-adrenal antibodies — <u>not</u> available in Singapore.
- o AMH is **not** recommended as a diagnostic test for POI.

<u>**General health screening:**</u>

Baseline screening including BP, BMI, HbA1c, lipid panel and BMD screening via DEXA scan.

Implications of POI:

- Loss of fertility — up to 5–10% of POI patients may experience spontaneous ovulation.
- If the woman is <u>not</u> keen on fertility, she will still need contraception.
  - o The majority will need oocyte or embryo donation and conception via IVF.

    - o Alternatives are adoption or choosing not to pursue fertility.
    - o IVF-preimplantation genetic testing (IVF-PGT) is a possible option for women with Fragile X syndrome. The updated terminology for PGT for monogenic disorders, e.g., Fragile X syndrome, is PGT-M.
- Oestrogen-deficiency problems — short- and long-term complications include
    - o Osteoporosis.
    - o Cardiovascular disease.
    - o Sexual dysfunction.
    - o Cognitive impairment.
    - o Stroke.
    - o Parkinson's disease.
- Potential for genetic inheritance.
- Psychosocial issues — depression and anxiety.
- Premature mortality — mainly due to cardiovascular disorders if POI is left untreated.

Management of POI

Multidisciplinary care: Endocrinologist, reproductive medicine specialist, psychologist/psychiatrist and medical social worker for support.

Goals of management:

- o Oestrogen therapy improves cardiovascular risk factors, reduces the risk of osteoporosis, urogenital atrophy and cognitive impairment and maintains sexual health and quality of life.
- o General health.
- o Fertility issues.
- o Psychosocial aspects.
- o Management of underlying causes, e.g., Turner syndrome.

Lifestyle modifications include regular exercise and a healthy diet.

- o Maintain a healthy weight, stop smoking and abstain from/reduce alcohol intake.
- o Calcium and vitamin D supplements are recommended if serum levels are low.

- o Annual check: BP, OGTT, lipid panel, ± thyroid function test (if deranged), BMD screen (repeat in 2–3 years in women with osteoporosis).

Oestrogen therapy:

- o All women with POI should be treated with oestrogen therapy regardless of whether symptoms are present.
- o Oestrogen therapy reduces cholesterol levels and cardiovascular disease and helps in fracture prevention. It also reduces vaginal atrophy and dryness — now known as GSM.
- o For GSM, women can use topical oestrogen therapy with lubricating gel.
- o Types of oestrogen therapy:
  1. Systemic sex steroid hormone replacement therapy (HRT or MHT).
  2. Combined oral contraceptive pills (COCPs).
- o Currently, there is no evidence to recommend COCPs over MHT in women with POI. MHT may improve cardiovascular markers and bone health more than COCP. Women on MHT who do not desire fertility will still require contraception. There is no increased risk of breast cancer with MHT before the natural age of menopause.
- o MHT should be the first line for preventing/treating osteoporosis in POI.
- o Recommended duration of MHT

  Treat women with POI till the age of natural menopause between 50 and 51 years old.
  - ▪ If the uterus is present, the woman needs combined oestrogen and progestogen therapy to reduce the risk of endometrial hyperplasia and cancer.
  - ▪ If the uterus is absent, oestrogen-only therapy can be given except in women with endometriosis. For women with endometriosis, combined oestrogen and progesterone therapy is recommended to reduce the chance of recurrence of endometriosis.
- o Consider a transdermal route of oestradiol in women with VTE risk factors.

CHAPTER 54

Menopausal Hormone Therapy (Also Known as Hormone Replacement Therapy)

Background

Since the Women's Health Initiative (WHI) was released in 2002, there has been confusion about the role of menopausal hormone therapy (MHT) in women. Twenty years have passed, and more studies have emerged to guide us in providing symptomatic patients with appropriate individualised treatment options.

Indications for MHT

- **Symptomatic relief for menopausal symptoms**, which adversely affect the **quality of life**.
- Women with **primary ovarian insufficiency (POI)** and **early menopause**. These patients use MHT until at least the natural age of menopause (50–51 years old).
- Women who had **early surgical menopause** before the age of 45 years (bilateral oophorectomy).
- For women with menopausal symptoms, aged <60 years old or within 10 years of menopause, MHT will also aid in osteoporosis treatment.
- MHT may also be considered in women unable to tolerate other osteoporosis treatments.
- Topical or local therapy for treating **genitourinary syndrome of menopause (GSM) or atrophic vaginitis.**

MHT is *not* recommended to prevent coronary heart disease, osteoporosis, cognitive function or dementia.

Absolute Contraindications of MHT

- History of breast cancer
- History of high-risk endometrial cancer or other hormone-dependent cancers
- History of coronary heart disease
- Previous stroke or transient ischaemic attack (TIA)
- Unexplained vaginal bleeding that has *not* been evaluated
- Known hypersensitivity to active components of MHT
- Liver disease/liver failure

Relative contraindications of MHT — transdermal route is preferred

- BMI >30 kg/m^2
- Previous or family history of venous thromboembolism (VTE)
- Patients at moderate risk of cardiovascular disease (10-year risk: 5–10%)
- Hypertension with variable control
- Migraine
- Women on medications that are enzyme inducers
- Gallbladder disease

Risks of MHT

***Breast cancer*:**

- Oestrogen-alone MHT is associated with little or no change in breast cancer risk.
- Combined MHT can be associated with an increased breast cancer risk, but the risk varies with the duration of MHT and the progestogen type.
- In the WHI study, the breast cancer risk was increased in the combined hormone therapy arm with conjugated equine oestrogen and medroxyprogesterone acetate (MPA) and decreased in the oestrogen-only arm. In addition, dydrogesterone and micronised progesterone have lower risks than norethisterone and medroxyprogesterone when used in combined hormone therapy.
- Continuous combined MHT has a higher risk than sequential MHT, but the absolute excess risk is small — i.e., 10 additional diagnoses per 1,000 women aged 50–59 with up to 14 years of use.

- In women with a low background risk of breast cancer, the benefits of using MHT to treat symptoms for up to 5 years outweigh the risks.
- Vaginal oestrogen is *not* associated with an increased risk of breast cancer.
- There is *no* increase in breast cancer risks in women (up to 50 years old) who are BRCA carriers taking MHT after risk-reducing bilateral salpingo-oophorectomy. After 50 years of age, use non-hormonal alternatives.

***Ovarian cancer*:**
- Some meta-analyses and epidemiological studies have shown a possible increase in serous and endometrioid ovarian cancer risks.
- *No* adverse effects in women with epithelial ovarian cancer who take MHT.

***Cardiovascular risk*:**
- The benefits of systemic MHT (oestrogen-alone or combined MHT) outweigh the risks if **used within 10 years from the onset of menopause or at age <60**. It is associated with reducing the progression of atherosclerosis, the risk of coronary heart disease, death from cardiovascular disease and all-cause mortality.
- *No benefits* are shown in women who start MHT >10 years after menopause, with no difference in coronary heart disease or mortality. There is *no increase* in cardiovascular events, cardiovascular mortality or all-cause mortality in women who start MHT >10 years after menopause.

***Stroke*:**
- There is an absolute risk of stroke if used after 10 years from the onset of menopause or at age >60.
- Transdermal oestradiol is *unlikely* to increase the risk of stroke.

***Venous thromboembolism (VTE)*:**
- The background VTE risk is 1.7 per 1,000 women >50 years old.
- Oral MHT is associated with an increased VTE risk by 2–4 times and is highest in the first year after starting MHT.
  - The VTE risk varies based on the type and dose of oral oestrogens and progestogens. For example, conjugated equine oestrogen is more pro-thrombotic than oestradiol. Micronised progesterone and dydrogesterone are *unlikely* to increase the VTE risk.

- Transdermal oestradiol is ***unlikely*** to increase the VTE risk.
- There is an absolute risk of VTE if used after 10 years from the onset of menopause or at age >60.

***Dementia*:**

- *Unlikely* to increase dementia risk or adversely affect cognitive function in women who start MHT <60 years old.
- There is an absolute risk of dementia if used after 10 years from the onset of menopause or at age >60.

***Initiating hormone therapy (Refer to Figures 54.1 and 54.2)*:**

- Evaluate for contraindications, cardiovascular and breast cancer risks.
- Menstrual history to exclude unexplained abnormal uterine bleeding (AUB) that may need evaluation.
- Order a mammogram if not up to date.
- Consider screening for hyperlipidaemia and diabetes.
- The **lowest effective dose** that can control symptoms and therapy for >5 years should be individualised based on risk factors for breast cancer and cardiovascular events.
- For women with an intact uterus, **combined MHT** must be used to protect against the risk of unopposed oestrogen on the endometrium.
- Oestrogen-only therapy/tibolone can be used in women who have Mirena® IUCD or women who have had hysterectomy.
- Mirena® can be used for endometrial protection for 4 years (as per FDA 2022)

***Special considerations*:**

- *Indications of transdermal therapy*
    - Patient's preference
    - Symptoms are not well controlled despite oral hormone replacement therapy (HRT)
    - Gastrointestinal (GI) conditions that affect oral absorption — transdermal HRT; avoid the first-pass metabolism
    - Previous or family history of VTE
    - BMI >30 kg/m^2
    - Patients at moderate risk of cardiovascular disease (10-year risk: 5–10%)
    - Poorly controlled hypertension
    - Migraine ± aura
    - On medications that are enzyme inducers
    - Gallbladder disease

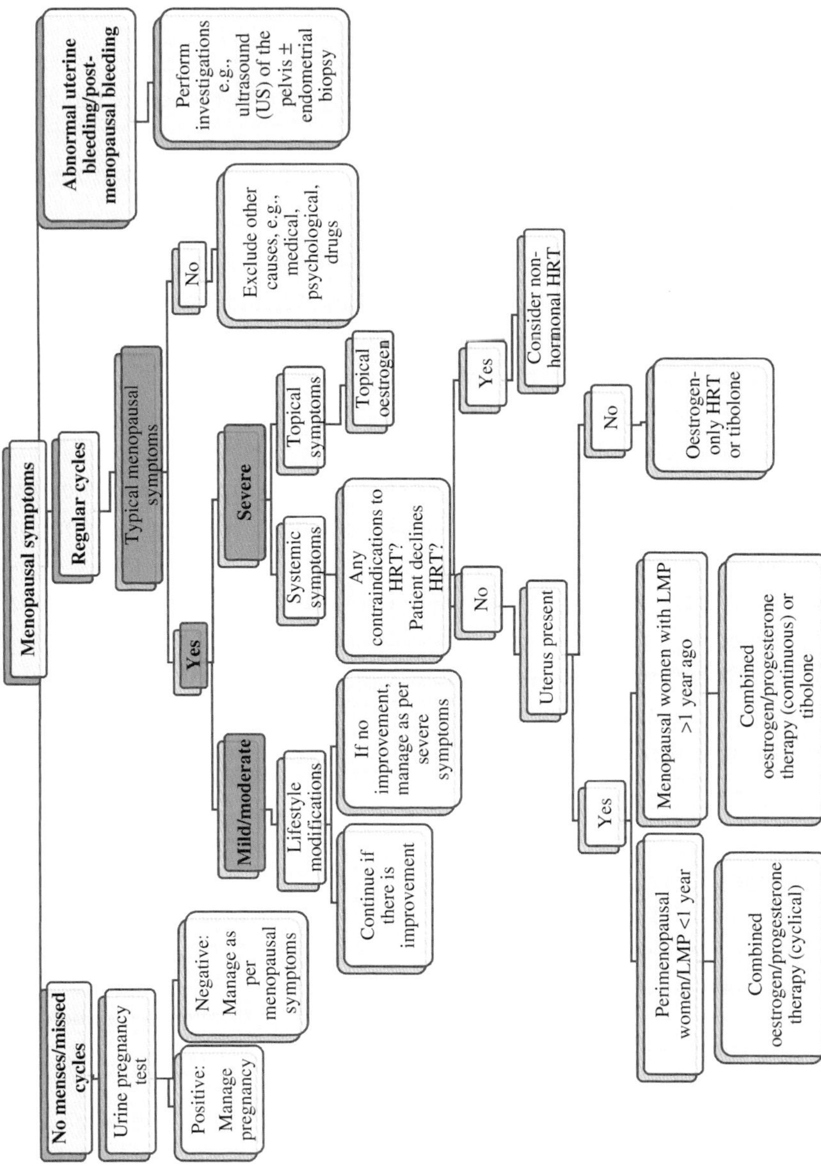

Fig. 54.1 Treatment of menopausal symptoms.

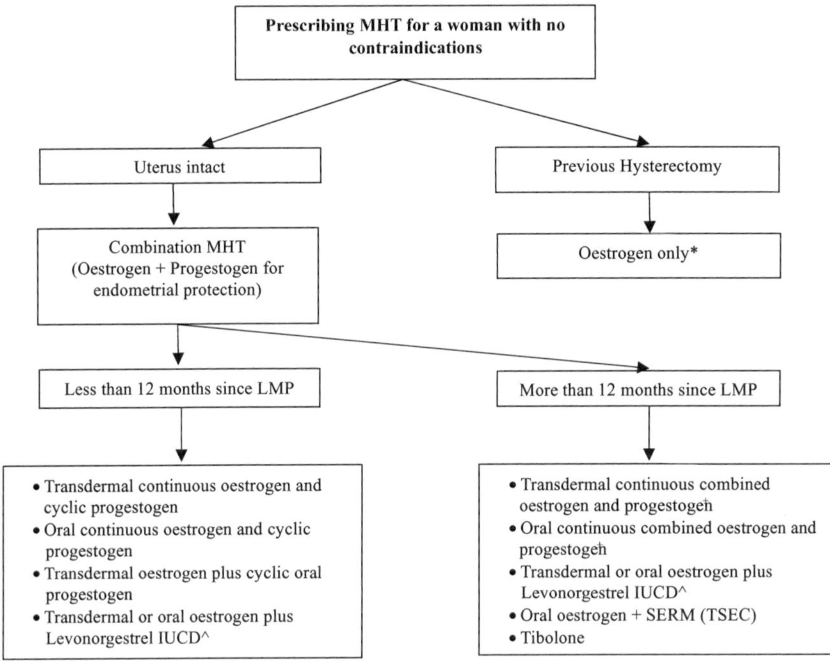

Fig. 54.2 Prescribing MHT.

****Exception:*** Women who have residual endometriosis following hysterectomy.
†***Alternatively***, women can continue continuous oestrogen and cyclical progestogen.
^Levonorgestrel IUCD can be used up to 4 years for endometrial protection.
IUCD — intrauterine contraceptive device; LMP — last menstrual period; SERM — selective oestrogen receptor modulator; TEC — tissue-selective oestrogen complex.

- A lower dose of oestrogen use in MHT also lowers the risk of VTE.

Women with a history of breast cancer:

- Multidisciplinary team (MDT) care approach with a menopause specialist, a breast surgeon and a medical oncologist.
- For vasomotor symptoms: Initiate lifestyle changes and non-hormonal MHT. <u>Avoid</u> paroxetine and fluoxetine in women on tamoxifen, as these medications reduce the efficacy of tamoxifen. Likewise,

systemic MHT should *not* be used in women on aromatase inhibitors. Individualise treatment and discuss with the MDT team for severe and refractory symptoms.

- *For genitourinary syndrome of menopause (GSM)*, use vaginal moisturisers and lubricants. Avoid topical oestrogens in women taking aromatase inhibitors. Individualise treatment and discuss with the MDT team for severe and refractory symptoms. Ultra-low dose topical oestrogens may be required.

***Follow-up of women on MHT*:**

- Review at 3 months with a focus on bleeding pattern and compliance, especially for those on separate oestrogen and progestogen therapy.
- If persistent abnormal uterine bleeding (AUB) occurs after 4–6 months of MHT, check if patients take MHT appropriately and their compliance. Consider evaluating for AUB with an ultrasound scan of the pelvis ± endometrial biopsy if AUB persists for >6 months, bleeding occurs after amenorrhoea has been established or if there are risk factors for endometrial hyperplasia/cancer.
- Ensure regular mammograms, in line with current breast cancer screening guidelines.

Common Hormone Preparations

Oestrogen-Only Therapy

For women without a uterus

- *Side effects:* Fluid retention, breast tenderness, bloating, nausea, dyspepsia, headaches.

	Brand name	Active ingredient	Dose	Remarks
Oral oestrogen	Estrofem®	17β-Oestradiol	1 mg	
			2 mg	
	Progynova	Oestradiol valerate	1 mg	
			2 mg	
	Premarin	Conjugated equine oestrogen	0.3 mg	
			0.625 mg	

(Continued)

	Brand name	Active ingredient	Dose		Remarks
Transdermal oestrogen (lower risk of VTE)	Estraderm	17β-Oestradiol	25 μg/ 24 hours	Twice weekly application	– Apply the gel/ patch over arms/ shoulders/inner thighs. – Avoid breast and vulva areas. – Need progesterone in women with an intact uterus, e.g., Mirena® IUCD or cyclical progestin for 12–14 days in a sequential regimen or daily in a continuous combined regimen.
			50 mcg/ 24 hours		
	Estrogel	Oestradiol	0.75 mg (half ruler)		
			1.5 mg (full ruler)		
	Divigel	Oestradiol	0.5 mg (0.5 g sachet)		
			1 mg (1 g sachet)		

Progestogen

- To be used with oestrogen in women with an intact uterus as combined MHT.
- Natural progesterone is safer for the cardiovascular system with no adverse lipid effects.
- Side effects of oral progestogens: Fluid retention, breast tenderness, headaches, mood swings.

Active ingredient	Brand name	Dose	Remarks
Medroxyprogesterone	Provera	5 mg	Rarely used because of the higher risk of breast cancer compared to the other progestogens in MHT
Dydrogesterone	Duphaston	10 mg	Use at 5 mg or 10 mg daily for the first 12 days of each calendar month
Micronised progesterone	Utrogestan	100 mg	Use at 100 mg or 200 mg daily for the first 12 days of each calendar month
Levonorgestrel	Mirena IUCD	20 μg/24 hours	Off-label use Can be used for 4 years — change if needed

Combined MHT

For women with an intact uterus — a combination of oestrogen with progestogen or Mirena® IUCD.

Brand name	Active ingredient	Dose	Remarks
Cyclical MHT			
Femoston	Oestradiol Dydrogesterone	• Oestradiol 1 mg daily, dydrogesterone 10 mg (14 days)	
		• Oestradiol 2 mg daily, dydrogesterone 10 mg (14 days)	
Progyluton	Oestradiol Norgestrel	• 11 tablets of oestradiol 2 mg • 10 tablets of oestradiol 2 mg and norgestrel 500 µg	Symptoms may occur during the 7 days pill-free period. Expect withdrawal bleeding during the pill-free period.
Trisequens	Oestradiol Norethisterone	• 12 tablets of oestradiol 2 mg • 10 tablets of oestradiol 2 mg and norethisterone 1 mg • 6 tablets of oestradiol 1 mg	Triphasic HRT 100 mg or 200 mg daily for the first 12 days of each calendar month. Expect monthly withdrawal bleeding. Norethisterone has been associated with a higher risk of breast cancer.
Continuous combined MHT			
Femoston-conti	Oestradiol Dydrogesterone	• Oestradiol 1 mg daily • Dydrogesterone 5 mg daily	Sequential combined regimen. Expect monthly withdrawal bleeding.
Activelle®	Oestradiol Norethisterone	• Oestradiol 1 mg • Norethisterone 0.5 mg	Norethisterone has been associated with a higher risk of breast cancer.
Other hormones			
Livial (selective tissue oestrogenic activity regulator STEAR)	Tibolone	2.5 mg daily – Start at 1.25 mg daily or 2.5 mg every other day	To be used only in *postmenopausal women* who have had no menses for at least 1 year. It can increase libido and help in sexual response by increasing bioavailable testosterone. <u>Side effects:</u> Breast tenderness, headache, dizziness, vaginal spotting, weight gain. <u>Rare long-term side effects:</u> VTE, stroke, hypertension, breast or endometrial cancer.

(*Continued*)

Brand name	Active ingredient	Dose	Remarks
Ospemifene (selective oestrogen receptor modulator SERM)	Osphena	Oral 60 mg tablet daily	Indicated for treating moderate to severe vulvovaginal atrophy (VVA) and dyspareunia in postmenopausal women. <u>*Side effects:*</u> Mild increase in hot flushes, headache, night sweats, slightly increased VTE risk. It should be discontinued for at least 4 weeks before surgery or during periods of prolonged immobilisation.

Day of Cycle	1	2	3	4	5	6	7	8	9	10	11	12	13	14	15	16	17	18	19	20	21	22	23	24	25	26	27	28
Premarin **EstroFem** **Progynova**	•	•	•	•	•	•	•	•	•	•	•	•	•	•	•	•	•	•	•	•	•	•	•	•	•	•	•	•
	Unopposed estrogen therapy - recommended for women without a uterus																											
Activelle **Femoston Conti 1/5**	◊	◊	◊	◊	◊	◊	◊	◊	◊	◊	◊	◊	◊	◊	◊	◊	◊	◊	◊	◊	◊	◊	◊	◊	◊	◊	◊	◊
	Continuous Combined Therapy																											
Femoston 1/10 **Femoston 2/10**	•	•	•	•	•	•	•	•	•	•	•	•	•	•	◊	◊	◊	◊	◊	◊	◊	◊	◊	◊	◊	◊	◊	◊
	Continuous estrogen and cyclic progestogen therapy																											
Progyluton	•	•	•	•	•	•	•	•	•	•	•	◊	◊	◊	◊	◊	◊	◊	◊	◊	◊	*	*	*	*	*	*	*
	Cyclic estrogen and progestogen																					7 Tablet-free days (withdrawal bleed)						
Trisequens	•	•	•	•	•	•	•	•	•	•	•	•	◊	◊	◊	◊	◊	◊	◊	◊	◊	◊	•	•	•	•	•	•
	Triphasic therapy																											

• Estrogen ◊ Estrogen + Progestogen *Withdrawal bleed

Source: https://www.healthhub.sg/a-z/medications/160/hormone-replacement-therapy.

Local Oestrogen Therapy

Progestogen is <u>not</u> required for endometrial protection as systemic absorption is minimal.

Brand name	Active ingredient	Dose	Remarks
Vagifem	Oestradiol	10 μg pessary	Initiate treatment with one pessary daily for 2 weeks, followed by one pessary weekly for maintenance therapy. (Cumulative dose after 1 year of weekly usage is equivalent to 1 mg of oestradiol.)
Premarin	Conjugated oestrogen	0.625 mg/g cream	Initiate treatment with one application daily for 3 weeks, followed by followed by one or two applications per week for maintenance therapy, depending on severity of the condition.

Testosterone therapy — refer to Chapter 58: *Female Sexual Dysfunction*.

- Consider testosterone supplementation for menopausal women with low sexual desire if MHT alone is ineffective.
- Testosterone is effective for postmenopausal women with hypoactive sexual desire disorder.
- Check the baseline testosterone level before treatment to exclude a high baseline level.

When to stop MHT?

1. Once menopausal symptoms improve, continue lifestyle changes that can maintain symptom improvement for the patients. Discuss the risks and benefits of continuing MHT with the patient.
   - Current data are *inconclusive* to recommend either stopping MHT abruptly or a tapering approach to reduce rebound symptoms in the long term.
2. When *contraindications* develop during treatment with MHT, e.g., cardiovascular disease, cerebrovascular disease, breast cancer and uterine cancer.
3. Patients with POI and early menopause should use HRT until at least the average age of menopause and may be continued on HRT if indicated.

When to stop MHT before surgery?

- Limited evidence is available.
- HRT in postmenopausal women increases the risk of perioperative VTE, and most women have other risk factors for VTE because of age.
- For major surgeries in women with risk factors for VTE, consider stopping **oral** oestrogen-containing HRT **4 weeks** before the operation.
- There is *no need* to stop HRT if the woman is undergoing minor surgeries or using non-oral HRT.
- There should be an emphasis on perioperative mechanical or pharmacological VTE prophylaxis, e.g., adequate hydration, early ambulation, compression stockings, calf compressors or physiotherapy.

CHAPTER 55

Osteoporosis

Definition:

1) Osteoporosis

- A progressive systemic skeletal disease characterised by
  - ➢ Low bone mass.
  - ➢ Micro-architectural deterioration of bone tissue with a consequent increase in bone fragility and susceptibility to fractures.

2) Fragility fracture

- It is a fracture that occurs with minimal trauma, such as a fall from one's standing height with no other identifiable major forces. These fractures can occur in the spine, hip, wrist, humerus, ribs and pelvis.

Diagnosis:

- **Dual-energy X-ray absorptiometry (DEXA)** to measure bone mineral density (BMD) is the gold standard for diagnosing osteoporosis.
  - The WHO classification for osteoporosis is shown in Table 55.1. The *T-score* is based on the standard deviation (SD) between a woman's BMD and that of a young adult reference population. This should only be used in *postmenopausal* women.
  - For *premenopausal* women, the *Z-score* is recommended. The *Z*-score compares the woman's BMD to that of an age-matched population. A *Z*-score of 2.0 or less below the mean is low.

Qualitative ultrasound of the heel (QUS) has been shown to predict fragility fractures. However, because of varied results, it *cannot* be used for following up patients on medical treatment for osteoporosis. Consider adding a vertebral fracture assessment (VFA) or a thoracolumbar X-ray to look for vertebral fractures in women with loss of height or low back pain.

Table 55.1 WHO Criteria for Osteoporosis

WHO diagnostic category	BMD *T*-score (SD) (at either spine or hip)	Description
Normal	≥–1.0	Spinal or hip BMD within 1.0 SD below the young adult female reference mean (*T*-score ≥–1.0)
Low bone mass (osteopenia)	<–1 to >–2.5	Spinal or hip BMD between 1.0 SD and 2.5 SD below the young adult female reference mean
Osteoporosis	≤–2.5	Spinal or hip BMD >2.5 SD below the young adult female reference mean
Severe/established osteoporosis	≤–2.5 plus one or more fragility fractures	BMD >2.5 SD below the young adult female reference mean and the presence of one or more fragility fractures

Investigations to Exclude Secondary Causes of Osteoporosis

Commonly performed tests:

- *Renal panel*: For baseline renal function to rule out chronic kidney disease.
- *Full blood count*: To rule out malignancies or malabsorptive disorders.
- *Corrected serum calcium*: Hypercalcaemia might indicate hyperparathyroidism or malignancy; hypocalcaemia might indicate malabsorption or vitamin D deficiency.
- *Serum 25-hydroxy vitamin D level*: For baseline and to identify vitamin D deficiency (the optimal level is >20–30 ng/ml or 50–75 nmol/L).

Others if indicated:

- *Thyroid-stimulating hormone*: To rule out hyperthyroidism.
- *Erythrocyte sedimentation rate (ESR)*: Very high levels can indicate rheumatological conditions.
- *Alkaline phosphatase*: High levels are found in liver conditions, Paget disease, recent fractures or bone disorders.
- *Serum phosphate*: High levels are associated with vitamin D deficiency or renal phosphate wasting.
- *Spot urine calcium/creatinine ratio*: Levels will be high in idiopathic hypercalciuria.

Optimising Bone Health

- 10% increase in peak bone mass delays the onset of osteoporosis in a woman by 13 years.
- 80% of peak bone mass is genetically determined.
- *Factors in pregnancy that positively influence fetal bone accretion*:
  - Higher maternal intake of calcium and calcium-rich products, phosphorus and magnesium.
  - Low fat intake.
  - High-dose vitamin D supplements between 1,000–2,800 IU, especially if maternal deficiency present.
  - Avoid alcohol and stop smoking.
- Factors during infancy, childhood and adolescence that positively influence bone accretion:
  - Adequate calcium intake.
  - Vitamin D supplements for those who are deficient.
  - Increased physical activity, especially pre-puberty.

***Aim of treatment of osteoporosis*:**

- Prevent fractures.
- Management of **risk factors for osteoporosis and fractures** (refer to Table 55.2).
- Manage **falls risk** (refer to Table 55.3).

Table 55.2 Risk Factors for Osteoporosis and Fractures

Family history of osteoporosis or fragility fractures
Previous fragility fracture
Ageing [high risk on the osteoporosis self-assessment tool for Asians (OSTA)]
Low body weight (high risk on OSTA)
Height loss (>2 cm within 3 years)
Early menopause (≤45 years old)
Certain medications (such as prednisolone or its equivalent for >5 mg/day for ≥3 months)
Low calcium intake (<500 mg/day)
Excessive alcohol intake (>2 units/day)
Smoking (any)
Prolonged immobility
History of falls
Presence of disease that can lower bone density or increase fracture risks (e.g., hyperthyroidism, diabetes mellitus or any inflammatory rheumatic disease)

Adapted from MOH ACG 2018.

Table 55.3 Falls Risk

Intrinsic factors	Extrinsic factors
• Age • Female • Not married, including single and widowed • Living alone • Osteoarthritis of the knee • Stroke • Parkinson's disease • Hypertension • Diabetes • Osteoporosis • Chronic conditions • Urinary incontinence • Cognitive impairment • Depressive symptoms • Poor vision • Postural hypotension • Weak handgrip strength • Self-perceived poor health • Previous history of falls • Fear of falling	• Four or more prescribed drugs • Use of hypnotics, anti-depressants or tranquillisers • Use of a walking aid • Mobility impairment • Balance deficit • Gait deficit • Inappropriate footwear and foot problems • Environmental and home hazards

Adapted from HPB-MOH CPG 2015.

Tools for Osteoporosis Screening

- ***OSTA*** (refer to Table 55.4).
  - OSTA score = age in years — weight in kg.
  - *Measure BMD if*:
    - High risk on OSTA (>20).
    - Medium risk on OSTA (0–20) and risk factors present.
  - For patients considered low risk (<0), reassess risks if there is significant weight loss or development of risk factors or if the last assessment was at least 5 years ago.
- ***FRAX***® *fracture risk assessment tool.*
  - Available online from https://www.sheffield.ac.uk/FRAX/.
  - Computes the 10-year probability of hip fracture or a major osteoporotic fracture.
  - A *major* osteoporotic fracture is a clinical spine, hip, forearm or humerus fracture.
  - It can calculate fracture risk based on BMI and clinical risk factors without BMD. By using this tool, BMD can be ordered when the treatment threshold is reached.

Table 55.4 OSTA

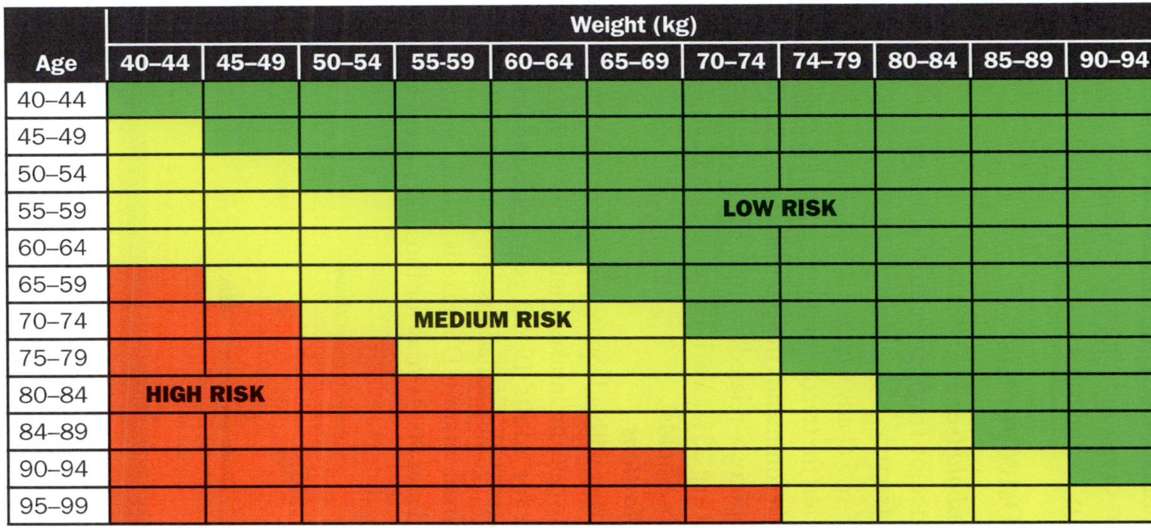

Adapted from Koh LK, Sedrine WB, Torralba TP, *et al*. (2001) A simple tool to identify Asian women at increased risk of osteoporosis. *Osteoporos Int*. **12**(8):699–705. doi:10.1007/s001980170070.

Screening Strategy

It encompasses a combination of a population-wide approach screening all women above 65 years of age and high-risk population screening with tools such as FRAX® and OSTA and those with clinical risk factors. See Fig. 55.1.

Management of Osteoporosis

- ***Treatment threshold*** **(see Fig. 55.1)**
  - Any presence of fragility requires treatment to prevent the subsequent fracture.
  - *T*-score of ≤–2.5 at any site.
  - FRAX® reaches the treatment threshold (thc National Osteoporosis Foundation recommends treatment for a 10-year probability of any major osteoporosis-related fracture ≥20% or a 10-year probability of hip fracture ≥3%. Various countries have developed their treatment thresholds).
- ***Lifestyle modifications***
  - A balanced diet with adequate protein, calcium and vitamin D.
    - Adequate calcium intake is defined as 800 mg/day of elemental calcium for adults 19–50 years old and 1,000 mg/day of elemental calcium for adults ≥51 years old.
    - The optimal vitamin D intake is 600 IU/day for those 51–70 years old and 800 IU/day for those ≥71 years old.

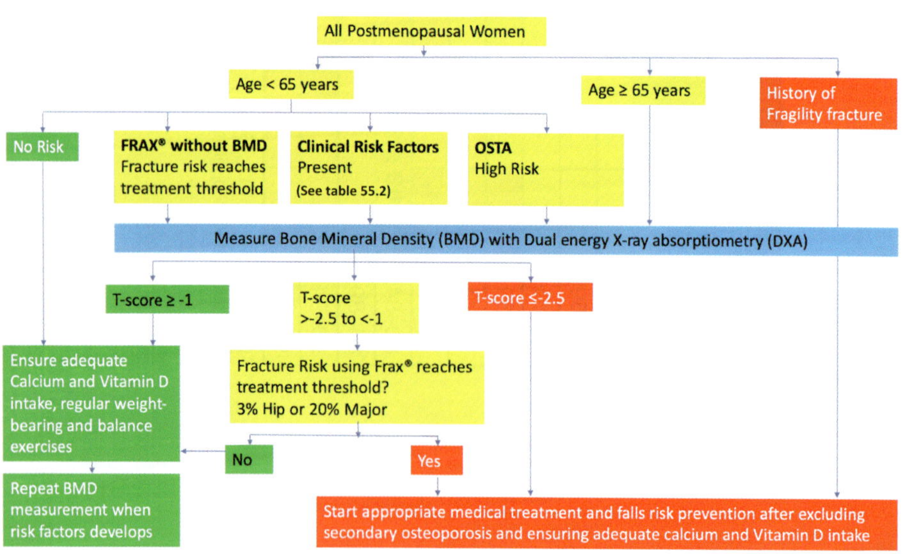

Fig. 55.1 Screening strategy and treatment threshold.

  - Avoid excessive alcohol and caffeine intake.
  - Stop smoking.
  - Adopt an active lifestyle with appropriate weight-bearing and balance exercises.
  - Fall prevention, e.g., home safety and footwear.
    - Addressing intrinsic and extrinsic factors. See Table 55.3.
- ***Pharmacotherapy***
  - Ensure adequate calcium and vitamin D. Replace vitamin D if deficient before treatment.
  - Individualise the treatment to patients based on their medical history and discuss the risk/benefit of each treatment.
  - Specific pharmacological treatment is shown in Table 55.5.
  - Osteoporosis is a chronic disease, and patients must be managed lifelong to reduce fracture risks, which increase with age.
  - ***Drug holiday***:
    - Drug holidays have been shown to lower the risks of osteonecrosis of the jaw (ONJ) and atypical femoral fractures (AFFs).
    - For those with a prior fracture or high fracture risk (ie. fractures during treatment hip-T-score ≤−2.5 or other significant risk factors determined by a risk assessment tool e.g. FRAX), continuing oral bisphosphonates for 10 years and IV bisphosphonates for 6 years has greater benefits versus risks.
    - For those without a prior fracture or low to moderate risk patients, one can consider a drug holiday after 5 years of oral bisphosphonates or 3 years of IV bisphosphonates. Reassess after 2–4 years. Consider resuming treatment if there are new fractures, additional risk factors or significant decrease in BMD.
    - A drug holiday is *not* recommended for denosumab because of the risk of rebound fracture and increased risk of rapid bone loss.
  - Look for significant DEXA BMD deterioration of >4–5% from the previous measurement and any fractures that occur while on medications.

When to repeat BMD?

- 1–2 years after initiation of pharmacological treatment and every 2–3 years thereafter.
- 2–3 years for those on drug holiday from bisphosphonates.
- For those near the treatment threshold or have conditions and treatment that may result in rapid bone loss, repeat in about 1–2 years.
- For those with normal BMD, one could repeat in 15 years.

Table 55.5 Pharmacological Treatment of Osteoporosis

Medication	Evidence of effectiveness in osteoporosis	Contraindications	Clinical considerations/precautions
Oral bisphosphonates: Alendronate Risedronate Ibandronate	√ Vertebral fracture √ Non-vertebral fracture (alendronate, risedronate) √ Hip fracture (alendronate, risedronate) • Preferred initial treatment or • After anabolic treatment or Denosumab	• CrCl <30 ml/min. • Hypocalcaemia. • Oesophageal or gastric abnormalities such as gastric ulcers, achalasia, uncontrolled gastro-oesophageal reflux. • Inability to remain upright for 30 minutes. • Aspiration risk and difficulty in swallowing liquids.	*When taking alendronate or risedronate, advise patients to*: • Swallow the tablet whole with plain water at least 30 minutes before taking food, beverages or other medications (especially antacids, calcium, iron or mineral supplements). • Remain upright until after eating. *When taking ibandronate, advise patients to*: • Swallow the tablet whole with plain water at least 60 minutes before taking food, beverages or other medications (especially antacids, calcium, iron or mineral supplements). • Remain upright until after eating. • Do note the small increase in risks of ONJ and AFF after prolonged therapy.
Intravenous zoledronic acid (bisphosphonate)	√ Vertebral fracture √ Non-vertebral fracture √ Hip fracture • Preferred initial treatment or • After anabolic treatment or Denosumab	• CrCl <35 ml/min. • Hypocalcaemia.	• Give IV infusion for at least 15 minutes. • Ensure the patient is adequately hydrated before use. • Use with caution in patients with significant vitamin D deficiency. • Check serum calcium and phosphate at 9–14 days after infusion if the patient shows symptoms of hypocalcaemia or hypophosphataemia. • A small increase in risks of ONJ and AFF after prolonged therapy.
Subcutaneous denosumab (RANKL inhibitor)	√ Vertebral fracture √ Non-vertebral fracture √ Hip fracture • For women unable to tolerate bisphosphonates • Patients with breast cancer at high risk of fracture	Hypocalcaemia.	• Ensure adequate calcium and vitamin D intake. • Use with caution in patients with pre-existing eczema, renal impairment or recurrent infections. • Do note the small increase in risks of ONJ and AFF after prolonged therapy. • Denosumab cessation must be followed with bisphosphonates to prevent the risk of rebound fracture. • Has been studied for use up to 10 years.

Medication	Evidence of effectiveness in osteoporosis	Contraindications	Clinical considerations/precautions
Subcutaneous teriparatide (recombinant parathyroid hormone)	√ Vertebral fracture √ Non-vertebral fracture X Hip fracture • Consider for postmenopausal women at very high risk of fracture with T-score of ≤–3.0 or multiple risk factors or on antiresorptive treatment who continue to sustain fracture or have persistent bone loss	• CrCl <30 ml/min. • Hyperparathyroidism or hypercalcaemia. • Paget disease of bone or unexplained increased alkaline phosphatase levels. • History of bone radiation.	• Daily subcutaneous injection. • Should not use for longer than 2 years and should be followed by an anti-resorptive agent.
Subcutaneous romosozumab (sclerostin-binding analogue)	√ Vertebral fracture √ Non-vertebral fracture √ Hip fracture • For postmenopausal women who are not at increased risk of cardiovascular disease/stroke and have a very high risk of fracture due to T-score of ≤3.0 or multiple risk factors or if other treatment options fail	• History of myocardial infarction or stroke. • Hypocalcaemia.	• Monthly S/C injection. • Switch to anti-resorptive after 12 months of administration. • Nasopharyngitis is a very common adverse reaction. • Hypersensitivity reactions, rashes and dermatitis are common adverse reactions. • Rare cases of ONJ and AFF have been reported.
Raloxifene (selective oestrogen receptor modulator, SERM)	√ Vertebral fracture X Non-vertebral fracture X Hip fracture • Use in postmenopausal women with high risk of breast cancer and low risk of VTE and no significant vasomotor symptoms	CrCl <30 ml/min History of or current VTE (including DVT, pulmonary embolism and retinal vein thrombosis).	• To be used at least 12 months from the last menstrual period. • Studied up to 8 years of use • Consider starting an antiresorptive agent after discontinuation

(*Continued*)

(Continued)

Medication	Evidence of effectiveness in osteoporosis	Contraindications	Clinical considerations/precautions
Calcitonin (nasal spray)	√ Increases spine BMD? The effect on the vertebral fracture risk is small and inconsistent.	It is *not* recommended for osteoporosis treatment as it is *not* as effective as the other medications and has potential risks. May consider in post menopausal women with no other alternative treatment options and are at least 5 years postmenopause.	– Use for acute pain relief in patients with vertebral fractures. – <u>*Side effects:*</u> Hypersensitivity reactions, hypocalcaemia and rhinitis. – Long-term use is associated with an increased risk of cancer, e.g., basal cell carcinoma.
Menopausal hormone therapy (MHT) (including tibolone) can be considered to prevent osteoporosis or fragility fractures in postmenopausal women before 60 years old or within 10 years after menopause. In addition, MHT can prevent osteoporosis in women who menopause before the age of 45. The risks/benefits of treatment need to be weighed and discussed.			
MHT Refer to Chapter 54: *Menopausal Hormone Therapy (Also Known as Hormone Replacement Therapy)*	√ Vertebral fracture √ Non-vertebral fracture √ Hip fracture	• History of breast cancer. • History of high-risk endometrial cancer or other hormone-dependent cancers. • History of coronary heart disease. • Previous stroke or transient ischaemic attack (TIA). • Unexplained vaginal bleeding that has not been evaluated. • Known hypersensitivity to active components of MHT. • Liver disease/liver failure.	– Increased risk of cardiovascular events if started after 60 years old or after 10 years from menopause. – The risk of VTE is lower with transdermal oestrogen compared to oral. – Slight increase in breast cancer risk in combined MHT.
Tibolone Refer to Chapter 54: *Menopausal Hormone Therapy (Also Known as Hormone Replacement Therapy)*	√ Vertebral fracture √ Non-vertebral fracture **X** Hip fracture		Increased risk of stroke in older postmenopausal women ≥60 years.

√, effective for; **X**, *in*effective for.

CHAPTER 56

Subfertility, Semen Analysis and Management of Azoospermia

Definition:

Subfertility is defined as the failure to conceive after 1 year of regular unprotected sexual intercourse in the absence of known reproductive pathology. It affects 10–15% of couples trying to conceive.

Over 80% of couples will conceive within 1 year with regular unprotected sexual intercourse if the woman is below 40 years old. About half of those who do not conceive in the first year will do so in the second year (cumulative rate of 90%).

The American Society for Reproductive Medicine (ASRM) recommends initiating fertility evaluation after failure to achieve a pregnancy within 12 months of unprotected regular intercourse or therapeutic insemination in women younger than 35 years old or within 6 months in women ≥35 years old.

**Prior to embarking on fertility evaluation for couples, EXCLUDE any absolute contraindications for pregnancy, and aim to OPTIMISE any pre-existing medical conditions — refer to Chapter 1: *Pre-Conception Preparation.*

In all cases of infertility, the prognosis of pregnancy is greatly influenced by:

1. Age of woman
2. Duration of infertility
3. Occurrence of a previous pregnancy (primary versus secondary subfertility)

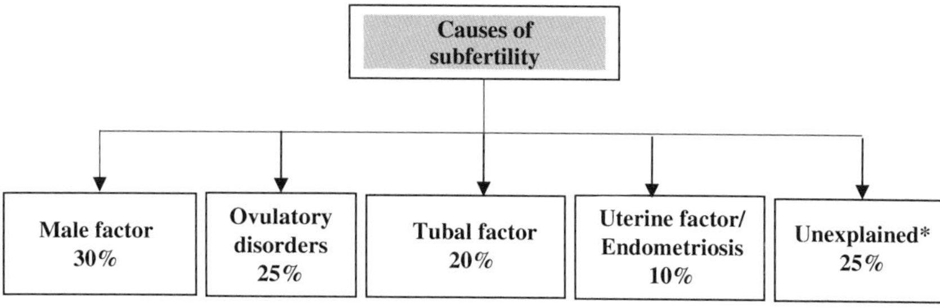

*Not identifying a cause for infertility does *not* necessarily mean that the couple is normal or has no cause.
**Combined male and female subfertility occurs in about 40% of couples.

History

Female	Male
■ Age ■ Marital status and duration ■ Previous pregnancies o With current or previous partner o Spontaneous or assisted conception — clomid/letrozole/intrauterine insemination (IUI)/*in vitro* fertilisation (IVF) o Year, mode of delivery o Antenatal/postnatal issues (gestational diabetes, hypertension) ■ Occupation ■ Drug allergy ■ Medical conditions (e.g., diabetes, hypertension and gynaecological cancers) ■ Past surgeries ■ History of chemotherapy/radiation ■ Smoker ■ Consumes alcohol ■ Menstrual history o Average cycle length o Menstrual flow o Intermenstrual bleeding o Postcoital bleeding o Dysmenorrhoea ■ Sexual history o Duration of trying o Frequency of sexual intercourse o Dyspareunia: Superficial/deep o Sexual dysfunction: Vaginismus/low libido o Previous contraception used ■ Previous fertility investigations and treatment (if any)	■ Age ■ Previous paternity o With the current partner or previous partner o Spontaneous or assisted conception (clomid/letrozole/IUI/IVF) ■ Occupation ■ Drug allergy ■ Medical conditions (e.g., diabetes, hypertension and cancers) ■ Past surgeries ■ History of chemotherapy/radiation ■ Smoker ■ Consumes alcohol ■ Sexual history o Sexual dysfunction: Erectile dysfunction/premature ejaculation/ low libido o Testicular injuries/surgeries ■ Previous fertility investigations and treatment (if any)

***Physical examination*:**

- Vitals — BMI, BP, heart rate.
- General inspection — dysmorphism.
- Breast examination.
- Abdomen — scars, masses.
- Speculum and vaginal examination — vulva, vagina, cervix pathology. Any abnormal discharge, Müllerian abnormalities.

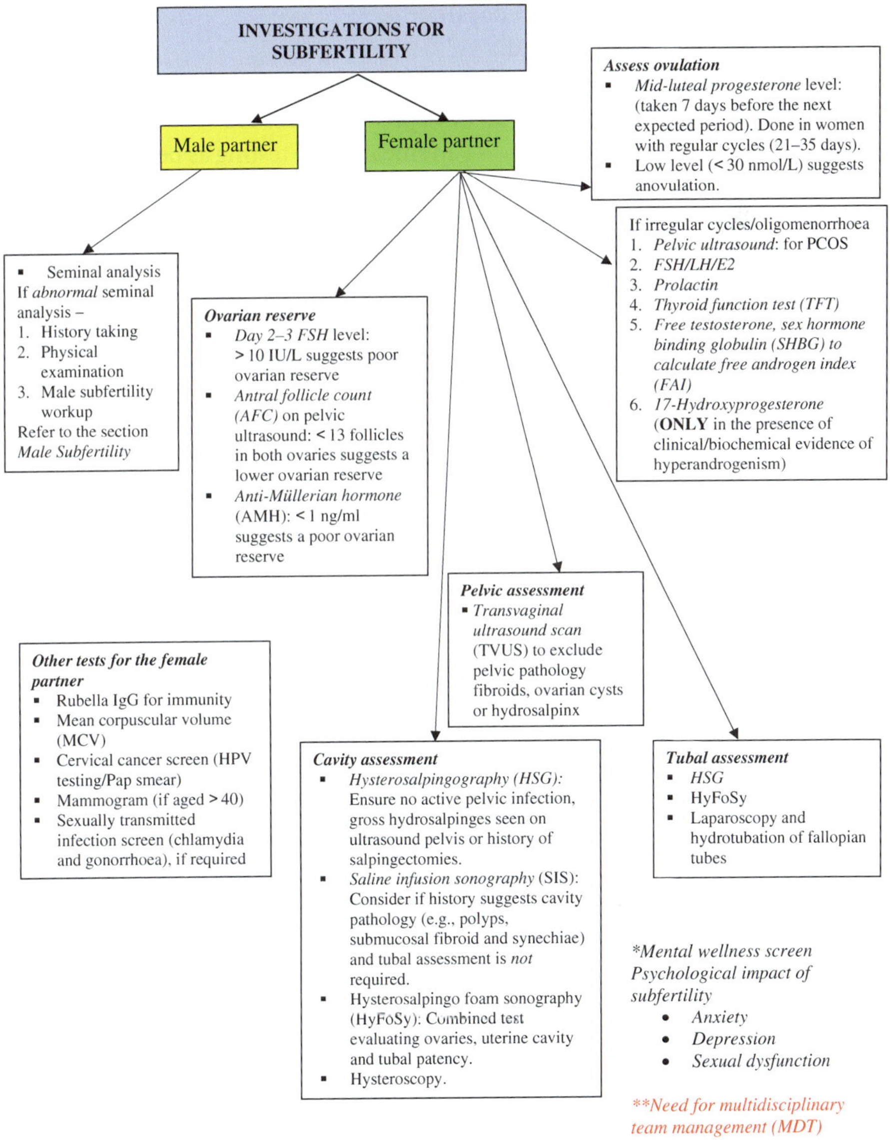

Management of Subfertility

General advice

- Stop smoking or alcoholic binging.
- Weight
  - Reduce weight if BMI >30 kg/m^2.
  - Increase weight if BMI <18.5 kg/m^2.
- Moderate exercise for 30 minutes, 5 times/week.
- Timed coitus (every 2–3 days).
- Pre-conception folic acid.
- Screening for rubella/varicella immunity. Vaccinate if non-immune and avoid pregnancy for 28 days post vaccination.
- Cervical cancer screening — Pap smear/HPV testing as per screening guidelines.
- Thalassaemia screen (ensure MCV ≥80 fl).
- Optimise medical conditions and review teratogenic drugs (if applicable).

Refer to an OBGYN if

- Woman's age ≥35 years.
- Woman's age >30 and after trying for >1 year.
- Woman's age <30 and after trying for >2 years.
- Duration of subfertility >2 years.
- Known history of reproductive pathology, e.g., amenorrhoea/oligomenorrhoea, pelvic inflammatory disease (PID), endometriosis and galactorrhoea.
- Known history or reason for infertility, e.g., tubal ligation/vasectomy, primary ovarian insufficiency (POI).
- Follicle-stimulating hormone (FSH) >10 IU/L.
- Sexual dysfunction (e.g., vaginismus, erectile dysfunction and premature ejaculation).
- Pelvic abnormalities on ultrasound scan, e.g., congenital Müllerian abnormalities, large fibroids or endometriotic cysts.
- Blocked fallopian tubes or abnormal uterine cavity on cavity imaging (e.g., HSG).
- Male conditions, e.g., history of urogenital surgery, varicocele and significant systemic illness.
- Abnormal human semen analysis (HSA)

Principles of Subfertility Treatment

Ovulation Induction (OI)

- Given to women who are anovulatory (WHO group 2 ovulation disorder).
- Types
  - Clomiphene citrate (clomid).
  - Letrozole.
- Starting the medication
  - Start with the lowest dose on days 2–6 of menses.
    - Pregnancy should be excluded ***prior*** to OI.
    - Women may need a course of oral progestins (dydrogesterone or medroxyprogesterone acetate 10 mg OM × 1 week) to induce periods prior to starting on OI medications.
  - Advise couples to have sexual intercourse every other day from day 8 to 18.
  - Check serum progesterone levels on day 21 for ovulation (ovulatory levels are >30 nmol/L).
  - Increase the OI medication dose if serum progesterone is <30 nmol/L, and repeat day 21 serum progesterone.
  - Unsuccessful, prolonged use of OI agents should be avoided because of poor success rates (usually used for 6 months or less).

OI drugs	Letrozole	Clomiphene citrate (clomid)
Mechanism of action	Aromatase inhibitor	Anti-oestrogen — selective oestrogen receptor modulator (SERM)
Indication	First line	Second line
Starting dose	2.5 mg OM × 5 days Stepwise increment — 5 mg, 7.5 mg OM	50 mg OM × 5 days Stepwise increment — 100 mg, 150 mg OM
Side effects	• Hot flushes • Mood swings	Generally well tolerated • Mood swings — most common • Hot flushes — 10% • Visual — blurred/double vision, light sensitivity <2%/optic neuropathy • Nausea • Breast tenderness • Pelvic discomfort
Pregnancy rates	Comparable	

(Continued)

(Continued)

OI drugs	Letrozole	Clomiphene citrate (clomid)
Pros	▪ Monofollicular development — lower chance of multiple pregnancies ▪ ***Fewer*** side effects	▪ Improves hirsutism and hyperandrogenism
Cons	▪ ***Teratogenic*** if taken when already pregnant	• Thins the endometrium ▪ Relatively higher multiple pregnancy rate

- Laparoscopic/microsurgical surgery for tubal blockage or peritubal adhesions.
- In women who are obese (BMI ≥30 kg/m^2), a combination of clomiphene and metformin can be considered to improve ovulation, pregnancy and live birth rates in women with polycystic ovarian syndrome (PCOS) who are clomiphene-resistant.
  - Metformin should be started at a low dose, with incremental doses of 500 mg every 1–2 weeks to minimise gastrointestinal side effects.
- Metformin *alone* can be considered for women with PCOS and anovulatory subfertility, although women should be informed that there are other more effective OI agents (as shown in the table above).
- Gonadotrophins and laparoscopic ovarian surgery (ovarian drilling) can be used as second-line agents in anovulatory women who have failed oral first-line OI agents, particularly women with PCOS who are clomiphene-resistant (refer to Chapter 36: *Polycystic Ovarian Syndrome*).

Intrauterine Insemination (IUI)

- Types
  - Natural IUI.
    - Based on the woman's menstrual cycle *without* any usage of medications.
  - Clomid/letrozole IUI.
    - Monofollicular development.
    - Lower success rates compared to super-ovulatory (SO) IUI (~10%).
  - Superovulation and intrauterine Insemination (SO IUI) — with gonadotrophins.

    - Aims for 2–3 follicles, resulting in a higher chance of multiple pregnancies and a potential need for multifetal pregnancy reduction.
    - Highest success rates compared to natural or clomid/letrozole IUI (~15%).
- Prerequisites
  - Adequate concentration of sperm after washing ($>1 \times 10^6$/ml).
  - ≥1 patent fallopian tube.
  - Patient preference.
- ***Indications***
  - Unexplained subfertility.
  - Mild endometriosis.
  - "Mild" male factor.
  - Disability (physical or psychological) preventing vaginal sexual intercourse (e.g., sexual dysfunction).
  - Same-sex relationship.
  - Condition requiring specific considerations in relation to the method of conception, e.g., after sperm washing where the male partner is HIV positive.

In Vitro Fertilisation (IVF)

- Two types of fertilisation — either natural (conventional IVF) or intra-cytoplasmic sperm injection (ICSI)
  - **IVF** — allowing the oocyte to fertilise naturally.
  - **ICSI** — injecting a single sperm into an egg. ICSI typically has higher fertilisation rates.
- ***Indications***
  - >35 years old and trying for 6 months.
  - Decreased ovarian reserve.
  - Primary ovarian insufficiency (POI) requiring donor eggs.
  - Tubal factor — history of tubal ligation, bilateral salpingectomy, bilateral hydrosalpinx.
  - Unexplained subfertility with previous IUI attempts.
  - Moderate to severe endometriosis.
  - Severe male factor — including use of surgically extracted sperms and donor sperms.

  - o Pre-implantation genetic testing (PGT) — for certain hereditary genetic disorders, e.g., thalassaemia.
  - o Fertility preservation — freezing of gametes (oocytes/sperms) or embryos for medical indications (e.g., before chemotherapy for cancer) or social reasons.

Success rates of various fertility methods

- o The spontaneous pregnancy rate in fertile couples is 20–30% per menstrual cycle.
- o The spontaneous pregnancy rate in couples with unexplained subfertility is 2–4% per menstrual cycle. Of these couples, 15% will conceive without treatment in 1 year and 35% in 2 years.
- o OI — 4% per month (no significant difference in live births per woman with OI use compared to expectant management).
- o *IUI*: 10–15% per cycle.
- o *IVF*: 30% per cycle.

Treatment of Endometriosis — Associated Subfertility

- Women who cannot attempt or decide to conceive immediately after surgery may be offered hormonal therapy as it does *not* negatively impact their fertility while improving the immediate outcome of surgery for pain.
- Postoperative hormone suppression should *not* be prescribed solely to enhance future pregnancy rates.
- In women with ASRM stage 1 or 2 endometriosis, operative laparoscopy can be offered as it improves ongoing pregnancy rates.
- Women with endometrioma-associated subfertility may be offered surgery as it increases their chances of natural pregnancy.
- There is *no* evidence that surgery improves fertility in women with deep infiltrating endometriosis, but it may represent a treatment option in symptomatic women wanting to conceive.
- Before surgery, the woman should be counselled on the risks and benefits and their chances of pregnancy post-operatively. Results of other fertility investigations (e.g., partner's semen analysis) should be considered. The endometriosis fertility index (EFI) should be used as it is validated — refer to Chapter 46: *Endometriosis and Adenomyosis*.

Tubal Factors

Condition	Management of tubal factor
Unilateral blocked tube	• Conservative • IUI — focus on the patent side • IVF • Management depending on proximal or distal blockage (as shown below)
Bilateral blocked tubes	• Conservative • IVF • Management depending on proximal or distal blockage (as shown below)
Proximal blockage	Tubal recannulation • Fallopian tube recanalisation (FTR) — interventional radiology (IR) guided — Refer to chapter 63 • Surgery — diagnostic laparoscopy, hydrotubation, tubal recanalisation
Distal blockage (hydrosalpinx)	• Conservative and proceed with IUI/IVF o Hydrosalpinges may affect embryo implantation and hence pregnancy rates • Salpingectomy/tubal clipping before IVF • Surgery — diagnostic laparoscopy KIV therapeutic, neosalpingostomy

***Complications of fertility treatment*:**

1) Miscarriage
2) Ectopic pregnancy — refer to Chapter 8: *Approach to Ectopic Pregnancy*
3) Higher-order multiple pregnancies and need for fetal reduction — refer to Chapter 12: *Multiple Pregnancy*
4) Ovarian hyperstimulation syndrome (OHSS)
5) Complications related to IVF procedure:

Ovarian stimulation	• Pain, bruising • *Side effects of gonadotrophins* — nausea, bloating, mood swings, headache • Too many follicles → OHSS risks • Too few follicles → longer stimulation period/ cycle cancellation

(*Continued*)

(*Continued*)

Egg retrieval/ oocyte pick-up (OPU)	• Sedation risks
	• OPU risks
	  • Bleeding
	  • Infection
	  • Injury to other organs — bladder, bowel, vessels
	• No eggs collected
	• Too many eggs collected — OHSS risks

Fertilisation	No/failed fertilisation → no embryos
Embryo transfer (ET)	• No embryos for transfer (does not survive thawing) • Postponement of ET (e.g., OHSS — freeze all) • Failed transfer (vaginismus, stenotic cervical os) • Bleeding • Infection • Uterine perforation (rare)

Ovarian Hyperstimulation Syndrome (OHSS)

OHSS is an iatrogenic complication of the luteal phase and early pregnancy after ovarian stimulation and ART treatment, particularly IVF. It is a systemic disease resulting from the production of vasoactive products [vascular endothelial growth factor (VEGF)] released by hyperstimulated ovaries. The pathophysiology is characterised by increased capillary permeability, leading to fluid leakage from the vascular compartment, with third-space fluid accumulation and intravascular dehydration. Its occurrence depends on the administration of human chorionic gonadotrophin (HCG).

Early and Late Forms of OHSS

The early form of OHSS (<10 days after the ovulation trigger injection of HCG) is related to an exaggerated ovarian response to gonadotrophin stimulation, while the late form (≥10 days after HCG) is mainly related to pregnancy and the secretion of placental HCG. Cases that constitute both early OHSS and followed by pregnancy can potentially be serious and long-lasting.

Mild ovarian hyperstimulation occurs in up to 33% of stimulated cycles, while 3–8% of IVF cycles are complicated by *moderate to severe forms* of OHSS.

Symptoms of OHSS

Common symptoms:
- Abdominal bloatedness and pain
- Weight gain over a short period of time
- Nausea and vomiting prevent the intake of food and fluids
- Diarrhoea
- Increase in thirst
- Decrease in appetite

More severe symptoms:
- Decreased or no urine output
- Shortness of breath, chest pain — respiratory distress due to an elevated diaphragm from ascites and/or pleural effusion
- Pain in upper or lower limbs — deep vein thrombosis (DVT)

***Signs of OHSS*:**
- Ascites — clinical or on ultrasound scan
- Abdominal distension — increase in abdominal girth (abdominal circumference measured at the level of the umbilicus)
- Lower limb oedema
- Enlarged ovaries on ultrasound scan

***More severe signs*:**
- Tense ascites requiring paracentesis
- Hypovolaemia, hypotension
- Pleural effusion (more frequently on the right side)
- Pericardial effusion
- Adult form of respiratory distress syndrome
- Oliguria or anuria

- DVT — pain either in the upper limb (more common) or in the lower limb
- Multiple organ failure
- Death (1/500,000 cycles)

***Laboratory findings*:**

- Electrolyte disorders (hyponatraemia or hyperkalaemia)
- Haemoconcentration (haematocrit >45%)
- Leucocytosis >15,000/mm^3
- Creatinine clearance (CrCl) <50 ml/min; serum creatinine >1.2 mg/dl
- Elevated liver enzymes
- Hypercoagulability

Differentials of OHSS:

- Procedure (egg retrieval) related complications
  - Infection and its complications, e.g., tubo-ovarian abscess (TOA), PID, endometritis
  - Bleeding
  - Organ injury: Bladder, bowel injury
- Ovarian cyst accidents → torsion
- Non-gynaecological causes of pain, e.g., appendicitis
- Pregnancy: Ectopic

Complications related to OHSS:

- *Ovarian torsion*
  - Causes sudden, extreme abdominal pain and nausea. The incidence of ovarian torsion is 1 in 5,000 stimulation cycles but more frequent if OHSS and pregnancy are present.
  - To rule out other differentials of abdominal pain if present (as stated above).
- *Ovarian bleeding*
  - Hyperstimulated ovaries are very vascular, and intraovarian bleeding may be caused by pressure, excessive movement or bimanual examination.
  - Signs of acute haemorrhage include hypotension, nausea and a sudden drop in haematocrit count.
- *Thromboembolic symptoms*

- Both venous (65.7%) and arterial localisations have been described; 83% of these occur in the neck, arm and head veins (60%); thrombosis also occurs in arteries and veins of the lower body; pulmonary embolism occurs in 4–12%.

Semen Analysis and Management of Azoospermia

Semen Analysis

	Normal range (WHO decision limits 2021)	Pathological term
Abstinence (days)	2–7	
pH	≥7.2	
Volume (ml)	>1.4	Aspermia (no semen)
Density ($\times 10^6$/ml)	≥16	Azoospermia (no sperm) Oligozoospermia/oligospermia
Motility (%)	Total motility (a + b) ≥42 OR Progressive motility (a) ≥30	Asthenozoospermia
(a) Rapid/moderate		
(b) Slow/*in situ*		
(c) Immotile		
Morphology (%)	≥4	Teratozoospermia
WBC ($\times 10^6$/ml)	<1	Leukospermia

Patient's name label

SEMEN ANALYSIS REPORT

Husband's name label

Semen Analysis		
Date sample received:	**Time sample received:**	**Received by:**
Time sample produced:	**Method of production:** Masturbation / Coitus Withdrawal / Male Factor Condom	**Days abstained:** (2-7)
Date analysed:	**Time analysed:**	**Spillage** Y / N

Parameters		**WHO (2021) Decision Limits**	**Analysed by**
Colour		Grey-Opalescent	
Viscosity	Normal / ______ *(increased)	Normal	
Liquefaction	Complete / Incomplete	Complete	
pH		7.2 - 7.8	
Volume (ml)		≥ **1.4**	
Motility (%): (a+b)		≥ **30** (a) or (a+b) ≥ **42**	
a) Rapid / Moderate			
b) Slow / In-situ			
c) Immotile			
Vitality (%)		≥ **54**	
Agglutination		< 10 sperm/agglutinate	
Debris			
Density (x 10^6/ml)		≥ **16**	
Round cells (x 10^6/ml)			
Sperm morphology (%)		≥ 4	
WBC		< 5/100 sperm	

Comments: ______________________________

____

____

____

- Semen analysis is **not** a test of fertility but a component of the investigation for subfertility.
- Semen specimens can be obtained by (i) masturbation, (ii) coitus withdrawal or (iii) using a male condom.
- At least 3 days of abstinence before collection of the semen specimen is advised.
- A repeat semen analysis should be performed only if the result of the first analysis is abnormal.
- *A repeat semen analysis may also be indicated if*:
  - o Significant time has lapsed since the first test (e.g., 2 years).
  - o The man has developed new significant medical conditions since the last test (e.g., diabetes mellitus).
  - o The man has had testicular/pelvic surgeries or treatment (e.g., radiation therapy), injuries and infections since the last test.
  - o The man has developed sexual dysfunction since the last test (e.g., erectile dysfunction).

***Abnormal semen analysis:* What to do?**

- *Review the man for*:
  - o Collection difficulties, e.g., spillage.
  - o Recent stressors, e.g., recent illness.
  - o Medication/traditional medication use, e.g., anabolic steroids.
  - o Occupational and environmental exposures to teratogens.
  - o Excessive exercise or weight changes.
- Repeat the test in 3 months if the first sample is abnormal because the cycle of spermatozoa formation takes about 3 months to complete. However, it can be repeated as early as 8 weeks, based on the man's preferences as this may cause anxiety.
- For men with azoospermia or severe oligozoospermia, a repeat test should be repeated *immediately* or within 2–4 weeks of the initial test.

Investigations for azoospermia or severe oligoasthenoteratozoospermia (OATS):

- FSH, LH, total testosterone (done early morning)
- Prolactin
- Male karyotype

- ± Y chromosome microdeletion
- Ultrasound scrotum (including the urogenital tract)

Causes of male subfertility:

- Unexplained: 40–50%
- Testicular disease (primary hypogonadism): 30–40%
- Sperm transport problems: 10–20%
- Hypothalamic pituitary (secondary hypogonadism): 1–2%

The most important parameters of the semen analysis are *sperm concentration* and *motility*.

Non-obstructive	***Hypothalamic pituitary (secondary hypogonadism)*** *Congenital* – Kallmann syndrome – Genetic disorders affecting multiple organs — Prader–Willi syndrome – Haemochromatosis *Acquired* – Tumours – Trauma – Infection – Radiation therapy/chemotherapy/surgery – Systemic disorders — chronic illness, malnutrition – Morbid obesity – Vascular – Endocrine disorders — acromegaly, Cushing's, hyperprolactinaemia – Infiltrative diseases — sarcoidosis, tuberculosis
	Testicular *Congenital* – Chromosomal — Klinefelter syndrome, Y chromosome deletions

(*Continued*)

	– Defective androgen synthesis/response [5-alpha reductase deficiency, androgen insensitivity syndrome (AIS)] – Cryptorchidism *Acquired* – Varicocele – Atrophy – Torsion – Trauma – Infection — mumps, gonorrhoea, chlamydia – Systemic illness – Cancer – Radiation – Chemotherapy – *Drugs* — anabolic steroids – Environmental toxins — heavy metal – Hyperthermia – Auto-sperm antibodies
Obstructive	– Retrograde ejaculation – Erectile dysfunction – Premature ejaculation – Congenital absence of vas deferens – Prior vasectomy – Previous surgeries on the scrotum, seminal duct, epididymis, prostate or seminal vesicles
Unexplained 40–50%	

Predictive value of sperm morphology in determining the pregnancy rate is low.

Enhancing male sperm quality:

Prevention

- Avoid tight trousers and underwear or heat, such as frequent sauna visits.
- Avoid excessive ejaculation or prolonged abstinence.
- Avoid drugs that affect sperm, i.e., anabolic steroids and testosterone.
- Stop smoking and limit alcohol use.
- Prevent STDs by adopting safer sexual practices and using condoms.
- Adopt a healthy diet and regular exercise to prevent obesity, which is associated with higher oestrogen levels.

Therapeutic — potentially treatable

- Antioxidant and micronutrient supplements to improve sperm parameters (L-carnitine/arginine, co-enzyme Q10, vitamin E, selenium, zinc, myo-inositol) — refer to Figure 56.1
- Varicocele surgery
- Antibiotics for infection
- Surgery for genital tract obstructions
- Hormonal therapy for gonadotrophin deficiency
- Reversible drug or toxin effects

Drugs that can affect sperm production or function:

• Alcohol • Alkylating agents • Allopurinol • Anabolic steroids • Cyclosporine	• Cimetidine • Colchicine • Erythromycin • Gentamicin • Neomycin	• Nitrofurantoin • Spironolactone • Sulfasalazine • Tetracyclines

Azoospermia

The diagnosis of azoospermia requires two or more centrifuged semen samples to confirm the complete absence of sperms. Baseline investigations, as stated above, should be done.

Improved sperm parameter*	Micronutrient (dose/day)	Study citation
• Sperm volume • Sperm concentration • Sperm motility • Sperm morphology	Coenzyme Q10 (30 mg), vitamin E (120 mg), folic acid (800 mg), selenium (60 μg), zinc (40 mg), L-carnitine (440 mg), L-arginine (250 mg), glutathione (160 mg)	Imhof *et al.* [*E-SPEN J* 2012;**7**(1)]
	L-carnitine (1,000 mg)	Lipovac *et al.* [*Reprod Biol Endocrinol* 2016;**14**(1)]
• Sperm motility • Sperm morphology • Either sperm volume or sperm concentration	Zinc sulphate (440 mg)	Hadwan *et al.* [*Int J Vitam Nutr Res* 2015;**85**:165–173]
	Myoinositol (1 g), L-carnitine (30 mg), L-arginine (30 mg), vitamin E (30 mg), selenium (55 μg), folic acid (200 μg)	Montanino Oliva *et al.* [*Int J Endocrinol* 2016;1674950]
• Sperm morphology • One other sperm parameter	Coenzyme Q10 (100 mg), zinc (10 mg), L-carnitine (680 mg), lycopene (5 mg), astaxanthin (16 mg)	Singh *et al.* [*J Clin Diagn Res* 2016;**10**(7)]
	L-carnitine (1,000 mg), fumarate (725 mg), acetyl-L-carnitine (500 mg), fructose (1,000 mg), coenzyme Q10 (20 mg), vitamin C (90 mg), zinc (10 mg), folic acid (200 μg), vitamin B12 (1.5 μg), selenium (50 μg), citric acid (50 mg)	Busetto *et al.* [*Andrologia* 2018;**50**(3)]
		Micic *et al.* [*Andrologia* 2019;e13267]
	Coenzyme Q10 (120 mg), vitamin C (80 mg), vitamin E (40 mg)	Kobori *et al.* [*Arch Ital Urol Androl* 2014;**86**:1]
	Vitamin E (400 IU), selenium (200 μg)	Mohammad and Tavanbakhsh [*Int J Gen Med* 2011;99–104]
	Myoinositol (4 g), folic acid (400 μg)	Calogero *et al.* [*Andrology* 2015;**3**:491–495]
	Coenzyme Q10 (300 mg)	Safarinejad [*J Urol* 2009;**182**:237–248]
	Alpha-lipoic acid (600 mg)	Haghighian *et al.* [*Fertil Steril* 2015;**104**:318–324]
• Sperm motility only	Myoinositol (2 g), L-carnitine (60 mg), L-arginine (60 mg), vitamin E (60 mg), selenium (110 μg), folic acid (400 μg)	Dinkova *et al.* [*Eur Rev Med Pharmacol Sci* 2017;**21**(2 Suppl):62–65]
	Zinc (400 mg), vitamin E (20 mg), vitamin C (10 mg)	Omu *et al.* [*Med Princ Pract* 2008;**17**:108–116]
	Vitamin E (400 mg)	ElSheikh *et al.* [*Andrology* 2015;**3**:864–867]
• No effect observed	Coenzyme Q10 (200 mg)	Nadjarzadeh *et al.* [*J Endocrinol Invest* 2011;**34**:224–228]
	Folic acid (10 mg), zinc sulphate (400 mg)	Raigani *et al.* [*Andrologia* 2014;**46**(9):956–962]
	Folic acid (400 μg)	Calogero *et al.* [*Andrology* 2015;**3**:491–495]

Fig. 56.1 Summary of effects of different micronutrients/antioxidant formulations on sperm parameters.

*Significant improvement (p<0.05) compared with pre-treatment or control.

Source: Tan TC, Chew YJ, Tung J. Antioxidant and micronutrient supplementation on the sperm parameters of male patients with idiopathic infertility: An updated literature review: Latest news for doctors, nurses and pharmacists: Pharmacy. MIMS News. https://specialty.mims.com/topic/antioxidant-and-micronutrient-supplementation-on-the-sperm-parameters-of-male-patients-with-idiopathic-infertility–an-updated-literature-review. Published June 9, 2020. Accessed August 28, 2022.

Table 56.1 Evaluation of the Azoospermic Patient

History	Examination	Investigations
Previous paternity	BMI	FSH, LH, prolactin levels
Medical history, including childhood illnesses, STI	General inspection — dysmorphism	Total testosterone level (done early morning)
Surgery — genital, pelvic or inguinal surgery or trauma	Secondary sexual characteristics (Tanner staging, hair distribution and gynaecomastia)	Ultrasound imaging of the urogenital tract and testes
Exposure to gonadotoxins/heat	Presence of abdominal, inguinal or scrotal scars or masses	Karyotyping Y chromosome microdeletion
Medications	Testicular size, consistency (normal = 4–5.5 cm long/12–25 ml) *An orchidometer is used to measure the testicular size*	± MRI pituitary gland
Family history of birth defects, mental retardation, reproductive failure or cystic fibrosis	Epididymis (any masses) *Previous epididymitis may cause fibrosis and thickening of the epididymis*	
Developmental history — pubertal development	Presence of vas deferens *Absence of vas deferens could be congenital or due to cystic fibrosis*	
Smoking, alcohol intake	Presence of varicoceles	
Sexual history — any sexual dysfunction, low libido Previous partners and any issues		
Previous investigations, treatment (if any)		

Management of Azoospermia

1. *Hypogonadotrophic hypogonadism* — low FSH, LH and testosterone levels. Pituitary MRI to exclude pathological lesions. If the pituitary MRI is normal, gonadotrophins (HCG or FSH) may be given to initiate spermatogenesis. It may take up to 1 year to induce sufficient spermatogenesis resulting in acceptable semen parameters. Refer to an endocrinologist and a reproductive andrologist.
2. *Primary testicular failure (hypogonadism)* — high FSH, LH and low testosterone levels. There is no known upper limit of FSH levels that implies testicular failure. Usually, we use a cut-off of 2 times above

the normal limit. However, they may still have sperms in the testis, which could be retrieved surgically. Refer to urology or a reproductive andrologist for assessment and counselling.

3. *Obstructive causes — normal FSH, LH and testosterone levels*

   The treatment option is dependent on the cause. This includes a surgical correction to bypass the obstruction, allowing for natural conception or surgical sperm retrieval followed by ICSI.

Approach to Azoospermia

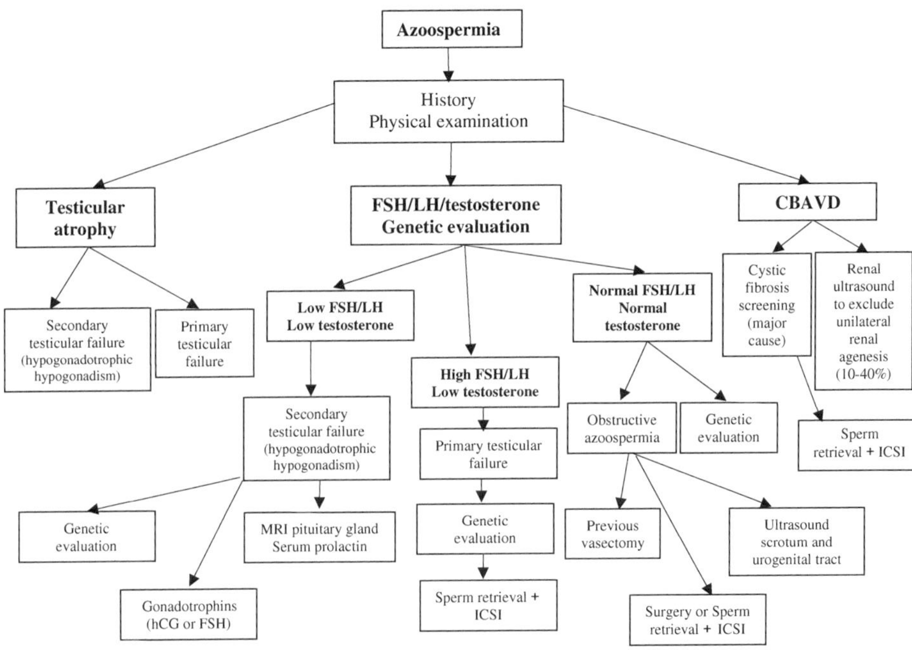

**Genetic evaluation* should be offered as obstructive azoospermia and impaired spermatogenesis secondary to genetic causes are *not* mutually exclusive.
ICSI, intracytoplasmic sperm insemination; CBAVD, congenital bilateral absence of vas deferens.

Alternatives:

1) Donor sperm
2) Adoption
3) Child-free life

CHAPTER 57

Approach to Galactorrhoea and Hyperprolactinaemia

Galactorrhoea is defined as excessive lactation unrelated to breastfeeding and postpartum.

Physiological lactation usually occurs in the immediate postpartum period and is caused by a sudden drop in progesterone in the presence of high prolactin levels.

Most patients present with nipple discharge.

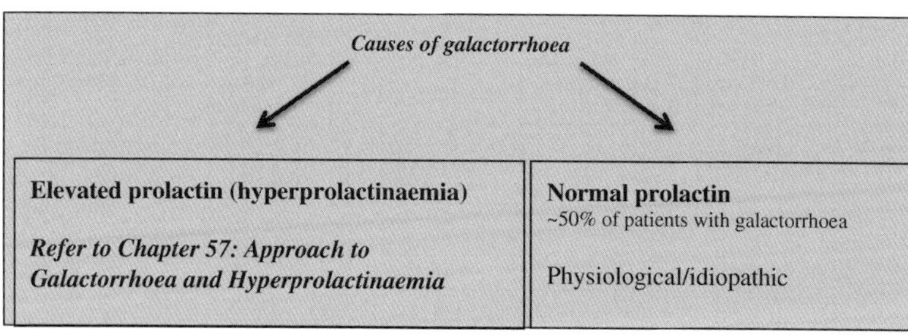

The normal prolactin level is usually quoted as <25 ng/ml. The normal prolactin level used in KKH is 6.98–32.94 ng/ml

Hyperprolactinaemia is the most common cause of galactorrhoea.

Up to 90% of women with hyperprolactinaemia have galactorrhoea.

Aetiology of galactorrhoea:

1) Physiological causes:

a. Pregnancy — can start as early as the second trimester.
b. Lactation — may continue for up to 2 years after cessation of breastfeeding.
c. Puberty and menopause — due to fluctuating hormone levels.

d. Neonatal — exposure to *in utero* maternal hormones.
e. Nipple stimulation and suckling.

2) **Non-physiological causes — refer to Chapter 57: *Approach to Galactorrhoea and Hyperprolactinaemia.***
3) **Normoprolactinaemic cause — no cause is found (idiopathic galactorrhoea) — conservative management.**

Approach to Galactorrhoea

History

- **Details of discharge:**
  - Unilateral or bilateral
  - Colour (clear, white, green, bloody)
  - Amount
  - Duration
  - Odour
- **Associated symptoms:**
  - Nipple/skin changes
  - Breast pain
  - Breast lumps
  - Fever
- **Medication history (drugs causing high prolactin levels)**
- **LMP, pregnant or postpartum**
- **Signs and symptoms of high prolactin and thyroid disorders**
- **Visual disturbances/headache**
- **± Details suggestive of hyperprolactinaemia — refer to Chapter 57: *Approach to Galactorrhoea and Hyperprolactinaemia***

Physical examination:

- **Vital parameters**
  - Thyroid signs
  - Visual fields
  - Abdominal exam
- **Bilateral breast exam:**
  - Unilateral or bilateral
  - Uniductal or multiductal
  - *Discharge*: Colour, consistency, blood, amount, smell

- *Associated signs*: Nipple/skin changes, tenderness, lumps
- *Axillary examination*: Enlarged lymph nodes

***Pathological nipple discharge*:**
- Unilateral, uniductal, persistent, spontaneous
- May be blood-tinged
- It is important to identify and refer to a breast surgeon expediently as malignancies may occur in 10% of pathological nipple discharge

Approach to galactorrhoea

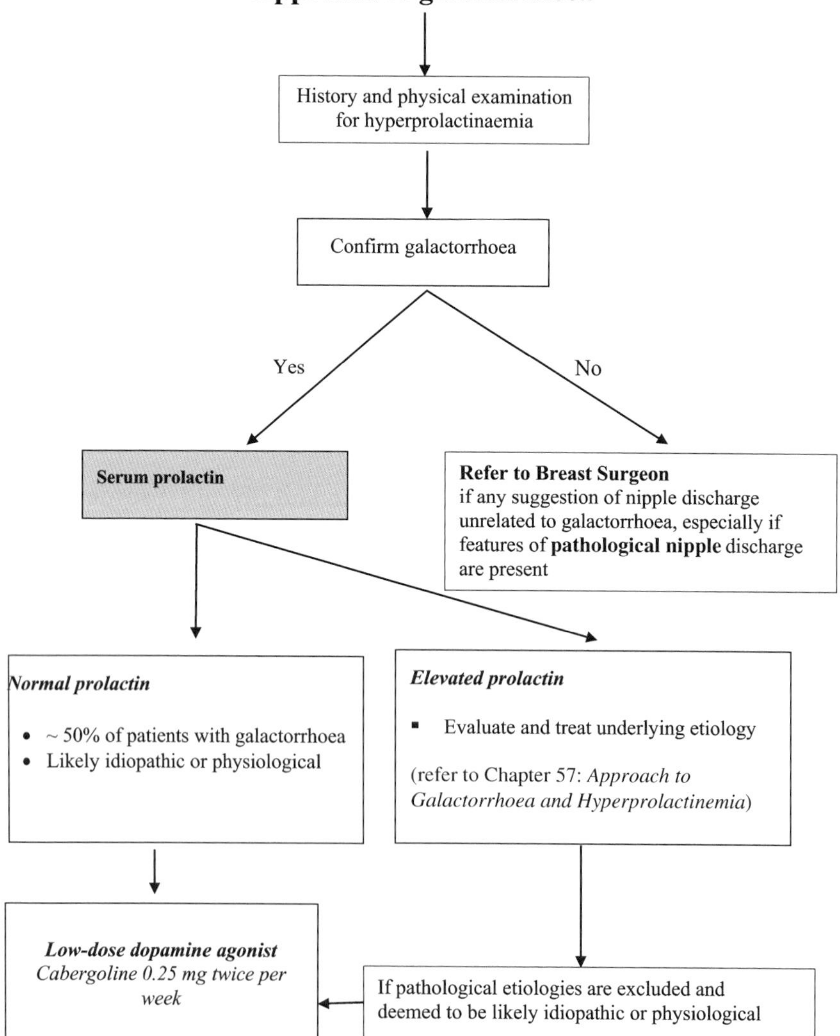

Approach to Hyperprolactinaemia

Causes of Hyperprolactinaemia

No cause is found in about one-third of hyperprolactinaemia.

Physiological	Pharmacological	Pathological
Lactation Pregnancy Stress Coitus Exercise Nipple stimulation Sleep Seizures	***Drugs — dopamine — antagonists*** *(mechanism of action)* ***Anti-psychotics*** ➢ ***Typical*:** o Haloperidol o Phenothiazine o Butyrophenone ➢ ***Atypical*:** o Risperidone o Olanzapine ***Anti-depressants:*** o Tricyclic anti-depressants o Selective serotonin reuptake inhibitors (SSRIs) o Serotonin and norepinephrine reuptake inhibitors (SNRIs) **Anti-convulsants** **Anti-emetics** o Metoclopramide o Domperidone **Anti-hypertensives** o Methyldopa o Verapamil **Opioids** **Monoamine oxidase (MAO) inhibitors** **Cimetidine** **Oestrogens**	***Hypothalamic–pituitary disorders*** **Pituitary stalk section** **Infiltrative** ■ Sarcoidosis ■ Granulomas ■ Tuberculosis ■ Histiocytosis **Trauma** **Cranial irradiation** **Previous surgery** **Tumours** ■ Craniopharyngioma ■ Meningioma ■ Germinoma **Pituitary diseases** o Empty sella syndrome o Tumours ■ *Pituitary adenoma* – Prolactinoma – Non-functioning adenoma o Acromegaly o Cushing disease **Systemic diseases** o Chronic renal disease o Liver cirrhosis o Hypothyroidism o PCOS **Irritation/injuries of the chest wall**, e.g., severe burns, shingles

Symptoms of hyperprolactinaemia:
- Galactorrhoea
- Oligo or amenorrhoea
- Subfertility
- Sexual dysfunction

Additional history to screen for underlying etiology:
- LMP, pregnant or breastfeeding
- Medication history
- Neurological symptoms, e.g., visual disturbances, headaches
- Other medical diseases, e.g., hypothyroidism, chronic renal or hepatic disease
- Previous neurological surgery or irradiation
- Excessive exercise or stress

⬇

Physical examination:
- **Breast examination**

  *Refer to Chapter 57: *Approach to Galactorrhoea and Hyperprolactinaemia*
- **Gynaecological examination**
- **Neurological examination/visual fields**
  - Bitemporal hemianopia
  - Signs of space occupying lesions
- **Systemic review**
  - Chronic renal failure
  - Liver cirrhosis
  - Hypothyroidism
  - Acromegaly

⬇

Investigations:
- **Serum prolactin**
  - Normal <25 ng/ml.
  - To exclude macroprolactin as the cause of hyperprolactinaemia by performing the PEG precipitation test.
- **MRI pituitary to exclude pituitary tumour**

  Endocrine screen
  - Thyroid function test (TFT).
  - Growth hormone, adrenocorticotropic hormone (ACTH).

⬇

Management of hyperprolactinaemia:

- Drug-induced hyperprolactinaemia.
  - Assess indications of medication.
  - Discontinue medication and re-assess serum prolactin levels.
  - Do not need to treat asymptomatic drug-induced hyperprolactinaemia.
  - If possible, switch to a drug with less dopamine-antagonist side effects.
  - If not possible — cautious administration with close surveillance of the patient.
- **Dopamine agonists**, e.g., cabergoline or bromocriptine — first-line medical treatment.
  Treatment with dopamine agonists can regulate the patient's menses and induce ovulation when prolactin levels normalise. After normalisation of prolactin levels – about 80% of patients will ovulate and pregnancy rates of 70–80% can be achieved. Dopamine agonists have ***not*** been associated with miscarriages, fetal anomalies or other adverse pregnancy outcomes, e.g., preterm deliveries.
  <u>*Side effects*</u> include light-headedness, nausea and headache.
- Systemic or endocrine disorders.
  Treat the underlying chronic disease, e.g., thyroxine replacement for hypothyroidism.

MANAGEMENT OF PROLACTINOMA (MICRO AND MACRO)

Medical (first-line)
Dopamine agonists (bromocriptine or ****cabergoline**)
**Preferred drug

↓

Surveillance
- Serial prolactin levels to assess return to normal
- Repeat MRI scan in 1 year

↓

Stop dopamine agonists
After 1 year of treatment if serum prolactin returns to normal and no evidence of the remnant tumour on MRI scan

Surgery
- Failure of medical therapy.
- Expanding prolactinoma (patient with neurological and visual deficits <u>*not*</u> responding to dopamine agonists).
- Infarction/haemorrhage into prolactinoma with visual disturbances, severe headache, altered consciousness, vascular collapse.
- Resistant or malignant prolactinoma

Radiotherapy
- *Rarely used*
- Resistant to medical and surgical therapy

Management of pituitary adenomas/prolactinomas in pregnancy:

- Pituitary microadenoma <10 mm diameter
- Pituitary macroadenoma >10 mm diameter

  Co-manage with an endocrinologist.

  Refer to a neurosurgeon if surgery is needed.

Risk of enlargement of microprolactinomas in pregnancy:

- Low risk of tumour expansion
- Usually, dopamine agonists are discontinued in pregnancy

Risk of enlargement of macroprolactinomas in pregnancy:

- Higher risk (30%) of tumour expansion
- Continue medical treatment (dopamine agonist)
- Monitor visual fields in each trimester
- Warn the patient to look out for headaches and visual symptoms

10% of pituitary macroadenoma in pregnancy may require surgery. Surgery is usually performed in the second trimester if tumour expansion occurs despite treatment with a dopamine agonist.

CHAPTER 58

Female Sexual Dysfunction

- ***Sexual dysfunction*** is defined as having a sexual problem that is associated with personal distress.
- Both males and females may have sexual dysfunction.
- **For males, please refer to a urologist for evaluation.**
- About 40% of women worldwide report sexual problems.
- One in eight women experiences personal or interpersonal distress with it.
- For married couples, sexual dysfunction is associated with marital distress, which is more apparent for males.
- Sexual problems may be uncovered during history-taking by asking further questions.
  - For example, when asked about postcoital bleeding, the woman may say that she has not had sex for a long time → prompt by asking, "Do you have any concerns regarding sexual intercourse?"
- Patients may present with pain with sexual activity, non-consummation of marriage and subfertility.
- Female sexual dysfunction may take the form of:

Disorders with pain (refer to the Section on *Female Sexual Pain*)	**Disorders without pain**
Vaginismus	Low libido
Dyspareunia (superficial/deep)	Impaired arousal
	Anorgasmia

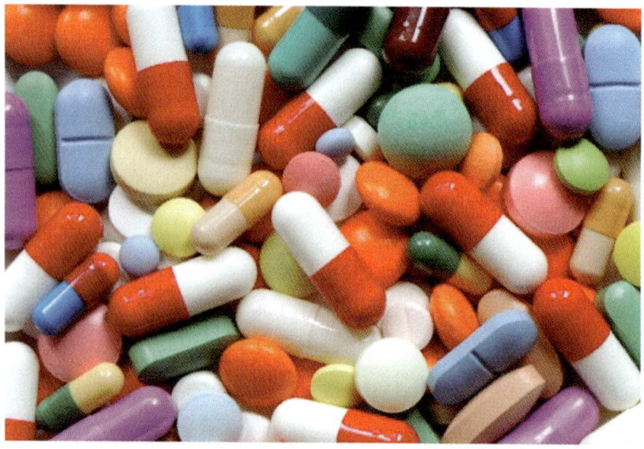

Fig. 58.1 Drugs.

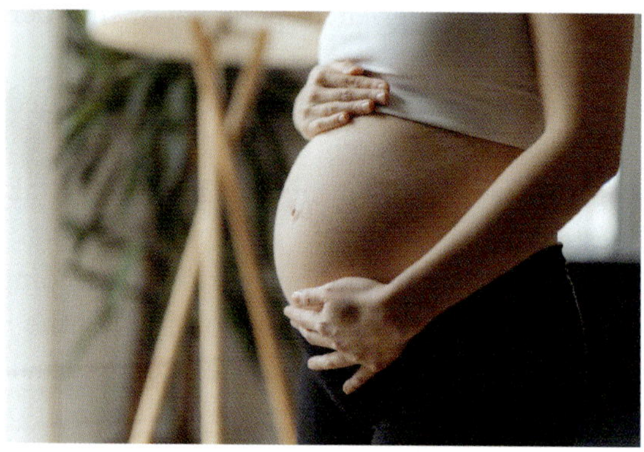

Fig. 58.2 Pregnancy.

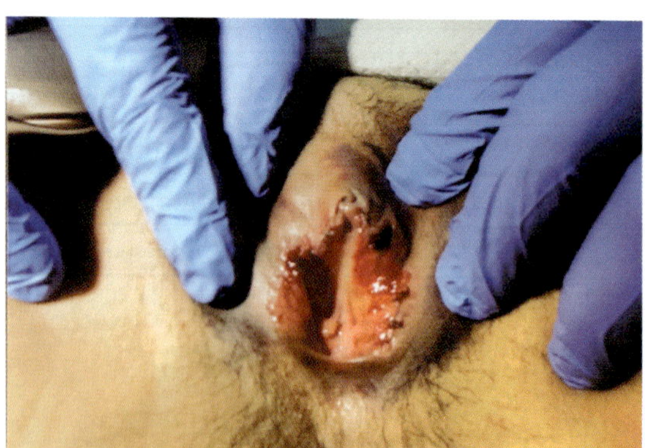

Fig. 58.3 Female genital mutilation (FGM).

Risk Factors for Sexual Dysfunction

Lifestyle/social	Relationship factors — marriage issues Fatigue and stress Obesity Substance use — nicotine, alcohol, opioids
Medication (Figure 58.1)	GnRH agonists Selective serotonin reuptake inhibitors (SSRIs) Anti-psychotics Benzodiazepines Beta-blockers Anti-epileptics Aromatase inhibitors
Gynaecological	Pregnancy (Figure 58.2) Childbirth Lactation Subfertility Pelvic organ prolapse (POP) Incontinence Endometriosis Uterine fibroids Genitourinary syndrome of menopause (GSM) Female genital mutilation (FGM) — refer to Figure 58.3
Medical illness	Endocrine disorders — hyperthyroidism, hyperprolactinaemia Hypertension Neurological disease Bladder pain syndrome (BPS) Rheumatoid arthritis, fibromyalgia (chronic pain) Renal failure and dialysis Cancer
Psychiatric disorders	Depression — 17–26% report a low sexual desire Anxiety Psychosis
Hypoestrogenic states	Primary ovarian insufficiency (POI) Pregnancy Functional hypothalamic amenorrhoea, e.g., anorexia nervosa, excessive exercise, low BMI Medications, e.g., GnRH agonists
Menopause	Menopausal symptoms

History:

- Type of symptom — pain with sex, low libido, impaired arousal, unable to achieve orgasm → usually a combination of symptoms.
- Duration of symptoms, whether there was a triggering event.
- Methods tried so far, e.g., vaginal lubricant, previous consultations with other doctors or therapists.
- Medical/surgical/obstetric history.
- Social history — the quality of the relationship with the partner.
- History of sexual abuse.
- Substance use, e.g., nicotine, recreational drugs.
- Medication history.
- Menopausal status, menstrual history.
- Fertility status — if trying to conceive and the duration of trying.
- <u>*History of gynaecological conditions*:</u>
  Fibroids/endometriosis/pelvic inflammatory disease (PID).
  Incontinence/POP (pelvic organ prolapse).
- *History of vulvovaginal or pelvic injury*, e.g., FGM.
- Presence of vulvovaginal/pelvic pain.
- Presence of vulvovaginal itch/dryness/discharge.

Examination:

- Ensure normal pelvic anatomy.
- Assess for genital or pelvic tenderness.
- Vulval/vaginal/cervical lesions.
- POP.
- Pelvic floor hypertonus.
- Vulvovaginal atrophy.
- Vaginal discharge.

Investigations:

- Indicated by history and/or physical examination.
- Serum androgen level has <u>*no*</u> role — it does not predict sexual function in women.
- FSH and E2 are <u>*not*</u> warranted — menopause is a clinical diagnosis unless there is suspicion of POI in women <40 years old.

Management of Females With Sexual Dysfunction

General advice:

- Multidisciplinary and multimodal approach — a sexual health clinic is available at KKH with a team comprising a gynaecologist, a family medicine specialist with an interest in sexual dysfunction, a psychologist and a physiotherapist.
- Individualised to the patient/couple.
- Assess the patient's goals.
- Consider partner's issues — refer to urology for male partners as indicated.
- Screen for psychological issues — such as depression and anxiety.
- Refer to a psychiatrist and/or a psychologist as needed.
- Treat associated conditions, e.g., arthritis, urinary/faecal incontinence and gynaecological conditions such as endometriosis and PID.
- Switch or reduce dosages of medications that may be the cause of the problem.

Lifestyle modification:

- Use of vaginal lubricants and moisturisers.
- Management of stress and fatigue, introducing novelty to sex life.
- Healthy weight loss.

Allied healthcare professionals:

- Refer to a sex therapist if concerns are specifically related to sex and organic conditions have been treated or excluded.
- Refer the couple for counselling if concerns are about improving communication and reducing conflict.
- Physiotherapy for vaginismus.

Pharmacological:

- Pharmacological treatment — to start only when sexual problems are <u>*not*</u> improving with non-pharmacological interventions.
- *Pre*menopausal patients — efficacy is seen with non-hormonal therapy.
- *Post*menopausal patients — hormonal therapy is beneficial.

Medications	Premenopausal	Postmenopausal
Hormonal		
Vaginal oestrogens ▪ Vagifem® (oestradiol) 10 mcg vaginal tablet ON × 2 weeks, then 1 night/ week for maintenance ▪ Premarin® cream 1 application ON × 3 weeks, then 1–2 nights/ week for 3 months for maintenance	Not helpful unless hypoestrogenic state or POI	Improves GSM
Androgen therapy ▪ Treatment *not* approved by the US FDA — to document in medical records regarding off-label use ▪ ***Contraindicated*** in women with cardiovascular disease, hepatic disease, endometrial hyperplasia/ malignancy, breast cancer ▪ Use with caution in women at high risk of the above disorders	▪ No significant improvement ▪ Consider the significant potential risk of inadvertent exposure of a developing fetus to androgens — genital tract formation begins in the fourth week of pregnancy	▪ Serum concentrations of androgens at the upper limit of normal have been shown to improve female sexual function ▪ **Testosterone 1% ointment (100 g)** is available at KKH — this is an extemporaneous/ compounded preparation (use is *not* recommended by an expert panel) ▪ Consider commercial preparation **androgel** (*not* available at KKH but is available in Singapore) ▪ **Androgel 1% gel (sachet)** — 1 sachet to use over 10 days and applied to the skin of arms, legs or abdomen (the dose is 1/10 of the dosage for males) ▪ **Androfeme 1% —** licensed for women but *not* available in Singapore — dose is 0.5 ml (5 mg) and comes with an applicator marked with 0.25 ml graduations in a carton ▪ *Adverse effects:* Cosmesis, i.e., hirsutism and acne, decreased HDL levels, "oestrogenic" effects as most androgens are aromatised to oestrogens
Systemic oestrogens	No improvement	No improvement
Tibolone	No information	Modest improvement
Non-hormonal		
Flibanserin ▪ PO 100 mg ON ▪ FDA approved but with a black box warning ▪ *Not* available in Singapore — need to bring in via NPNP* and exemption⁺ if required	▪ Improvement seen ▪ Centrally-acting serotonin receptor agonist/antagonist ▪ *Side effects* — somnolence, dizziness ▪ Safety concerns when taken with alcohol or certain medications such as anti-depressants, fluconazole (CYP P450 inhibitors)	*Not* indicated for use in these women

(Continued)

Medications	Premenopausal	Postmenopausal
Bupropion ▪ Off-label use for SSRI-induced sexual dysfunction ▪ Sustained-release 300 mg/day dosing in the morning	▪ Low cost ▪ *Not* available in KKH ▪ Available in CGH, SGH, SKH ▪ NPNP* required	No information
Bremelanotide ▪ FDA approved ▪ SC 1.75 mg at least 45 minutes before anticipated sexual activity ▪ *Contraindicated* in uncontrolled hypertension (HTN) or known cardiovascular disease	▪ Treatment of hypoactive sexual desire disorder ▪ *Side effects* — nausea, vomiting, flushing, headache, hyperpigmentation ▪ *Not* available in Singapore ▪ Need to bring in via NPNP* and exemption⁺ if required	Not approved for use in these women
Phosphodiesterase (PDE-5) inhibitors, e.g., sildenafil ▪ Not FDA approved	▪ Effective only for women with sexual dysfunction associated with SSRI use ▪ Available in KKH	Limited information
Herbal supplements	Avoid (*un*proven safety and efficacy)	Avoid (*un*proven safety and efficacy)

*NPNP — named-physician-named-patient medication assistance request form.
⁺Exemption — drug not available in Singapore, have to import from overseas.

Follow-Up of Females with Sexual Dysfunction

- Every 3 months till improvement, then every 6–12 months.
- Review for side effects of pharmacological therapy.
- Assess treatment efficacy via improvement of patient's symptoms and achievement of treatment goals.
- Review mental state and quality of relationship with a partner — refer to a therapist/psychologist/psychiatrist as required.
- Refer to a fertility specialist if keen to conceive for consideration of assisted reproductive techniques, e.g., IUI and IVF.

Female Sexual Pain

- *Definition:* Vulvovaginal or pelvic pain that is triggered by or exacerbated during sexual contact.
- Incidence of painful intercourse ranges from 8–22%.

- Women with genital–pelvic pain dysfunction experience the persistence of:
  - Pain with vaginal penetration.
  - Marked vulvovaginal or pelvic pain during genital contact.
  - Marked fear or anxiety about vulvovaginal or pelvic pain in anticipation of, during or as a result of genital contact.
  - Marked hypertonicity or over-activity of pelvic floor muscles with or without genital contact (i.e., vaginismus).

(a) ***Superficial (distal) dyspareunia*** — pain limited to the vulva or vaginal entrance.

Causes include:
- ***Vaginismus:*** Involuntary muscle spasm with vaginal penetration. Incidence increased by 60% in 2020 compared to 2017.
- *Decreased oestrogen levels*: During the postpartum period, when lactating and during menopause.
- *Decreased lubrication*: Decreased physiologic arousal because of medical conditions such as hypothyroidism and diabetes mellitus.
- *Myofascial pelvic pain syndrome*: Characterised by short, tight, tender pelvic floor muscles that can be localised/diffuse.
- *Vulvodynia*: Vulvar pain of unknown cause.
- *Alterations of vaginal anatomy*: Congenital anomalies (e.g., vaginal septae), skin diseases (e.g., lichen sclerosus), post-procedure changes (e.g., perineal tear following vaginal birth or FGM).

(b) ***Deep (proximal) dyspareunia*** — deep vaginal, uterine or pelvic pain.

Causes include:
- Endometriosis.
- Adnexal masses.
- PID or other abdominopelvic infections.
- Fibroids.
- Myofascial pelvic pain syndrome.
- Chronic female pelvic pain syndrome.
- *Malignancy*: Cancer itself, as well as its treatment (e.g., radiation therapy), hormone-blocking therapies (e.g., letrozole, GnRH agonists).
- Surgery, e.g., hysterectomy, salpingo-oophorectomy.

Management of Female Sexual Pain

- Sexual pain is often multifactorial.
- Take a detailed **history**: To evaluate for possible physical, sexual and psychosocial causes of pain.
  - When? Where? Any association with specific events?
  - Character and pattern of pain.
  - Methods tried to alleviate pain.
- ***Careful physical examination***:
  - Before the examination, ask about previous experiences with pelvic examination.
  - Obtain verbal consent.
  - Begin by explaining the order of examination and the purpose of each component of the examination.
  - Take measures to reduce anxiety and discomfort, such as:
    - Agreeing that the examination will be stopped at the patient's request.
    - The patient may be accompanied by someone or have a device for calming music.
    - Offering the patient a hand mirror so that she may observe the examination, completing the examination over a few visits or pre-treatment with an anxiolytic.
  - Visual inspection.
  - Check for possible causes, e.g., skin changes, congenital anomalies, post-procedure changes.
  - Determine areas of pain.
  - Pressure point testing with Q-tip. Starting from the distal, i.e., the medial aspect of the thighs towards the genital region.
  - Palpation.
  - ***Speculum examination***: May use a narrow speculum and/or application of topical anaesthetic agents such as lidocaine gel about 10 minutes before the examination.
  - Abdominal, bimanual and recto-vaginal examination.
- ***Investigations***:
  - Guided by examination findings.
  - Swabs if discharge seen.

  - Biopsy of any lesions that are found.
  - Urine FEME and culture if urinary symptoms are accompanied by suprapubic or bladder tenderness.
  - Imaging, such as an ultrasound scan of the pelvis, if an adnexal mass is felt on examination.
- ***Refer immediately to the relevant medical speciality/authority if:***
  - The patient is in an unsafe relationship, e.g., domestic/sexual abuse.
  - FGM is found.
  - Vulvar dermatoses are present and you are <u>*not*</u> familiar with the diagnosis or treatment.
  - There is graft-versus-host disease of the genital tissues in patients who have received stem cells/bone marrow from a donor.

Treatment of Female Sexual Pain

- Treat identifiable causes, e.g., lichen sclerosus, with high-potency steroid creams and refer to a vulval specialist and local oestrogen therapy for GSM.
- Refer to a physiotherapist for vaginismus and myofascial pelvic pain syndrome.
- Refer to a psychiatrist/psychologist for any issues with mental well-being.
- Refer to a medical social worker (MSW) if required.
- Refer to a sex therapist as indicated.

CHAPTER 59

Breast Cancer Screening and Diagnostic Tests

Breast Cancer Screening

Screening Mammogram Schedule in Singapore

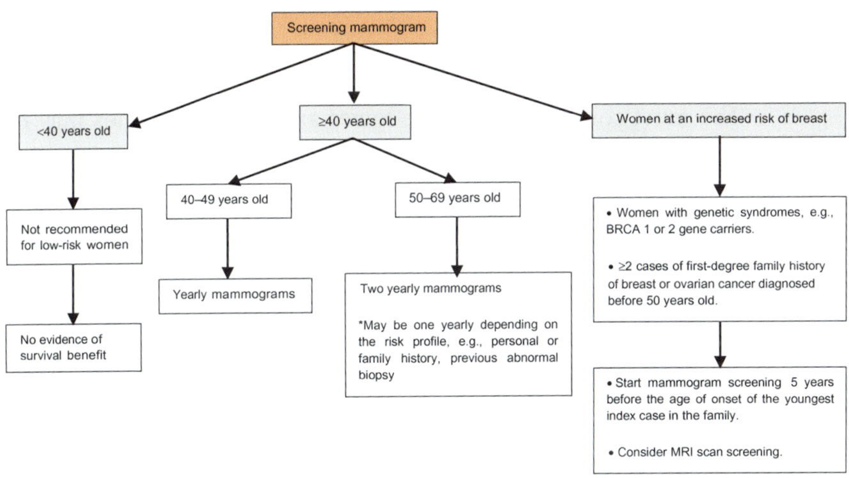

- Do monthly breast self-examination (BSE) if ≥30 years old.
- Women ≥70 years old may continue with screening mammograms in accordance with the guidelines for ≥50–69 years old, depending on the presence of other medical history and life expectancy.

Introduction

- *Anatomical variations*
  - **<u>Polymastia:</u>** (Figure 59.1) Accessory breast tissues. They affect 2–6% of females. They can occur at any point along the milk line

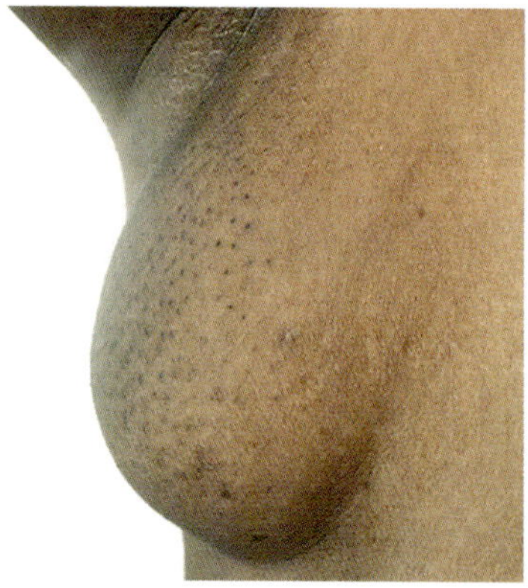

Figure 59.1 Polymastia.
Source: https://www.amaris-b.com/conditions/armpit-fat-axillary-accessory-breast.

from the axilla to the groin. Rarely found on the face, back or thigh. The most common site is the lower axilla. These tissues may or may not have a nipple or areola. The tissues can become swollen or tender, especially during the onset of puberty or pregnancy. Surgical resection may be required if there is painful swelling or the development of a benign/malignant tumour in the accessory breast tissues.

- **Polythelia (Figure 59.2) (also known as accessory nipples/ supernumerary nipples):** They can occur at any point along the milk line from the axilla to the groin, as regression of these

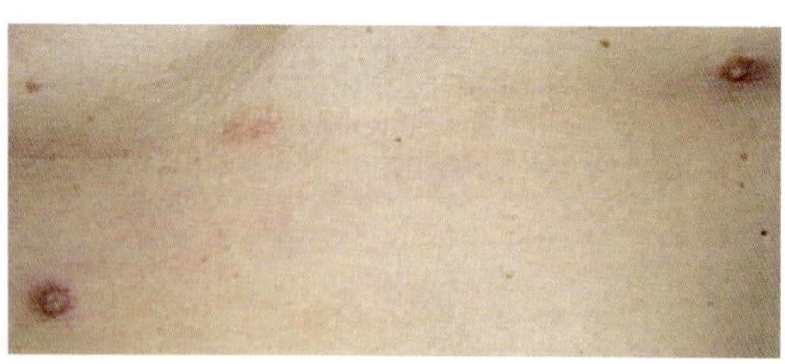

Figure 59.2 Polythelia.
Source: https://www.atlasdermatologico.com.br/disease.jsf?diseaseId=333.

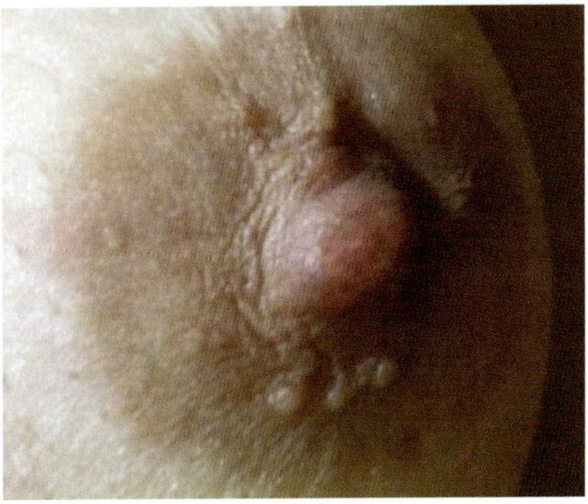

Figure 59.3 Montgomery's tubercles.
Source: https://ph.theasianparent.com/montgomerys-tubercles.

nipples did not occur during embryonic development. The most common site is inferior to the normal breast. They are usually asymptomatic. Excision is usually done for cosmesis and rarely for medical indications. Rarely, polythelia may be associated with renal abnormalities, especially if the patient has other congenital abnormalities. Suggest performing an ultrasound scan of the kidneys, bladder and ureters for these patients.

- **Montgomery's tubercles/Morgagni tubercles (Figure 59.3):** Sebaceous glands that appear as small non-pigmented nodules at the edge of the nipple's areola. They secrete lubricating oil with antibacterial properties to keep the nipples and areolas soft during breastfeeding. However, if the glands get obstructed, it can result in inflammation, infection or a Montgomery cyst (i.e., a retroareolar cyst). A Montgomery cyst usually resolves spontaneously. Rarely, the cyst may require drainage or resection.

- *Common benign conditions of the breast:* Fibrocystic change and benign tumours such as fibroadenomas, papillomas and phyllodes tumours.
- *Common malignant lesions: in situ* cancers such as ductal carcinoma *in situ* (DCIS) and infiltrative cancers.

Mammogram (MMG)

- *Mammographic features suspicious for cancer*:
  1. Spiculated or ill-defined masses.
  2. Clusters of heterogeneous or pleomorphic microcalcifications with a linear, branching or casting configuration.
  3. Architectural distortion.
  4. *Others* — lymph node enlargement, skin thickening, nipple retraction.
- Using standard nomenclature and terminology, mammograms are reported using the **BIRADS** scoring system (***B**reast **I**maging **R**eporting and **D**ata **S**ystem*) — refer to **Table 59.1**.
- BIRADS has a scale to classify breast tissue density.
- Dense breast density is defined as categories C or D.
  A — almost entirely fatty.
  B — scattered areas of fibroglandular density.
  C — heterogeneously dense.
  D — extremely dense.

Table 59.1 BIRADS Classifications

BIRADS final assessment categories			
Category		Management	Likelihood of cancer
0	Incomplete assessment Need additional imaging or prior MMG for comparison	Recall for additional imaging or await prior MMG for comparison	N/A
1	Negative	Routine screening	Essentially 0%
2	Benign	Routing screening	Essentially 0%
3	Probably benign	Short-interval follow-up (6 months) or continued surveillance MMG	≤2%
4	Suspicious	Tissue diagnosis Refer to a breast surgeon	4a. *Low* suspicion of malignancy (2–9%) 4b. *Moderate* suspicion of malignancy (10–49%) 4c. *High* suspicion of malignancy (50–94%)
5	Highly suggestive of malignancy	Tissue diagnosis Refer to a breast surgeon	95–100%
6	Known biopsy-proven	Surgical excision, when clinically appropriate	N/A

- The risk of malignancy can be estimated based on the BIRADS score.
- The false-negative rate of MMG is around 10–30%, most commonly in patients with dense breast tissue.
- Up to 15% of cancers detected on clinical breast examination are *not* visible on diagnostic MMG. Therefore, adding a breast ultrasound scan decreases the false-negative rate but does *not* exclude breast cancer.
- If both MMG and ultrasound are negative, the chance of malignancy is 0–3%.

Breast Ultrasound Scan

- An ultrasound scan of the breast is a useful adjunct to distinguish between cystic and solid masses seen on mammograms.
- It is the preferred investigation in patients whose breasts contain dense glandular tissue, such as those aged <35 years or in lactating mothers.
- *Ultrasound scans of the breasts are useful for the following indications*:
  - Evaluating palpable lumps in breasts.
  - Evaluating breast symptoms in young women — in whom MMG is less useful because of the density of their breasts.
  - Evaluating a mass detected on MMG, allowing the mass to be characterised as solid or cystic.
  - Localising and characterising mass lesions detected by MRI screening, enabling them to be biopsied or localised before surgery.
  - As an adjunct to the evaluation of the mammographically dense breast, even when no focal lesion is seen on the MMG.
  - Evaluating the integrity of breast implants.
- Lesions that are solid, hypoechoic, irregular and taller than wide and have shadowing or increased vascularity have an increased risk of malignancy. Therefore, these lesions should be followed up closely for interval change if a biopsy is *not* performed.
- *Breast density* is now recognised as an important consideration in breast cancer screening. This is because dense breast tissue lowers the sensitivity of mammographic screening. In the West, breast density is thought to be associated with an increased breast cancer risk, although this could *not* be proven in an Asian population.

- For women with *dense breasts*, the following are the options to improve breast cancer detection rates:
  1) 3D mammograms (also termed breast tomosynthesis) instead of a conventional 2D mammogram.
  2) Supplemental ultrasound scan of the breasts.
  3) Supplemental MRI breasts.

Breast Biopsy

- When assessing for biopsy, in addition to radiological features, consider other factors such as the age of the patient, the duration of the lesion, family and personal history of breast cancer.
- In the presence of a palpable mass, normal radiological imaging should *not* deter the clinician from performing a biopsy.
- For lesions seen on mammography and/or ultrasound but are *not* palpable, image guidance (using X-rays or ultrasound scans) may be necessary to guide the clinician during the biopsy procedure.

Part 4
Investigations in Gynaecology

CHAPTER 60

Tumour Markers in Gynaecology and Pregnancy

Tumour markers are used to screen, diagnose, guide and monitor response to cancer treatment and to determine recurrences. Some tumour markers are used to stage and prognosticate cancers.

Tumour Markers in Gynaecological Cancers

Type of tumour	Serum tumour marker
Epithelial ovarian cancer	Cancer antigen 125 (CA125)
Mucinous cystadenocarcinoma	CEA and CA19-9
Endodermal sinus tumour/yolk sac tumour	AFP
Choriocarcinoma	βHCG
Embryonal cell carcinoma	βHCG and AFP
Dysgerminoma	LDH
Granulosa cell tumour	Inhibin

Tumour marker	Indication	Management
CA125 (<35.0 U/ml)	To exclude epithelial ovarian cancer or primary peritoneal cancer. Used for monitoring of women with ovarian cancer (to monitor the response to treatment and to detect recurrence). **Not recommended* as routine screening for ovarian cancer because of low specificity and positive predictive value. It has also <u>not</u> been shown to reduce mortality from ovarian cancer.	CA 125 is derived from the pericardium, pleura and peritoneum and can be increased in conditions relating to these areas. ***<u>Causes of raised CA 125</u>*** ***Physiological/benign causes:*** Pregnancy, menstruation, smoking. ***Gynaecological conditions:*** Pelvic inflammatory disease (PID), uterine fibroids, endometriosis, adenomyosis, benign ovarian tumours, functional ovarian cysts, ovarian hyperstimulation syndrome (OHSS), Meigs syndrome. ***Non-gynaecological causes:*** Appendiceal abscess, diverticulitis, colitis, pancreatitis, liver cirrhosis, pleural/pericardial effusion, myocardial infarction, cardiomyopathy, cardiac failure, pneumonia, pulmonary embolism, renal insufficiency, systemic lupus erythematosus (SLE), cystic fibrosis, urinary tract infection (UTI), tuberculosis, peritonitis, recent surgery. ***Malignant causes:*** Ascites due to malignancy. ***Gynaecological cancers:*** Epithelial ovarian cancers (most commonly serous, endometrioid and clear cell carcinoma), fallopian tube and primary peritoneal cancers, endometrial cancer. CA125 may <u>not</u> be raised in early-stage ovarian cancer — it can be normal in 50% of stage 1 ovarian cancer. It is less frequently raised in mucinous ovarian tumours. ***Non-gynaecological cancers:*** Breast, colon, gallbladder, pancreas, liver, lung, haematological malignancies. Perform an *ultrasound pelvis* to exclude pelvic pathology. *Refer to a gynae-oncologist* if a gynaecological malignancy is suspected.
CEA (≤5.0 μg/L)	To exclude primary colorectal cancer. As a tumour marker, to identify recurrences after surgical resection, to localise cancer spread. Not so useful as a screening tool.	CEA is expressed in adenocarcinomas. ***<u>Causes of raised CEA</u>*** ***<u>Benign causes:</u>*** Cirrhosis of the liver. Ulcerative colitis, Crohn's disease. Chronic obstructive lung disease. Pancreatitis. ***<u>Malignant causes:</u>*** **Gynaecological cancers:** Borderline and malignant mucinous ovarian cancer. **Non-gynaecological cancers:** Colorectal, gastrointestinal (GIT), pancreatic, lung, breast cancer. Refer to a general surgeon/colorectal surgeon for oesophagogastroduodenoscopy (OGD) + colonoscopy. Do a mammogram ± ultrasound scan of the breasts.

(*Continued*)

Tumour marker	Indication	Management
βHCG (<5 IU/L) Refer to Chapter 29: *An Overview of Serum Human Chorionic Gonadotrophin*	To exclude germ cell tumours (GCTs).	***Causes of raised βHCG*** ***Benign causes:*** Pregnancy. *Aneuploidy screening* — elevated in trisomy 21 but reduced in trisomies 18 and 13. Exogenous HCG injections. Pituitary HCG in menopause. In response to or recovery from chemotherapy-induced gonadal suppression. Laboratory errors. ***Malignant causes:*** GCT of the ovary, e.g., embryonal carcinoma. Gestational trophoblastic neoplasia (GTN), e.g., invasive mole or choriocarcinoma (refer to Chapter 9: *Approach to Gestational Trophoblastic Disease*).
AFP (≤9 μg/L)	To exclude liver cancer or GCT.	***Causes of raised AFP in non-pregnant women*** ***Benign causes:*** Cirrhosis, hepatitis. ***Malignant causes:*** *Gynaecological*: GCTs, e.g., immature teratoma, endodermal sinus tumour (yolk sac tumour), embryonal carcinoma. Hepatocellular carcinoma (HCC). ***Causes of raised AFP in pregnancy*** *Wrong dates* — pregnancy dating is more accurate (8–10 weeks) using a first-trimester ultrasound scan via the crown-rump length (CRL) than the LMP. *Multiple pregnancies.* *Neural tube defects,* e.g., anencephaly, spina bifida, sacrococcygeal teratoma (SCT). *Abdominal wall defects*, e.g., omphalocele, gastroschisis, complete eventration. *Intrauterine death (IUD).* ***Causes of low AFP in pregnancy*** Wrong dates. Trisomies 21 and 18. Diabetes mellitus.
LDH (120–260 U/L)	To exclude dysgerminoma.	– Raised in dysgerminoma of the ovary. – Pregnancy — can be elevated in pre-eclampsia; haemolysis, elevated liver enzymes and low platelets (HELLP); pulmonary embolism; haemolytic anaemia; infections; adnexal masses. – Non-gynaecological causes: Haemolytic/ megaloblastic anaemia, infections, liver disease, acute myocardial infarction (AMI), muscle damage, cancer (lymphoma, melanoma, renal cell carcinoma), some medications.

(*Continued*)

(*Continued*)

Tumour marker	Indication	Management
Inhibin A/inhibin B Levels of inhibin are *higher* in *pre-menopausal* women and fluctuate during the menstrual cycle. ***Inhibin A*** **Premenopausal:** <97.5 pg/ml **Postmenopausal:** <2.1 pg/ml ***Inhibin B*** **Premenopausal** *Follicular*: <139 pg/ml *Luteal*: <92 pg/ml **Postmenopausal:** <10 pg/ml	To exclude granulosa cell tumour.	– Raised in granulosa cell tumour (inhibin is superior to oestradiol as a tumour marker for granulosa cell tumour). – Can be increased in some epithelial mucinous ovarian tumours. – Inhibin A is also part of the second-trimester quadruple screening for aneuploidy — inhibin levels increase in T21. – High inhibin is also associated with abnormal placentation — higher risk of pre-eclampsia, fetal growth restriction and iatrogenic preterm birth.
Oestradiol (E2) Premenopausal: ≤2,382 pmol/L		May be raised in feminising sex-cord stromal cell tumours, e.g., granulosa cell tumours. ***Please note:*** Oestradiol is **not** a sensitive tumour marker.
Testosterone (nmol/L) 21–49 years: 0.5–1.9 ≥50 years: 0.4–1.2	Abnormal if total testosterone (TT) is >5 nmol/L; needs further evaluation.	May be raised in androgen-secreting sex-cord stromal cell tumours, e.g., Sertoli–Leydig tumours. Perform an ultrasound scan of the pelvis and an androgen profile.
CA 19-9 <34.1 U/ml	*Not useful* as a screening tool. Can have prognostic significance in evaluating the effectiveness of treatment of cancer of exocrine pancreas/GIT cancers.	***Causes of raised CA 19-9*** ***Benign causes:*** Pancreatitis. Liver cirrhosis. Biliary tract disease/obstruction. ***Malignant causes:*** ***Gynaecological:*** Borderline and malignant mucinous ovarian tumours. ***Non-gynaecological:*** Pancreatic, oesophageal, colorectal, hepatocellular, gallbladder, bile duct, gastric cancers. – May need to refer to a hepatobiliary surgeon.
CA 15-3 <30 U/ml	Used in the evaluation of **metastatic** breast cancer and measuring response to treatment.	***Causes of raised CA 15-3*** ***Benign causes:*** Vitamin B12 deficiency. Megaloblastic anaemia. Thalassaemia/sickle cell disease. Endometriosis. Breast conditions. ***Malignant causes:*** Raised especially in advanced breast cancer. Other cancers: Ovary, colon, liver, pancreatic and lung.

Tumour Markers in Pregnancy

Altered by PREGNANCY	Not altered by PREGNANCY
CA125 Elevated in most cases of **epithelial ovarian cancer**. The level of CA 125 rises and peaks in the first trimester and slowly declines with advancing gestation (CA 125 is produced by decidua in pregnancy). **CA 125 level after 16 weeks** is generally **not** affected by *pregnancy*. The evaluation of CA 125 is still advised in the presence of a suspicious adnexal mass. 1. As a baseline test. 2. Indicates potential malignancy when it is grossly elevated. 3. For monitoring treatment response and to detect recurrences in subsequent management.	***LDH*** Elevated in cases of **dysgerminoma** of the ovary. Certain other conditions in *pregnancy* may result in elevated LDH, e.g., pre-eclampsia and HELLP syndrome. Otherwise, LDH is a reliable tumour marker for diagnosing dysgerminomas and follow-up of these tumours during pregnancy.
AFP **Limited role of AFP** in *pregnancy* as it is altered by *pregnancy*. ***Causes of raised AFP:*** 1. *Pregnancy*: – Physiologically up to 2.5 MoM. – Multiple pregnancies. 2. *Fetal/placental abnormality* – Placental abruption. – Neural tube defects, e.g., anencephaly, spina bifida, SCT. – Abdominal wall defects, e.g., omphalocele, gastroschisis, complete eventration. 3. *Malignancy* – GCTs. – Hepatocellular cancer. *In pregnancy*, it can be used as part of the second-trimester aneuploidy screening test for Down syndrome (trisomy 21, T21). – **↓AFP <0.5 MoM** is associated with T21 and trisomy 18. May be of value when the level is grossly elevated — AFP levels **>9 *MoM*** should prompt concern for GCT (gonadal/non-gonadal origin), especially in the absence of *fetal* anomalies (the level associated with NTD is usually much lower). **Screening for NTD is usually performed via a detailed ultrasound scan rather than serum AFP in Singapore.*	***CEA and CA 19-9*** Serum levels are increased during the third trimester of pregnancy. However, despite the elevations, the majority remain within the normal range. ***Causes of raised CEA:*** • Mucinous ovarian tumour (most common). • Serous ovarian tumour. • Colorectal cancer. **CA 19-9** has been found to be raised in *mucinous ovarian tumours* (both borderline and malignant).
βHCG **No role of** βHCG in pregnancy as it is physiologically elevated in pregnancy except for monitoring of pregnancy of unknown location (PUL), ectopic pregnancy and gestational trophoblastic disease (GTD)/GTN.	***CA 15-3*** Elevated in *advanced* breast cancer. A reliable tumour marker in monitoring breast cancer in pregnancy.

βhCG, AFP and CA125 may be physiologically **elevated** in pregnancy.

CHAPTER 61

Female Hormonal Profile in Obstetrics and Gynaecology

- Measurement of follicle-stimulating hormone (FSH), luteinising hormone (LH) and oestradiol (E2) should be done on days 2–4 of menses if there has been a recent menstrual cycle.
- In cases of prolonged amenorrhoea, the testing can be performed anytime.
- The measurement of serum androgens [total testosterone (TT), DHEA-S] is *not useful* in women on combined oral contraceptive pills (COCPs) as COCPs suppress serum gonadotrophins and ovarian androgens, especially testosterone.
- If an evaluation of hormones is needed, COCPs need to be discontinued for at least 8–12 weeks before hormonal testing.

FSH	LH	Oestradiol	Testosterone (total)	Prolactin	Condition
↔/↓	↔/↓	↓	↓	↔	**Hypothalamic amenorrhoea (HA)/ (functional)** – Weight tends to be low or lean. – Ovaries may appear polycystic but with a normal volume. Small uterus and thin endometrium. – The biochemical picture is either low or inappropriately "normal" — in a hypo-oestrogenic state, the appropriate physiological response is stimulation of FSH and LH. Hence, "normal" FSH/LH is actually low. – Serum FSH is typically higher than LH (helps to distinguish HA from PCOS).
↓	↓	↓	↓	↔	**Hypogonadotrophic hypogonadism (HH)** – Weight normal/high. – Ovaries are small/multicystic. – Small uterus and thin endometrium.
↓	↓	↓	↓	↔/↑	**Hypopituitarism (HP)** – A decrease in prolactin is rare. – Ovaries are small. – Small uterus and thin endometrium.
↔	↔/↑	↔	↔/↑	↔/↑	**PCOS** – ≥20 follicles per ovary in either ovary or increased ovarian volume ≥10 ml or follicle number per section ≥10 in either ovary. – Serum LH typically > FSH in PCOS.
↑	↑	↓	↓	↔	<40 years old: **Primary ovarian insufficiency (POI).**
					40–45 years old: **Early menopause (EM).**
					>45 years old: **Menopause (average age in SG is 50–51 years old).**
↔	↔	↔	↔	↔	If amenorrhoea, exclude anatomical defects in the outflow tract, e.g., Müllerian agenesis (absent uterus) or imperforate hymen.
↓	↓	↓	↑↑	↔	**Adrenal tumour**
↓	↓	↓	↔	↑	**Hyperprolactinaemia**

Clinical Interpretation of Female Hormonal Profile

	PCOS	HA, e.g., anorexia, stress, extreme exercise	HH, e.g., craniopharyngioma	HP	Hypergonadotrophic hypogonadism (e.g., POI or menopause)
FSH	Normal	Normal/low	Low	Low	High (>30 IU/ml)
LH	Normal/high	Normal/low	Low	Low	High
E2	Normal	Low	Low	Low	Low (<88 pg/ml)
Anti-Müllerian hormone (AMH)	High	Normal/low	Normal/low	Low	Very low
Testosterone	Normal/high	Low	Low	Low	Low
Body weight	High/normal/low	Low	Normal/high	Any	Any
Uterus	Normal	Normal	Small	Small/normal	Small/normal
Endometrial thickness	Thick	Thin	Thin	Thin	Thin
Morphology of ovaries	Polycystic ovaries (PCO)	PCO	Quiescent/small	Small	Small
Ovarian volume (average volume 5 ml3)	High ≥10 ml	Normal	Normal/low	Low	Low antral follicle count (AFC)
Amenorrhoea	Secondary	Secondary	Primary	Primary/secondary	Primary/secondary

1+A — Hypothalamic Amenorrhoea
1+H — Hypothalamic Hypopituitarism
1+P — Hypopituitarism

Hormone	Result	Implications and actions
Prolactin (7.0–32.9 μg/L)	↑	Refer to Chapter 57: *Approach to Galactorrhoea and Hyperprolactinaemia.*
Prolactin	↓	An isolated hypoprolactinaemia usually does *not* have significant implications.
Total Testosterone (TT) (range: 0.5–1.9 nmol/L) **If TT is >5 nmol/L, further investigations are needed.**	↑	***Causes of elevated TT:*** 1. PCOS (testosterone level can be *mildly* elevated in PCOS, **usually TT <5 nmol/L**). 2. Cushing's syndrome.* 3. Congenital adrenal hyperplasia (CAH).* 4. Androgen-secreting ovarian tumours,* e.g., Leydig, Sertoli–Leydig cell tumours. 5. Androgen-secreting adrenal tumours.* 6. Drugs, e.g., exogenous androgens. Free testosterone can be calculated from TT and SHBG. SHBG testing is *rarely* required, except when there are abnormalities of sex hormone binding (as in this case, TT level can be misleading). Examples include hyperthyroidism, anticonvulsant use and severe obesity.
DHEA-S	↑	DHEA-S is an *adrenal* androgen. Level >700 μg/dl → to evaluate for androgen-secreting ovarian tumours with US pelvis. If US pelvis is negative, the patient will require further evaluation with an **adrenal CT scan** to exclude an androgen-secreting adrenal tumour.
17 Hydroxyprogesterone (17-OHP)	↑	Must be done at 8 a.m. Morning value of >200 ng/dl suggests a diagnosis of non-classical CAH.
AMH	↑	AMH reflects the size of the primordial follicle pool. It is used as a biochemical marker of ovarian function. Different laboratories use different units; our laboratory uses ng/ml, and some use pmol/L. To convert into pmol/L = multiply value in ng/ml with 2.247. To convert into ng/ml = divide the value in pmol/L by 7. **<u>AMH varies according to age.</u>** **It also determines the fertility potential:** **<0.5 ng/ml:** Reduced ovarian reserve <3 follicles in an IVF cycle. **<1.0 ng/ml:** Baseline ovarian reserve with a likelihood of limited eggs at retrieval. **>1.0 but <3.5 ng/ml:** Good response to stimulation. **>3.5 ng/ml:** Vigorous response to ovarian stimulation. High AMH is found in patients with PCOS. Caution should be exercised to avoid OHSS. **AMH levels in women without infertility *do not correlate* with future fertility potential or the time to pregnancy.** **AMH *should <u>not</u>* be used to predict the reproductive status or the onset of menopause.** **If FSH is >10 in a young woman, refer to a fertility specialist to discuss ovarian preservation/assisted reproductive techniques (ARTs).**

(Continued)

(*Continued*)

Hormone	Result	Implications and actions
Progesterone	↑/↓	**Role in gynaecology** is usually in fertility investigation — to confirm the presence of ovulation. It should be done at the mid-luteal phase, i.e., 7 days before the ***next expected period***. E.g., day 21 of a 28-day cycle, day 28 of a 35-day cycle. In women with *prolonged irregular menstrual cycles*, serial measurements may be needed. For example, starting from day 28 of a 35-day cycle and repeated weekly thereafter until the next menstrual cycle. ***<u>Interpretation of serum progesterone results:</u>*** ***>30 nmol/L*: Ovulation has occurred.** ***3–30 nmol/L*:** Either ovulation has not occurred, or the blood test was taken at an inappropriate time. ***<3 nmol/L*:** No ovulation in the previous 14 days. Ovulation induction agents (e.g., letrozole or clomiphene) given on days 2–6 of the menstrual cycle can be considered in women who are anovulatory. However, as letrozole is teratogenic, *pregnancy must be excluded before initiation*. Therefore, a urine pregnancy test is mandatory on day 1 of the menstrual cycle before starting letrozole to induce ovulation. ***<u>Role of serum progesterone in obstetrics is usually in cases of threatened miscarriage:</u>*** **A level of ≥35 nmol/L** indicates a low risk of miscarriage (<10%), and the patient can be reassured. **A level of <35 nmol/L** indicates a higher risk of miscarriage (70–80%); oral progesterone is usually recommended as stated below (KKH regime). ○ **Loading dose** of oral (PO) dydrogesterone (Duphaston) 40 mg once followed by PO Duphaston 10 mg TDS for 2 weeks. ○ ***Alternative*:** PO Utrogestan 200 mg ON × 2 weeks.

CHAPTER 62

Imaging Modalities in Obstetrics and Gynaecology

- Always remember to exclude *pregnancy* — check the last menstrual period (LMP), especially for imaging with ionising radiation. Pregnancy can only be *excluded* by a negative, highly sensitive urine pregnancy test (UPT) that can detect a βHCG level of around 20 mIU/ml if performed *at least 21 days from the last unprotected sexual intercourse* (UPSI).
- Information to be provided on the radiological request form includes — age, pregnancy status, LMP, previous gynaecological surgery (e.g., previous oophorectomy/hysterectomy/polypectomy), any significant medical problems [diabetes mellitus (DM), renal disease, asthma], presenting symptoms, pertinent physical findings, contrast allergy, presence of any foreign body, e.g., intrauterine contraceptive device (IUCD), implants and urgency of the investigation.
- It is also important to mention the differential diagnoses when ordering radiology investigations so that the most appropriate imaging can be ordered.
- If in doubt, the clinician should discuss it with a radiologist to obtain maximum diagnostic yield.
- For an ultrasound (US) scan of the pelvis — to indicate transabdominal (TA) only or both TA and transvaginal scan (TV), depending on the patient's virginity status or preference. TA/TV scan imaging is superior to TA scan alone.
- ***Ionising radiation:*** X-rays, computed tomography (CT) and PET scans, fluoroscopic procedures and nuclear medicine examinations.
- ***Non-Ionising radiation:*** Ultrasound scans and magnetic resonance imaging (MRI) are the preferred imaging modalities in pregnancy.

Radiation Exposures Associated with Common Radiological Investigations

Examination	Typical effective dose (mSv)	Equivalent number of chest X-rays (CXRs)
X-ray		
Limbs and joints (except hip)	<0.01	<0.5
Chest (single PA)	0.02	1
Lumbar spine	1.3	65
Hip	0.3	15
Pelvis	0.7	35
Abdomen	1.0	50
Intravenous urogram (IVU)	2.5	125
Barium meal	3	150
CT head	2.3	115
CT chest	8	400
CT abdomen or pelvis	10	500
MMG	0.21	10
HSG	1.2	60
DEXA bone densitometry	0.01	<0.5
Ultrasound	**No radiation exposure**	
MRI	**No radiation exposure**	

The US Nuclear Regulation Commission (USNRC) recommends total fetal exposure during pregnancy of **<5.0 mSv.**

CT, computed tomography scan; MMG, mammogram; HSG, hysterosalpingogram; MRI, magnetic resonance imaging scan.

Benefits and Limitations of Common Imaging Modalities

Imaging modality	Benefits	Limitations
US scan	• Portable • Relatively inexpensive • Widely available • No radiation risk (suitable for use in pregnancy) • Quick to perform • Can be used in interventional radiology to guide the placement of drains/tubes/ lines or for biopsy	• Highly operator-dependent, *most* operator-dependent imaging modality. • Patient-dependent, e.g., habitus. • Limited diagnostic accuracy in certain conditions.

(*Continued*)

Imaging modality	Benefits	Limitations
X-ray	• Portable • Inexpensive • Widely available — often used as a screening test • Quick to perform	• Radiation risk (can be reduced with shielding). • Limited diagnostic accuracy in certain conditions.
CT scan	• Widely available • Excellent depiction of anatomic detail, e.g., bone • Very fast exam time (5–20 minutes) • Can be used for guided biopsy	• Increases lifetime radiation burden and increases the risk of subsequent carcinogenesis. • May require contrast (caution in renal impairment, DM and dehydration because of the risk of contrast-induced nephropathy). • May need pre-medication for special patient groups (asthma/DM/multiple drug allergies).
MRI	• Superior depiction of soft tissue, e.g., cervical/endometrial cancer staging • No radiation risk (suitable for use in pregnancy)	• Expensive. • May require contrast (see above). • Risk of nephrogenic systemic fibrosis. • May require sedation in patients. • Longer imaging time. • Claustrophobia/patient anxiety. • *Contraindicated* in patients with metal implants, metallic intraocular foreign bodies, hearing aids, cardiac implantable electronic devices (CIEDs), e.g., pacemakers, and tattoos. Nowadays, MRI-conditional CIEDs are widely available. Hence, it is important to clarify the type of CIED and its compatibility with MRI. • *Contraceptive devices*: ▪ Filshie® clips are made of titanium and are hence safe for MRI scans up to 3T. ▪ Essure® device consists of a stainless-steel coil wrapped within a nickel–titanium alloy outer coil. It is conditionally safe for MRI scans up to 3T, based on the manufacturer. ▪ IUCD: – All plastic IUCDs, e.g., Mirena®, are MRI-safe. – Copper IUCDs are safe for imaging up to 3T. – ***Unsafe:*** Stainless-steel ring-shaped devices used exclusively in China between 1988 and 2000 are *not* safe for MRI.

Radiological Evaluation of a Patient Presenting With Acute Abdominal Pain

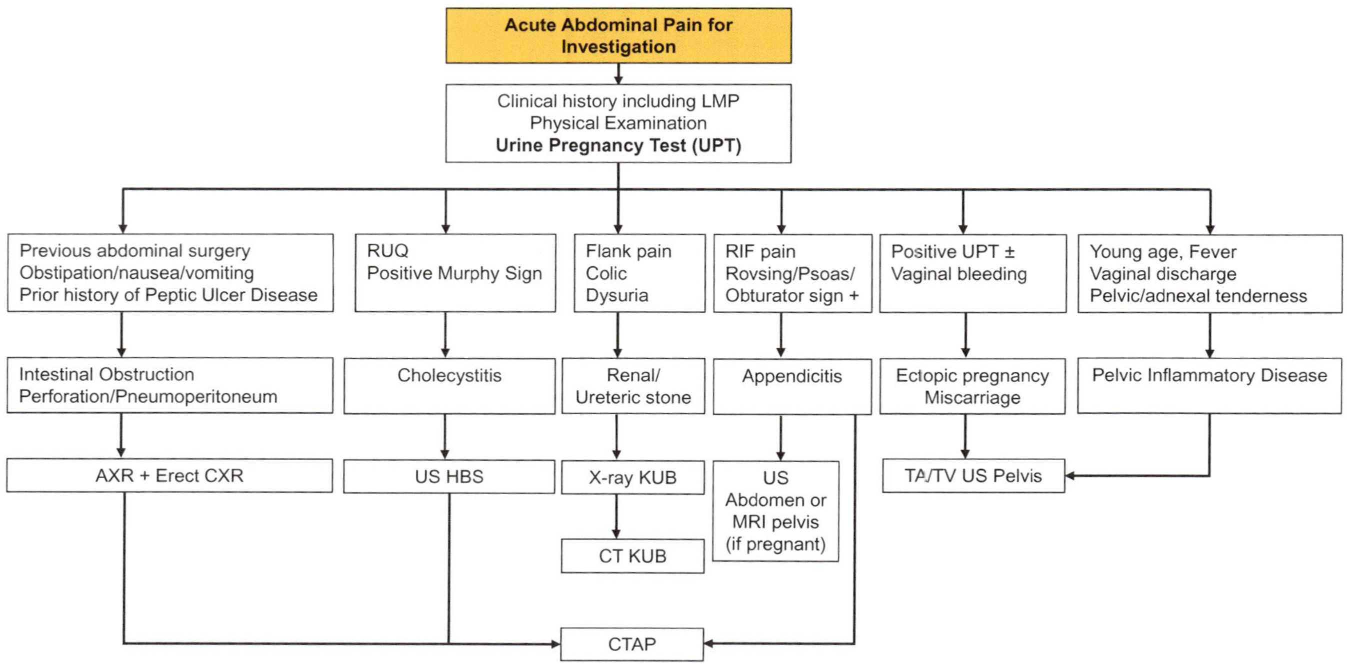

Diagnostic imaging modality	Follow-up action
Chest X-ray (CXR) • Ideally, posteroanterior (PA) erect. • Portable anteroposterior (AP) erect is not equivalent to PA erect. • Supine AP radiographs should only be performed for very ill patients who cannot stand or sit up. • **Safe in pregnancy in all trimesters (with an abdominal shield).**	To assess respiratory, cardiac and chest wall pathology. Indications for CXR: • Pre-op assessment for selected patients, e.g., age ≥70, history of chronic lung disease (for a full list, refer to the section *Pre-Operative Investigations* in Chapter 64: *Pre-Operative Anaesthetic Information*). • As part of septic work-up to exclude lung pathology, e.g., pneumonia. • Chest symptoms, e.g., shortness of breath (SOB), chronic cough, fever, chest pain or trauma, desaturation. • Correlate for patients with clinical signs suggestive of cardiac failure/ pulmonary oedema. • Diagnosis and follow-up of pulmonary tuberculosis. • Check tube placement, e.g., a nasogastric tube (NGT), a chest tube, an endotracheal tube (ETT), a central venous catheter (CVC), a peripherally inserted central catheter (PICC). • Assess for rib fractures (need oblique views correlating to the side of pain). • Detection of foreign bodies. • Follow up to monitor response to treatment, e.g., antibiotics for pneumonia. • Part of the investigations to detect perforated viscus — subdiaphragmatic free gas on the erect CXR. *Action*: • When in doubt, please consult the duty radiologist for an opinion. • Multidisciplinary management — may need further imaging: US chest if pleural or pericardial effusion is suspected, CT thorax for further characterisation of lung pathology, CT pulmonary angiogram (CTPA) in suspected pulmonary embolism (PE). • Treatment is dependent on the pathology found.
Abdominal X-ray (AXR) ***Supine AXR*** — coverage from the diaphragm to the abdomen. May *not* include pubic symphysis. AXR is useful in detecting intestinal obstruction and ileus or in locating sizeable (>5 mm) radio-opaque foreign bodies. ***Erect or decubitus AXR*** is useful in tandem with a supine radiograph to confirm the presence of free gas. Erect AXR is *not* a substitute for a supine radiograph.	• To look for "gas", masses and stones. • The presence of gas–fluid levels is seen in intestinal obstruction or postoperative ileus. • The absence of gas-fluid levels does not exclude intestinal obstruction, as the intestines may be distended with fluid. • Mural thickening of the bowel wall and the presence of tiny mural gas pockets suggest ischaemic bowel and impending perforation. • Look for a sudden change in bowel calibre — points to the level of obstruction. • While perforation of a viscus is associated with free abdominal air (better demonstrated on erect or decubitus projection), the absence of free air does *not* completely exclude perforation. • To look for foreign bodies, e.g., a missing IUCD, retained surgical gauze. • To check the placement of radio-opaque tubes and abdominal catheters. • Depending on the clinical condition, the patient's BMI and the location of pain, an abdominal or pelvic ultrasound scan may be useful as the next line of investigation. • *CT scan of the abdomen and pelvis* is the next investigation tool for abdominal pain, able to localise the level of transition for post-surgical ileus and identify and characterise masses, foreign bodies and other pathologies.
X-ray of kidney, ureter and bladder (KUB) Includes pubic symphysis (c.f. AXR, see above).	• Indicated in cases of renal or ureteric colic but can also be used to investigate intestinal obstruction as it allows visualisation of rectal gas. • 80–90% sensitivity if radio-opaque stones >3 mm. • Can assess symphysis pubis diastasis and sacroiliac joints in postnatal patients.

(*Continued*)

(*Continued*)

Diagnostic imaging modality	Follow-up action
Ultrasound pelvis (either TA scan alone or TA + TV scan). **TA scan only:** Need a full bladder. For patients *without* sexual history or vaginismus or who decline a TV scan. **TA scan** is useful for evaluating the abdomen and upper pelvis, i.e., for large masses. **TV scan** is in direct/close apposition to the genital organs. Useful for obese patients and early pregnancy evaluation. Evaluates pelvic structures better, i.e., uterine size, endometrial thickness and polyps. **TA + TV scan:** For patients with sexual history. TA/TV scan imaging is superior to TA scan alone.	Most ordered imaging modality by gynaecologists. Important ultrasound scan findings include: **Gynaecological scan:** to assess the uterus, endometrial cavity, ovaries and adnexa. *Indications* • Assess the menstrual cycle, e.g., endometrial thickness (ET varies with the cycle; tamoxifen use may increase the ET), follicular tracking. • Evaluate symptoms, i.e., abnormal uterine bleeding, postmenopausal bleeding, postcoital/intermenstrual bleeding, dysmenorrhoea, pelvic pain. • Assess and follow up on pelvic masses/previously detected abnormalities, e.g., fibroids, ovarian cysts/masses. • Assess for ovarian torsion, e.g., whirlpool sign. • Assess and follow up for pelvic infections and their complications, e.g., hydrosalpinx, tubo-ovarian abscesses. • Evaluate endocrine abnormalities, e.g., polycystic ovarian syndrome (PCOS). • Evaluate Müllerian anomalies of the uterus or vagina, e.g., uterine didelphys, bicornuate or septate uterus. • Assess for haematometra/pyometra. • Locate an IUCD. • Evaluate the pelvic floor in women with urogynaecological issues, e.g., pelvic organ prolapse and urinary incontinence and check post-void residual volume. • Evaluate women with subfertility/infertility. • Screen or investigate for gynaecological malignancies. • Pre- and postoperative assessment of pelvic organs. • Assess post-surgical complications. • Assess post-pregnancy/miscarriage/termination complications. **Recommended to scan on days 2–10 to follow up on functional ovarian cysts.** **Obstetrics:** *First trimester* — usually done by obstetricians. To send for a scan by a radiologist if a second opinion is needed. *Ultrasound scan:* • To confirm the location of the fetus, viability, dating, number of fetal poles, chorionicity for multiple gestations (between 11 and 14 weeks of gestation). • To check the presence of other masses such as fibroids or ovarian cysts in pregnancy. • Presence of multiple cystic spaces in the endometrium suggestive of molar pregnancy. • FTS scan at 11 to 13 + 6 weeks is part of the aneuploidy screening test — assesses nuchal translucency (NT) and presence of nasal bone (NB). *Second to third trimesters* • Screening scan for fetal structural anomalies at about 20 weeks. • Growth and Doppler scans, if applicable. Ultrasound is also used as an adjunct for procedures such as chorionic villus sampling (CVS), amniocentesis and oocyte pick-up. **If any abnormalities are detected, consult an obstetrician for further management.**

(Continued)

Diagnostic imaging modality	Follow-up action
Ultrasound Doppler of lower limbs	To exclude deep vein thrombosis (DVT). To map venous anatomy for varicose veins. In cases of suspected PE (pulmonary embolism) with confirmed DVT on US Doppler, CTPA is *not* required for a diagnosis of PE. Anticoagulation should be commenced immediately.
Ultrasound kidney, ureter, bladder (KUB) (focused on KUB)	**Indications for ultrasound KUB:** • Evaluation of renal parenchyma and cystic kidney disease. • Diagnosis of hydronephrosis. • Measurement of kidney size and echogenicity as part of an evaluation of chronic kidney disease. • Cysts, tumours, abscesses, obstructions, fluid collection and infections within or around the kidneys. • Urinary tract obstruction. • In patients with uterine anomalies, to exclude co-existing renal tract malformations. Renal anomalies are found in 20–30% of patients with Müllerian defects.
Ultrasound abdomen Assesses hepatobiliary system (HBS), gallbladder, spleen, pancreas, portal venous system, free fluid in abdomen and kidneys.	• To evaluate non-specific abdominal pain or masses (first-line imaging in pregnancy). • 6–8 hours of fasting is required to distend the gallbladder. • May need to drink water before the ultrasound scan if the stomach is distended with gas.
Ultrasound hepatobiliary system (HBS)	**Indications for ultrasound HBS:** • Biliary colic • Acute cholecystitis • Jaundice and biliary duct dilatation • Gallstones • Sepsis • Ascites • Hepatic abnormalities (e.g., transaminitis) **Management:** Treatment depends on the cause; refer to a gastroenterologist or a hepatobiliary surgeon.
CT scan abdomen/pelvis (CTAP) Coverage of scan includes from the level of the diaphragm to pubic symphysis. Routine scans are performed in the portovenous phase (please discuss with the radiologist if looking for a bleeding source or characterising liver lesions as they may require different scan protocols).	• Commonly used to investigate abdominal pain or pelvi-abdominal mass and guide further management. • CTAP is superior to AXR for the investigation of abdominal pain and can be used for: o Detection of appendicitis, diverticulitis and colitis. o Diagnosis of abdominal/pelvic collections in patients with persistent sepsis. o Confirmation of suspected postoperative complications, e.g., haemorrhage, infection/collection, visceral injuries (bladder, bowel, ureter) and ileus/intestinal obstruction. • A multiphasic scan (including plain, arterial, venous and delayed phases) is important to diagnose arterial bleed and differentiate it from venous bleed. • Venous bleeds, if significant and prolonged, are <u>not</u> treatable by embolisation.

(Continued)

(*Continued*)

Diagnostic imaging modality	Follow-up action
CT scan Thorax/abdomen /pelvis (CTTAP) Coverage from the thoracic inlet to the pubic symphysis. Different scan trigger time than for assessment of PE (pulmonary embolism).	Used as part of staging for gynaecological cancers, especially ovarian cancer.
CT Pulmonary Angiogram (CTPA) Triggered for maximum enhancement within the pulmonary trunk. *Not* to withhold in pregnancy if clinically indicated.	To detect PE (pulmonary embolism). Other lung pathology may also be demonstrated *if confirmed PE*: MDT care. Resuscitate patient and therapeutic anticoagulation with low-molecular-weight heparin (LMWH). ***Other treatment considerations:*** US Doppler scan of the lower limbs to look for DVT. Thrombolytics. IVC *Filter* if there is DVT, but the patient is <u>*not*</u> suitable for thrombolytics. Catheter or surgical embolectomy (transfer to Singapore General Hospital as there is no cardiothoracic support setup at KKH).
CT brain Can be done if indicated in pregnancy.	Readily available in the acute setting and useful for diagnosing intracranial haemorrhage, acute infarct and space-occupying lesions. May need to supplement with an MRI brain.
MRI brain	Preferred brain imaging modality in *pregnancy* as there is <u>*no*</u> ionising radiation with MRI.
MRI pelvis	MRI is a superior imaging modality for the evaluation of soft tissue masses (e.g., fibroids with an atypical appearance on US pelvis). Used to characterise and stage endometrial and cervical cancers. Also, for evaluation of abdominal pain in *pregnancy* when the US scan is inconclusive and appendicitis or other gastrointestinal pathology is suspected.
MRI in pregnancy A fetal MRI scan may be indicated to characterise findings detected on antenatal ultrasound.	*Safety in pregnancy* MRI is safe for the mother and fetus in the second and third trimesters. During the first trimester, it should be restricted to maternal indications for which the information is considered clinically imperative. Inadvertent exposure to magnetic resonance imaging during the first trimester has **not** been associated with any long-term sequelae. Gadolinium contrast may be used in pregnant women when the benefits outweigh the potential risks. It is safe to continue breastfeeding after receiving a gadolinium contrast agent. Gadolinium crosses the placenta and is excreted by the fetal kidneys into the amniotic fluid. Concerns of nephrogenic systemic fibrosis. No reported adverse human fetal effects. <u>***Clinical uses of MRI in pregnancy***</u> **1. <u>Fetal</u>** • **MRI brain** (e.g., to evaluate abnormalities seen on the US or following fetal infections or an intrauterine demise of one twin in monochorionic twins). • **Oropharynx or face** — assess oropharyngeal anatomy where airway patency may be compromised by masses or mandibular or other facial malformations.

(Continued)

Diagnostic imaging modality	Follow-up action
	• **Neck** — neck masses relative to the fetal airway can be assessed, which can assist in managing delivery when an EXIT (*ex utero* intrapartum treatment) procedure is being considered, e.g., fetal goitre and thyroid. • **Thoracic** — e.g., bronchopulmonary sequestration (BPS), congenital pulmonary airway malformation (CPAM), congenital diaphragmatic hernia (CDH). • Assessment and characterisation of vascular tumours or malformations. If rapidly growing, a trial of sirolimus to shrink the lesion *in utero* may be attempted. • **Intra-abdominal** — presence of bowel within the thorax in CDH. It can also confirm suspected bowel obstruction and anorectal malformations. • **MRI spine** — can be used to confirm/characterise suspected spinal cord anomalies. **2. *Maternal*** • **Evaluate abdominal pain or masses**, e.g., bowel, kidneys, bladder, ovarian and adnexal masses. • **Placental accreta spectrum** — MRI is the imaging method of choice when there is a risk of posterior placenta increta or percreta.
MRI abdomen	Evaluation of abdominal pain in *pregnancy* when the US scan is inconclusive.
Mammogram (MMG) **Ultrasound breast**	Refer to Chapter 59: *Breast Cancer Screening and Diagnostic Tests.*
Hysterosalpingogram (HSG) *X-ray* + iodine-based dye. Consider azithromycin 1 g as antibiotic prophylaxis before any tubal patency test, especially in women with a history of pelvic inflammatory disease or known abnormal tubes (administered as a single dose to be consumed with sips of water on the morning of the procedure). ***Disadvantages of HSG:*** Ionising radiation risk. Pain/syncope. Contrast allergy. Perforation.	This test evaluates tubal patency and endometrial pathology: • Cavity — shape, pathology, e.g., endometrial polyps, fibroids, uterine synechiae/septum. • Tubal — patency and pathology, e.g., hydrosalpinx, cornual block, salpingitis isthmica nodosa. It does ***not*** evaluate uterine (e.g., fibroids) and ovarian pathology and antral follicle count (AFC). HSG is performed between **days 6 and 11** of the menstrual cycle. *Indications for HSG:* • Recurrent miscarriages • Routine work-up for subfertility • Suspected uterine anomalies • Suspected intrauterine adhesions (Asherman syndrome) *Contraindications for HSG:* • Pregnancy • Undiagnosed vaginal bleeding • Active pelvic infection • History of severe reaction to iodinated contrast
Hysterosalpingo foam contrast sonography (Hyfosy) *Ultrasound* + saline infusion followed by ExEm foam gel. Antibiotic prophylaxis as per HSG. No ionising radiation risk.	This test evaluates: • Uterus — pathology, e.g., uterine anomalies • Cavity — shape, pathology, e.g., endometrial polyps, submucosal fibroids, intrauterine adhesion (Asherman syndrome) • Ovaries — pathology, AFC • Tubal — patency, pathology **Timing:** Within 10 days after the period has cleared, i.e., perform between days 10 and 15 of the menstrual cycle.

(Continued)

(Continued)

<table>
<tr><th>Diagnostic imaging modality</th><th>Follow-up action</th></tr>
<tr><td>Bone mineral densitometry (BMD)
<u>Indications for BMD:</u>
(Adapted from the National Osteoporosis Foundation).
1. Age >65 years.
2. Age 50–69 years with clinical risk factors for fractures.
3. Adults aged >50 years with fractures.
4. Adults with co-morbidities that increase the risk of osteoporosis e.g., rheumatoid arthritis or prednisolone use (>5 mg for more than 3 months duration).</td>
<td>Purpose: to screen for osteoporosis
<table>
<tr><th>Diagnosis</th><th>T-score criteria on BMD</th></tr>
<tr><td>Normal</td><td>≥−1.0</td></tr>
<tr><td>Low bone mass (osteopenia)</td><td>Between −1.0 and −2.5</td></tr>
<tr><td>Osteoporosis</td><td>≤−2.5</td></tr>
<tr><td>Severe (established) osteoporosis</td><td>≤−2.5 and fragility fracture</td></tr>
</table>
Consider repeating BMD testing 1–2 years after starting pharmacological therapy, and every 2–3 years thereafter or as soon as 6 months after initiating steroid therapy or perhaps never if very little change is expected or the results of testing are unlikely to influence patient management decisions.
<u>Management of osteoporosis:</u> (Refer to Chapter 55: Osteoporosis for more information)
1) Lifestyle measures
a. Diet, exercise
b. Reduce or stop smoking/alcohol
c. Fall precautions
d. Correct reversible causes, e.g., reviewing medications causing osteoporosis
2) Pharmacological therapy
a. Calcium/vitamin D3
b. Bisphosphonates (PO or IV)
c. Denosumab injection — 6 monthly
d. Recombinant parathyroid hormone
e. Romosozumab
f. Selective oestrogen receptor modulator
g. Menopausal Hormone Therapy (MHT)
h. Calcitonin (rarely recommended)
3) MDT
a. Menopause specialist
b. Physiotherapists
c. Orthopaedics — if fractures are present</td></tr>
</table>

CHAPTER 63

Role of Interventional Radiology (IR) in Obstetrics and Gynaecology

Interventional radiology (IR) refers to minimally invasive, image-guided medical interventions. IR procedures utilise real-time imaging modalities such as ultrasound (US), computed tomography (CT) scans or magnetic resonance imaging (MRI) to guide the radiologist. IR can be used as an alternative to some traditional surgery, resulting in better outcomes as it is less invasive, thus resulting in a shorter hospital stay and faster recovery.

Imaging Modalities Used for IR

1. US Scan

a) *Most frequently used because of the following advantages*
- Real-time imaging enables the tracking of needle trajectory.
- Detailed characterisation of cystic collections.
- Colour and pulse Doppler to identify vessels and vascularity.
- Non-ionising radiation.
- Availability of different probes for different regions — transcutaneous, transvaginal (TV), transrectal (TR).
- Quick start-up time.
- Equipment is relatively inexpensive.

b) *Conditions that are limited by penetration of the US*
- Deep-seated lesions.
- Overlying lung, gas-filled bowels, calcifications, calculi, bone.
- Obese patients.
- Not all lesions seen on CT or MRI are visible on US scan.

c) *Portability*
- The flexibility of performing location, though it would be best to be in a sterile environment.
- Possibility of intraoperative assessment and localisation of lesions that may be occult on palpation.

CT Scan

a) *Frequently used for*
- Deep-seated lesions/collections, structures such as retroperitoneal masses/nodes and pelvic masses beyond the reach of the TV/TR approach.
- Pulmonary/thoracic applications.
- Bone biopsy/ablation.

b) *Easier and better appreciation of anatomy*
- Easier to appreciate the relationship of structures with a complete view of the section.
- Accurate needle placement in experienced hands.

c) *Limitations of CT scan*
- Ionising radiation to patients and staff.
- CT fluoroscopy, when used intermittently, has the potential for a shift of needle position between imaging.
- Need time to warm up the machine.
- Vessels may not be delineated from adjacent structures on an unenhanced CT scan.

MRI Scan

a) *Uses of MRI*
- For biopsy of lesions that are occult on ultrasound and CT scans.
- It can be used for pregnant women where ionising radiation is to be avoided.

b) *Limitations of MRI*
- High cost.
- Specialised magnetic-resonance-compatible equipment, e.g., monitoring devices and needles, is required.

General Risks of IR Procedures

1. *Anxiety/discomfort/pain*
   - Most procedures are performed with the patient still conscious.
   - Occasionally, patients who are sensitive may feel the passage of the needle or catheter into the body.
   - Prolonged procedure or inability to adequately anaesthetise the needle/catheter tract because of limitation of needle length or proximity of the major vessel to the site
2. *Haemorrhage*
   - Usually related to inadvertent puncture of an artery and may *not* be immediately noticed because of small incisions
   - Haematoma may take days to weeks to resolve.
   - May require transfusion with blood or blood products
3. *Infection*
   - Usually very rare as skin preparation follows surgical standards and incisions are tiny
   - Related to an inadvertent transgression of infected collections
   - Immunocompromised patients
4. *Radiation exposure (fluoroscopy and CT-guided procedures)*
   - Local skin discolouration/burns
   - Long-term carcinogenic risks

Common IR procedures done at KK Hospital — refer to the table below:

1. Aspiration and drainage
2. Biopsy
3. Vascular access devices
4. Prophylactic placement of bilateral internal iliac artery balloons
5. Angio-embolisation
6. Percutaneous nephrostomy
7. Antegrade ureteric stenting
8. Varicose vein ablation
9. Fallopian tube recanalisation (FTR)

Procedure	Indications/modality	Pre-procedure preparation	Post-procedure care/risks
1. *Aspiration/drainage* Aspiration • Usually with an 18/19 G sheathed needle or a 21/22 G Chiba needle. • The tract is usually *not* dilated. • May safely transgress structures with minimal or no significant damage. • May be considered as an alternative to drainage if the bleeding risk is increased, but a fluid sample or decompression of a collection is necessary. • For small collections (<3 cm diameter) — unsuitable for drain insertion. • Reduced recovery time of aspiration compared to drainage. Drainage • A pigtail drainage catheter is usually inserted, directly or after tract dilatation, over a guidewire to allow further fluid egress. • Used when the volume is large.	*Indications* 1. *Diagnostic* – For microbiological investigations – Cytology 2. *Therapeutic* (i) Abscess drainage For complex/inspissated collections a. Allow time for liquefaction b. Allow daily flushing to thin out fluid for easier drainage (ii) Decompress → relieve pressure symptoms *Modality* 1. Ultrasound — most used 2. CT scan — for deep-seated collections or collections complicated by the presence of a large amount of gas 3. Fluoroscopy — usually used in combination with a US scan to delineate the extent of the collection	– Similar pre-operative investigations because of the risk of bleeding or damage to adjacent structures, which may require surgery. – Discussion of the case with an interventional radiologist (IR). – Completed procedure forms with relevant history and details. – Informed consent. *Blood tests:* 1. Full blood count (FBC) — haemoglobin/platelet count. 2. Coagulation panel (PT/APTT). 3. Type and screen (T&S) if there is a low bleeding risk. Group and crossmatch (GXM) if deranged blood parameters or coagulopathy present. – *Fasting:* At least 3–6 hours before the procedure to avoid risks associated with reflux/vomiting and aspiration. – Commence intravenous (IV) fluids containing dextrose if diabetic or prolonged fasting. – IV sedation is usually required for TV/TR procedures. – *Antibiotic cover for:* 1. Infected/likely infected collections. 2. Possibility of the transgression of the bowel. 3. Obstructed ductal systems. – Cessation of antiplatelet and anticoagulation therapy to reduce the risk of prolonged/profuse bleeding. – Appropriately filled and labelled specimen forms and bottles.	i. Vital signs — a surrogate marker for haemorrhage. Peripheral pulse quality may hint at extrinsic compression on pelvic vessels by a haematoma. The first 4–6 hours are crucial to identify arterial bleeding. ii. Observe the wound site (open dressing to inspect) — bleeding, infection. iii. Observe the patient for pain and other unexpected symptoms such as increasing swelling/girth around the biopsy site. iv. Maintain IV access or IV fluids to replace the blood loss. v. Low threshold for imaging if massive blood loss is suspected, including arterial phase if a CT scan is performed.

(Continued)

Procedure	Indications/modality	Pre-procedure preparation	Post-procedure care/risks
2. *Biopsy* *Routes* i. The transabdominal route is less invasive, although some pelvic masses may be better accessed via TV or TR routes ii. Transthoracic for pulmonary lesions	<u>*Indications*:</u> 1. Histological confirmation of disease before definitive treatment 2. Imaging findings are atypical or inconclusive 3. To exclude a secondary pathology <u>*Modality*:</u> 1. Ultrasound guidance (90%) 2. CT guidance for lungs, bones and deep-seated soft tissue lesions or complex anatomy 3. MR guidance for lesions that are occult on ultrasound and CT scans	– Discussion of the case with an IR. – Completed procedure forms with relevant history and details. – Informed consent. – *Blood tests*: FBC, PT/APTT, T&S if low bleeding risk. GXM if deranged blood parameters or coagulopathy present. – <u>*Fasting*:</u> At least 3–6 hours to avoid risks associated with reflux/vomiting and aspiration. – Commence IV fluids containing dextrose if diabetic or prolonged fasting. – IV sedation is usually required for TV/TR procedures. – Antibiotic prophylaxis is <u>*not*</u> routinely required. – Cessation of antiplatelet and anticoagulation therapy to reduce the risk of prolonged/profuse bleeding. – Appropriately filled and labelled specimen forms and bottles.	i. Similar to that of aspiration and drainage ii. Angiography and embolisation if arterial bleeding or large pseudo-aneurysm identified on imaging subsequently <u>*Specific Risks*:</u> i. Collateral injury — bowel, bladder, vessels (depending on the location of the biopsy target) ii. Pseudo-aneurysm — apposition of the artery to the vein with subsequent healing iii. Haemorrhage — especially if the artery transgressed iv. Spillage of bowel contents v. Urine leakage
3. *Vascular access devices* ***Types*** **A. *Peripherally inserted central catheter (PICC)*** • *Normal versus power injectable* a. Power-injectable PICC may withstand the high flow rates and injection pressures required for contrast administration for future CT scans. b. Slightly more costly compared to regular PICC	<u>*Indications*:</u> 1. Difficult venous access. 2. Parenteral nutrition. 3. Administration of medications: Chemotherapy agents, blood clotting factors, prolonged antibiotic use. 4. Frequent blood sampling. <u>*Modality*:</u> 1. Ultrasound-guided needle access.	– Prior discussion of the case with an IR. – Completed procedure forms with relevant history and details. – Informed consent. – <u>*Fasting*</u> — 4 hours (in consideration of the potential for a contrast reaction and the possible need for sedation). – *Blood tests* — FBC, PT/PTT (for CVC and ports). – Blood tests are <u>*not*</u> needed for PICCs.	i. Weekly change of dressing, or earlier whenever soiled, including a Statlock device ii. Sterile technique when accessing a vascular access device iii. Flush with normal saline before heparinisation/ Taurolock to clear the residual drug from a catheter

(Continued)

(Continued)

Procedure	Indications/modality	Pre-procedure preparation	Post-procedure care/risks
• <u>*Cuffed versus uncuffed*</u> (i) Fibrous cuff buried under the skin at the catheter entry site; usually takes 2–3 weeks; thereafter, does *not* slip easily or dislodge (ii) Fibrous ingrowth around the cuff potentially excludes the catheter from ascending infection, secures the catheter *in situ* and reduces chances of accidental pull-out of the catheter. (iii) Requires blunt dissection to loosen the cuff at removal • <u>Single-, double- or triple-lumen options</u> (i) Normally, external diameters of the catheters do *not* differ very much; as such, more lumens generally mean smaller lumen sizes and a potentially higher likelihood of blockage of each lumen. (ii) Catheters are usually cut to length, and both lumens are flush (at the same level). **B. *Central venous catheter (CVC)*** • <u>*Tunnelled*</u> (i) Usually inserted via an infra-clavicular subcutaneous tunnel into the internal jugular vein with a catheter tip positioned within the superior vena cava (SVC). The external jugular vein is sometimes used if the internal jugular vein is stenosed/occluded.	2. Fluoroscopy to confirm guidewire location in IVC. Measuring the Mandrel wire tip location helps determine the catheter length required. 3. Venogram — useful to delineate venous anatomy, especially when unable to advance catheter because of stenosis/spasm. <u>*Routes*</u> i. <u>*PICC*</u> — usually basilic or brachial vein in the arm. Cephalic vein when medial arm veins are exhausted. Seldom placed in the forearm. Very rarely in the lower limb veins (great saphenous). ii. <u>*CVC and ports*</u> — internal jugular vein, subclavian vein.	– *Local anaesthesia*: Topical EMLA cream is applied to the skin of the puncture site 20–30 minutes before the procedure.	iv. Urokinase/recombinant tissue plasminogen activator (rTPA) to dissolve fibrin sheath <u>*Specific Risks:*</u> i. Collateral injury to the adjacent artery, resulting in thromboembolism, pseudo-aneurysm, arteriovenous shunt ii. Pneumothorax iii. Thrombophlebitis/phlebitis iv. Haematoma v. Fibrin sheath formation vi. Thrombus formation within the catheter or in the vein around the catheter vii. Catheter slippage/pull out

(Continued)

Procedure	Indications/modality	Pre-procedure preparation	Post-procedure care/risks
(ii) Fibrous ingrowth around the cuff (~2 weeks) has advantages and disadvantages such as cuffed PICCs. • *<u>Non-tunnelled</u>* (i) May be inserted via the subclavian, internal or external jugular and femoral veins (ii) Easily removed at the end of therapy (iii) Possible slippage/accidental pull-out (iv) Ascending infection if patient's dressing is not optimally maintained • *<u>Dialysis versus non-pheresible</u>* (i) Dialysable catheters are of a larger calibre to ensure adequate flow for dialysis and harvesting of stem cells. **C. *Implanted vascular access port system (port-a-cath)*** • Single- or dual-port reservoirs a. Different sizes available b. Insertion is like tunnelled CVC, with an additional step of creating a subcutaneous pocket for the port reservoir • Different materials a. Silastic/plastic variants with a radio-opaque marker base b. Metallic — titanium • Surgical incision to create and remove the port a. Larger scar than that of a tunnelled CVC b. Infection control considerations • Trained personnel to access and manage • Skin puncture for every access			

(Continued)

(*Continued*)

Procedure	Indications/modality	Pre-procedure preparation	Post-procedure care/risks
4. *Prophylactic placement of bilateral internal iliac artery balloons* *If used for obstetric cases:* – Vascular sheaths and balloon catheter secured to the skin. – Patient transferred to the operating room for a caesarean section. – Bilateral occlusion balloons are inflated as soon as the umbilical cord is ligated. – Balloons deflated after haemostasis is secured to inspect for any residual ooze/bleed. – Balloon catheters are then deflated and removed. – The left groin sheath is removed, leaving the right groin sheath to maintain access overnight, with a view for emergent angio-embolisation should there be unexpected heavy bleeding PV/from the surgical drain or sudden precipitous/unexplained drop in haemoglobin level. – Proceed for angio-embolisation if the placenta remains *in situ.* – Removal of left groin sheath if placenta delivered or subtotal hysterectomy performed.	*Indications* 1. Placenta accreta spectrum (PAS) 2. Placenta praevia 3. Any other obstetric or gynaecological conditions with the potential for severe haemorrhage *Modalities* 1. Ultrasound-guided access into bilateral common femoral arteries 2. Fluoroscopy – Low dose, minimal exposure – Confirm the location of the balloon catheter and the volume needed to occlude internal iliac arteries – Ensure balloons are deflated and in a good position	– Prior consultation at the IR clinic (for a thorough explanation of the procedure and to obtain informed consent) – Prior discussion of the case with an IR – Completed procedure forms with relevant history and details – *Blood tests*: FBC, PT/PTT, GXM – Cessation of antiplatelet and anticoagulation therapy to reduce the risk of prolonged/profuse bleeding – Fasting for 6 hours (anaesthesia, contrast reaction) – Shaving (optional in emergent situations) – Bladder catheter (decompress bladder, monitor intake and output)	– Monitor for 24 hours in an ICU – IV pump infusion of normal saline at 10 ml/hour to *in situ* right common femoral artery sheath to prevent thromboembolism – Monitor dorsalis pedis and posterior tibial pulses *Risks:* i. Groin haematoma ii. Infection iii. Arterial dissection iv. Contrast allergy/reaction v. Vascular dissection/rupture
5. *Angio-embolisation* *Embolic agents used* **(i) *Gelfoam slurry*** – Used in emergency haemorrhage. – Temporary, dissolves in days to weeks. – Inexpensive.	*Indications* 1. PAS with placenta left *in situ* after caesarean delivery. 2. Uterine fibroids (as a standalone procedure). 3. Bleeding tumour (either standalone for palliation or as	– *Consultation at the IR clinic* (for a thorough explanation of the procedure, counsel on risks and provide alternative treatments before obtaining informed consent) – *Baseline US/MRI scan to document*	i. *Post-embolisation syndrome* o First 72 hours o Pain — need for opiate patient-controlled analgesia (PCA) pump o Nausea and vomiting

(Continued)

Procedure	Indications/modality	Pre-procedure preparation	Post-procedure care/risks
– Low risk of non-target collateral embolisation. – Permanent particulate agents. **b. *Polyvinyl alcohol (PVA)*** – Variable size range. – Least expensive permanent embolic agent. – Some reports of long-term recanalisation of vessels. **c. *Embospheres*** – Uniform size and shape → possible better/closer packing. – Costlier than PVA. **d. *Drug-eluting beads*** – May be coated with a chemotherapeutic agent for slow release into the target organ. – Currently used for hepatic tumours. **e. *Metallic coils*** a. Stainless-steel coils. b. Nitinol coils — MRI compatible. c. Fibre-lined coils — better thrombogenesis. d. Controlled release coils — able to remove if noted to be unsuitable after initial deployment. **f. *Amplatzer plugs*** – Variety of shapes and sizes for different applications. – Controlled release — final deployment only when certain. – Rapid action. – Relative cost may be “cheaper” if multiple coils are required.	part of a staged procedure for large tumours before surgical resection). *Modalities* 1. Ultrasound-guided common femoral artery access. 2. Fluoroscopy. a. Angiogram to detail vascular anatomy. b. Angiogram and fluoroscopy to confirm catheter tip placement in the appropriate artery. c. Continuous fluoroscopy during injection of an embolic agent to avoid reflux into the non-target vessel.	1. Size, number and location of fibroids 2. Confirm placenta accreta, increta or percreta *Consultation with the women's pain anaesthesia team:* – Counselling on pain management after embolisation – Fasting for 6 hours (anaesthesia, contrast reaction) – Shaving (optional in emergent situations) – Bladder catheter (decompress bladder, monitor urine output)	o Fever o Per vaginal discharge ii. *Infection* — due to ischaemia and necrosis, especially if tissue is retained or a large polypoidal fibroid iii. *Primary ovarian insufficiency (POI)* — collateral reflux embolisation of the ovarian artery iv. Bleeding related to tumour necrosis v. May take 6–18 months for the fibroid/placenta to resorb *Risks:* i. Groin haematoma ii. Infection iii. Arterial dissection iv. Contrast allergy/reaction v. Vascular dissection/rupture

(Continued)

(Continued)

Procedure	Indications/modality	Pre-procedure preparation	Post-procedure care/risks
g. *Glue* – Liquid agent, radiolucent. – Mixed with lipiodol or tantalum, which affects setting time and provides radio-opacity. – Sets when in contact with ionic substances. – Rapid action. – Ideal for arteriovenous malformations where small vascular feeders are difficult to reach but need to be closed off. – Leaves a solid cast. **h. *Onyx*** – Gel-to-paste-like agent. Sets to become a solid cast. – Grey colouration — may be useful for tracing vessels during subsequent surgical resection for complex tumours.			
6. Percutaneous nephrostomy (PCN)	<u>*Indications*</u> 1. Urinary outflow tract obstruction with moderate to severe hydronephrosis causing renal impairment 2. Pyonephrosis 3. Stone removal <u>*Modalities*</u> 1. Ultrasound-guided percutaneous access 2. Fluoroscopy	– Consultation at the IR clinic (for a thorough explanation of the procedure and to obtain informed consent) – <u>Fasting</u> for 4 hours (potential contrast reaction) – Appropriate IV antibiotic prophylaxis	<u>*Risks:*</u> i. Acute sepsis ii. Haemorrhage iii. Perforation/rupture of renal pelvis/ureter iv. Contrast reaction v. Urine leakage (catheter drainage holes are obstructed) vi. Urosepsis (if not draining well)

(Continued)

Procedure	Indications/modality	Pre-procedure preparation	Post-procedure care/risks
7. Antegrade ureteric stenting *Technique* i. Antegrade nephrostogram to determine the level of obstruction ii. Tight stenosis may need balloon plasty iii. Soft versus stiff (tumour) stent	a. Antegrade nephrostogram to determine the level of obstruction b. Confirm the catheter loop position *Indications* 1. Obstruction to the ureteric outflow tract (tumour, stones) 2. Aids surgical resection (palpable and marks the ureter position) 3. Provides patients with "normality" compared to PCN	– Fasting for 6 hours (IV sedation, potential contrast reaction) – Appropriate IV antibiotic prophylaxis (similar to PCN) – Ensure urine culture from PCN is negative and no further features of urosepsis	e. Follow-up i. Regular 3–6 monthly change ii. Proceed to antegrade ureteric stenting in 3–7 days when urine clears of blood and no bacterial growth *Risks:* i. Pain and discomfort ii. Perforation/rupture of renal pelvis/ureter iii. Contrast reaction iv. Tight tumoural stenosis may result in persistent hydronephrosis, renal impairment and recurrent urosepsis v. Obstruction of draining side holes from crystalline encrustation *Follow-up:* i. US kidneys and review in the IR clinic in 1 month ii. 3–6 monthly changes of the ureteric stent
8. Varicose vein ablation ***CEAP classification*** *i. Clinical categories (C):* C0: No visible or palpable signs of venous disease C1: Telangiectasias or reticular veins C2: Varicose veins C3: Oedema C4: Changes in skin and subcutaneous tissue secondary to chronic venous disease C4a: Pigmentation or eczema	*Indications* 1. Symptomatic varicose veins 2. Cosmesis *Modalities:* 1. Chemical sclerosant (sodium tetradecyl sulphate) 2. Endovascular ablation (laser, radiofrequency)	– Fasting for 6 hours (IV sedation, potential contrast reaction)	*Outcomes:* i. Bruising. ii. Skin discolouration. iii. Pressure bandage or compression stocking to be worn for 7–10 days. *Risks:* i. Pulmonary embolism. ii. Phlebitis.

(Continued)

(*Continued*)

Procedure	Indications/modality	Pre-procedure preparation	Post-procedure care/risks
C4b: Lipodermatosclerosis or atrophie blanche C5: Healed venous ulcer C6: Active venous ulcer ii. *Etiologic (E)* Ec: Congenital Ep: Primary Es: Secondary (post-thrombotic) En: No venous cause identified iii. *Anatomic (A)* As: Superficial veins Ap: Perforator veins Ad: Deep veins An: No venous location identified iv. *Pathophysiologic (P)* Pr: Reflux Po: Obstruction Pr&Po: Reflux and obstruction Pn: No venous pathophysiology identifiable	*Technique* 1. Ultrasound-guided access into the great saphenous vein 2. Local and tumescent anaesthetic ± IV sedation		*Follow-up:* i. At 3–7 postoperative days with a Doppler ultrasound scan to exclude DVT and to confirm closure of the treated vein. ii. At 6 weeks, confirm closure of the treated vein. For sclerotherapy, if the vein is still patent.

(Continued)

Procedure	Indications/modality	Pre-procedure preparation	Post-procedure care/risks
9. *Fallopian tube recanalisation (FTR)*	<u>Indications</u> 1. Proximal tubal occlusion/ tubal obstruction caused by muscular/tubal/cornual spasms, mucus aggregates, secretions, amorphous debris or stromal oedema → success rates ~70% to 90%. <u>Modality:</u> – Done under fluoroscopic guidance: unblock the fallopian tubes by passing a guidewire and a catheter through the obstructed segment of the tube. – Takes ~30 minutes to 1 hour. May take longer depending on the extent of the blockage and the structure of the fallopian tube.	– Performed after menses have ended for that cycle and before day 14 of the cycle – <u>Fasting</u> for 6 hours (IV sedation, potential contrast reaction) – Empty bladder – Local anaesthetic spray to the cervix	<u>Outcomes:</u> – 30–40% of women have successful pregnancies post-FTR. Most pregnancies occur within the first year of FTR. – Risk of ectopic pregnancy 3% → the woman should be advised to have an early dating scan for subsequent pregnancies. <u>Risks of FTR:</u> – Pain. – Vaginal bleeding. – Infection. – Re-occlusion 25% → FTR can be repeated. – Failure to unblock the tube (could be due to occlusion from fibrosis, salpingitis or salpingitis isthmica nodosa). – Tubal perforation 2%.

CHAPTER 64

Pre-Operative Anaesthetic Information

Aims of pre-operative assessment:

- Determine the impact of surgical pathology on the patient's condition.
- Optimise underlying co-morbidities through further testing, therapy and other sub-speciality consultation → reduce day-of-surgery cancellations and delays.
- Take informed consent for anaesthesia, including options available and risks/benefits of various options.
- Provide patient education on postoperative pain management, peri-operative medication use, fasting and other peri-operative issues.

Patients may be recalled to the anaesthetic clinic for repeat and/or admission for correction of abnormal pre-admission testing (PAT) results, e.g., if haemoglobin (Hb) is <10 g/dl. She may be given oral iron or intravenous (IV) Ferinject to optimise her pre-op Hb and to ensure group and crossmatched blood is available for the surgery.

Indications for Ordering Pre-Admission Tests (PATs) and Validity Period of Results

Blood investigations are valid for **4 weeks** unless there is an acute change in the clinical or physiological condition.

Electrocardiogram (ECG) and chest X-ray (CXR) may be valid for **6 months** with a *stable baseline.*

Hence, if an operation is deferred to a later date, there is **no need** to repeat PAT if the tests are still valid by the above criteria.

Type and Screen (T+S)

Scheduled for *moderate-risk* elective operations and **Hb >10 g/dl** — refer to the Operation Risk Reference Table.
Type and screen (T&S) is required in obstetric patients to determine if anti-D (Rhogam) is required for Rh-negative patients with a Rh-positive partner.

Group and Crossmatch (GXM)

Scheduled for *moderate-risk* operation and **Hb ≤10 g/dl.**
Scheduled for *high-risk* operations — refer to the Operation Risk Reference Table.

Pre-Operative Investigations

Urine pregnancy test (UPT): For all patients in the reproductive age group *except* postmenopausal, post-hysterectomy or those with bilateral salpingo-oophorectomy.

No pre-operative investigations are required if *all* of these conditions are fulfilled:

- ✓ No previous medical history, i.e., American Society of Anesthesiologists (ASA) status 1
- ✓ No history of abnormal bleeding
- ✓ Scheduled for low-risk elective operations except cancer staging* — refer to the Operation Risk Reference Table
- ✓ Age less than 50 years

*All patients with suspected or confirmed malignancy require a full blood count (FBC) at a minimum.

Condition	FBC	UECr	ECG	CXR	PT/APTT/INR	TFT	LFT	Cervical spine X-ray
Age <50	✓ if moderate/high-risk surgeries OR low-risk surgeries and the patient is bleeding							
Age ≥50	✓	✓	✓ for age ≥60	✓ for age ≥70				
For termination of pregnancy (TOP)	✓ if the patient is bleeding							
Anaemia/abnormal uterine bleeding (AUB)	✓							
Blood disorders or on antiplatelets/ anticoagulation	✓				✓			
Hypertension (HTN) or cardiac disease	✓	✓	✓	✓	✓ for high-risk surgeries			
Diabetes mellitus	✓	✓	✓	✓ for moderate/ high-risk surgeries	✓ for high-risk surgeries			
Malignancy/ moderate- to high-risk surgery (refer to the Operative Risk Reference Table)	✓	✓	✓	✓ (not needed if CTTAP was done)	✓		✓ for advanced cancer	

Condition	FBC	UECr	ECG	CXR	PT/APTT/INR	TFT	LFT	Cervical spine X-ray
Renal impairment (serum creatinine >153 µmol/L)	✓	✓	✓	✓ for moderate/ high-risk surgeries	✓ for moderate/ high-risk surgeries			
Chronic liver disease/jaundice (abnormal LFT)	✓	✓	✓	✓	✓		✓	
Thyroid disease	✓		✓			✓		
Lung disease: COPD/ bronchiectasis/ pneumonia in last 6 months Smoking history >10 pack-years	✓	✓	✓	✓				
Chronic use of diuretics or digoxin	✓	✓	✓	✓				
Rheumatoid arthritis	✓							✓ 3 views (open mouth, flexion and extension)

The above table only serves as a guide; Please correlate clinically and order investigations as appropriate for the patient based on her clinical condition.

Source: KKH Pre-Anaesthetic Clinic & Peri-Operative Patient Management, Updated October 2022.

FBC, full blood count; T&S, type and screen; GXM, group and crossmatch; RP, renal panel, i.e., urea, electrolytes and creatinine; ECG, electrocardiogram; CXR, chest X-ray; PT/APTT/INR, prothrombin time/activated partial thromboplastin time/international normalised ratio; TFT, thyroid function test; LFT, liver function test.

Operation Risk Reference Table

Low risk Blood loss ≤200 ml	Moderate risk Blood loss ≤1,000 ml	High risk Blood loss ≥1,000 ml
Evacuation of uterus TOP Dilatation and curettage Hysteroscopy with or without polypectomy Removal/insertion of intrauterine contraceptive devices (IUCDs) Laser vaporisation of cervical intraepithelial neoplasia (CIN) Cone biopsy Cancer staging Flexible or rigid cystoscopy Excision of Bartholin's cyst Oocyte pick-up (OPU)/embryo transfer (ET) Tension-free vaginal tape (TVT) insertion Pelvic floor repair without sacrospinous fixation Testicular sperm aspiration (TESA)/ microsurgical epididymal sperm aspiration (MESA) Excision biopsy of breast lumps Mastectomy ± axillary clearance	Minimally invasive surgery (MIS), including salpingostomy, salpingectomy, cystectomy, oophorectomy, myomectomy, hysterectomy, four-in-one laparoscopy Open salpingectomy, cystectomy, oophorectomy, myomectomy, hysterectomy Vaginal hysterectomy, sacrospinous fixation (SSF) Caesarean section Mastectomy with flap reconstruction	Tumour debulking surgery, including omentectomy, bowel surgery and lymphadenectomy Wertheim's operation Pelvic exenteration Caesarean hysterectomy Placenta praevia/accreta surgery

Requires FBC at a minimum.

High-Risk Patients for Surgery

High-risk indications for antiplatelet therapy

- <2 weeks percutaneous coronary intervention (PCI)
- <2 weeks stroke
- <6 weeks acute myocardial infarction (AMI)
- <6 weeks bare-metal stent (BMS)
- <6 months drug-eluting stent (DES)
- <12 months DES with a high risk of stent thrombosis

Laboratory Tests for Measurement of Anticoagulation Effect

Anticoagulant	Specific test	Availability
Warfarin	INR	24 hours.
Unfractionated heparin (UFH)	APTT	24 hours.
Low-molecular-weight heparin (LMWH)	Anti-Xa	Available only during office hours in KKH. For same-day results, the specimen must reach the specialised haematology laboratory by 3 p.m.
Dabigatran	Diluted thrombin time with dabigatran standards to calculate dabigatran concentration	**Unavailable in KKH.** Normal thrombin clotting time [available 24 hours, turnaround time (TAT) — 1 hour] excludes presence of significant dabigatran levels.
Direct Xa inhibitors: rivaroxaban, apixaban	Anti-Xa chromogenic assays using a product-specific calibrator	Available only during office hours. For same-day results, the specimen must reach the specialised haematology laboratory by 3 p.m. The assay for apixaban is currently **not available.**

If the results of tests are deranged — consult an anaesthetist or a haematologist.

Peri-Operative Management of Anticoagulants and Antiplatelets Before Procedures

Antiplatelets	Management	
Non-steroidal anti-inflammatory drugs (NSAIDs) COX-2 inhibitors	This is usually non-essential, to stop if possible, especially for high-bleeding-risk surgeries. Interruption duration variable, ≥1 day depending on the half-life of NSAIDs: Stop for five times the half-life. Generally safe.	
Aspirin (Cardiprin, Disprin)	Generally appropriate to continue if the risk of arterial thrombosis is moderate or high (e.g., if taken for secondary prevention of cardiovascular disease) unless the surgical bleeding risk is high. Consult an anaesthetist or a haematologist pre-operatively before surgery.	
Clopidogrel (Plavix)	Stop for 7 days. Can restart 24-48 hours post-op if no concerns of bleeding	
Prasugrel	Stop for 7 days.	
Ticlopidine (Ticlid)	Stop for 9 days.	
Ticagrelor	Stop for 5 days.	
Tirofiban	Stop for 8 hours — longer in patients with renal impairment.	
Eptifibatide	Stop for 8 hours — longer in patients with renal impairment.	
Abciximab	Stop for 48 hours.	
Dipyridamole (Presantin)	Stop for 1 day.	
Anticoagulants	**Management**	
Warfarin	Assess the need for bridging therapy. Consult an anaesthetist or a haematologist pre-operatively. Stop for 5 days (for those with a stable INR of 2–3).	
Rivaroxaban	Procedures with a low bleeding risk	CrCl >50: Stop for 24 hours CrCl 30–50: Stop for 24 hours CrCl <30: Stop for 48 hours
	Procedures with a moderate/high bleeding risk	CrCl >50: Stop for 48 hours CrCl 30–50: Stop for 48 hours CrCl <30: Stop for 96 hours
Dabigatran	Procedures with a low bleeding risk	CrCl >50: Stop for 24 hours CrCl 30–50: Stop for 48 hours CrCl <30: Stop for 96 hours
	Procedures with a moderate/high bleeding risk	CrCl >50: Stop for 48 hours CrCl 30–50: Stop for 96 hours CrCl <30: Stop for 144 hours
Apixaban	Procedures with a low bleeding risk	CrCl >50: Stop for 24 hours CrCl 30–50: Stop for 24 hours CrCl <30: Stop for 48 hours
	Procedures with a moderate/high bleeding risk	CrCl >50: Stop for 48 hours CrCl 30–50: Stop for 48 hours CrCl <30: Stop for 96 hours

If medication is ceased today, tomorrow is day 1.

Peri-Operative Management of Anticoagulants in Central Neuraxial Blocks (CNBs)

Anticoagulants	Minimum interval between the last dose of anticoagulant and CNB	Minimum interval between CNB or catheter removal and next dose of anticoagulant
Warfarin	When INR <1.2	2 hours
Unfractionated heparin (UFH)		
Heparin full dose Intravenous (IV) or subcutaneous (SC) >5,000 U twice a day (BD) or three times a day (TDS)	When APTT <40	
Heparin mini-dose SC 5,000 U BD or TDS	May be given; no time restriction for catheter placement or removal	
LMWH, e.g., enoxaparin (Clexane)		
Enoxaparin *prophylactic* dose Up to S/C 40 mg once daily	12 hours	2 hours
Enoxaparin *therapeutic* dose Up to S/C 1.5 mg/kg QDS	24 hours	2 hours

DVT prophylaxis:

To be considered in the presence of risk factors: Increased age, prolonged bed rest, malignancy, previous venous thromboembolism (VTE), obesity, inflammatory bowel disease.

SC enoxaparin 1 mg/kg or 0.01 U/kg once daily.

Reduce the dose in renal impairment.

Peri-Operative Management of Common Conditions

Condition	Management
1. Uncontrolled asthma defined as: • >2 attacks per week • Last serious attack <2 weeks ago • Evidence of increased airway resistance, i.e., prolonged expiratory phase, wheezing and rhonchi	• Refer to respiratory medicine for optimisation. • Postpone surgery for at least 2–4 weeks for stabilisation. • *Exceptions:* Time-sensitive surgeries: Termination of pregnancy at the end of the first trimester, cancer surgery. • In these cases, consult an anaesthetic consultant.

(Continued)

(Continued)

Condition	Management
2. Hypertension • Take repeated blood pressure (BP) readings 15 minutes apart	
BP >140/90 but <160/110	• Refer to a general practitioner (GP)/outpatient polyclinics (OPS). • Allow at least 1 week of anti-hypertensives before surgery.
Hypertensive emergency **BP ≥160/110 + signs of acute target organ damage** • *Cardiovascular system (CVS)*: Dyspnoea, chest pain • *Central nervous system (CNS)*: Neurologic deficit, headache, epistaxis, giddiness, psychomotor agitation, blurring of vision • *Renal*: Oliguria	• Admit to a high-dependency unit (HDU)/intensive care unit (ICU) for acute stabilisation. • Allow **at least 4 weeks of** anti-hypertensives before surgery. • Assess the extent of chronic target organ damage [ischaemic heart disease (IHD), h/o transient ischaemic attack (TIA)/cerebrovascular accident (CVA), renal impairment]. • Advise to do home BP monitoring. • Warn the patient that surgery may be cancelled if BP is high on the day of surgery.
Hypertensive urgency **BP ≥160/110 + no signs of acute target organ damage**	• Refer to a GP/OPS within 24–48 hours. • Advise to seek help if symptoms or signs of target organ damage. • Allow at **least 4 weeks of** anti-hypertensives before surgery. • Assess the extent of chronic target organ damage (IHD, history of TIA/CVA, renal impairment). • Advise to do home BP monitoring. • Warn the patient that surgery may be cancelled if BP is high on the day of surgery.
White coat hypertension BP >140/90, but the patient's BP is usually normal at home	• Continue anti-hypertensives with sips of water on the day of operation. • May cause peri-operative hypotension. • Consider cessation if the patient is on ≥2 concurrent anti-hypertensive drugs, one of which is angiotensin-converting-enzyme inhibitors (ACEi)/angiotensin receptor blockers (ARBs) (consult an anaesthetic consultant for advice).
3. Diabetes mellitus (DM) • Stress from surgery increases cortisol and catecholamine, resulting in hyperglycaemia and ketosis. • This is a risk factor for postoperative sepsis, impaired wound healing and diabetic ketoacidosis (DKA) or hyperosmolar hyperglycaemic syndrome (HHS).	Steps to consider in the peri-operative management of diabetes. • Ensure that the patient is booked first on the operating list to minimise the period of fasting. • Hypocount monitoring 4–6 hourly while on nil by mouth (NBM), with sliding scale insulin therapy used to maintain glycaemic goals (aim hypocount 8–10). • Start IV 5% dextrose solution when the patient is NBM (especially if the patient is on insulin). • Consider postponing/cancelling non-emergency procedures if the patient presents with metabolic abnormalities (DKA, HHS, etc.) or HbA1c >8.5%. • Oral hypoglycaemic agents should be recommenced at pre-operative doses once the patient is taking well orally. They should continue to be withheld if the food intake is likely to be reduced. • In type 1 DM, basal insulin should not be withheld while NBM, whereas in patients with type 2 DM (T2DM) on insulin, insulin can be withheld or given in reduced doses — for dose adjustment of diabetic medications, please consult the family medicine service, an anaesthetist or an endocrinologist. • Refer to the Section on the management of T2DM patients while NBM.

(*Continued*)

Condition	Management
4. Hyperthyroidism or hypothyroidism	• Order and trace free thyroxine (FT4)/thyroid-stimulating hormone (TSH). Exclude a goitre and difficult airway. • In large goitres, do a **neck X-ray** to assess for any retrosternal extension. • Refer to an endocrinologist if **FT4 is abnormal**. (TSH takes longer to revert to normal.)
5. Morbid obesity (defined as BMI >37.5)	• Screen for difficult airway and systemic complications, including hypertension, IHD, obstructive sleep apnoea (OSA) and glucose intolerance. • May undergo a minor procedure (e.g., dilatation and curettage, evacuation of the uterus, TOP, breast lump excision) in day surgery if no OSA. • If OSA is present, admit the patient electively the day before or as a same-day-admission (SDA) case.
6. Obstructive Sleep Apnoea (OSA)	• Use the STOP-BANG questionnaire for OSA assessment. • *For high-risk patients*: o Assess for systemic complications related to including a difficult airway. o Determine if an alternative surgical approach may be feasible, e.g., open surgery rather than MIS. o Convert day surgery to SDA or inpatient admission. o Explore regional anaesthesia. o Advocate peri-operative continuous positive airway pressure (CPAP) therapy. o Discuss the possibility of ICU admission for postoperative monitoring.
7. Rheumatoid arthritis (RA)	• **Order cervical spine X-rays:** Three views (open mouth, flexion and extension views to assess for atlantoaxial dislocation). • Order a lung function test if severe restrictive pulmonary disease is present (dyspnoea of grade 3–4) in patients scheduled for major surgery. • Continue steroid and anti-rheumatic drugs peri-operatively (discuss with a rheumatologist regarding the need to adjust medications pre-operatively).

Gynaecology Elective Procedures

For: T2DM patients on insulin or oral hypoglycaemic agents (OHGAs) when NBM.

***Exclude*: Type 1 DM, pregnancy and labour, DKA, HHS, total parenteral nutrition (TPN), ICU settings and palliative patients.**

Please consult the family medicine service (FMC)/endocrinology team if:

1. Patients are on **insulin therapy.**
2. Patients are on **sodium-glucose cotransporter-2 inhibitors** (**SGLT2i**), **e.g., dapagliflozin, empagliflozin, canagliflozin, ertugliflozin.**

3. There is difficulty in controlling glucose within the target range — ideal range: 8–10 mmol/L, acceptable range: 6–12 mmol/L.

KKH protocol:

OHGAs only#	Insulin treated or OHGAs#
If only a short duration of fasting is expected (i.e., miss one meal) **Omit SGLT2 inhibitors 2–3 days before surgery *(refer to **SGLT2i omission)*** **Omit all OHGAs on the day of surgery** ***If prolonged fasting is expected (i.e., miss two or more meals)*** **Omit SGLT2 inhibitors 2–3 days before surgery *(refer to **SGLT2i omission)*** **Omit all OHGAs on the day of surgery** • If needed (e.g., blood glucose >12), start S/C glargine based on 0.1 U/kg on the morning of the procedure • Start dextrose 5%-containing drip Interim basal insulin may not be required for patients with well-controlled DM on diet control, single OHGA or elderly patients (>75 years old)	**Omit SGLT2 inhibitors 2–3 days before surgery *(refer to **SGLT2i omission)*** **On the day of surgery**, • **Omit all OHGAs and SGLT2 inhibitors** • **Omit short or rapid-acting insulin** • Continue the usual dose of basal insulin (glargine, Levemir, Insulatard) • Omit combination insulin, e.g., Mixtard/NovoMix o Mixtard/NovoMix. Calculate 70% of AM dose as a basal requirement: Order as glargine in the morning • Start dextrose 5%-containing drip ***Note:*** When NBM, the basal component can be reduced by 25–50% if: 1. The total daily dose of insulin requirement is very high (>1 U/kg/day) 2. The patient has a high risk of hypoglycaemia/ previous hypoglycaemic episodes

#Refer to examples.

↓

4–6 hourly capillary glucose monitoring and administering insulin if glucose is high, according to the ***T2DM (nil-by-mouth) sliding scale order set***

↓

1. **Continue IV 5% dextrose-containing drip with basal insulin until the patient can take a full diet.**
2. Capillary glucose monitoring can be switched to TDS + 10 p.m. once starting to eat.
3. When the patient can take a full diet, stop the drip and basal insulin and resume usual DM medications if there are no contraindications.
4. For patients previously on SGLT2 inhibitors, wait for at least 1–2 weeks postoperatively before starting.

Refer to a GP/OPS for review before restarting the medications.

↓

*****SGLT2i omission***

Omit SGLT2 inhibitors 2 days before surgery and on the day of surgery (in total 3 days before surgery) — if taking ertugliflozin, *add an additional day.*

For example:

If the patient is taking dapagliflozin, empagliflozin or canagliflozin and the operation is scheduled for **Friday**, the last dose is to be taken on **Tuesday morning**.

If the patient is taking ertugliflozin and the operation is scheduled for **Friday**, the last dose is to be taken on **Monday morning**.

KKH Anaesthesia Review Form for Elective Surgeries

Reg No 198904227G

KK Women's and Children's Hospital
SingHealth

ANAESTHETIC REVIEW FOR ELECTIVE SURGERIES

Patient's name label

Date of referral : ____________ Referring doctor : ____________

Diagnosis : ____________ Operation : ____________

Op Date : ____________

Day Surgery / Same Day Admission / Inpatient * (delete accordingly)

Name of Anaesthetic doctor : ____________

Date of review : ____________

PLAESE TICK THE **INDICATION** FOR ANAESTHETIC REFERRAL :

CVS

- ☐ Abnormal ECG
- ☐ Irregular heart beat
- ☐ History of heart attack, chest pain or heart failure
- ☐ History of heart valve problems or heart murmur
- ☐ Shortness of breath on climbing one flight of stairs
- ☐ Pacemaker in-situ
- ☐ Uncontrolled BP (>150/90 for two readings)

RESPIRATORY

- ☐ Frequent asthma (≥ once a week)
- ☐ Abnormal chest x-ray

GASTRO/RENAL

- ☐ History of liver disease or jaundice
- ☐ Chronic renal disease

ENDOCRINE

- ☐ Poorly-controlled diabetes mellitus (hypocount > 15mmol/L)
- ☐ Abnormal thyroid function test
- ☐ Morbid obesity (BMI ≥ 38)

CNS/NEUROMUSCULAR

- ☐ Stroke or weakness or numbness of the arm, leg or face with onset in the last six months
- ☐ Rheumatoid arthritis / SLE

ANAESTHESIA

- ☐ Personal or family history of anaesthetic problems
- ☐ Previous difficult airway
- ☐ History of deep vein thrombosis / pulmonary embolism

MEDICATIONS

- ☐ On warfarin, heparin, ticlopidine or clopidogrel

OTHERS

- ☐ ____________

____

ANAE(W)-1001(JUL 2006)R1

Checklist for Referral to the Anaesthetic Clinic in the Antenatal Period for Obstetrics Patients

Obstetric

- Placenta accreta spectrum (PAS)

Anaesthetic

- Previous problems or complications with anaesthesia (e.g., intubation difficulties, malignant hyperthermia)
- Allergy to local anaesthetics or opioids

Haematological

- Clotting/platelet problems
- Sickle cell disease and variants
- Jehovah's Witness

Adverse drug reactions

- Severe drug reactions, e.g., anaphylaxis

Endocrine and metabolic disorders

- Poorly controlled DM

Musculoskeletal

- Back problems (including thoracic) and previous back surgery
- Severe neck or joint problems
- Congenital abnormalities, e.g., spina bifida, myelomeningocele
- Rheumatoid arthritis
- Chronic pain syndrome involving visits to pain clinics or neurologists

Medical disorders involving neurological, cardiovascular (e.g., uncontrolled BP), respiratory, renal system and autoimmune disorders

Miscellaneous

- Obesity (BMI >37.5)
- Transplant recipients
- Patient's request (e.g., worries about back pain associated with regional anaesthesia)

Cardiac Conditions Requiring Infective Endocarditis (IE) Prophylaxis

Prosthetic cardiac valve or material
Presence of a cardiac prosthetic valve
Transcatheter implantation of prosthetic valves
Cardiac valve repair with devices, including annuloplasty, rings or clips
Left ventricular assist devices or implantable heart
Previous, relapsed or recurrent IE
Congenital heart disease (CHD)
Unrepaired cyanotic congenital CHD, including palliative shunts and conduits
Completely repaired congenital heart defect with a prosthetic material or device, whether placed by surgery or by transcatheter during the first 6 months after the procedure
Repaired CHD with residual defects at the site of or adjacent to the site of a prosthetic patch or prosthetic device
Surgical or transcatheter pulmonary artery valve or conduit placement
Cardiac transplant recipients who develop cardiac valvulopathy

Antibiotic Regimen for IE Prophylaxis

Situation	Agent	Dose
Oral	Amoxicillin	2 g
Unable to take oral medication	Ampicillin	2 g intramuscular (IM) or IV
Allergic to penicillin or ampicillin and able to take oral medication	Cephalexin	2 g
	Azithromycin or clarithromycin	500 mg
	Doxycycline	100 mg
Allergic to penicillin or ampicillin and unable to take oral medication	Cefazolin or ceftriaxone	1 g IM or IV

Peri-Operative or Stress Steroid Cover

Glucocorticoid therapy (**prednisolone ≥ 5 mg per day in adults**) across all routes of administration (oral, inhaled, topical, intranasal, intra-articular) can cause suppression of the hypothalamic–pituitary–adrenal axis and is the most common cause of adrenal insufficiency peri-operatively.

(Guidelines from the Association of Anaesthetists, the Royal College of Physicians and the Society for Endocrinology, United Kingdom.)

Procedure type	Intraoperative dose	Postoperative dose
Major surgery, including caesarean section	• IV hydrocortisone 100 mg at induction, followed by immediate initiation of a continuous infusion of hydrocortisone at 200 mg/24 hours • *Alternative*: IV dexamethasone 6–8 mg (will suffice for 24 hours)	• IV hydrocortisone 200 mg/24 hours infusion while NBM • *Alternative*: IM hydrocortisone 50 mg every 6 hours • Resume enteral glucocorticoid at double the pre-surgical therapeutic dose for 48 hours if recovery is uncomplicated
Labour and vaginal delivery	• IV hydrocortisone 100 mg at the onset of labour, followed by immediate initiation of a continuous infusion of hydrocortisone 200 mg/24 hours • *Alternative*: IM hydrocortisone 100 mg followed by IM hydrocortisone 50 mg every 6 hours	

References

1. Abbassi-Ghanavati M, Greer LG, Cunningham FG. (2009) Pregnancy and laboratory studies: A reference table for clinicians. *Obstet Gynecol* **114**(6): 1326–1331. [Published correction appears in *Obstet Gynecol.* 2010 Feb; 115(2 Pt 1): 387.]
2. Adewuya AO, Ola BA, Dada AO, Fasoto OO. (2006) Validation of the Edinburgh Postnatal Depression Scale as a screening tool for depression in late pregnancy among Nigerian women. *J Psychosom Obstet Gynaecol* **27**(4): 267–272.
3. Adoni A, Ben Chetrit A. (1991) The management of intrauterine devices following uterine perforation. *Contraception* **43**(1): 77–81.
4. Akkurt MÖ, Yalçın SE, Akkurt İ, *et al.* (2015) The evaluation of risk factors for failed response to conservative treatment in tubo-ovarian abscesses. *J Turk Ger Gynecol Assoc* **16**(4): 226–230.
5. Alalade AO, Maraj H. (2017) Management of adnexal masses in pregnancy. *Obstet Gynaecol* **19**(4): 317–325.
6. Alexander EK, Pearce EN, Brent GA, *et al.* (2017) 2017 Guidelines of the American Thyroid Association for the Diagnosis and Management of Thyroid Disease During Pregnancy and the Postpartum. *Thyroid* **27**(3): 315–389. [Published correction appears in *Thyroid.* 2017 Sep; 27(9): 1212.]
7. Al-Husban N, Obeidat N, Al-Kuran O, *et al.* (2019) H1N1 Infection in Pregnancy; A Retrospective Study of Feto-Maternal Outcome and Impact of the Timing of Antiviral Therapy. *Mediterr J Hematol Infect Dis* **11**(1): e2019020.
8. American College of Obstetricians and Gynecologists (ACOG) Committee on Health Care for Underserved Women, American Society of Addiction Medicine. ACOG Committee Opinion No. 524 (2012): Opioid abuse, dependence, and addiction in pregnancy. *Obstet Gynecol* **119**(5): 1070–1076.
9. ACOG Committee Clinical Practice Guidelines — Gynecology Management of Postmenopausal Osteoporosis: ACOG Clinical Practice Gudieline No. 2 [Published correction appears in *Obstet Gynecol.* 2022 Jul 1; **140**(1): 138] *Obstet Gynecol.* 2022; **139**(4): 698–717.

10. ACOG Committee Opinion No. 455 (2010): Magnesium sulfate before anticipated preterm birth for neuroprotection. *Obstet Gynecol* **115**(3): 669–671.
11. ACOG Committee Opinion No. 495 (2011): Vitamin D: Screening and supplementation during pregnancy. *Obstet Gynecol* **118**(1): 197–198.
12. ACOG Committee Opinion No. 601 (2014): Tamoxifen and uterine cancer. *Obstet Gynecol* **123**: 1394–1397.
13. ACOG Committee Opinion No. 736 (2018): Optimizing Postpartum Care. *Obstet Gynecol* **131**(5): e140–e150.
14. ACOG Committee Opinion No. 797 (2020): Prevention of Group B streptococcal early-onset disease in newborns. *Obstet Gynecol* **135**: e51–e72.
15. ACOG Practice Bulletin No. 102 (2009): Management of stillbirth. *Obstet Gynecol* **113**(3): 748–761.
16. ACOG Practice Bulletin No. 147 (2014): Lynch syndrome. *Obstet Gynecol* **124**(5): 1042–1054.
17. ACOG Practice Bulletin No. 181 (2017): Prevention of Rh D Alloimmunization. *Obstet Gynecol* **130**(2): e57–e70.
18. ACOG Practice Bulletin 189 (2018): Nausea and Vomiting of Pregnancy. *Obstet Gynecol* **131**(5): 935.
19. ACOG Practice Bulletin No. 190 (2018): Gestational Diabetes Mellitus. *Obstet Gynecol* **131**(2): e49–e64.
20. ACOG Practice Bulletin No. 196 (2018): Thromboembolism in Pregnancy. *Obstet Gynecol* **132**(1): e1–e17. [Published correction appears in Obstet Gynecol. 2018 Oct; 132(4): 1068.]
21. ACOG Practice Bulletin No. 203 (2019): Chronic Hypertension in Pregnancy. *Obstet Gynecol* **133**(1): e26–e50.
22. ACOG Practice Bulletin, No. 223 (2020): Thyroid Disease in Pregnancy. *Obstet Gynecol* **135**(6): e261–e274.
23. Advisory Committee on Immunization Practices Centers for Disease Control and Prevention (CDC). (2008) Guiding principles for development of ACIP recommendations for vaccination during pregnancy and breastfeeding. *MMWR Morb Mortal Wkly Rep* **57**(21): 580.
24. American Diabetes Association. (2021) 14. Management of Diabetes in Pregnancy: *Standards of Medical Care in Diabetes-2021. Diabetes Care* **44**(Suppl. 1): S200–S210.
25. Anand M. (2022) Female sexual pain: Differential diagnosis. In: Sharp HT, Eckler E, eds. *UpToDate.* Waltham, MA: UpToDate Inc. Available online at: https://www.uptodate.com (updated May 13, 2022; accessed September 10, 2022).

26. Ang SB. (2019) Postmenopausal osteoporosis: Diagnosis, Frax® and Management. *Singap Fam Physician* **45**(7): 8–15.
27. Arab H, Alharbi AJ, Oraif A, *et al.* (2020) The role of progestogens in threatened and idiopathic recurrent miscarriage [published correction appears in *Int J Womens Health.* 2020 Apr 08;12:253]. *Int J Womens Health* **11**:589–596. Published 2019 Nov 7. doi:10.2147/IJWH.S224159.
28. Arroll B, Khin N, Kerse N. (2003) Screening for depression in primary care with two verbally asked questions: cross sectional study. *BMJ* **327**(7424): 1144–1146.
29. Azziz R. (2021) Epidemiology, phenotype, and genetics of the polycystic ovary syndrome in adults. In: Barbieri RL, Martin KA, eds. *UpToDate.* Waltham, MA: UpToDate Inc. Available online at: https://www.uptodate.com (updated June 16, 2021; accessed February 10, 2022).
30. Baber RJ, Panay N, Fenton A, *et al.* (2016) 2016 IMS Recommendations on women's midlife health and menopause hormone therapy. *Climacteric* **19**(2): 109–150.
31. Bachnas MA, Akbar MIA, Dachlan EG, Dekker G. (2021) The role of magnesium sulfate ($MgSO_4$) in fetal neuroprotection. *J Matern Fetal Neonatal Med* **34**(6): 966–978.
32. Bacha E, Hijazi ZM. (2020) Management of coarctation of the aorta. In: Fulton DR, Connolly HM, eds. *UpToDate.* Waltham, MA: UpToDate Inc. Available online at: https://www.uptodate.com (updated November 13, 2020; accessed March 20, 2022).
33. Bainbridge SA, Roberts JM. (2008) Uric acid as a pathogenic factor in preeclampsia. *Placenta* **29**(Suppl. A): S67–S72.
34. Bakour SH, Timmermans A, Mol BW, Khan KS. (2012) Management of women with postmenopausal bleeding: Evidence-based review. *Obstet Gynaecol* **14**(4): 243–249.
35. Barbieri R, Ehrmann D. (2022) Clinical manifestations of polycystic ovary syndrome in adults. In: Synder PJ, Martin KA, eds. *UpToDate.* Waltham, MA: UpToDate Inc. Available online at: https://www.uptodate.com (updated September 7, 2022; accessed September 18, 2022).
36. Barbieri R, Ehrmann D. (2022) Diagnosis of polycystic ovary syndrome in adults. In: Crowley WF, Martin KA, eds. *UpToDate.* Waltham, MA: UpToDate Inc. Available online at: https://www.uptodate.com (updated May 2, 2022; accessed September 18, 2022).
37. Bates SM, Greer IA, Middeldorp S, *et al.* (2012) VTE, thrombophilia, antithrombotic therapy, and pregnancy: Antithrombotic Therapy and Prevention of Thrombosis, 9th ed: American College of Chest Physicians

Evidence-Based Clinical Practice Guidelines. *Chest* **141**(2 Suppl.): e691S–e736S.

38. Bates SM, Rajasekhar A, Middeldorp S, *et al.* (2018) American Society of Hematology 2018 guidelines for management of venous thromboembolism: Venous thromboembolism in the context of pregnancy. *Blood Adv* **2**(22): 3317–3359.
39. Bauer ME, Balistreri M, MacEachern M, *et al.* (2019) Normal Range for Maternal Lactic Acid during Pregnancy and Labor: A Systematic Review and Meta-Analysis of Observational Studies. *Am J Perinatol* **36**(9): 898–906.
40. Bayer Pte Ltd (2023). Mirena Product Leaflet (16 November 2023) [Brochure]. Accessed at https://eservice.hsa.gov.sg/prism/common/enquirepublic/SearchDRBProduct.do?action=getProductDetails on 20 December 2023.
41. Beavis AL, Gravitt PE, Rositch AF. (2017) Hysterectomy-corrected cervical cancer mortality rates reveal a larger racial disparity in the United States. *Cancer* **123**(6): 1044–1050.
42. Becker CM, Bokor A, Heikinheimo O, *et al.* (2022) ESHRE guideline: Endometriosis. *Hum Reprod Open* **2022**(2): hoac009.
43. Berlanda N, Vercellini P, Fedele L. (2010) The outcomes of repeat surgery for recurrent symptomatic endometriosis. *Curr Opin Obstet Gynecol* **22**(4): 320–325.
44. Belgi RH. (2022) Epidemiology, clinical manifestations, and diagnosis of tuboovarian abscess. In: Sharp HT, Marrazo J, Chakrabarti A, eds. *UpToDate*. Waltham, MA: UpToDate Inc. Available online at: https://www.uptodate.com (updated February 7, 2022; accessed September 18, 2022).
45. Belgi RH. (2022) Management and complications of tuboovarian abscess. In: Sharp HT, Marrazo J, Chakrabarti A, eds. *UpToDate*. Waltham, MA: UpToDate Inc. Available online at: https://www.uptodate.com (updated April 19, 2022; accessed September 18, 2022).
46. Bell KJ, Hayen A, Macaskill P, *et al.* (2009) Value of routine monitoring of bone mineral density after starting bisphosphonate treatment: Secondary analysis of trial data. *BMJ* **338**: b2266.
47. Berghella V, Figueroa D, Szychowski JM, *et al.* (2010) 17-alpha-hydroxyprogesterone caproate for the prevention of preterm birth in women with prior preterm birth and a short cervical length. *Am J Obstet Gynecol* **202**(4): 351.e1–351.e6.
48. Bernhard LM, Klebba PK, Gray DL, Mutch DG. (1999) Predictors of persistence of adnexal masses in pregnancy. *Obstet Gynecol* **93**(4): 585–589.
49. Bhatla N, Denny L. (2018) FIGO Cancer Report 2018. *Int J Gynaecol Obstet* **143**(Suppl. 2): 2–3.

50. Bhutia K, Ng QJ, Puri M. (2022) Diabetes Mellitus in Pregnancy. In: Trivedi SS, Puri M, Agrawal S, eds. *Management of High-Risk Pregnancy: A Practical Approach*, 3rd ed. New Delhi, India: Jaypee Brothers Medical Publishers (P) Ltd. 218–235.
51. Blavier F, Blockeel C, Cools W, *et al.* (2020) Serum progesterone levels could predict diagnosis, completion and complications of miscarriage. *J Gynecol Obstet Hum Reprod* **49**(5): 101721. doi:10.1016/j.jogoh.2020.101721.
52. Blondon M, Harrington LB, Righini M, *et al.* (2014) Racial and ethnic differences in the risk of postpartum venous thromboembolism: A population-based, case-control study. *J Thromb Haemost* **12**(12): 2002–2009.
53. Body C, Christie JA. (2016) Gastrointestinal Diseases in Pregnancy: Nausea, Vomiting, Hyperemesis Gravidarum, Gastroesophageal Reflux Disease, Constipation, and Diarrhea. *Gastroenterol Clin North Am* **45**(2): 267–283.
54. Briggs GG, Freeman RK, Yaffe SF. (2011) *Drugs in Pregnancy and Lactation*, 8th ed. Philadelphia, PA: Lippincott Williams & Wilkins.
55. Briggs Pregnancy and Lactation [Internet]. (accessed January 30, 2022).
56. British Association for Sexual Health and HIV (BASHH). Guidelines for Sexually Transmitted Infections. Available online at: https://www.bashh.org/guidelines (accessed May 7, 2022).
57. British HIV Association. British HIV Association guidelines for the management of HIV in pregnancy and postpartum 2018 (2020 third interim update). Available online at: https://www.bhiva.org/file/5f1aab1ab9aba/BHIVA-Pregnancy-guidelines-2020-3rd-interim-update.pdf (accessed December 29, 2021).
58. British Thoracic Society, Scottish Intercollegiate Guidelines Network. SIGN 158: British guideline on the management of asthma. Revised edition published on July 2019. Available online at: https://www.sign.ac.uk/media/1773/sign158-updated.pdf (accessed May 1, 2022).
59. Brown JP, Josse RG, Scientific Advisory Council of the Osteoporosis Society of Canada. (2002) 2002 clinical practice guidelines for the diagnosis and management of osteoporosis in Canada. *CMAJ* **167**(10 Suppl.): S1–S34.
60. Bruijn MM, Vis JY, Wilms FF, *et al.* (2016) Comparison of the Actim Partus test and the fetal fibronectin test in the prediction of spontaneous preterm birth in symptomatic women undergoing cervical length measurement. *Eur J Obstet Gynecol Reprod Biol* **206**: 220–224.
61. Bruni L, Barrionuevo-Rosas L, Albero G, *et al.* ICO Information Centre on HPV and Cancer (HPV Information Centre). Human papillomavirus and related diseases in the world: Summary report. 22 October 2021. Available

online at: http://www.hpvcentre.net/statistics/reports/XWX.pdf (accessed January 4, 2022).

62. Buyon JP. (2022) Neonatal lupus: Epidemiology, pathogenesis, clinical manifestations, and diagnosis. In: Klein-Gitelman M, Triedman JK, Garcia-Prats JA, Tepas E, eds. *UpToDate.* Waltham, MA: UpToDate Inc. Available online at: https://www.uptodate.com (updated January 7, 2022; accessed March 23, 2022).
63. Buyon JP. (2020) Neonatal lupus: Management and outcomes. In: Klein-Gitelman M, Triedman JK, Garcia-Prats JA, Tepas E, eds. *UpToDate.* Waltham, MA: UpToDate Inc. Available online at: https://www.uptodate.com (updated August 11, 2020; accessed March 23, 2022).
64. Carusi DA. (2021) Condylomata acuminata (anogenital warts): Treatment of vulvar and vaginal warts. In: Barbieri RL, Eckler K, eds. *UpToDate.* Waltham, MA: UpToDate Inc. Available online at: https://www.uptodate.com (updated September 6, 2022; accessed September 18, 2022).
65. Carp H. A systematic review of dydrogesterone for the treatment of threatened miscarriage. *Gynecol Endocrinol* 2012; **28**(12): 983–990. doi:10.3109/09513590.2012.702875.
66. Castleman J, Gurney L, Kilby M, Morris RK. (2021) Identification and management of fetal anaemia: A practical guide. *Obstet Gynaecol* **23**(3): 196–205.
67. Centers for Disease Control and Prevention. Lactational Amenorrhea method. Available online at: https://www.cdc.gov/reproductivehealth/contraception/mmwr/mec/appendixg.html (accessed May 5, 2022).
68. Centre for Metabolic Bone Diseases, University of Sheffield, UK. WHO Fracture Risk Assessment Tool (FRAX). Available online at: http://www.shef.ac.uk/FRAX/.
69. Cervical Screen Singapore Advisory Committee. (2019) Management Guidelines for Cervical Screening and Preinvasive Disease of the Cervix. Available online at: https://www.sccps.org/wp-content/uploads/2019/03/CSS-Clinical-Mgt-Guidelines-2019_March-Release.pdf (accessed June 10, 2022).
70. Chan LY, Tam WH, Lau TK. (2001) Venous thromboembolism in pregnant Chinese women. *Obstet Gynecol* **98**(3): 471–475.
71. Chan WS, Rey E, Kent NE, *et al.* (2014) Venous thromboembolism and antithrombotic therapy in pregnancy. *J Obstet Gynaecol Can* **36**(6): 527–553.
72. Chapter of Haematologists, College of Physicians, College of Obstetricians and Gynaecologists, Singapore. Joint Consensus Statement — Venous Thromboembolism in Pregnancy. Recommendations for Prevention,

Treatment and Investigation. Available online at: https://www.ams.edu.sg/view-pdf.aspx?file=media%5C6016_fi_257.pdf&ofile=CPS-COGS+VTE+Consensus+Statement+2021+0326.pdf (accessed February 21, 2022).

73. Chee C, Lee D, Chong Y, *et al.* (2005) Confinement and other psychosocial factors in perinatal depression: A transcultural study in Singapore. *J Affect Disord* **89**: 157–166.
74. Chen CP, Hsu TC, Wang W. (1998) Ileal penetration by a Multiload-Cu 375 intrauterine contraceptive device. A case report with review of the literature. *Contraception* **58**(5): 295–304. [Published correction appears in Contraception 1998 Dec; 58(6): following 389.]
75. Chen LM, Berek JS. (2021) Borderline ovarian tumors. In: Groff B, Dizon DS, Chakrabarti A, Vora SR, eds. *UpToDate.* Waltham, MA: UpToDate Inc. Available online at: https://www.uptodate.com (updated July 31, 2021; accessed September 5, 2022).
76. Chi CC, Kirtschig G, Aberer W, *et al.* (2017) Updated evidence-based (S2e) European Dermatology Forum guideline on topical corticosteroids in pregnancy. *J Eur Acad Dermatol Venereol* **31**(5): 761–773.
77. CLOTS (Clots in Legs Or sTockings after Stroke) Trial Collaboration. (2010) Thigh-length versus below-knee stockings for deep venous thrombosis prophylaxis after stroke: A randomized trial. *Ann Intern Med* **153**(9): 553–562. [Published correction appears in Ann Intern Med. 2010 Dec 21; 153(12): 851.]
78. Coomarasamy A, Williams H, Truchanowicz E, *et al.* (2015) A Randomized Trial of Progesterone in Women with Recurrent Miscarriages. *N Engl J Med* **373**(22): 2141–2148.
79. Coomarasamy A, Devall AJ, Cheed V, *et al.* (2019) A Randomized Trial of Progesterone in Women with Bleeding in Early Pregnancy. *N Engl J Med* **380**(19): 1815–1824.
80. Cohen K, Rathod M, Ferriman E. (2010) Twin pregnancy. *Obstet Gynaecol Reprod Med* **20**(9): 259–264.
81. Cohen LS, Altshuler LL, Harlow BL, *et al.* (2006) Relapse of major depression during pregnancy in women who maintain or discontinue antidepressant treatment. *JAMA* **295**(5): 499–507. [Published correction appears in JAMA. 2006 Jul 12; 296(2): 170.]
82. Communicable Diseases Division, Ministry of Health, Singapore. Communicable Diseases Surveillance in Singapore 2017. Available online at: https://www.moh.gov.sg/resources-statistics/reports/communicable-diseases-surveillance-in-singapore-2017 (accessed December 31, 2021).

83. College of Obstetricians and Gynaecologists, Singapore. (2018) Guidelines for the Management of Gestational Diabetes Mellitus. Available online at: https://www.ams.edu.sg/view-pdf.aspx?file=media%5C4163_fi_430.pdf&ofile=COGS+GDM+Guidelines+2018.pdf (accessed February 22, 2022).
84. Corominas AI, Medina Y, Balconi S, *et al.* (2022) Assessing the Role of Uric Acid as a Predictor of Preeclampsia. *Front Physiol* **12**: 785219.
85. Cox JL, Holden JM, Sagovsky R. (1987) Detection of postnatal depression. Development of the 10-item Edinburgh Postnatal Depression Scale. *Br J Psychiatry* **150**: 782–786.
86. Cox JT, Palefsky JM. (2021) Human papillomavirus vaccination. In: Hirsch MS, ed. UpToDate. Waltham, MA: UpToDate Inc. Available online at: https://www.uptodate.com (updated December 17, 2021; accessed January 7, 2022).
87. Daroszewska A. (2012) Prevention and treatment of osteoporosis in women: An update. *Obstet Gynaecol Reprod Med* **22**(6): 162–169.
88. Dave FG, Adedipe T, Disu S, *et al.* (2019) Unscheduled bleeding with hormone replacement therapy. *Obstet Gynaecol* **21**(2): 95–101.
89. Davis SR, Lambrinoudaki I, Lumsden M, *et al.* (2015) Menopause. *Nat Rev Dis Primers* **1**: 15004.
90. Dawson-Hughes B. (2022) Vitamin D deficiency in adults: Definition, clinical manifestations, and treatment. In: Rosen CJ, Rubinow K, eds. *UpToDate.* Waltham, MA: UpToDate Inc. Available online at: https://www.uptodate.com (updated September 6, 2022; accessed September 19, 2022).
91. Delle Marchette M, Ceppi L, Andreano A, *et al.* (2019) Oncologic and fertility impact of surgical approach for borderline ovarian tumours treated with fertility sparing surgery. *Eur J Cancer* **111**: 61–68.
92. Delmas PD. (2002) Treatment of postmenopausal osteoporosis. *Lancet* **359**(9322): 2018–2026.
93. Depka M, Döpke S, Henkel-Klene A, *et al.* (2013) Management of Pregnancy in Patients with Antithrombin Deficiency. *Blood* **122**(21): 216.
94. Desmonts G, Couvreur J. (1984) Congenital toxoplasmosis. Prospective study of the outcome of pregnancy in 542 women with toxoplasmosis acquired during pregnancy. *Ann Pediatr (Paris)* **31**(10): 805–809.
95. Devaseelan P, Ong S. (2010) Twin pregnancy: Controversies in management. *Obstet Gynaecol* **12**(3): 179–185.
96. De Vries LS, Gunardi H, Barth PG, *et al.* (2004) The spectrum of cranial ultrasound and magnetic resonance imaging abnormalities in congenital cytomegalovirus infection. *Neuropediatrics* **35**(2): 113–119.
97. Dewick L, Jayaprakasan K, Raouf S. (2020) Syphilis in pregnancy: Identifying and managing a historic problem on the rise. *Obstet Gynaecol* **22**(3): 209–216.

98. Dockree S, Brook J, James T, *et al.* (2021) A pregnancy-specific reference interval for procalcitonin. *Clin Chim Acta* **513**: 13–16.
99. Dotters-Katz SK, Kuller JA, Hughes BL. (2021) Society for Maternal-Fetal Medicine Consult Series #56: Hepatitis C in pregnancy-updated guidelines: Replaces Consult Number 43, November 2017. *Am J Obstet Gynecol* **225**(3): B8–B18.
100. Dowdy SC, Mariani A, Lurain JR. (2011) Uterine cancer. In: Berek JS, ed. *Berek & Novak's Gynecology*, 15th ed. Baltimore: Lippincott, Williams & Wilkins. 1250–1253.
101. Doyle T, Kavanaugh-McHugh A, Fish FA. (2021) Management and outcome of tetralogy of Fallot. In: Connolly HM, Triedman JK, Armsby C, eds. *UpToDate.* Waltham, MA: UpToDate Inc. Available online at: https://www.uptodate.com (updated April 15, 2021; accessed May 10, 2022).
102. Doyle T, Kavanaugh-McHugh A. (2021) Pathophysiology, clinical features, and diagnosis of tetralogy of Fallot. In: Connolly HM, Triedman JK, Armsby C, eds. UpToDate. Waltham, MA: UpToDate Inc. Available online at: https://www.uptodate.com (updated April 5, 2021; accessed 23 March 2022).
103. Drukker L, Cavallaro A, Salim I, *et al.* (2020) How often do we incidentally find a fetal abnormality at the routine third-trimester growth scan? A population-based study. *Am J Obstet Gynecol* **223**(6): 919.e1–919.e13.
104. Drutz JE. (2022) Hepatitis B virus immunization in infants, children, and adolescents. In: Duryea TK, Edwards MS, Torchia MM, eds. *UpToDate.* Waltham, MA: UpToDate Inc. Available online at: https://www.uptodate.com (updated May 5, 2022; accessed June 10, 2022).
105. Eastell R, Rosen CJ, Black DM, *et al.* (2019) Pharmacological Management of Osteoporosis in Postmenopausal Women: An Endocrine Society* Clinical Practice Guideline. *J Clin Endocrinol Metab* **104**(5): 1595–1622.
106. Egemen D, Cheung LC, Chen X, *et al.* Risk estimates supporting the 2019 ASCCP risk-based management consensus guidelines. *J Low Genit Tract Dis.* 2020; **24**(2): 132–143.
107. El-Zibdeh MY, Yousef LT. Dydrogesterone support in threatened miscarriage. *Maturitas* 2009; **65** Suppl 1: S43–S46. doi:10.1016/j.maturitas.2009.11.013.
108. Enders M, Daiminger A, Exler S, *et al.* (2017) Prenatal diagnosis of congenital cytomegalovirus infection in 115 cases: A 5 years' single center experience. *Prenat Diagn* **37**(4): 389–398.
109. Er B, Chua YX. (2018) *Cervical Cancer Epidemiology and Screening Behavior in Singapore.* Statistics Singapore Newsletter. Available online at: https://www.singstat.gov.sg/-/media/files/publications/society/ssnmar18-pg7-9.pdf (accessed January 7, 2022).

110. ESHRE Guideline Group on RPL, Bender Atik R, Christiansen OB, *et al.* (2018) ESHRE guideline: Recurrent pregnancy loss. *Hum Reprod Open* **2018**(2): hoy004.
111. Exacoustòs C, Rosati P. (1993) Ultrasound diagnosis of uterine myomas and complications in pregnancy. *Obstet Gynecol* **82**(1): 97–101.
112. Exercise in Pregnancy Committee. Lee R, Thain Serene, *et al.* (2022) Perinatal society of Singapore: Guidelines on physical activity & exercise in pregnancy. Available online at: http://perinatal.sg/exercise.pdf (accessed June 20, 2022).
113. Feldman S, Goodman A, Peipert J. (2022) Screening for cervical cancer in resource-rich settings. In: Goff B, Elmore JG, Chakrabati A, Kunins L, eds. *UpToDate.* Waltham, MA: UpToDate Inc. Available online at: https://www.uptodate.com (updated July 26, 2022; accessed August 10, 2022).
114. Fine P, Mathé H, Ginde S, *et al.* (2010) Ulipristal acetate taken 48–120 hours after intercourse for emergency contraception. *Obstet Gynecol* **115**(2 Pt. 1): 257–263.
115. Fleishman CE, Tugertimur A. (2022) Clinical manifestations and diagnosis of atrioventricular (AV) canal defects. In: Triedman JK, Armsby C, eds. *UpToDate.* Waltham, MA: UpToDate Inc. Available online at: https://www.uptodate.com (updated July 18, 2022; accessed August 10, 2022).
116. Fleishman CE, Tugertimur A. (2022) Management and outcome of atrioventricular (AV) canal defects. In: Triedman JK, Armsby C, eds. *UpToDate.* Waltham, MA: UpToDate Inc. Available online at: https://www.uptodate.com (updated July 18, 2022; accessed August 10, 2022).
117. Foley E, Clarke E, Beckett VA, *et al.* Management of Genital Herpes in Pregnancy. Available online at: https://www.rcog.org.uk/media/5t0nborx/management-genital-herpes.pdf (accessed December 1, 2022).
118. Foong SC, Tan ML, Foong WC, *et al.* (2020) Oral galactagogues (natural therapies or drugs) for increasing breast milk production in mothers of non-hospitalised term infants. *Cochrane Database Syst Rev* **5**(5): CD011505.
119. Fonseca EB, Celik E, Parra M, *et al.* (2007) Progesterone and the risk of preterm birth among women with a short cervix. *N Engl J Med* **357**(5): 462–469.
120. Fraser IS, Parke S, Mellinger U, *et al.* (2011) Effective treatment of heavy and/or prolonged menstrual bleeding without organic cause: Pooled analysis of two multinational, randomised, double-blind, placebo-controlled trials of oestradiol valerate and dienogest. *Eur J Contracept Reprod Health Care* **16**(4): 258–269.
121. Fraser IS, Romer T, Parke S, *et al.* (2011) Effective treatment of heavy and/or prolonged menstrual bleeding with an oral contraceptive containing estradiol

valerate and dienogest: A randomized, double-blind Phase III trial. *Hum Reprod* **26**(10): 2698–2708.

122. Friedman AJ, Barbieri RL, Doubilet PM, *et al.* (1988) A randomized, double-blind trial of a gonadotropin releasing-hormone agonist (leuprolide) with or without medroxyprogesterone acetate in the treatment of leiomyomata uteri. *Fertil Steril* **49**(3): 404–409.
123. Fulton DR, Kane DA. (2020) Pathophysiology, clinical manifestations, and diagnosis of D-transposition of the great arteries. In: Triedman JK, Armsby C, eds. *UpToDate*. Waltham, MA: UpToDate Inc. Available online at: https://www.uptodate.com (updated February 25, 2020; accessed March 20, 2022).
124. Fulton DR, Kane DA. (2021) Management and outcome of D-transposition of the great arteries. In: Triedman JK, Armsby C, eds. *UpToDate.* Waltham, MA: UpToDate Inc. Available online at: https://www.uptodate.com (updated August 13, 2021; accessed March 20, 2022).
125. Fulton DR, Saleeb S. (2022) Isolated ventricular septal defects in infants and children: Anatomy, clinical features, and diagnosis. In: Triedman JK, Armsby C, eds. *UpToDate.* Waltham, MA: UpToDate Inc. Available online at: https://www.uptodate.com (updated August 1, 2022; accessed August 20, 2022).
126. Fulton DR, Saleeb S. (2022) Management of isolated ventricular septal defects in infants and children. In: Triedman JK, Armsby C, eds. *UpToDate.* Waltham, MA: UpToDate Inc. Available online at: https://www.uptodate.com (updated August 1, 2022; accessed August 20, 2022).
127. Gan E. Painful sex need not tear marriages apart. Doctors urge couples to seek help early. Available online at: https://www.todayonline.com/singapore/painful-sex-need-not-tear-marriages-apart-doctors-urge-couples-seek-help-early (accessed January 30, 2022).
128. Gershenson DM. (2017) Management of borderline ovarian tumours. *Best Pract Res Clin Obstet Gynaecol* **41**: 49–59.
129. Giachè S, Borchi B, Zammarchi L, *et al.* (2021) Hand, foot, and mouth disease in pregnancy: 7 years Tuscan experience and literature review. *J Matern Fetal Neonatal Med* **34**(9): 1494–1500.
130. Gilson R, Nugent D, Werner RN, *et al.* (2020) 2019 IUSTI-Europe guideline for the management of anogenital warts. *J Eur Acad Dermatol Venereol* **34**(8): 1644–1653.
131. Glasier AF, Cameron ST, Fine PM, *et al.* (2010) Ulipristal acetate versus levonorgestrel for emergency contraception: A randomised non-inferiority trial and meta-analysis. *Lancet* **375**(9714): 555–562.

132. Global Initiative for Asthma (GINA). (2021) Global Strategy for Asthma Management and Prevention. Available online at: www.ginaasthma.org (accessed January 29, 2022).
133. Gotlib IH, Whiffen VE, Mount JH, *et al.* (1989) Prevalence rates and demographic characteristics associated with depression in pregnancy and the postpartum. *J Consult Clin Psychol* **57**(2): 269–274.
134. Gould MK, Garcia DA, Wren SM, *et al.* (2012) Prevention of VTE in nonorthopedic surgical patients: Antithrombotic therapy and prevention of thrombosis: American college of chest physicians evidence-based clinical practice guidelines. *Chest* **141**(2): e227S–e277S.
135. Gourlay ML, Fine JP, Preisser JS, *et al.* (2012) Bone-density testing interval and transition to osteoporosis in older women. *N Engl J Med* **366**(3): 225–233.
136. Grimes DA. (2000) Intrauterine device and upper-genital-tract infection. *Lancet* **356**: 1013–1019.
137. Laufer MR. (2022) Ovarian and fallopian tube torsion. In: Sharp HT, Levine D, Chakrabarti A, eds. *UpToDate.* Waltham, MA: UpToDate Inc. Available online at: https://www.uptodate.com (updated May 17, 2020; accessed June 10, 2022).
138. Hale's Medications and Mother's Milk. Available online at: https://www.halesmeds.com/.
139. Hall V, Talbot PR, Stubbs SL, *et al.* (2001) Identification of clinical isolates of actinomyces species by amplified 16S ribosomal DNA restriction analysis. *J Clin Microbiol* **39**(10): 3555–3562.
140. Hamoda H, Panay N, Pedder H, *et al.* (2020) The British menopause society & women's health concern 2020 recommendations on hormone replacement therapy in menopausal women. *Post Reprod Health* **26**(4): 181–209.
141. Harden CL, Hopp J, Ting TY, *et al.* (2009) Practice parameter update: Management issues for women with epilepsy — focus on pregnancy (an evidence-based review): Obstetrical complications and change in seizure frequency: Report of the quality standards subcommittee and therapeutics and technology assessment subcommittee of the American academy of neurology and American epilepsy society. *Neurology* **73**(2): 126–132.
142. Harlow SD, Lin X, Ho MJ. (2000) Analysis of menstrual diary data across the reproductive life span applicability of the bipartite model approach and the importance of within-woman variance. *J Clin Epidemiol* **53**(7): 722–733.
143. Harrington K, Kurdi W, Aquilina J, *et al.* (2000) A prospective management study of slow-release aspirin in the palliation of uteroplacental insufficiency predicted by uterine artery Doppler at 20 weeks. *Ultrasound Obstet Gynecol* **15**(1): 13–18.

144. Hauptmann S, Friedrich K, Redline R, *et al.* (2017) Ovarian borderline tumors in the 2014 WHO classification: Evolving concepts and diagnostic criteria. *Virchows Arch* **470**(2): 125–142.
145. Hay D, Kieran E. (2009) Non-HIV sexually transmitted infections. *Obstet Gynaecol Reprod Med* **19**(8): 210–214.
146. Hayes EJ. (2022) Triplet pregnancy. In: Simpson LL, Barss VA, eds. *UpToDate.* Waltham, MA: UpToDate Inc. Available online at: https://www.uptodate.com (updated May 16, 2022; accessed June 15, 2022).
147. Hazra A, Collison MW, Davis AM. (2022) CDC sexually transmitted infections treatment guidelines, 2021. *JAMA* **327**(9): 870–871.
148. Healthhub. Recommended Dietary Allowances. Available online at: https://www.healthhub.sg/live-healthy/192/recommended_dietary_allowances (accessed January 6, 2022).
149. Hennessy M, Dennehy R, Meaney S, *et al.* (2021) Clinical practice guidelines for recurrent miscarriage in high-income countries: A systematic review. *Reprod Biomed Online* **42**(6): 1146–1171.
150. Hijazi ZM. (2021) Clinical manifestations and diagnosis of coarctation of the aorta. In: Fulton DR, Connolly HM, Armsby C, Yeon SB, eds. *UpToDate.* Waltham, MA: UpToDate Inc. Available online at: https://www.uptodate.com (updated March 22, 2021; accessed March 22, 2022).
151. Hoffman M. (1995) Primary ovarian carcinoma during pregnancy. *Clin Consul Obstet Gynecol* **7**: 237.
152. Hughes BL, Clifton RG, Rouse DJ, *et al.* (2021) A trial of hyperimmune globulin to prevent congenital cytomegalovirus infection. *N Engl J Med* **385**(5): 436–444.
153. Jacquemard F, Yamamoto M, Costa JM, *et al.* (2007) Maternal administration of valaciclovir in symptomatic intrauterine cytomegalovirus infection. *BJOG* **114**(9): 1113–1121.
154. James AH, Bates SM, Bauer KA, *et al.* (2017) Management of hereditary antithrombin deficiency in pregnancy. *Thromb Res* **157**: 41–45.
155. Jaya-Bodestyne SL, Lee LH, Tan LK, *et al.* (2020) Risk factors for pregnancy-associated venous thromboembolism in Singapore. *J Perinat Med* **49**(2): 153–158.
156. Jensen JT, Lukkari-Lax E, Schulze A, *et al.* (2022) Contraceptive efficacy and safety of the 52-mg levonorgestrel intrauterine system for up to 8 years: findings from the Mirena Extension Trial. *Am J Obstet Gynecol* **227**(6): 873.e1-873.e12. doi:10.1016/j.ajog.2022.09.007.
157. Jeremiah MP, Unwin BK, Greenawald MH, *et al.* (2015) Diagnosis and management of osteoporosis. *Am Fam Physician* **92**(4): 261–268.

158. Jo's Cervical Cancer Trust. *HPV FAQs*. Available online at: https://www.jostrust.org.uk/information/hpv/faqs (accessed January 5, 2022).
159. Joint Formulary Committee. (2011) *British National Formulary*, 62nd ed. London: BMJ Group and Pharmaceutical Press.
160. Joint Formulary Committee. (2011) *Immunological Products and Vaccines. British National Formulary*, 62nd ed. London: BMJ Group and Pharmaceutical Press.
161. Jones ER, O'Flynn H, Njoku K, *et al.* (2021) Detecting endometrial cancer. *Obstet Gynaecol* **23**(2): 103–112.
162. Kane DA. (2022) L-transposition of the great arteries: Anatomy, physiology, clinical features, and diagnosis. In: Fulton DR, Armsby C, eds. *UpToDate*. Waltham, MA: UpToDate Inc. Available online at: https://www.uptodate.com (updated September 19, 2022; accessed September 22, 2022).
163. Kane DA. (2021) L-transposition of the great arteries: Management and outcome. In: Fulton DR, Connolly HM, Armsby C, eds. *UpToDate*. Waltham, MA: UpToDate Inc. Available online at: https://www.uptodate.com (updated March 3, 2021; accessed September 22, 2022).
164. Kakkos SK, Caprini JA, Geroulakos G, *et al.* (2016) Combined intermittent pneumatic leg compression and pharmacological prophylaxis for prevention of venous thromboembolism. *Cochrane Database Syst Rev* **9**(9): CD005258.
165. Keppel KG, Taffel SM. (1993) Pregnancy-related weight gain and retention: Implications of the 1990 Institute of Medicine guidelines. *Am J Public Health* **83**: 1100–1103.
166. Khalil A, Sotiriadis A, Chaoui R, *et al.* (2020) ISUOG Practice Guidelines: Role of ultrasound in congenital infection. *Ultrasound Obstet Gynecol* **56**(1): 128–151.
167. Kilby MD. (2016) Bricker L on behalf of the Royal college of obstetricians and gynaecologists. Management of monochorionic twin pregnancy. *BJOG* **124**: e1–e45.
168. Kilpatrick CC. (2022) Approach to abdominal pain/pelvic pain in pregnant and postpartum women. In: Berghella V, Weiser M, Barss VA, eds. *UpToDate*. Waltham, MA: UpToDate Inc. Available online at: https://www.uptodate.com (updated July 21, 2022; accessed August 1, 2022).
169. Kimberlin DW, Jester PM, Sánchez PJ, *et al.* (2015) Valganciclovir for symptomatic congenital cytomegalovirus disease. *N Engl J Med* **372**(10): 933–943.
170. Kingsberg S, Spadt SK. (2022) Female sexual pain: Evaluation. In: Barbieri RL, Eckler K, eds. *UpToDate*. Waltham, MA: UpToDate Inc. Available online at: https://www.uptodate.com (updated February 18, 2022; accessed March 3, 2022).

171. Kim KR, Lee HI, Lee SK, *et al.* (2007) Is stromal microinvasion in primary mucinous ovarian tumors with "mucin granuloma" true invasion? *Am J Surg Pathol* **31**(4): 546–554.
172. KK Women's and Children's Hospital, Department of Gynaecological Oncology. (2019) Treatment Guidelines for Gynaecological Cancers.
173. KK Women's and Children's Hospital, Department of Maternal Fetal Medicine. (2019) Identification and management of Rhesus negative patients in pregnancy.
174. Klingensmith ME, Chen LE, Glasgow SC, *et al.* (2008) *The Washington Manual of Surgery*, 5th ed. Saint Louis: Washington University.
175. Knight M, Bunch K, Tuffnell, *et al.* (2021) Saving lives, improving mothers' care: Lessons learned to inform maternity care from the UK and Ireland confidential enquiries into maternal deaths and morbidity 2017–19. MBRRACE-UK.
176. Ko BS, Choi SH, Shin TG, *et al.* (2021) Impact of 1-hour bundle achievement in septic shock. *J Clin Med* **10**(3): 527.
177. Ku CW, Zhang X, Zhang VR, *et al.* (2021) Gestational age-specific normative values and determinants of serum progesterone through the first trimester of pregnancy. *Sci Rep* **11**(1): 4161. Published 202.
178. Ku CW, Allen JC Jr, Malhotra R, *et al.* (2015) How can we better predict the risk of spontaneous miscarriage among women experiencing threatened miscarriage?. *Gynecol Endocrinol* **31**(8): 647–651. doi:10.3109/09513590.2015.1031103.
179. Kubeček O, Laco J, Špaček J, *et al.* (2017) The pathogenesis, diagnosis, and management of metastatic tumors to the ovary: A comprehensive review. *Clin Exp Metastasis* **34**(5): 295–307.
180. Kuponiyi O, Alleemudder DI, Latunde-Dada A, *et al.* (2014) Nerve injuries associated with gynaecological surgery. *Obstet Gynaecol* **16**(1): 29–36.
181. Lam AYR, Lim W, McMicking J, *et al.* *Glob. libr. women's med.* doi: 10.3843/GLOWM.416423.
182. Larsson A, Palm M, Hansson L-O, *et al.* (2008) Reference values for clinical chemistry tests during normal pregnancy. *BJOG* **115**(7): 874–881.
183. Lau HY, Chen YJ, Yen MS, *et al.* (2013) Primary fallopian tube carcinoma: A clinicopathologic analysis and literature review. *J Chin Med Assoc* **76**(10): 583–587.
184. Lee HJ, Park TC, Kim JH, *et al.* (2017) *Norwitz E, Lee B.* The influence of oral dydrogesterone and vaginal progesterone on threatened abortion: A systematic review and meta-analysis. *Biomed Res Int* 2017: **3616875**. doi:10.1155/2017/3616875.

185. Lee KH. (2007) *Survival Guide to Acute Medicine*, 2nd ed. Singapore: Ridge Books.
186. Lee LH, Liu TC, Kuperan P, *et al.* (2011) Hereditary thrombophilia in an unselected cohort of venous thrombosis patients in Singapore. *J Clin Pathol* **64**(9): 814–817.
187. Lee LH, Gu KQ, Heng D. (2002) Deep vein thrombosis is not rare in Asia — the Singapore general hospital experience. *Ann Acad Med Singap* **31**(6): 761–764.
188. Lee NC, Rubin GL, Borucki R. (1988) The intrauterine device and pelvic inflammatory disease revisited: New results from the women's health study. *Obstet Gynecol* **72**(1): 1–6.
189. Lee YC, Min D, Holcomb K, *et al.* (2000) Computed tomography guided core needle biopsy diagnosis of pelvic actinomycosis. *Gynecol Oncol* **79**(2): 318–323.
190. Leiserowitz GS, Xing G, Cress R, *et al.* (2006) Adnexal masses in pregnancy: How often are they malignant? *Gynecol Oncol* **101**(2): 315–321.
191. Lek SM, Ku CW, Allen JC Jr, *et al.* (2017) Validation of serum progesterone <35nmol/L as a predictor of miscarriage among women with threatened miscarriage. *BMC Pregnancy Childbirth* **17**(1): 78. Published 2017 Mar 6. doi:10.1186/s12884-017-1261-41 Feb 18. doi:10.1038/s41598-021-83805-w.
192. Leruez-Ville M, Ghout I, Bussières L, *et al.* (2016) In utero treatment of congenital cytomegalovirus infection with valacyclovir in a multicenter, open-label, phase II study. *Am J Obstet Gynecol* **215**(4): 462.e1–462.e10.
193. Levine JC, Alexander ME. (2022) Fetal arrhythmias. In: Levine D, Wilkins-Haug L, Triedman JK, Barss VA, eds. *UpToDate.* Waltham, MA: UpToDate Inc. Available online at: https://www.uptodate.com (updated May 11, 2022; accessed May 22, 2022).
194. Li L, Zhang Y, Tan H, *et al.* (2020) Effect of progestogen for women with threatened miscarriage: a systematic review and meta-analysis. *BJOG* **127**(9): 1055–1063. doi:10.1111/1471-0528.16261.
195. Li M, Lee AX, Wong WL, *et al.* (2022) Benign metastasising leiomyoma: A rare disease and a diagnostic challenge. *BMJ Case Rep* **15**(7): e248575.
196. Li XY, Chao XP, Leng JH, *et al.* (2019) Risk factors for postoperative recurrence of ovarian endometriosis: Long-term follow-up of 358 women. *J Ovarian Res* **12**(1): 79.
197. Tang L, Hu Y. (2015) Ethnic diversity in the genetics of venous thromboembolism. *Thromb Haemost* **114**(5): 901–909.
198. Lijfering WM, Brouwer JL, Veeger NJ, *et al.* (2009) Selective testing for thrombophilia in patients with first venous thrombosis: Results from a

retrospective family cohort study on absolute thrombotic risk for currently known thrombophilic defects in 2479 relatives. *Blood* **113**(21): 5314–5322.
199. Lim BH, Mahmood TA. (2010) Pandemic H1N1 2009 (swine flu) and pregnancy. *Obstet Gynaecol Reprod Med* **20**(4): 101–106.
200. Lim K, Butt K, Crane JM, *et al.* (2011) SOGC Clinical Practice Guideline. Ultrasonographic cervical length assessment in predicting preterm birth in singleton pregnancies. *J Obstet Gynaecol Can* **33**(5): 486–499.
201. Lim LC, Tan HH, Lee LH, *et al.* (1999) Activated protein C resistance: A study among 60 thromboembolic patients in the Singapore population. *Ann Acad Med Singap* **28**(2): 252–255.
202. Liu Y, Ma L, Yang X, *et al.* (2019) Menopausal hormone replacement therapy and the risk of ovarian cancer: A meta-analysis. *Front Endocrinol* **10**: 801.
203. Lippes J. (1999) Pelvic actinomycosis: A review and preliminary look at prevalence. *Am J Obstet Gynecol* **180**(2): 265–269.
204. Lockwood CJ, Julien S. (2022) Nonimmune hydrops fetalis. In: Wilkins-Haug L, Levine D, Garcia-Prats JA, Barss VA, eds. *UpToDate.* Waltham, MA: UpToDate Inc. Available online at: https://www.uptodate.com (updated August 17, 2022; accessed September 6, 2022).
205. Longmore M, Wilkinson IB, Rajagopalan S. (2004) *Oxford Handbook of Clinical Medicine*, 6th ed. Oxford: Oxford University Press.
206. Lowe SA, Steinweg KE. (2022) Review article: Management of hyperemesis gravidarum and nausea and vomiting in pregnancy. *Emerg Med Australas* **34**(1): 9–15.
207. Luesley DM, Baker PN. (2010) *Obstetrics and Gynaecology: An Evidence-based Text for MRCOG*, 2nd ed. London: Hodder Arnold.
208. Mackillop L. Vitamin D Supplementation in Pregnancy Guideline 1. Available online at: https://www.oxfordshireccg.nhs.uk/professional-resources/documents/clinical-guidelines/endocrinology/Vitamin-D-supplementation-in-pregnancy-guideline.pdf (accessed October 16, 2021).
209. Mahendru A, Gajjar K, Eddy J. (2010) Diagnosis and management of tuberculosis in pregnancy. *Obstet Gynaecol* **12**(3): 163–173.
210. Mai PL, Best AF, Peters JA, *et al.* (2016) Risks of first and subsequent cancers among TP53 mutation carriers in the National Cancer Institute Li-Fraumeni syndrome cohort. *Cancer* **122**(23): 3673–3681.
211. Malinowski DP, Broache M, Vaughan L, *et al.* (2021) Cotesting in cervical cancer screening. *Am J Clin Pathol* **155**(1): 150–154.
212. Mannucci PM, Franchini M. (2015) Classic thrombophilic gene variants. *Thromb Haemost* **114**(5): 885–889.

213. Markovitch O, Klein Z, Gidoni Y, Holzinger M, *et al.* (2002) Extrauterine mislocated IUD: is surgical removal mandatory? *Contraception* **66**(2): 105–108.
214. Martin KA, Barbieri RL. (2022) Treatment of menopausal symptoms with hormone therapy. In: Crowley WF, Mulder JE, eds. *UpToDate.* Waltham, MA: UpToDate Inc. Available online at: https://www.uptodate.com (updated August 23, 2022; accessed September 5, 2022).
215. Martone S, Troìa L, Luisi S. (2021) Adnexal masses during pregnancy: Management for a better approach. *Gynecol Surg* **18**(1): 3.
216. Mason A, Goldacre M, Meddings D, *et al.* (2006) Use of case fatality and readmission measures to compare hospital performance in gynaecology. BJOG **113**(6): 695–699.
217. Mayeaux EJJ, Cox JT. (2014) *Modern Colposcopy Textbook & Atlas*, 3rd ed. Philadelphia, PA: Lippincott Williams and Wilkins.
218. McCarthy FP, Jones C, Rowlands S, *et al.* (2009) Primary and secondary cytomegalovirus in pregnancy. *Obstet Gynaecol* **11**(2): 96–100.
219. McLearn KT, Minkovitz CS, Strobino DM, *et al.* (2006) Maternal depressive symptoms at 2 to 4 months post partum and early parenting practices. *Arch Pediatr Adolesc Med* **160**(3): 279–284.
220. McLintock C, Brighton T, Chunilal S, *et al.* (2012) Recommendations for the prevention of pregnancy-associated venous thromboembolism. *Aust N Z J Obstet Gynaecol* **52**(1): 3–13.
221. Miller JC, Phil D. (2017) Recanalization of Fallopian Tubes. Massachusetts General Hospital Radiology Round. Available online at: https://www.massgeneral.org/assets/mgh/pdf/imaging/radiology-rounds/radiology-rounds-february-2017.pdf (accessed January 17, 2022).
222. Ministry of Health, Singapore. (2018) Gestational diabetes mellitus: An update on screening, diagnosis, and follow-up. Available online at: https://www.ace-hta.gov.sg/docs/default-source/acgs/gdm — an-update-on-screening-diagnosis-and-follow-up-(may-2018).pdf (accessed February 22, 2022).
223. Ministry of Health, Singapore. (2018) Osteoporosis: Identification and Management in Primary Care. Available online at: https://www.ace-hta.gov.sg/docs/default-source/acgs/osteoporosis — identification-and-management-in-primary-care-(nov-2018).pdf (assessed March 13, 2022).
224. MIMS Singapore. (2022) Available online at: https://www.mims.com/singapore (accessed February 1, 2022).
225. Montoya JG, Remington JS. (2008) Management of *Toxoplasma gondii* infection during pregnancy. *Clin Infect Dis* **47**(4): 554–566.

226. Moore Simas TA, Doyle Curiale DK, Hardy J, *et al.* (2010) Efforts needed to provide Institute of Medicine-recommended guidelines for gestational weight gain. *Obstet Gynecol* **115**(4): 777–783.
227. Mulik V, Dad N, Buhmaid S. (2021) Dengue in pregnancy: Review article. *Eur J Obstet Gynecol Reprod Biol* **261**: 205–210.
228. Munro K, Gharaibeh A, Nagabushanam S, *et al.* (2018) Diagnosis and management of tubo-ovarian abscesses. *Obstet Gynaecol* **20**(1): 11–19.
229. Murray D, Cox JL. (1990) Screening for depression during pregnancy with the Edinburgh Depression Scale (EDDS). *J Reprod Infant Psychol* **8**(2): 99–107.
230. Namuduri R. (2019) *Practical Atlas of Vulvar Disease*. Singapore: KK Women's and Children's Hospital.
231. National Center for Immunization and Respiratory Diseases. (2011) General recommendations on immunization—recommendations of the Advisory Committee on Immunization Practices (ACIP). *MMWR Recomm Rep* **60**(2): 1–64. [Published correction appears in MMWR Recomm Rep. 2011 Jul 29; 60: 993.]
232. National Library of Medicine. Drugs and Lactation Database (LactMed). Available online at: https://www.ncbi.nlm.nih.gov/books/NBK501922/ (accessed October 5, 2021).
233. National Registry of Diseases Office. (2022) Singapore Cancer Registry Annual Report 2019.
234. Neriishi K, Hirata T, Fukuda S, *et al.* (2018) Long-term dienogest administration in patients with symptomatic adenomyosis. *J Obstet Gynaecol Res* **44**(8): 1439–1444.
235. NICE Guidelines. (2019) Ectopic pregnancy and miscarriage: Diagnosis and initial management (NG126). Last updated November 24, 2021. Available online at: https://www.nice.org.uk/guidance/ng126/resources/ectopic-pregnancy-and-miscarriage-diagnosis-and-initial-management-pdf-66141662244037 (accessed September 11, 2021).
236. NICE Guidelines. (2015) Menopause: Diagnosis and management (NG23). Available online at: https://www.nice.org.uk/guidance/ng23/resources/menopause-diagnosis-and-management-pdf-1837330217413 (accessed December 5, 2021).
237. NICE Guidelines. (2018) Heavy menstrual bleeding (NG88). Available online at: https://www.nice.org.uk/guidance/ng88/resources/heavy-menstrual-bleeding-assessment-and-management-pdf-1837701412549 (accessed December 15, 2021).
238. NICE Guidelines: (2019) Ectopic pregnancy and miscarriage: diagnosis and initial management (NG126). Published April 17, 2019. Last updated November 24, 2021 https://www.nice.org.uk/guidance/ng126/resources/

ectopic-pregnancy-and-miscarriage-diagnosis-and-initial-management-pdf-66141662244037. Accessed September 11, 2021.

239. NICE Guidelines. (2019) Hypertension in pregnancy: Diagnosis and management (NG133). Available online at: https://www.nice.org.uk/guidance/ng133/resources/hypertension-in-pregnancy-diagnosis-and-management-pdf-66141717671365 (accessed November 10, 2021).

240. NICE Guidelines. (2019) Multiple Pregnancy: Twin and triplet pregnancies (NG137). Available online at: https://www.nice.org.uk/guidance/ng137/resources/twin-and-triplet-pregnancy-pdf-66141724389829 (accessed February 1, 2022).

241. NICE Guidelines. (2014) Antenatal and Postnatal Mental Health: Clinical Management and Service Guidance (CG 192). Last updated February 11, 2020. Available online at: https://www.nice.org.uk/guidance/cg192/resources/antenatal-and-postnatal-mental-health-clinical-management-and-service-guidance-pdf-35109869806789 (accessed March 12, 2021).

242. NICE Guideline. (2021) Postnatal care (NG 194). Available online at: https://www.nice.org.uk/guidance/ng194/resources/postnatal-care-pdf-66142082148037 (accessed December 5, 2021).

243. NICE. (2014) Vitamin D: Increasing supplement use in at-risk groups. Available online at: https://www.nice.org.uk/guidance/ph56/resources/vitamin-d-supplement-use-in-specific-population-groups-pdf-1996421765317 (accessed October 5, 2021).

244. Nelson-Piercy C. (2020) *Handbook of Obstetric Medicine*, 6th ed. Boca Raton, FL: CRC Press.

245. Ng QJ, Koh KM, Tagore S, Mathur M. (2020) Perception and Feelings of Antenatal Women during COVID-19 Pandemic: A Cross-Sectional Survey. *Ann Acad Med Singap* **49**(8): 543–552.

246. Nonacs R, Cohen LS. (2002) Depression during pregnancy: Diagnosis and treatment options. *J Clin Psychiatry* **63**(Suppl. 7): 24–30.

247. O'Neill S, Eden J. (2017) The pathophysiology of menopausal symptoms. *Obstet Gynaecol Reprod Med* **27**(10): 303–310.

248. O'Hara MW, Swain AM. (1996) Rates and risk of postpartum depression — A meta-analysis. *Int Rev Psychiatry* **8**(1): 37–54.

249. O'Hara MW. (1986) Social support, life events, and depression during pregnancy and the puerperium. *Arch Gen Psychiatry* **43**(6): 569–573.

250. Olawaiye AB, Cotler J, Cuello MA, *et al.* (2021) FIGO staging for carcinoma of the vulva: 2021 revision. *Int J Gynaecol Obstet* **155**(1): 43–47.

251. Oliver SE, Cloud GA, Sánchez PJ, *et al.* (2009) Neurodevelopmental outcomes following ganciclovir therapy in symptomatic congenital cytomegalovirus infections involving the central nervous system. *J Clin Virol* **46** (Suppl. 4): S22–S26.

252. Omar MH, Mashita MK, Lim PS, Jamil MA. (2005) Dydrogesterone in threatened abortion: pregnancy outcome. *J Steroid Biochem Mol Biol* **97**(5): 421–425. doi:10.1016/j.jsbmb.2005.08.013.
253. Ong A, Goh K. (2011) A Guide on Infectious Diseases of Public Health Importance in Singapore, 7th ed. Singapore: Ministry of Health.
254. Oon HH, Wong SN, Aw DCW, *et al.* (2019) Acne Management Guidelines by the Dermatological Society of Singapore. *J Clin Aesthet Dermatol* **12**(7): 34–50.
255. Otify M, Fuller J, Ross J, Shaikh H, *et al.* (2015) Endometrial pathology in the postmenopausal woman — an evidence based approach to management. *Obstet Gynaecol* **17**(1): 29–38.
256. Otto CM. (2021) Etiology, clinical features, and evaluation of tricuspid regurgitation. In: Zoghbi WA, Yeon SB, eds. *UpToDate.* Waltham, MA: UpToDate Inc. Available online at: https://www.uptodate.com (updated August 6, 2021; accessed September 22, 2022).
257. Otto CM. (2022) Management and prognosis of tricuspid regurgitation. In: Zoghbi WA, Yeon SB, eds. *UpToDate.* Waltham, MA: UpToDate Inc. Available online at: https://www.uptodate.com (updated August 31, 2022; accessed September 22, 2022).
258. Owen J, Hankins G, Iams JD, *et al.* (2009) Multicenter randomized trial of cerclage for preterm birth prevention in high-risk women with shortened midtrimester cervical length. *Am J Obstet Gynecol* **201**(4): 375.e1–375.e8.
259. Ozenne A, De Berti M, Body G, *et al.* (2022) Risk Factors for Recurrence of Borderline Ovarian Tumours after Conservative Surgery and Impact on Fertility: A Multicentre Study by the Francogyn Group. *J Clin Med* **11**(13): 3645.
260. Panay N. (2011) Management of premenstrual syndrome: Evidence-based guidelines. *Obstet Gynaecol Reprod Med* **21**(8): 221–228.
261. Package Insert. Duphaston® (Dydrogesterone). Abbott. Health Sciences Authority, Singapore. Last revision June 25, 2021.
262. Package Insert. Utrogestan® (Micronised Progesterone). Besins Healthcare Benelux SA. Health Sciences Authority, Singapore. Last revision April, 2018.
263. Pandian RU. (2009) Dydrogesterone in threatened miscarriage: a Malaysian experience. *Maturitas* **65** Suppl (1): S47–S50. doi:10.1016/j.maturitas.2009.11.016.
264. Pangarkar MA. (2022) The Bethesda System for reporting cervical cytology. *Cytojournal* **19**: 28.
265. Parker WH, Fu YS, Berek JS. (1994) Uterine sarcoma in patients operated on for presumed leiomyoma and rapidly growing leiomyoma. *Obstet Gynecol* **83**(3): 414–418.

266. Paul C, Zénut M, Dorut A, *et al.* (2015) Use of Domperidone as a Galactagogue Drug: A Systematic Review of the Benefit-Risk Ratio. *J Hum Lact* **31**(1): 57–63.
267. Pavord S, Myers B, Robinson S, *et al.* (2012) UK guidelines on the management of iron deficiency in pregnancy. *Br J Haematol* **156**(5): 588–600.
268. Pearl JP, Price RR, Tonkin AE, *et al.* (2017) SAGES guidelines for the use of laparoscopy during pregnancy. *Surg Endosc* **31**(10): 3767–3782.
269. Peipert J, Madden T. (2021) Long-term complications of pelvic inflammatory disease. In: Barbieri RL, Chakrabarti A, eds. *UpToDate*. Waltham, MA: UpToDate Inc. https://www.uptodate.com (updated July 26, 2021; accessed August 29, 2021).
270. Perkins RB, Guido RS, Castle PE, *et al.* (2020) 2019 ASCCP Risk-Based Management Consensus Guidelines for Abnormal Cervical Cancer Screening Tests and Cancer Precursors. *J Low Genit Tract Dis* **24**(2): 102–131. [Published correction appears in J Low Genit Tract Dis. 2020 Oct; 24(4): 427.]
271. Price GA, Bash MC. (2019) Epidemiology and pathogenesis of *Neisseria gonorrhoeae* infection. In: Marrazzo J, Bloom A, eds. *UpToDate*. Waltham, MA: UpToDate Inc. Available online at: https://www.uptodate.com (updated October 19, 2019; accessed January 4, 2022).
272. Pritts EA, Parker WH, Olive DL. (2009) Fibroids and infertility: An updated systematic review of the evidence. *Fertil Steril* **91**(4): 1215–1223.
273. Public Health England. (2021) Screening in pregnancy: 20-week screening scan. Available online at: www.gov.uk (accessed March 12, 2022).
274. Qureshi H, Massey E, Kirwan D, *et al.* (2014) BCSH guideline for the use of anti-D immunoglobulin for the prevention of haemolytic disease of the fetus and newborn. *Transfus Med* **24**(1): 8–20.
275. Queenan J, Hobbins J, Spong, C. (2010) *Protocols for High-Risk Pregnancies*, 5th ed. Chichester: Wiley-Blackwell.
276. Rathod RH. (2022) Hypoplastic left heart syndrome: Anatomy, clinical features, and diagnosis. In: Fulton DR, Armsby C, eds. *UpToDate*. Waltham, MA: UpToDate Inc. Available online at: https://www.uptodate.com (updated February 16, 2022; accessed March 13, 2022).
277. Rathod RH. (2022) Hypoplastic left heart syndrome: Management and outcome. In: Fulton DR, Armsby C, eds. *UpToDate*. Waltham, MA: UpToDate Inc. Available online at: https://www.uptodate.com (updated September 1, 2022; accessed September 13, 2022).
278. Ravindran F, Choudhary B. (2021) Ovarian Cancer: Molecular Classification and Targeted Therapy. In: Ho G, Webber K, eds. *Ovarian Cancer — Updates in Tumour Biology and Therapeutics*. London: IntechOpen.

279. Regan L, Rai R, Saravelos S, Li TC; (2023) Royal College of Obstetricians and Gynaecologists. Recurrent MiscarriageGreen-top Guideline No. 17 [published online ahead of print, 2023 Jun 19]. BJOG. 2023;10.1111/1471-0528.17515. doi:10.1111/1471-0528.17515.
280. Regitz-Zagrosek V, Roos-Hesselink JW, Bauersachs J, *et al.* (2019) 2018 ESC Guidelines for the management of cardiovascular diseases during pregnancy. *Kardiol Pol* 77(3): 245–326.
281. Reid RL. (2000) Premenstrual Dysphoric Disorder (Formerly Premenstrual Syndrome) [Updated 2017 Jan 23]. In: Feingold KR, Anawalt B, Boyce A, *et al.* eds. *Endotext* [Internet]. South Dartmouth, MA: MDText.com, Inc. Table 1, Diagnostic Criteria for Premenstrual Dysphoric Disorder (PMDD).
282. Rendi MH. Epithelial carcinoma of the ovary, fallopian tube, and peritoneum: Histopathology. In: Groff B, Garcia RL, Dizon DS, Chakrabarti A, eds. *UpToDate*. Waltham, MA: UpToDate Inc.
283. Revello MG, Lazzarotto T, Guerra B, *et al.* (2014) A randomized trial of hyperimmune globulin to prevent congenital cytomegalovirus. *N Engl J Med* **370**(14): 1316–1326.
284. Ross DS. (2020) Hyperthyroidism during pregnancy: Treatment. In: Cooper DS, Lockwood CJ, Mulder JE, eds. *UpToDate.* Waltham, MA: UpToDate Inc. Available online at: https://www.uptodate.com (updated September 3, 2020; accessed February 22, 2022).
285. Ross DS. (2021) Hypothyroidism during pregnancy: Clinical manifestations, diagnosis, and treatment. In: Cooper DS, Lockwood CJ, Mulder JE, eds. *UpToDate.* Waltham, MA: UpToDate Inc. Available online at: https://www.uptodate.com (updated April 15, 2021; accessed February 22, 2022).
286. Ross J, Chacko MR. (2022) Pelvic inflammatory disease: Clinical manifestations and diagnosis. In: Marrazzo J, Bloom A, eds. *UpToDate.* Waltham, MA: UpToDate Inc. Available online at: https://www.uptodate.com (updated April 20, 2022; accessed April 30, 2022).
287. Ross J, Chacko MR. (2020) Pelvic inflammatory disease: Pathogenesis, microbiology, and risk factors. In: Marrazzo J, Bloom A, eds. *UpToDate.* Waltham, MA: UpToDate Inc. Available online at: https://www.uptodate.com (updated December 20, 2020; accessed April 30, 2022).
288. Royal College of Obstetricians and Gynaecologists. Coronavirus (COVID-19) Infection in Pregnancy Version 14.2. Available online at: https://www.rcog.org.uk/globalassets/documents/guidelines/2021-12-06-coronavirus-covid-19-infection-in-pregnancy-v14.2.pdf (accessed January 1, 2022).
289. Royal College of Obstetricians and Gynaecologists. (2015) Chickenpox in Pregnancy: Green-top Guideline 13.

290. Royal College of Obstetricians and Gynaecologists. (2016) Diagnosis and Management of Ectopic Pregnancy: Green-top Guideline No. 21.
291. Royal College of Obstetricians and Gynaecologists. (2017) Prevention of Early-onset Neonatal Group B Streptococcal Disease: Green-top Guideline No. 36. *BJOG* **124**(12): e280–e305.
292. Royal College of Obstetricians and Gynaecologists. (2015) Reducing the risk of venous thromboembolism during pregnancy and the puerperium: Green Top Guideline No. 37a.
293. Royal College of Obstetricians and Gynaecologists. (2015) Thromboembolic Disease in Pregnancy and the Puerperium: Acute Management: Green Top Guideline No. 37b.
294. Royal College of Obstetricians and Gynaecologists. (2017) Management of Premenstrual Syndrome: Green-top Guideline No. 48. *BJOG* **124**(3): e73–e105.
295. Royal College of Obstetricians and Gynaecologists. (2008) Preventing Entry-Related Gynaecological Injuries: Green-top Guideline No. 49.
296. Royal College of Obstetricians and Gynaecologists. (2010) Malaria in Pregnancy, Prevention: Green-top Guideline No. 54a.
297. Royal College of Obstetricians and Gynaecologists. (2010) The diagnosis and treatment of malaria in pregnancy: Green-top Guideline No. 54b.
298. Royal College of Obstetricians and Gynaecologists. (2010) Late Intrauterine Fetal Death and Stillbirth: Green-top Guideline No. 55.
299. Royal College of Obstetricians and Gynaecologists. (2011) Management of Sickle Cell Disease in Pregnancy: Green-top Guideline No. 61.
300. Royal College of Obstetricians and Gynaecologists. (2011) Antepartum Haemorrhage: Green-top Guideline No. 63.
301. Royal College of Obstetricians and Gynaecologists. (2012) Bacterial Sepsis following Pregnancy: Green-top Guideline No. 64b.
302. Royal College of Obstetricians and Gynaecologists. (2016) Epilepsy in Pregnancy: Green-top Guideline No. 68.
303. Royal College of Obstetricians and Gynaecologists. (2016) The Management of Nausea and Vomiting of Pregnancy and Hyperemesis Gravidarum: Green-top Guideline No. 69.
304. Royal College of Obstetricians and Gynaecologists. (2013) Scientific Impact Paper No. 1 Air Travel and Pregnancy.
305. Royal College of Obstetricians and Gynaecologists. (2015) Scientific Impact Paper No. 48 Management of Women with a Genetic Predisposition to Gynaecological Cancers.

306. Rowland AG, Brady J. (2020) Colposcopy and cervical intraepithelial neoplasia. *Obstet Gynaecol Reprod Med* **30**(5): 133–138.
307. Runowicz CD, Brewer M. (2022) Adnexal mass in pregnancy. In: Barbara G, Chakrabarti A, eds. *UpToDate*. Waltham, MA: UpToDate Inc. Available online at: https://www.uptodate.com (updated May 13, 2022; accessed June 3, 2022).
308. Ryan NA, McMahon RF, Ramchander NC, *et al.* (2021) Lynch syndrome for the gynaecologist. *Obstet Gynaecol* **23**(1): 9–20.
309. Sachdeva A, Dalton M, Lees T. (2018) Graduated compression stockings for prevention of deep vein thrombosis. *Cochrane Database Syst Rev* **11**(11): CD001484.
310. Sang CQ, Zhao N, Zhang J, *et al.* (2018) Different combination strategies for prophylaxis of venous thromboembolism in patients: A prospective multicenter randomized controlled study. *Sci Rep* **8**(1): 8277.
311. Sauer WH, Walsh EP. (2021) Congenital third degree (complete) atrioventricular block. In: Link MS, Yeon SB, eds. *UpToDate*. Waltham, MA: UpToDate Inc. Available online at: https://www.uptodate.com (updated December 3, 2021; accessed January 15, 2022).
312. Samartzis EP, Labidi-Galy SI, Moschetta M, *et al.* (2020) Endometriosis-associated ovarian carcinomas: Insights into pathogenesis, diagnostics, and therapeutic targets — a narrative review. *Ann Transl Med* **8**(24): 1712.
313. Sedlacek TV, Lindheim S, Eder C, *et al.* (1989) Mechanism for human papillomavirus transmission at birth. *Am J Obstet Gynecol* **161**(1): 55–59.
314. Selçuk I, Bozdağ G. (2013) Recurrence of endometriosis; risk factors, mechanisms and biomarkers; review of the literature. *J Turk Ger Gynecol Assoc* **14**(2): 98–103.
315. Serrano B, Alemany L, Tous S, *et al.* (2012) Potential impact of a nine-valent vaccine in human papillomavirus related cervical disease. *Infect Agent Cancer* **7**(1): 38.
316. Cleveland Clinic. Sexual Dysfunction. Available online at: https://my.clevelandclinic.org/health/diseases/9121-sexual-dysfunction (accessed January 15, 2022).
317. Sheffield JS, Suresh BB. (2022) Cytomegalovirus infection in pregnancy. In: Wilkins-Haug L, Hirsch MS, Barss VA, eds. *UpToDate*. Waltham, MA: UpToDate Inc. Available online at: https://www.uptodate.com (updated May 2, 2022; accessed May 15, 2022).
318. Shehata H, Elfituri A, Doumouchtsis SK, *et al.* (2023) FIGO Good Practice Recommendations on the use of progesterone in the management of recurrent

first-trimester miscarriage. *Int J Gynaecol Obstet* **161** Suppl (1): 3–16. doi:10.1002/ijgo.14717.

319. Shen MC, Lin JS, Tsay W. (1997) High prevalence of antithrombin III, protein C and protein S deficiency, but no factor V leiden mutation in venous thrombophilic Chinese patients in Taiwan. *Thromb Res* **87**(4): 377–385.
320. Shifren JL. (2022) Overview of sexual dysfunction in women: Epidemiology, risk factors, and evaluation. In: Barbieri RL, Chakrabarti A, eds. *UpToDate*. Waltham, MA: UpToDate Inc. Available online at: https://www.uptodate.com (updated May 4, 2022; accessed May 15, 2022).
321. Shifren JL. (2022) Overview of sexual dysfunction in women: Management. In: Barbieri RL, Chakrabarti A, eds. *UpToDate*. Waltham, MA: UpToDate Inc. Available online at: https://www.uptodate.com (updated April 4, 2022; accessed May 15, 2022).
322. Singapore Ministry of Health. (2009) *Management of Genital Ulcers and Discharges: Clinical Practice Guidelines Volumes 1–2009 of MOH clinical practice guidelines*. Singapore: Ministry of Health.
323. Sizzi O, Rossetti A, Malzoni M, *et al.* (2007) Italian multicenter study on complications of laparoscopic myomectomy. *J Minim Invasive Gynecol* **14**(4): 453–462.
324. Society for Maternal-Fetal Medicine (SMFM), Dionne-Odom J, Tita AT, *et al.* (2016) #38: Hepatitis B in pregnancy screening, treatment, and prevention of vertical transmission. *Am J Obstet Gynecol* **214**(1): 614.
325. Somigliana E, Vigano' P, Parazzini F, *et al.* (2006) Association between endometriosis and cancer: A comprehensive review and a critical analysis of clinical and epidemiological evidence. *Gynecol Oncol* **101**(2): 331–341.
326. Summary of Product Characteristics (SmPC). (2020) Dostinex Tablets. Pfizer Limited.
327. Stanley AY, Durham CO, Sterrett JJ, *et al.* (2019) Safety of over-the-counter medications in pregnancy. *MCN Am J Matern Child Nurs* **44**(4): 196–205.
328. Stevenson JC, Collins P, Hamoda H, *et al.* (2021) Cardiometabolic health in premature ovarian insufficiency. *Climacteric* **24**(5): 474–480.
329. Strowitzki T, Marr J, Gerlinger C, *et al.* (2010) Dienogest is as effective as leuprolide acetate in treating the painful symptoms of endometriosis: A 24-week, randomized, multicentre, open-label trial. *Hum Reprod* **25**(3): 633–641.
330. Sultan AA, West J, Tata LJ, *et al.* (2012) Risk of first venous thromboembolism in and around pregnancy: A population-based cohort study. *Br J Haematol* **156**(3): 366–373.
331. Taylan E, Oktay K. (2019) Fertility preservation in gynecologic cancers. *Gynecol Oncol* **155**(3): 522–529.

332. Taylor D, Paton C, Kapur S. (2012) Use of psychotropic drugs in special patient groups. In: Taylor DM, Paton C, Kapur S, eds. *The Maudsley Prescribing Guidelines in Psychiatry*, 11th ed. Chichester: Wiley-Blackwell. 419–586.
333. Teoh D, Musa F, Salani R, *et al.* (2020) Diagnosis and management of adenocarcinoma in situ: A society of gynecologic oncology evidence-based review and recommendations. *Obstet Gynecol* **135**(4): 869–878.
334. Tan TC, Goh CMY, Tan SSX, *et al.* (2021) Epidemiology of pregnancy-associated pulmonary embolism in South Asian multi-ethnic country: Mortality trends over the last four decades. *JOGR* **47**(1): 174–183.
335. Tan TC, Ku CW, Kwek LK, *et al.* (2020) Novel approach using serum progesterone as a triage to guide management of patients with threatened miscarriage: A prospective cohort study. *Sci Rep* **10**(1): 9153. Published 2020 Jun 4. doi:10.1038/s41598-020-66155-x.
336. Tan TC, Tan KT, Tan HH, *et al.* (2008) *New Art And Science Of Pregnancy And Childbirth, The: What You Want To Know From Your Obstetrician.* Singapore: World Scientific Publishing Co. Pte. Ltd.
337. "The 2022 Hormone Therapy Position Statement of The North American Menopause Society" Advisory Panel. (2022) The 2022 hormone therapy position statement of The North American menopause society. *Menopause* **29**(7): 767–794.
338. The Faculty of Sexual & Reproductive Healthcare of the Royal College of Obstetricians & Gynaecologists. (2012) FSRH Clinical Guideline: Barrier Methods for Contraception and STI Prevention. Clinical Effectiveness unit (Updated October 2015).
339. The Faculty of Sexual & Reproductive Healthcare of the Royal College of Obstetricians & Gynaecologists. (2019) FSRH Clinical Guideline: Combined Hormonal Contraception. (Amended November 2020).
340. The Faculty of Sexual & Reproductive Healthcare of the Royal College of Obstetricians & Gynaecologists. (2017) FSRH Clinical Guideline: Contraception After pregnancy (Amended October 2020).
341. The Faculty of Sexual & Reproductive Healthcare of the Royal College of Obstetricians & Gynaecologists. (2017) FSRH Clinical Guideline: Contraception for Women aged over 40 Years. (Amended September 2019).
342. The Faculty of Sexual & Reproductive Healthcare of the Royal College of Obstetricians & Gynaecologists. (2022) FSRH Clinical Guideline: Drug Interactions with Hormonal Contraception.
343. The Faculty of Sexual & Reproductive Healthcare of the Royal College of Obstetricians & Gynaecologists. (2017) FSRH Clinical Guideline: Emergency Contraception. (Amended December 2020).

344. The Faculty of Sexual & Reproductive Healthcare of the Royal College of Obstetricians & Gynaecologists. (2014) FSRH Clinical Guideline: Male and Female Sterilisation. Clinical Effectiveness Unit.
345. The Faculty of Sexual & Reproductive Healthcare of the Royal College of Obstetricians & Gynaecologists. (2023) FSRH Clinical Guideline: Intrauterine Contraception. Clinical Effectiveness Unit (Amended July 2023).
346. The Faculty of Sexual & Reproductive Healthcare of the Royal College of Obstetricians & Gynaecologists. (2021) FSRH Clinical Guideline: Progestogen-only Implant.
347. The Faculty of Sexual & Reproductive Healthcare of the Royal College of Obstetricians & Gynaecologists. (2014) FSRH Clinical Guideline: Progestogen-only Injectable Contraception. Clinical Effectiveness Unit (Amended October 2020).
348. The Faculty of Sexual & Reproductive Healthcare of the Royal College of Obstetricians & Gynaecologists. (2015) FSRH Clinical Guideline: Progestogen-only Pills. Clinical Effectiveness Unit (Amended April 2019).
349. The Faculty of Sexual & Reproductive Healthcare of the Royal College of Obstetricians & Gynaecologists. (2017) FSRH Clinical Guideline: Switching or Starting Methods of Contraception. Clinical Effectiveness Unit (Amended March 2021).
350. The Faculty of Sexual & Reproductive Healthcare of the Royal College of Obstetricians & Gynaecologists. (2016) UK Medical Eligibility Criteria for contraceptive use. UKMEC (Amended September 2019).
351. The Fetal Medicine Foundation. Fetal abnormalities. Available online at: https://fetalmedicine.org/education/fetal-abnormalities (accessed March 10, 2022).
352. Thomson AJ, Royal College of Obstetricians and Gynaecologists. (2019) Care of women presenting with suspected preterm prelabour rupture of membranes from 24+0 weeks of gestation: Green-top guideline No. 73. *BJOG* **126**(9): e152–e166.
353. Tidy C. (2016) 'Hydrops Fetalis'. Patient. 1 April 2016 (accessed Feb 13, 2022).
354. Tien Dat T, Kotani T, Yamamoto E, *et al.* (2018) Dengue fever during pregnancy. *Nagoya J Med Sci* **80**(2): 241–247.
355. To M, Kidd M, Maxwell D. (2009) Prenatal diagnosis and management of fetal infections. *Obstet Gynaecol* **11**(2): 108–116.
356. Toriyabe K, Taniguchi H, Senda T, *et al.* (2016) Pregnancy and cesarean delivery after multimodal therapy for vulvar carcinoma: A case report. *Mol Clin Oncol* **5**(5): 583–586.

357. Turok D. (2022) Emergency contraception. In: Schreiber C, Eckler K, eds. *UpToDate*. Waltham, MA: UpToDate Inc. Available online at: https://www.uptodate.com (updated August 9, 2022; accessed August 26, 2022).
358. van Gelder MM, van Rooij IA, Miller RK, *et al.* (2010) Teratogenic mechanisms of medical drugs. *Hum Reprod Update* **16**(4): 378–394.
359. Vanaparthy R, Mahdy H. (2022) Hydrops Fetalis. [Updated 2022 Feb 26]. In: *StatPearls [Internet]*. Treasure Island, FL: StatPearls Publishing.
360. Vasanwala RF, Gani L, Ang SB. (2022) It starts from the womb: Maximizing bone health. *Climacteric* **25**(1): 11–21.
361. Vasquez P, Schreiber CA. (2010) The missing IUD. *Contraception* **82**: 126–128.
362. Vercellini P, Viganò P, Buggio L, *et al.* (2018) Perimenopausal management of ovarian endometriosis and associated cancer risk: When is medical or surgical treatment indicated? *Best Pract Res Clin Obstet Gynaecol* **51**: 151–168.
363. Verghese TS, Futaba K, Latthe P. (2015) Constipation in pregnancy. *Obstet Gynaecol* **17**(2): 111–115.
364. Verhaegen J, Gallos ID, van Mello NM, *et al.* (2012) Accuracy of single progesterone test to predict early pregnancy outcome in women with pain or bleeding: meta-analysis of cohort studies. *BMJ* **345**: e6077. Published 2012 Sep 27. doi:10.1136/bmj.e6077.
365. Verma V, Shree P, Kumar S. (2021) Genital wart during pregnancy: A rare case. *J Clin Diagn Res.* **15**(4): 1–2.
366. Vinogradova Y, Coupland C, Hippisley-Cox J. (2020) Use of hormone replacement therapy and risk of breast cancer: Nested case-control studies using the QResearch and CPRD databases. *BMJ* **371**: m3873.
367. Visser GHA, Thommesen T, Di Renzo GC, *et al.* (2021) FIGO committee for safe motherhood, newborn health. FIGO/ICM guidelines for preventing Rhesus disease: A call to action. *Int J Gynaecol Obstet* **152**(2): 144–147.
368. Wahabi HA, Fayed AA, Esmaeil SA, *et al.* (2018) Progestogen for treating threatened miscarriage. *Cochrane Database Syst Rev* **8**(8): CD005943.
369. Wang XX, Luo Q, Bai WP. (2019) Efficacy of progesterone on threatened miscarriage: Difference in drug types. *J Obstet Gynaecol Res* **45**(4): 794–802. doi:10.1111/jog.13909.
370. Workowski KA, Bachmann LH, Chan PA, *et al.* (2021) Sexually Transmitted Infections Treatment Guidelines, 2021. *MMWR Recomm Rep* **70**(4): 1–187.
371. Whitecar MP, Turner S, Higby MK. (1999) Adnexal masses in pregnancy: A review of 130 cases undergoing surgical management. *Am J Obstet Gynecol* **181**(1): 19–24.

372. World Health Organisation (WHO). (2021) Guidelines for the management of symptomatic sexually transmitted infections. Available online at: https://www.who.int/publications/i/item/9789240024168 (accessed December 17, 2021).
373. World Health Organisation (WHO). (1994) WHO study group on assessment of fracture risk and its application to screening for postmenopausal osteoporosis. Assessment of fracture risk and its application to screening for postmenopausal osteoporosis. Report of a WHO study group. *World Health Organ Tech Rep Ser* **843**: 1–129.
374. Wiesenfeld H. (2022) Pelvic inflammatory disease: Treatment in adults and adolescents. In: Marrazzo J, Bloom A, eds. *UpToDate*. Waltham, MA: UpToDate Inc. Available online at: https://www.uptodate.com (updated March 14, 2022; accessed April 19, 2022).
375. Wise J. (2021) NICE recommends progesterone to prevent early miscarriage. *BMJ* **375**: n2896.
376. Won HS, Kim DY, Yang MS, *et al.* (2011) Pregnancy-induced hypertension, but not gestational diabetes mellitus, is a risk factor for venous thromboembolism in pregnancy. *Korean Circ J* **41**(1): 23–27.
377. Woolcock JG, Critchley HO, Munro MG, *et al.* (2008) Review of the confusion in current and historical terminology and definitions for disturbances of menstrual bleeding. *Fertil Steril* **90**(6): 2269–2280.
378. Yao M, Tulandi T. (1997) Current status of surgical and nonsurgical management of ectopic pregnancy. *Fertil Steril* **67**(3): 421–33.
379. Yamanishi Y, Koshiyama M, Ohnaka M, *et al.* (2011) Pathways of metastases from primary organs to the ovaries. *Obstet Gynecol Int* **2011**: 612817.
380. Yang S, Liu Y, Wen J, *et al.* (2022) Clinical efficacy of dienogest versus levonorgestrel-releasing intrauterine system for adenomyosis. *Evid Based Complement Alternat Med* **2022**: 1995472.
381. Yawetz S. (2022) Immunisations during pregnancy. In: Lockwood CJ, Weller PF, eds. *UpToDate*. Waltham, MA: UpToDate Inc. Available online at: https://www.uptodate.com (updated September 2, 2022; accessed September 10, 2022).
382. Yedema CA, Kenemans P, Wobbes T, *et al.* (1992) Use of serum tumor markers in the differential diagnosis between ovarian and colorectal adenocarcinomas. *Tumour Biol* **13**(1–2): 18–26.
383. Yip SK, Sahota D, Pang MW, *et al.* (2004) Postpartum urinary retention. *Acta Obstet Gynecol Scand* **83**(10): 881–891.

384. Yonkers K, Casper R. (2022) Clinical manifestations and diagnosis of premenstrual syndrome and premenstrual dysphoric disorder. In: Barbieri RL, Crowley WF, Martin KA, eds. *UpToDate*. Waltham, MA: UpToDate Inc. Available online at: https://www.uptodate.com (updated March 25, 2022; accessed May 20, 2022).
385. Yu CK, Papageorghiou AT, Parra M, *et al.* (2003) Randomized controlled trial using low-dose aspirin in the prevention of pre-eclampsia in women with abnormal uterine artery Doppler at 23 weeks' gestation. *Ultrasound Obstet Gynecol* **22**(3): 233–239. doi: 10.1002/uog.218.
386. Zakin D, Stern WZ, Rosenblatt R. (1981) Complete and partial uterine perforation and embedding following insertion of intrauterine devices. II. Diagnostic methods, prevention, and management. *Obstet Gynecol Surv* **36**(8): 401–417.
387. Zanetta G, Mariani E, Lissoni A, *et al.* (2003) A prospective study of the role of ultrasound in the management of adnexal masses in pregnancy. *BJOG* **110**(6): 578–583.
388. Zuhair M, Smit GSA, Wallis G, *et al.* (2019) Estimation of the worldwide seroprevalence of cytomegalovirus: A systematic review and meta-analysis. *Rev Med Virol* **29**(3): e2034.